In the memory of
Dr. Eldon J. Gardner

Joji Utsunomiya Henry T. Lynch (Eds.)

Hereditary Colorectal Cancer

Proceedings of the Fourth International Symposium on Colorectal Cancer (ISCC-4)
November 9-11, 1989, Kobe JAPAN

With 97 Figures

Springer Japan KK

Joji Utsunomiya, M.D.
Professor and Chairman
Second Department of Surgery
Hyogo College of Medicine
1-1 Mukogawa-cho, Nishinomiya
Hyogo, 663 Japan

Henry T. Lynch, M.D.
Professor and Chairman
Department of Preventive Medicine
Creighton University School of Medicine
Hereditary Cancer Center
California at 24th Street
Omaha, NE 68178, USA

ISBN 978-4-431-68339-1 ISBN 978-4-431-68337-7 (eBook)
DOI 10.1007/978-4-431-68337-7

Originally published by Springer-Verlag Tokyo 1990
Softcover reprint of the hardcover 1st edition 1990

Foreword

Since the success in chemical induction of cancer in rabbit's ear skin by K. Yamagiwa in 1915, oncologists of the world have come to believe that they can only solve their problems by means of animal experimentation. The importance of environmental factors became more evident in 1935 when T. Yoshida and T. Sasaki introduced azodye hepatocarcinogenesis in rats. In the domain of the gastrointestinal tract, T. Sugimura has more recently accumulated enough evidence to indicate that locally active chemical mutagens are carcinogenic.

In contrast, principal approaches to colorectal tumors have been quite different: emphasis has been placed on gene identification. Long before cancer of the large bowel was recognized, importance of the roles of adenomatosis coli and its familial occurrence attracted the attention of epidemiologists and geneticists. Morphological characterization and analysis of hereditary trends of human material have already had a long history, and recently detailed analysis of genetic material has become feasible in the wake of rapid development in our knowledge of the oncoviruses, oncogenes, suppressor genes, chromosomal and DNA mapping, molecular mutation and so on. It is true that in colorectal pathology, and in no other field, these areas of research have been explored more extensively and decisively. The identification of previously ill-defined lesions such as precancers and benign neoplasms have been improved because sequential changes can be observed in multiple samples spread over a wide area and followed up in due course.

Multidisciplinary approaches with close cooperation of surgeons, pathologists, molecular biologists, geneticists, and epidemiologists among others, have contributed greatly to recent developments and will surely continue to do so in the immediate future. The organization of the present conference and gathering of global experts owe much to the efforts of Prof. J. Utsunomiya who has dedicated many years to the compilation of genetic-epidemiological data in Japan, especially with reference to the adenomatosis. This publication coedited by Prof. J. Utsunomiya and Prof. H.T. Lynch represents another step foreward toward solving remaining problems in this field.

Kunio Oota, M.D.
President, Japanese Association
of Medical Sciences

Preface

Three International Symposia on Colorectal Cancer, organized under the Chairmanship of Dr. Sydney J. Winawer, and held at New York (1979). Washington (1981), and Boston (1983) respectively, had the following topics as their themes: (1) Prevention, Epidemiology, and Screening, (2) Risk Factors and Screening, and (3) Policy for Prevention.

As a sequel to this series of meetings, we had the opportunity of organizing the Fourth International Symposium on Colorectal Cancer, held in Kobe, Japan, on November 9–11, 1989 with the specific theme of "Hereditary Colorectal Cancer." This topic is very timely, because of the imminent convergence of the fields of clinicoepidemiology and molecular genetics: the knowledge of colorectal cancer, accumulated through patient and persistent observations over many decades, has now reached a level at which the merging of incisive ideas and updated technology developed recently in molecular genetics promises to spark breakthroughs in major problems in cancer.

Under the term "Hereditary Colorectal Cancer," we include the presently recognized heritable conditions known to be predisposed to colorectal cancer, which can be roughly classified into the polyposis syndromes and hereditary nonpolyposis colorectal cancer (HNPCC). We have particularly focussed upon: (1) identification, surveillance, and management of HNPCC especially; (2) chemoprevention in theory; research, and practice; and (3) clinicopathological and cytomolecular aspects for better understanding of the etiology and pathogenesis of the conditions; these aspects include: (a) clinical spectra; (b) histopathological diversity; (c) genetic heterogeneity; (d) genetic markers and linkage studies; (e) markers for presymptomatic diagnosis; and (f) cloning and characterization of relevant gene sequences.

The aim of the symposium was to create and maintain an active workshop spirit throughout the meeting in order to generate in-depth discussions between experts in the range of disciplines which have impact upon the field. Spontaneity was encouraged so that new frontiers of knowledge might be developed freely in an intellectually challenging atmosphere.

The three-day symposium began with two plenary sessions which included 10 "state-of-the-art" lectures. This was followed by the workshops, which comprised 75 papers in 6 sessions, organized as two parallel series: one focussed upon genetic epidemiology and clinical features, while the other delved more heavily into basic science, particularly biomolecular genetics and pathology. Finally, these workshops were summarized by the respective chairpersons, with the primary intent of forecasting future research.

The program and content of this meeting were planned after painstaking discussions among the members of the several planning committees. These interdisciplinary interactions representing diverse fields contributed to the truly eclectic atmosphere which permeated the meeting. The symposium was attended by 70 distinguished speakers from an array of disciplines, including 18 from medicine, gastroenterology, and radiology, 18 from medical and biomolecular genetics, 16 from surgery and gynecology, 10 from pathology and biology, and 4 from epidemiology and biostatistics. These colleagues are from 15 different countries: 25 from the United States, 15 from Japan, 7 from the United Kingdom, 5 from Italy, 3 from the Netherlands, 2 from Denmark, and 1 each from Australia, Canada, Finland, France, Greece, Israel, New Zealand, Poland, and Sweden. Approximately 50 observers, mainly Japanese, joined in active discussion throughout the symposium.

This symposium was dedicated to the memory of Dr. Eldon J. Gardner, who contributed so much during most of his lifetime to the study of hereditary colorectal cancer. Dr. Gardner passed away during the period of conception of this symposium, and his contributions are greatly missed.

JOJI UTSUNOMIYA
HENRY T. LYNCH

Organization of the Fourth International Symposium on Colorectal Cancer

International Committee:

Chairman: Joji Utsunomiya, Japan
Co-chairman: Henry T. Lynch, USA

Sidney J. Winawer, USA
Paul Rozen, Israel
Sir Walter F. Bodmer, UK
Giuseppe Cristofaro, Italy
P. Meera Khan, The Netherlands
Bruce M. Boman, USA
Martin Lipkin, USA
Yusuke Nakamura, Japan
Stig Kullander, Sweden
Raymond L. White, USA

Local Organizing Committee:

Shozo Baba
Junichi Furuyama
Shinzo Isojima
Keiichi Kawai
Kozaburo Kimura
Yoshio Mishima
Takesada Mori
Tetsuichiro Muto
Masao Sasaki
Takehiko Sasazuki
Takashi Shimoyama
Akira Tonomura
Kei Takebe
Ryukichi Tobe
Masayuki Yasutomi
Yutaka Yoshida

Local Consultant Board:

Takeshi Hirayama
Shuji Kimura
Isamu Kinoh
Goro Kosaki
Kyoichi Nakamura
Yasuaki Nishizuka
Kunio Oota
Haruo Sugano
Takashi Sugimura
Shuji Tsuchiya
Hidenobu Watanabe

Sponsored by:

The International Committee or ISCC-4 at Hyogo College of Medicine

Co-sponsored by:

WHO Collaborative Center for Prevention of Colorectal Cancer at Memorial Sloan-Kettering Cancer Center, New York, USA

Imperial Cancer Research Fund London, UK
Creighton University, Omaha, USA
University of Utah Medical Center, USA
Dutch Colorectal Genetics Group, University of Leiden Medical Center, The Netherlands
The Hereditary Gastrointestinal Cancer Prevention Center, Brindisi, Italy
Japanese Association of Medical Sciences
Japanese Research Society for Colorectal Cancer

List of Contributors*

NIKI AGNANTIS, M.D.
National Hellenic Research Foundation, Biological Research Center,
48, Vas, Constantinou Avenue, Athens 11635, Greece

SHOZO BABA, M.D.
Second Department of Surgery, Hamamatsu College of Medicine,
3600, Handa-cho, Hamamatsu-shi, Sizuoka-ken, 431-31 Japan

LUCIO BERTARIO, M.D.
Institution Nazionale per lo Studio e la cura dei Tumori,
Via Venezian 1, 20133 Milan, Italy

TIM BISHOP, PH.D.
Genetic Epidemiology Laboratory, Imperial Cancer Research Fund,
3K Springfield House, Hyde Terrace, Leeds LS2 9LU, UK

SIR WALTER BODMER, PH.D.
Imperial Cancer Research Fund, P.O. Box 123, Lincoln's Inn Fields,
London WC2A 3PX, UK

C. RICHARD BOLAND, M.D., PH.D.
Department of Internal Medicine, University of Michigan,
Medical Center, Veterans Administration Hospital,
3912 Taubman Center, Box 0362, Ann Arbor, MI 48109-0362, USA

BRUCE M. BOMAN, M.D., PH.D.
Creighton Cancer Center, Department of Medicine, Creighton
University School of Medicine, The Hereditary Cancer Center,
Criss III, Room 353, California at 24th Street, Omaha, NE 68178, USA

PHILIP BRALOW, M.D.
Graduate Hospital, University of Pennsylvania, Graduate Hospital,
Philadelphia, PA 19146, USA

PANTALEO BUFO, M.D.
Instituto di Anatomia e istologia Patologica, Bari University,
70100 Bari, Italy

*First-mentioned author only

Steffen Bülow, M.D., Ph.D.
The Danish Polyposis Register, Deptartment of Surgery, Gastroenterology, Hvidovre University Hospital, DK 2650, Hvidovre, Denmark

Randall W. Burt, M.D.
Department of Medicine, Division of Gastroenterology, University of Utah, 4R118 Medical Center, Salt Lake City, UT 84132, USA

Mitsuro Chiba, M.D.
First Department of Internal Medicine, University of Akita, 1-1-1, Honmichi, Akita, 010 Japan

James Church, M.D., Ch.B.
Department of Colorectal Surgery, Desk A-111, The Cleveland Clinic Foundation, 9500 Euclid Avenue, Cleveland, OH 44195, USA

Giuseppe Cristofaro, M.D.
Hereditary Gastrointestinal Cancer Prevention Center, Via de Terrible 9, 72100 Brindisi, Italy

Jerome J. DeCosse, M.D., Ph.D.
Department of Surgery, Hospital Cornell Medical Center, Cornell University Medical College, 525 E 68 Street, New York, NY 10021, USA

Emilio Di Giulio, M.D.
Institute of Surgery, University of Rome "La Sapienza", Viale Regina Elena 324, 00161 Rome, Italy

David L. Ernest, M.D.
University of Arizona, 1515, N. Campbell Avenue, Tucson, AZ 85724, USA

Andrew P. Feinberg, M.D., M.P.H.
Howard Hughes Medical Institute, University of Michigan Medical Center, MSRBI Room 4520, 1150 W. Medical Campus Drive, Ann Arbor, MI 48109, USA

Robert J. Fitzgibbons Jr., M.D.
Department of Surgery, Creighton University School of Medicine, The Hereditary Cancer Center, 601 N. 30 Steet, Omaha, NE 68131, USA

Eileen A. Friedman, Ph.D.
Department of Gastroenterology, Memorial Sloan-Kettering Cancer Center, 1275 York Avenue, Box 244, New York, NY 10021, USA

Anna-Maria Frischauf, Ph.D.
Molecular Analysis of Mammalian Lab., Imperial Cancer Research Fund, P.O. Box 123, Lincoln's Inn Fields, London WC2A 3PX, UK

GERRIT GRIFFIOEN, M.D.
Department of Gastroenterology, University Hospital,
Rynsburger Weg 10, 2333AA, Leiden, The Netherlands

STANLEY R. HAMILTON, M.D.
Department of Pathology and Oncology Center, The Johns Hopkins
Medical Institute, Baltimore, MD 21205, USA

LEMUEL HERRERA, M.D., M.AQ., F.A.C.S.
Roswell Park Memorial Institute, State University of N.Y at Buffalo,
666 Elm Street, Buffalo, NY 14263, USA

TAKESHI HIRAYAMA, M.D.
Institute of Preventive Oncology, 1-2, Ichigaya Sadohara-cho,
Shinjuku-ku, Tokyo, 162 Japan

TATSURO IKEUCHI, M.D.
Tokyo Medical and Dental University, Medical Research Institute,
1-5-45, Yushima, Bunkyo-ku, Tokyo, 113 Japan

TAKEO IWAMA, M.D.
Tokyo Medical and Dental University, The Research Center for
Polyposis and Intestinal Disease, 1-5-45, Yushima, Bunkyo-ku,
Tokyo, 113 Japan

JEREMY R. JASS, M.D.
University of Auckland School of Medicine, Private Bag, Auckland,
New Zealand

P. MEERA KHAN, M.D., PH.D.
Human Genetics Institute, University of Leiden, Sylvius Laboratories,
Wassenaarseweg 72, P.B. 9503, 2300 RA Leiden, The Netherlands

YOUNG S. KIM, M.D.
Gastroint. Research Laboratory, University of California,
Medical Center, 4150 Clement Street, San Francisco, CA 94121, USA

LEVY KOPELOVICH, PH.D.
VA Medical Center, Bay Pines, Florida, University of South Florida,
College of Medicine, Research Service (151), Bay Pines, FL 33504, USA

PIOTR KROKOWICZ, M.D.
Newton Street 16a/4260-161, Poznan, Poland

STIG KULLANDER, M.D.
Department of Obstetrics and Gynecology, University of Lund,
Malmo General Hospital, Malmo, Sweden

STEPHEN J. LANSPA, M.D., F.A.C.P.
Department of Medicine-Gastroenterology, Creighton University,
School of Medicine and Hereditary Cancer Consultation Center,
California at 24th Street, Omaha, NE 68178, USA

BERNARD LEVIN, M.D.
Gastrointestinal Oncology, MD Anderson Cancer Center,
The University of Texas, 1515 Holcombe, Blvd., Houston, TX 77030,
USA

MARTIN LIPKIN, M.D.
Memorial Sloan Kettering Cancer Center, Cornell University Medical
College, 1275 York Avenue, New York, NY 10021, USA

HENRY T. LYNCH, M.D.
Department of Preventive Medicine, Creighton University School of
Medicine, The Hereditary Cancer Center, California at 24th Street,
Omaha, NE 68178, USA

JANE F. LYNCH, B.S.N.
Department of Preventive Medicine, Creighton University School of
Medicine, The Hereditary Cancer Center, California at 24th Street,
Omaha, NE 68178, USA

PATRICK M. LYNCH, M.D.
Department of Gastroenterology, MD Anderson Hospital and
Tumor Institute, 1515 Holcombe Blvd., Houston, TX 77030, USA

FINLEY MACRAE, M.D., F.R.A.C.P., M.R.C.P.
Department of Gastroenterology, The Royal Melbourne Hospital,
Post Office, Royal Melborne Hospital 305D, Victoria, Australia

PIETRO L. MINGAZZINI, M.D.
Department of Biopathology, University of Rome "La Sapienza",
Viale Regina Elena 324, 00161 Rome, Italy

YOSHIO MISHIMA, M.D.
Second Department of Surgery, Tokyo Medical and Dental University,
1-5-45, Yushima, Bunkyo-ku, Tokyo, 113 Japan

MICHIKO MIYAKI, M.D.
The Tokyo Metropolitan Institute of Medical Science,
3-18-22, Honn-Komagome, Bunkyo-ku, Tokyo, 113 Japan

TETSUICHIRO MUTO, M.D.
First Department of Surgery, The University of Tokyo,
7-3-1, Hongo, Bunkyo-ku, Tokyo, 113 Japan

YUSUKE NAKAMURA, PH.D.
Cancer Institute, 1-37-1, Kamiikebukuro, Toshima-ku, Tokyo,
170 Japan

TOMIO NARISAWA, M.D.
First Department of Surgery, University of Akita, 1-1-1, Honmichi,
Akita, 010 Japan

CHRISTOS PARASKEVA, PH.D.
Department of Pathology, The Medical School, University Walk,
Bristol BS8 1TD, UK

Gloria M. Petersen, ph.d.
Division of Medical Genetics, Cedars-Sinai Medical Center, 8700 Beverly Blvd., Los Angeles, CA 90048-1869, USA

Paul Rozen, m.b., b.s.
Department of Gastroenterology, Tel Aviv Medical Center, 6 Weizman Street, Tel Aviv 64239, Israel

Takehiko Sasazuki, m.d.
Kyushu University, Medical Institute of Bioregulation, 3-1-1, Maide, Higashi-ku, Fukuoka, 812 Japan

Peter Schlag, m.d.
Chirurgische Universitätsklinik, Im Neuenheimer Feld 110, 6900 Heidelberg, Federal Republic of Germany

Silvano Senatore, m.d.
"Di Summa" Brindisi Hospital, 72100 Brindisi, Italy

Joan Slack, d.m., f.r.c.p.
Royal Free Hospital School of Medicine, Pond Street, Hampstead, London NW3 2QG, UK

Thomas Smyrk, m.d.
Department of Pathology, Creighton University School of Medicine, 601N 30th Street, Omaha, NE 68131, USA

Ellen Solomon, ph.d.
Imperial Cancer Research Fund, Lincoln's Inn Fields, London WC2A 3PX, UK

Jens O. Søndergaard, m.d.
Department of Surgical, Gastroenterology, Hvidovre University, OK 2650, Hvidovre, Denmark

Hartley S. Stern, m.d., f.r.c.s.(c)
Mount Sinai Hospital, Suite 1225, 600 University Avenue, Toronto, Ontario, M5G 1X5, Canada

Hideho Takada, m.d.
Department of Surgery, Kansai Medical University, 1, Fumizono-cho, Moriguchi, Osaka, 570 Japan

Gilles Thomas, m.d.
The Institute Curie, 26, Rue D'Ulm, 75231, Paris, CX5 France

Carli M.J. Tops, m.sc.
Human Genetics Institute, Silvius Lab., University of Leiden, P.B. 9503, 2300 RA Leiden, The Netherlands

Yoshiyuki Tsuji, m.d.
Department of Obsterics and Gynecology, Hyogo College of Medicine, 1-1 Mukogawa-cho, Nishinomiya, Hyogo, 663 Japan

KYOSUKE USHIO, M.D.
National Cancer Center, 5-1-1, Tsukiji, Chuo-ku, Tokyo, 104 Japan

JOJI UTSUNOMIYA, M.D.
Second Department of Surgery, Hyogo College of Medicine,
1-1 Mukogawa-cho, Nishinomiya, Hyogo, 663 Japan

HANS F.A. VASEN, M.D.
Foundation for the Detection of Hereditary Tumors,
P.O. Box 12009, 3501 AA Utrecht, The Netherlands

BERT VOGELSTEIN, M.D.
Research Laboratories, Room 109, Johns Hopkins Oncology Center,
424 N. Bond Street, Baltimore, MD 21231, USA

MICHAEL J. WARGOVICH, PH.D.
Section of Gastrointestinal Oncology and Digestive Diseases,
Box 78, MD Anderson Hospital and Tumor Institute,
1515 Holcombe Blvd., Houston, TX 77030, USA

HIDENOBU WATANABE, M.D.
First Department of Pathology, Niigata University, 754, Ichiban-cho,
Asahimachi-dori, Niigata, 951 Japan

PATRICE WATSON, PH.D.
Department of Preventive Medicine, Creighton University School of
Medicine, The Hereditary Cancer Center, California at 24th Street,
Omaha, NE 68178, USA

RAYMOND L. WHITE, PH.D.
Howard Hughes Medical Institute, University of Utah,
631 Wintrobe Bldg., UUMC, Salt Lake City, UT 84132, USA

RODGER J. WINN, M.D.
Department of Medicine, The University of Texas, MD Anderson
Cancer Center, TX 77030, USA

ANDREW H. WYLLIE, M.D.
Department of Pathology, University Medical School, Teviot Place,
Edinburgh EH8 9AG, UK

Table of Contents

Chapter 4: Chemoprevention of Colorectal Cancer

Chapter 7: Cytomolecular Aspects of Colorectal Cancer

Chapter 1

General Aspects of Hereditary Colorectal Cancer

The Concept of Hereditary Colorectal Cancer and the Implications of Its Study

JOJI UTSUNOMIYA

ABSTRACT

Hereditary colorectal cancer (HCC) is roughly divided into 1) the polyposis syndrome including adenomatous polyposis coli (APC), Peutz-Jeghers syndrome and juvenile polyposis; and 2) hereditary nonpolyposis colorectal cancer (HNPCC) including Lynch syndrome I, II and hereditary soritary adenoma. They are rarely encountered in practice, but their importance are increasingly appreciated in cancer research. APC provided one of the best model for classical medelian dominant inheritance of desease in man which proved a single gene relates to cancer occurrence. Extensive clinicopathological and cytological observations suggest the gene is regulating cell proliferation of common tissue not only of the large bowel, and provided us with a clue for detecting locus of APC gene. Biostatistical analysis on age specific cancer rate of APC suggests several hits are required for colorectal cancer occurrence and the gene plays a role for the initial step of sequential events for it. The recent cytomolecular studies are going to prove this hypothesis. Chemical as well as surgical preventive measures for colorectal cancer are developing in this field. Experiences in the polyposis study are efficiently utilized for HNPCC study in clinical characterization as well as in detecting effective biomarker, and in estimating the proportion of HNPCC in general colorectal cancer.

Keywords: hereditary colorectal cancer, adenomatous polyposis coli, APC, familial adenomatous polyposis, FAP, Gardner syndrome, Peutz-Jeghers syndrome, Juvenile polyposis, hereditary nonpolyposis colorectal cancer, HNPCC, familial colorectal cancer.

1. INTRODUCTION

In the early part of this century, there were two important reports which initiated the traditional lines of genetic studies on large bowel cancer: one by Alfred Warthin (1913) on the cancer family which was developed by Hauser and Weller (1936) and further by H.T.Lynch (1967) in U.S.A.; and the another one by Lockhart-Mummery (1925) on the intestinal polyposis which has been inherited through Dukes (1952), Veal (1965), Bussey (1975), and Bodmer (1985), and extended by the formation of The Leed Castle Polyposis Group in 1982 in England. In U.S.A., Jeghers et al. (1949) and Gardner et al. (1951) also made many significant contributions to the study of polyposis. The former subject is now called "hereditary nonpolyposis colorectal cancer" (HNPCC) (Lynch et al., 1988), nonpolyposis familial large bowel cancer (Utsunomiya et al., 1981) or Lynch syndrome I and II, and the latter is hereditary polyposis syndromes. The newer concept of hereditary solitary adenoma of the colon proposed by Woolf (1955) and updated by Burt (1985) is included in the former. Under the term of hereditary colorectal cancer, all of these conditions are included.

In this article, I would like to discuss the significance of the polyposis study to the nonpolyposis study, and to elucidate further the value of the study of hereditary colorectal cancer in tackling the common cancer problem. The information used for this review was collected from a series of studies done by the author and/or his collaborators at the Polyposis Center (1975-1983), at the surgical departments of Tokyo Medical and Dental University (1970-1983) and of Hyogo College of Medicine (1983-1989), and during the interinstitutional collaborative cancer research projects on the polyposes and allied conditions, supported in part by a Grant-in-Aid from the Ministry of Education and from the Ministry of Health and Welfare of Japan.

2. CENTRAL REGISTER

Since the polyposis register was initiated in 1925 in St. Marks Hospital, England, similar activities have been established in many countries in the world. In Japan, the Center for Analyzing Familial Polyposis (the Polyposis Center) was established by the author at Tokyo Medical and Dental University in 1975. Since 1982 when the author left there, the activity has been maintained by T. Iwama under the name of the Research Center for Polyposes and Intestinal Diseases, headed by T. Mishima.

Information on the probands of the polyposis syndromes as well as nonpolypotic familial cancer has been collected through five different sources: inquiries to hospitals throughout the nation, autopsy records, published literature, voluntary visits by patients, and the Japanese Society for Large Bowel Cancer Research. For each family, an exact pedigree map, a "working pedigree," has been constructed using the koseki, the national family register which has been traditionally maintained for more than 80 years. In order to identify family members, a permanent coding system was devised (Utsunomiya, 1989[a]). The affected members are identified through hospital records, death certificates, and communication with their family members. The Center sent a list of these high risk people to local physicians who registered the cases in order to promote the examinations of relevant family members. By this means, an increasing frequency of linking two or more independently registered pedigrees has been recognized and this has accelerated confirmation of the pedigrees (Utsunomiya et al., 1977, 1980, 1989). In 1982, when the author moved to his present institution, Hyogo College of Medicine, the Center had registered 472 families (697 cases) of APC, 131 families (146 cases) of Peutz-Jeghers syndrome and many with other polyposes. A family survey had been completed on 327 APC families with 4,847 members, and had revealed the presence of 854 affected and 3,545 persons at high risk as possible APC gene carriers.

3. STUDIES ON HEREDITARY POLYPOSIS SYNDROMES

The polyposis syndrome includes APC and hamartomatous polyposes which consist of Peutz-Jeghers syndrome and juvenile polyposis coli. They have common principal characteristics which include familial occurrence, excessive risk for cancer, involvement throughout the GI tract, and association with other congenital lesions (Table 1). The polyposis syndrome has been accepted as the model for studies on the genetic high-risk approach and in genetic oncology because its characteristic manifestation provides us with an excellent marker of the relevant gene for constructing a strategy for management as well as for the basic genetic study. Among them, APC has been most cultivated because of its relatively frequent occurrence and of its nearly-100% risk of colorectal cancer.

Table 1 Classification of Polyposis Syndromes

Classification (Morson)		polyposis			Cancer	inheri-
Genetic and histological	Terminology	st.	si.	li.	risk	tance
Hereditary						
Neoplastic	Adenomatous polyposis coli	+	+	+	+++	AD
Hamartomatous	Peutz-Jeghers' syndrome	+	+	+	+	AD
	Juvenile polyposis	+	+	+	+	AD
Nonhereditary						
Inflammatory	Inflammatory polyposis	−	−	+	−	−
	Lymphoid polyposis	−	+	+	−	−
Unclassified	Metaplastic polyposis	−	−	+	−	−
	Cronkhite-Canada syndrome	+	+	+	±	−

st=stomach, si=small intestine, li=large intestine, AD=autosomal dominant

4. STUDIES ON FAMILIAL ADENOMATOUS POLYPOSIS COLI (APC)

APC, synonymously called familial adenomatous polyposis (FAP) or adenomatosis coli (AC), indicates all the conditions in which more than 100 adenomas are distributed throughout the large bowel, regardless of familial occurrence and of association with any extracolonic lesions.
(According to the recent letter from Sir Walter Bodmer, there is now a clear understunding from Human Gene Mapping Community, and particular its Nomemclature Committee, that the name for the polyposis gene should be APC. The confusion with Familial Amyloid Polyneuropathy and the redundancy of Familial in the name of Familial Adenomatous Polyposis (FAP) are convincing argument for APC terminology. He, however, think Familial Adenomatous Polyposis may remain for the syndrome, because of its world wide popularity in surgical and pathological field. As the chairman of the Fourth International Symposium of Colorectal Disease, the author would like to decide to use Adenomatous Polyposis Coli, APC in this text, because the study on this condition is increasingly focused on molecular biology)

4.1 Heterogeneity of manifestations of APC

Many of the diagnostic terms previously proposed as separate conditions in the classification of the polyposes have, in the past, made valuable contributions toward the development of the concept, but are now obsolete after the recent development of endoscopic and x-ray examination techniques, since which time gastric and duodenal polyps have been considered the essential traits of the APC gene. (Utsunomiya et al.,1974, Ushio et al.,1976)

Based on the number of polyps in the large bowel, APC has be categorized by T.Iwama into the <u>sparse polyps form</u>, and the <u>profuse polyps form</u> distinguished by 10 polyps per square cm on the colonic mucosa (cited in Maeda et al.1984, Utsunomiya 1989[a,b]).

Regarding the Gardner syndrome, there are different grades of expression of manifestations, from the occult osteomas of the jaw which were detected by the focused x-ray examination in nearly 90% of APC (Utsunomiya et al.,1975) to the cases with the classical full brown Gardner stigmata which were observed merely in 7%. An adverse correlation between the expressibility of Gardner stigmata and number of colonic adenomas (Table 2) suggests the gene responsible for the two manifestations may be almost identical but pleiotrophic (Utsunomiya 1989[b]).

Table 2 Correlation between Gardner stigmata and polyp density types of APC

	polyp density	
Garnder type	sparse	profuse
GS + 20	19(24.4%)	1 (1.3%)
GS - 58	37(47.5%)	21(27.0%)

By M.Tanimura cited in Utsunomiya (1989[b])

In addition to the rather common Gardner syndrome, there are some other rare syndromes. The peculiar features of the Turcot syndrome are expected to be elucidated by Hamilton at the symposium. Genetic association of adenomatous polyposis and multiple cartilaginous exostosis (so-called Zanca syndrome) has recently been confirmed in one Japanese family by Miura et al (Utsunomiya 1989[b]). Based on the evidence of manifest heterogeneity, APC could be tentatively subclassified as follows:

- common types
  - simple APC
    - profuse polyps form
    - sparse polyps form
  - Gardner type—(usually with sparse polyps)
- uncommon types—Turcot synd., Zanca synd., and may be others

On many other occasions, associations of neoplastic or non-neoplastic disorders have been observed. Clinical detailed observation on individual patients, through rare, provided us with the important lead to a solution of a general problem. The location of the APC gene in chromosome No.5 first demonstrated by Bodmer (1987), had been motivated by incisive observations by Herrera et al. (1986) on a patient afflicted with mental retardation and multiple anomalies.

4.2 Genetic background of APC

The accumulated informations on over 300 families at the Polyposis Center provided us with an excellent opportunity to perform classical medical genetic analysis in incidence, sex ratio, sporadic case rate, penetrance, and segregation ratio. The result confirmed the classical mode of autosomal dominant transmission of the traits and proved there is a single gene responsible for adenoma production in the large bowel mucosa. The surprising similarity in the genetic background observed between our series and that of St.Marks (Table 3) indicates the mutation of the gene is occur independently to racial differences.

Table 3 Genetic elements of APC in Japanese and western populations

Genetic element	Japanese[1]	British[2]	U.S.A.[3]
Incidence	1/17,422	1/23,930	1/7,437
Male/Female ratio	1.67	1.31	1.48
Familial case	56%	55%	–
Penetrance	93.7%	80%	90%
Segregation ratio (observed)	0.427	0.361	0.400
Segregation ratio (adjusted)	0.456	0.458	0.499

[1]Murata et al. (1981), Utsunomiya (1989)[b], [2]Veale (1965), [3]Reed (1955)

4.3 Natural history and colorectal cancer risk of APC

Age-specific prevalence rate analysis provided us with the information to enable estimation of average time spans each of the evolutional phases of the patients: incubation, adenoma, and cancer stages respectively. At the beginning, the polyps were estimated to achieve a clinically detectable size in 80% of the gene carriers at between 5 and 10 years of age (Utsunomiya, 1989[b]). The cancer stage was found to begin about 5 years younger in females than in males, suggesting that there might exist a significant influence of sex hormones on the course of disease (Utsunomiya, 1989[b]). We found that in the female siblings of the index patient, infant death was significantly increased over the control group of the same sex, while there was no such marked difference in the male siblings (Utsunomiya et al., 1975). The evidence suggested female infants carrying the APC gene may be less resistant than male gene carriers.

A comparison between the Japanese and English polyposis studies revealed that the duration of the adenoma phase was similar, but the Japanese series had a longer cancer phase which was estimated from the average age of cancer diagnosis and that of death (7.3 years in males and 9.6 years in females) than the British (3.6 years and 4.0 years). This may reflect that Japanese colorectal cancers are better differentiated than the British series. The Japanese nationwide survey report on colorectal cancer in 1977 revealed that 60% of cases were "well differentiated", 27% "moderately" and 3.8% "poorly", while the data in the British study were 20%, 60% and 20% respectively (Morson and Dowson, 1972). The APC-related cancers were found predominantly in the left colon, as observed in general colorectal cancer (Utsunomiya, 1989[a, b]). The time trend of increasing sigmoid colon predominancy observed in general colorectal cancer was also observed in the APC cancers (Utsunomiya 1989[a]).

4.4 Multi-hit theory for APC cancer

The age-specific incidences of almost all cancers show a straight line, if plotted logarithmically. Armitage & Doll (1954) presented a theory that cancer develops from sequential multiple hits and that the number of necessary hits can be calculated from the age specific incidence of cancer. The number of hits required for colorectal cancer occurrence in the general population was estimated to be five to six whereas it was estimated to be one or two hits less for cancer of APC (Ashley 1969). We have obtained essentially the same result using the Japanese series (Utsunomiya & Murata 1980) (Fig.1). This provided us with the evidence that alteration of a single gene plays a role equivalent to the initial step of the evolutional sequence of a cancer occurrence in the colon, and that cancer develops under the considerable influence of additional postzygotic factors (Knudson 1977). The hypothesis is now being confirmed by recent molecular genetic studies which will be described at this symposium.

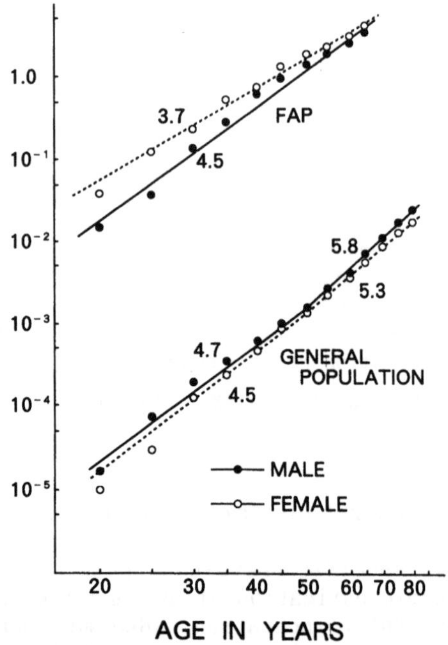

Fig.1 Number of hit required for colorectal cancer occurrence estimated in age specific prevalence in FAP(APC) and general population (Utsunomiya & Murata 1980)

4.5 Extracolonic cancers in APC

In cases where a patient live longer as a result of surgical prophylactic reatment, malignant lesions in other organs will acquire the chance to become manifest, presenting new problems. Gastric cancer was at least 10 times as likely to occur in APC patients than in the general population (Utsunomiya 1989[b]). In cancer incidence of the upper GI tract as a whole, there was no significant difference between Japanese and Western APC, but there was a striking difference in the site of cancer in the upper GI tract between the two groups. While Japanese APC produced gastric cancer 3 times more frequently than duodenal cancer, the latter was 5 times more than the former in the Western group (Table 4). The evidence suggest that the function of the APC gene could be modified to produce cancer also in the stomach under the relevant environmental circumstances. This leads to the speculation that there might exist a similar trend in the tumor spectrum of HNPCC in Japan or in other countries with a high risk of gastric cancer.

Table 4 Upper gastrointestinal cancer in APC: a comparison between Japanese and western populations

Upper GI cancer	Polyposis Center of Japan 1,564 cases, 1988*		Leed Castle Polyposis Group (10 registers of western countries) 1,255 cases, 1988**	
Gastric cancer	33	2.11%	7	0.56%
Duodenal cancer	10	0.64%	37	2.93%
Total	43	2.76%	44	3.49%

* report from the Polyposis Center, 1988
**Jagelman et al., 1988

4.6 Subclinical manifestation of APC

Investigations on phenotypic manifestations of APC at subclinical or subhistological levels contributed to the elucidation of the mechanism of the abnormal gene responsible for APC, and the development of methods for presymptomatic diagnosis.

In the background colon mucosa of APC patient, abnormal characteristics were observed by means of cytokinetic techniques (Lipkin et al., 1974, 1984 and Iwama et al., 1977) as well as by detecting the binding to epithelial cells of the specific glucoconjugates by PAT/KOH/PAS method (Muto et al.) and lectin UEA-1 (Kuroki et al., 1990). A similar histochemical difference was seen also in the gastric mucosa (Nishiura et al., 1984). The reason for the mysterious discrepancy observed in biochemical characteristics, as demonstrated by binding ability to some glucoconjugates, in the proximal and distal large bowel mucosa is to be clarified during the symposium.

Observations on the peculiar behavior of cultured somatic cells from the patient is of prime importance, as will be discussed by Kopelovich. In 1976, we observed that the cultured fibroblasts of the patients (APC and PJS) showed characteristics which resembled more an established cell line than the primary culture from normal persons: clonal morphology, growth rate and characteristics, and susceptibility to killing by mutagenesis (M. Sasaki cited in Utsunomiya et al., 1977). The study has been further extended productively by Miyaki et al. (1988). The above observations, in vivo as well as in vitro, suggested that the somatic cells of APC patients have already undergone some slight alteration towards eventual neoplastic change and the gene responsible for APC might act in controlling the essential function of growth and proliferation of the somatic cells.

4.7 Identification, surveillance and management of APC

Identification and surveillance: The central register is essential for promoting identification and surveillance of the patient and preservation of the information on the relevant pedigree over generations. Currently at the Polyposis Center, 600 families have been successfully registered, including 1,700 patients, deceased and living, over 14 years' activities (Table 5). The system is now being applied effectively to the nonpolyposis study.

Table 5 Number of APC family registered and patient identified at the Polyposis Center, Japan

	1972	1973	1974	1975	1977	1978	1981	1983	1989
Families registered	157	165	216	255	338	411	504	562	631
Patients identified	245	457	572	697	848	853	921	—	1738

The recent remarkable advances in identification of the gene responsible for APC and colorectal cancer promises a practical DNA diagnostic method, which will be hopefully developed as a result of the present symposium.

Management: Until the molecular genetic therapy for these conditions is realized, the approaches available for management are confined to prevention of colorectal cancer by chemical or surgical means. The important classical observation on the spontaneous regression of rectal polyps after total colectomy suggested that the APC patient is a sensitive model for testing preventive agents against colorectal cancer (DeCosse et al., 1989). Fruitful results on this line are eagerly expected in the symposium. At present, surgical elimination of the tissue at risk is the only available practical way of management for APC. Ideal function-restorative proctocolectomy has recently become feasible using the pelvic pouch procedures. Our J-pouch method (Utsunomiya et al.,1980) is now becoming most popular not only for treatment of APC but also for ulcerative colitis (Utsunomiya et al.,1989).

5. STUDIES ON HAMARTOMATOSIS POLYPOSES

5.1 Peutz-Jeghers Syndrome (PJS)

Peutz-Jeghers syndrome was encountered in clinical practice at a frequency of one quarter that of APC. The mode of transmission is classical autosomal dominant. In these patients, however, dissimilar to APC, the risk for cancer is less profound but distributed over various organs in addition to the intestine, therefore presenting us with a difficulty in proposing any useful preventive surgery (Utsunomiya et al.,1975). Cultured fibroblasts of the patient showed marked abnormalities as also seen in APC (Miyaki et al.1989) suggesting to us the importance of a cytomolecular study.

5.2 Juvenile Polyposis

Eighteen cases of juvenile polyposis were reported in Japan up to 1986 (Utsunomiya 1989[a]). This condition may be more closely related to APC than PJS, because it was occasionally associated with adenomas and cancer risk was rather localized in the large intestine. The association with variouscongenital abnormalities will provide good motivation for molecular geneticanalysis on this condition.

Identification of the gene responsible for these hamartomatous polyposes will contribute to the understanding of the genetic mechanism for the control stability of histological organization in the intestine.

6. STUDIES ON HEREDITARY NONPOLYPOSIS COLORECTAL CANCER (HNPCC)

Because of difficulty in confirmation of this trait, the lack of associated clinical markers such as adenomas, and insufficient clinical as well as pathological information, HNPCC has been less well understood, particularly regarding heterogeneity and mode of transmission. The information obtained and knowledge gained through the polyposis study will be effectively utilized for the study of HNPCC.

6.1 Characterization of family history positive nonpolyposis colorectal cancer

Currently, the diagnostic criteria proposed by Lynch can be applied exclusively to and selected rare large pedigrees. For most potential HNPCC patients, possibly over 80%, who are sporadic (non-familial) cases or constitute a small fragmental family, the criteria are not always practicable. There is an apparent necessity to establish clinical diagnostic criteria for these patients at present, since a DNA diagnostic method is not yet available. In order to elucidate clinical and epidemiological characteristics of HNPCC, we had an invaluable opportunity to compare colorectal cancer among the nonpolyposis patients with a positive family history (the patient who has one or more close relatives with colorectal cancer), those with a negative history, and those with APC patients. As a result, it was found that in the history-positive patient, the lesion was more frequently multiple, shifted to the right colon, and appeared at much younger ages than the history-negative patient (Table 6). The most impressive finding was that the history-positive cancer patient had relatives who died with other cancers three times more frequently than the history-negative patient. Moreover, the age of death of the relatives was much younger in the former than the latter (Table 7). We consider that this finding is useful for identification of HNPCC.

Table 6 Comparison of "polyposis cancer" and "familial nonpolyposis cancer"*

	Colorectal cancer patients		
	nonpolyposis group family history		APC group
	negative (n=241)	positive (n=60)	APC (n=229)
Average age	57.8yr	47.7yr	39.1yr
Right cancer	23.0%	39.0%	25.0%
Multiple cancer	3.0%	26.7%	37.6%

* Utsunomiya J., Iwama T., Matsumura T., et al. (1981)

Table 7 Association of extracolonic cancer in family members of nonpolyposis colorectal cancer patients with positive and negative colorectal cancer family history**

Cancer in family member	Colorectal cancer patients family history	
	negative (n**=122)	positive (n*=48)
Patient with other ca.	35	43
Number per family	0.28	0.90
Stomach	10 (29.0%)	17 (39.6%)
Uterine (origin unknown)	2 (5.8%)	5 (11.7%)
Endometrium	0	1 (2.4%)
Breast	0	4 (9.3%)
Other organs	23 (65.8%)	16 (37.2%)
Average age of death (yr.)	66.7	47.7

* Utsunomiya J., Iwama T., Matsumura T., et al. (1981)
**number of family

6.2 Heterogeneity of HNPCC

According to Lynch (1985), there are subsets of HNPCC, Lynch syndrome I or cancer family syndromes and Lynch syndrome II or hereditary site-specific colorectal cancer. They have common characteristics in early onset and proximal colon predominancy, except for an association with endometrial cancer in the former. In Japan, many similar pedigrees have been reported, which, however, are associated with a higher incidence of gastric cancer as will be further discussed by Sakiyama in this issue. The evidence may suggest that the expression of the gene responsible for HNPCC can be modified by environmental effects as seen in APC.

6.3 The proportion of HNPCC in general colorectal cancer

The family size specific frequency distribution was similar in APC, PJS and the family history positive colorectal cancer group (Table 8). The fact that about one half, 48.6%, of APC families did not show any positive family history indicates that there could exist a considerable number, possibly same number, of cancers associated with HNPCC hidden in the general colorectal cancer population. On the other hand, we could reasonably speculate that in the families such as Lynch descrived, we are looking at the extreme portion of the frequency distribution of individuals who manifest the more common HNPCC.

The frequency of family history positive cases in the general colorectal cancer population has been consistent among investigators from different areas; from 8.6% to 3.4% and 4.5% in our series. The purely coincidental association of colorectal cancer in one of the parents was estimated to be 0.5%, because the prevalence of colorectal cancer in the Japanese general population at the age of 50-60 which corresponds to the average age of HNPCC patients, was 0.25%. Therefore, the relative proportion of genetically determined familial colorectal cancer would be approximately 4.0%. Then, we assumed that the hereditary compartment, familial and sporadic, might occupy about 8% of the whole colorectal cancer population.

Table 8 Family size specific frequency distribution : nonpolyposis colorectal cancer compared to APC and PJS*

No. affected in a pedigree	APC No. (%)	PJS No. (%)	Familial non-polypotic cancer No.
Index pt only	120 (48.6)	60 (66.7)	—
2	50 (20.2)	18 (20.0)	21
3	32 (13.0)	4 (4.4)	8
4	14 (5.7)	2 (2.2)	3
5	8 (3.2)	4 (4.4)	4
6	9 (3.6)	—	2
7	3 (1.2)	—	1
8	4 (1.6)	—	—
9	4 (1.6)	1 (1.1)	—
10	1 (0.4)	—	—
11	1 (0.4)	1 (1.1)	—
12	1 (0.4)	—	—
Total	247	90	39

*(Utsunomiya J, Iwama T, Matsumura T, et al., 1981)

Lectin UEA-1 which did not bind usually to the rectal mucosa showed positive binding by a significantly increased level in the colorectal cancer family history positive individuals. This differential lectin binding may be useful for presymptomatic diagnosis (Kuroki).

7. CONCLUSION

APC has been intensively studied because of its characteristic manifestations with classical mendelian dominant inheritance which provided us with an excellent model for genetic implication for colorectal carcinogenesis. The information and knowledge thus accumulated were found to be applicable to the study of HNPCC. Hereditary colorectal cancer was estimated to occupy more or less 8% of general colorectal cancer. Nevertheless, the study was considered to be one of the most effective approaches to the elucidation of etiology, pathology and and management of colorectal cancer. Therefore, the author convice there is appearent and urgent needs to organize the international and interdisciprinary symposium on hereditary colorectal cancer in order to make a break through in general cancer problem.

REFERENCES

Armitage P, Doll R (1954) The age distribution of cancerand multi-stage theory of carcinogenesis.

Ashley DTB (1969) Colonic cancer arising in polyposis coli. J Med Genet 6: 376-378

Bodmer WF, Bailey CJ, Bodmer J, et al (1987) Localization of the gene for familial adenematous polyposis on chromosome 5. Nature 328: 614-616

Burt RW, Bishop DT, Cannon LA, Dowdle MA, Lee RG, Skolnick MH (1985) Dominant inheritance of adenomatous colonic polyps and colorectal cancer. N Engl J Med 312: 1540-1544

Bussey HJR (1975) Familial Polyposis Coli. Baltimore: Johns Hopkins University Press

DeCosse JJ, Miller HH, Lesser ML (1989) Effect of wheat fiber and Vitamins C and E on rectal polyps in patient with familial adenomatous polyposis. J Natl Cancer Inst 81: 1290-1297

Dukes CE (1952) Familial intestinal polyposis. Ann Eugenics 17: 1-29

Gardner EJ (1951) A genetic and clinical study of intestinal polyposis, a predisposing factor for carcinoma of the colon and rectum. Am J Hum Genet 3: 167-176

Hauser JJ, Weller CV (1936) A further report on the cancer family on Warthin. Am J Cancer 27: 434-449

Herrera L, Kakatis, Gibas L, Pietzak E, Sandberg AA (1986) Gardner's syndrome in a man with interstitial deletion of 5q. Am J Med Genet 25: 473-476

Iwama T, Utsunomiya J, Sasaki J (1977) Epithelial cell kinetics in the crypts of familial polyposis of the colon. Jap J Surg 7: 230-234

Jagelman DG, DeCosse JJ, Bussey HJR (1989) Upper gastrointestinal cancer in familial adenomatous polyposis. Lancet 1: 1149-1151

Jeghers H, McKusick VA, Katz KH (1949) Generalized intestinal polyposis and melanin spots of the oral mucosa, lips and digits: A syndrome of diagnostic significance. N Engl J Med 241: 933-1031

Knudson JR A G (1977) Genetic and environmental interaction in the origin of human cancer. In: Mulvihill JJ, Miller RW, Fraumeni Jr JF (ed.) Genetic of Human Cancer. Raven Press, New York

Kuroki T, Utsunomiya J, Miki Y, Yamamura T, Kubota A (1990) Histochemical detection of the colorectal cancer high risk group. to be submitted

Lipkin M (1974) Phase 1 and phase 2 proliferative lesions of colonic epithelial cells in disease leading to colonic cancer. Cancer 34: 878-888

Lipkin M, Blattner WA, Gardner EJ et al (1984) Classification and risk asessment of individuals with familial polyposis, Gardner syndrome and familial non-polyposis colon cancer from [^{3}H]dThd-labeling patterns in colonic epithelial cells. Cancer Res 44: 4201-4207

Lockhart-Mummery JP (1925) Cancer and hereditary. Lancet 1: 427

Lynch HT, Krush AJ (1967) Hereditary adenocarcinoma of the colon. Gastroent 53: 517-527

Lynch HT, Kimbering W, Albano WA et al (1985) Hereditary nonpolyposis colorectal cancer (Lynch Syndrome I and II), clinical description of resource. Cancer, 934-938

Maeda M, Iwama T, Utsunomiya J, Aoki N and Suzuki S (1984) Radiological features of familial polyposis coli: Grouping by polyp profusion. Brit J Radiol 57: 217-227

Miyaki M, Akamatsu N, Sato C, Utsunomiya J (1988) Chemical and viral transformation of cultured skin fibroblasts from patient with familial polyposis coli. Mutat Res 199: 399-414

Morson BC (1962) Precancerous lesions of the colon and rectum. Classification and controversial issues. JAMA 179: 316-321

Morson BC, Dawson IMP (1972) Gastrointestinal Pathology, Blackwell Scientific Pub. Oxford, London

Murata M, Utsunomiya J, Iwama T, Tanimura M (1981) Frequency of adenomatosis coli in Japan. Jap J Hum Genet 26: 19-30

Muto T, Kamiya J, Sawada T, Agawa S, Morioka, Utsunomiya J (1985) Mucin abnormality of colonic mucosa in patients with familial polyposis coli. Dis Colon Rectum 28: 147-148

Nishiura M, Hirota T, Itabashi M, Ushio K, Yamada T and Oguro Y (1984) A clinical and histochemical study of gastric polyps in familial polyposis coli. Am J Gastroent 79: 98-103

Ohsato K, Yao T, Watanabe H, Iida M, Itoh H (1977) Small-intestinal involvement in familial polyposis diagnosed by operative intestinal fiberscopy. Dis Colon Rectum 20: 414-420

Reed TE, Neel JV (1955) A genetic study of multiple polyposis of the colon (with an appendix deriving a method of estimating relative fitness). Am J Hum Genet 7: 236-263

Turcot J, Desperes JP and St.Pierre F (1959) Malignant tumors of the central nervous system associated with familial polyposis of the colon: Report of two cases. Dis Colon Rectum 2: 465-468

Ushio K, Sasagawa M, Doi H, Yamada T, Ichikawa H, Hojo K, Koyama Y, Sano R (1976) Lesions associated with familial polyposis coli: Studies of lesions of the stomach, duodenum, bones and teeth. Gastrointest Radiol 1: 67-80

Utsunomiya J, Maki T, Iwama T, Matsunaga Y, Ichikawa T, Shimomura T, Hamaguchi E, Aoki N (1974) Gastric lesions of familial polyposis coli. Cancer 34: 745-754

Utsunomiya J, Iwama T, Suzuki H (1975) Clinical and genetic study on familial polyposis coli: sex ratio. J J Hum Genet 20: 283, in Japanese

Utsunomiya J and Nakamura T (1975) The occult osteomatous changes in the mandible in patients with familial polyposis coli. Br J Surg 62: 45-51

Utsunomiya J, Gocho H, Miyanaga T, Hamaguchi H, Kashimura A, Aoki N (1975) Peutz-Jeghers syndrome. Johns Hopkins Med J 36: 71-82

Utsunomiya J (1977) Present status of adenomatosis coliin Japan In: Pathophysiology of Carcinogenesis in Digestive Organs (Farber E et al eds) University of Tokyo Press, Tokyo; Parks Press, Baltimore: 305-321

Utsunomiya J, Iwama T (1980) Adenomatosis coli in Japan. In: Winawer S, Schottenfeld D, Sherlock P, eds. Colorectal cancer: Prevention, epidemiology, and screening. NewYork: Raven Press: 83-95

Utsunomiya J, Iwama T, Imajo M, Matsuo S, Sawai S, Yaegashi K, Hirayama R (1980)[b] Total colectomy, mucosal proctectomy and ileoanal anastomosis. Dis Colon Rectum 23: 459-466

Utsunomiya J, Iwama T, Hirayama T (1980) Clinical and population genetics of the hereditary gastrointestinal polyposes. In: Rotter JI, Samloff and Rimoin DL (ed). Heterogeneity and Genetics of Common Gastrointestinal Disorders. Academic Press, New York, London, etc : 351-416

Utsunomiya J, Murata M and Tanimura M (1980) An analysis of the age distribution of colon cancer in adenomatosis coli. Cancer 45: 198-205

Utsunomiya J, Iwama T, Hirayama R (1981) Familial large bowel cancer In: De Cosse JJ (ed.) Large bowel cancer,Churchill Livingstone, Edinburgh, London, Melbourne and New York, PP. 16-36

Utsunomiya J, Iwama T, Matsumura T et al (1981) A study on nonpolyposis familial large bowel cancer. Gekka (Surgery) 43: 881-890 (in Japanese)

Utsunomiya J (1989)[a] Pathological and genetic aspects of adenomatosis coli in Japan. In: Takebe H and Utsunomiya J (ed.) Ganetics of Human Tumor in Japan. Japan Scientific Societies Press, Tokyo and Taylor & Francis LTD, London and Philadelphia, pp 45-64

Utsunomiya J (1989)[b] Pathology, genetics and management of hereditary gastrointestinal polyposes. In: Lynch HT and Hirayama T (ed.) Genetic epidemiology of cancer. CRC press, Inc. Boca Raton, Florida, pp 219-249

Utsunomiya J (1989)[a] J-pouch: Changes of the method over years. Germ J Gastroent 24: 249-251

Utsunomiya J, Yamamura T (1989)[b] Radikale chirurgie bei schrverer colitis ulcerosa: Dreizeitiges vorgehen ohne permanentes ileostoma. Der Chirurg 60: 565-572

Utsunomiya J, Miki Y, Kuroki T, Iwama T (1990) In:Herrera L(ed) Familial adenomatous polyposis. Alan R Lus, Inc. pp101-107

Veale AMO(1965) Intestinal Polyposis. Cambridge: Cambridge University Press

Warthin AS (1913) Hereditary with reference to carcinoma. Arch Intern Med 12: 546

Watanabe H, Enjoji M, Yao T, Ohsato K (1978) Gastric lesions in familial adenomatosis coli. Human Pathol 9: 269-283

Woolf CM, Richards RC, Gardner EJ (1955) Occasional discrete polyps of the colon and rectum showing an inherited tendency in a kindred. Cancer 8: 403-408

Zanca P (1953) Multiple hereditary cartilaginous exostosis with polyposis of the colon. U S Armed Forces M J.6,116-122

Historical and Natural Cancer History Facets of the Lynch Syndromes

HENRY T. LYNCH, STEPHEN J. LANSPA, THOMAS C. SMYRK, ROBERT J. FITZGIBBONS JR., PATRICE WATSON, BRUCE M. BOMAN, JANE F. LYNCH, and GIUSEPPE CRISTOFARO

ABSTRACT

Knowledge of cancer genetics, in concert with a thorough cancer family history, has the potential for providing one of the most powerful tools for the recognition of patients at high risk for cancer of specific anatomic sites. These facts have enabled the collection of a prodigious body of descriptive data dealing with the genetics of colorectal cancer. We shall discuss one facet of this problem; namely, the historical background and characteristics of the natural history, which has led to the recognition of hereditary nonpolyposis colorectal cancer (Lynch syndromes I and II). Since premonitory clinical signs of cancer risk are lacking in this disorder(s), it is clear that priority must now be given to the search for biomolecular markers of cancer risk.

Keywords: Lynch syndromes, genetics, history, diagnosis

INTRODUCTION

The study of patients at risk for hereditary colorectal cancer portends one of the most powerful and potentially cost-effective models for the elucidation of etiology, carcinogenesis, prevention, and control. However, success in such a venture will be contingent upon a meticulous compilation of the cancer family history. This should encompass a thorough documentation of genealogy, cancer (all sites), and extra-cancer phenotypic manifestations. For example, in the case of familial adenomatous polyposis (FAP) or its so-called Gardner's syndrome variant, multiple adenomatous colonic polyps, cutaneous signs such as epidermoid cysts, osteomas and congenital hypertrophy of the retinal pigment epithelium (CHRPE) will represent cardinal physical signs for the assessment of genetic risk status. On the other hand, when distinguishing signs are lacking, as is the case for the Lynch syndromes, one must then rely exclusively on pedigree interpretation in concert with knowledge of the natural history pattern of the cancer phenotype [Lynch & Lynch 1985].

Hereditary nonpolyposis colorectal cancer (HNPCC), referred to in the past as the Cancer Family Syndrome and more recently as the Lynch syndromes, has two major subdivisions: 1) hereditary site-specific nonpolyposis colorectal cancer (Lynch syndrome I), which is characterized by an autosomal dominantly inherited susceptibility to nonpolyposis colorectal carcinoma, with early age of onset, predilection to the proximal colon, and multiple primary colonic cancer; and 2) Lynch syndrome II, which shows all of the features of Lynch syndrome I, but is also associated with extracolonic cancer, particularly carcinoma of the endometrium and ovary [Lynch et al 1985a]. Recent studies have shown tumor heterogeneity in Lynch syndrome II, as evidenced by the presence of an excess of gastric [Cristofaro et al 1987], small bowel

[Lynch et al, in press-a], pancreatic [Lynch et al 1985b], urologic [Lynch et al, in press-b], and laryngeal cancers [Lynch et al 1988a] in specific extended kindreds.

Historical Perspective of the Lynch Syndromes

A formidable barrier to the comprehension of colorectal cancer genetics is frequently posed by incomplete pathologic verification of the cancer-prone phenotype among patients and their relatives. It was, therefore, fitting that a detailed clinical/pathologic investigation of a family with an exceedingly high incidence of colorectal cancer was launched in 1895 by Aldred Warthin, Chairman of the Department of Pathology at the University of Michigan School of Medicine at Ann Arbor [Warthin 1913]. This study was prompted by Warthin's intense interest in his seamstress' admonition that one day she was going to die of cancer of her "bowels or female organs" because "everbody in my family died of cancer." Soberingly, as she had predicted, she died of endometrial carcinoma. However, not everyone in her family died of cancer. Only half of the individuals in the cancer-prone lineage of this large family died of this disease. Males and females were equally affected, and the overall pattern of cancer transmission in this family was consistent with an autosomal dominant factor. The most common anatomic sites of cancer predilection were the colorectum (in the absence of florid colonic polyposis) and the endometrium. Thus, one of the hallmarks of genetic predisposition to cancer; namely, consistent anatomic site(s) of predilection, appeared almost monotonously in multiple generations of this large family.

Longitudinal followup with rigorous genealogic and pathologic documentation of cancer was subsquently pursued in this family by Warthin [1925], and later, by his colleagues Hauser and Weller [1936]. We began study of this family (now known as Family G) in 1965 and published an update of the pedigree in 1971, providing some 75 years (1895-1970) of followup experience [Lynch & Krush 1971].

The medical/genetic significance of HNPCC in association with endometrial cancer as a hereditary cancer syndrome was defined for the first time in 1966 [Lynch et al 1966]. This description emanated from our detailed observation of the unique familial clustering of these lesions in two extended midwestern kindreds, which we later referred to as the Cancer Family Syndrome [Lynch et al 1966]. Formal segregation analysis subsequently confirmed our original assumption of autosomal dominant inheritance [Bailey-Wilson et al 1986].

Hundreds of families which fit the criteria of Lynch syndromes I and II have now been described among virtually all nationalities and races [Lynch & Lynch 1985]. Its public health impact has been found to be enormous [Lynch & Lynch 1985; Lynch 1986; Mecklin 1987a]. For example, of the 151,000 patients in the United States who will be affected with cancer of the colon and rectum in 1989 [Silverberg & Lubera 1989], at least 6% will manifest the Lynch syndromes. In contrast, less than 1% of all colorectal cancers will fit its more well-known hereditary counterpart, FAP.

Natural History of the Lynch Syndromes: Its Cardinal Features

In order to comprehend the natural history of cancer expression in the Lynch syndromes, ten extened HNPCC kindreds from our resource were investigated [Fitzgibbons et al 1987]. Kindred members with colorectal cancer differed significantly ($p<0.05$) from patients with sporadic colorectal cancer, as evidenced by the following: a) the mean age of initial colon cancer diagnosis was 44.6 years; b) 72.3% of initial colon cancers were located in the right colon; and c) 18.1% had synchronous colon cancer, with a risk for metachronous colonic lesions in 10 years of 40%. Comprehension of these natural history characteristics of the Lynch syndromes are crucial for diagnosis, surveillance, and management.

Surveillance and Management

The above cardinal features of the Lynch syndromes form the basis for their management strategies. We recommend that all first degree relatives (parents, progeny, siblings) of syndrome cancer affecteds undergo meticulous education about their cancer risk and the natural history of cancer in the Lynch syndromes. Ideally, this educational experience should be provided by their primary physician, beginning in their mid to late teens. We prefer this early educational indoctrination so that these high risk patients might attain a more objective appreciation about their cancer risk status. This information could then have a positive impact on their need for lifelong compliance to our rigorous surveillance program.

At age 20, we recommend initiation of occult blood testing of stool. This should then be performed three times each year thereafter. Colonoscopy should be started at age 25, performed every other year through age 35, and then annually thereafter. Women should undergo pelvic examination, with vacuum aspiration curettage of the endometrium at the time of their initial colonoscopy, and then annually. Should colon cancer occur, a subtotal abdominal colectomy with ileorectal anastomosis is indicated because of the significant risk of synchronous and metachronous lesions. The rectum should receive careful lifetime surveillance [Lynch et al 1988b].

Women presenting with colon cancer and who have completed their families, or who are postmenopausal, should also be considered as candidates for prophylactic hysterectomy and bilateral salpingo oophorectomy. Great care should be given so that the consequences of this prophylactic surgery are clearly understood by these women. If there is a desire for future pregnancies, then this surgical prophylaxis should be deferred in favor of intensive surveillance [Lynch et al 1988c].

Differential Diagnosis of the Lynch Syndromes

Diagnosis of the Lynch syndromes must be made by recognizing a genetic predisposition to colorectal cancer in the absence of physical signs and/or biomarkers of acceptable sensitivity and specificity to the deleterious genotype [Lynch & Lynch 1985; Lynch et al 1985a; 1988c]. The cancer genetic diagnostician must rely almost exclusively on the pedigree, and his knowledge of hereditary colorectal cancer-prone syndromes. This task may be exceedingly difficult in certain circumstances, particularly when considering the several obstacles to genetic diagnosis. These are virtually the same types of problems which impact on family studies of all varieties. These include man's long generation intervals, inability to control or, in some circumstances, adequately ascertain matings, limited number of progeny, early deaths of at risk individuals, and in the case of cancer, difficulty in obtaining definitive clinical and pathologic documentation of cancer. In addition, key relatives may not comply with the investigation, thereby limiting disclosure of vital medical/genetic information.

Sorting out medical/genetic/epidemiologic clues for Lynch syndrome diagnosis will, therefore, require patient/family compliance, meticulous documentation of genealogic, medical, and pathologic information, and a sufficient number of relatives will require observation over a relatively long period of time.

In addition to the diagnostic distinction between Lynch syndromes I and II, the clinician must exclude their hereditary colorectal cancer counterparts. These include the several familial adenomatous polyposis (FAP) syndromes and the hereditary discrete colorectal polyp-cancer syndrome [Burt et al 1985]. Familial clusterings of colorectal cancer must also be considered [Lynch & Lynch 1985]. This may be due to chance and/or possible common environmental exposures.

Minimal diagnostic criteria, which may be observed in only a limited number of patients, may have to be relied on for syndrome assessment, particularly when dealing with small families. Nevertheless, certain clinical features of hereditary cancer should immediately alert the clinician to the possibility of the Lynch syndromes. For example, colon cancer diagnosed before age 45 should be suggestive of hereditary etiology. When the cancer is located in the cecum or ascending colon, or if there are synchronous or metachronous colorectal cancers or a history of early onset endometrial or ovarian carcinoma, the diagnostician's index of suspicion should increase significantly.

Clinical Example of Lynch Syndrome II in a Nuclear Family

An example of a putative Lynch syndrome II diagnosis in a nuclear family was entertained when a brother and sister at ages 25 and 27, respectively, developed proximal colon cancer in the absence of multiple colonic polyps. Each manifested a history of metachronous colonic cancers. The sister subsequently developed endomentrial carcinoma at age 35. Their mother was found to have had proximal colonic cancer, also in the absence of multiple colonic polyps, at age 30. She developed endometrial carcinoma at age 37, and at the time of hysterectomy and bilateral salpingo oophorectomy, was found to have a Stage I carcinoma of her ovary.

Since it would be highly unlikely on a statistical basis to find extremely early onset proximal and metachronous colorectal cancers, and carcinoma of the endometrium and ovary in these three patients to have occurred by chance, particularly in two generations, the diagnosis of Lynch syndrome II was given serious consideration. The presence of these findings, coupled with addition of colon and endometrial cancer, in a large, extended family, with a high degree of pathology verification, would clearly add more credibility to the strength of this diagnosis.

Probabilities of Early Onset Colon and Endometrial Cancer

In order to appreciate the probability of early onset colon and endometrial carcinoma prior to age 40, we compiled their likelihoods based on age-specific colon and endometrial cancer incidence from the SEER data. These studies indicate that the probability of manifesting colon cancer by age 40 is $7x10^{-4}$, and of endometrial carcinoma by age 40 is $4.4x10^{-4}$. The probability of a female having both colon and endometrial cancer onset prior to age 40, if these diseases are unrelated, is (0.00044)(0.0007), or 3 in 10 million. This same probabilistic approach was given to the assessment of proximal colon cancer, which occurs in about 35% of all patients with colonic cancer. Herein, the probability of proximal colon cancer in a patient less than age 40 would be (0.35)(0.0007) or 2.5×10^{-4}.

Another scenario would be a nuclear family of 8, comprised of both parents with a sibship of 6. If all cancer diagnoses in this family were considered as independent, then the probability of two cases of proximal colon cancer at less than age 40 would be equal to 1.7×10^{-6} or 2 in a million. The probability of 3 cases of proximal colon cancer at less than age 40 would equal 8.7×10^{-10}, or 1 in a billion.

While these age-specific cancer computations do not portend etiologic significance, they do nevertheless provide a basis for comprehending their relative frequencies. Therefore, assessing the clinical significance for early onset colorectal and endometrial cancer, including their combination in a single patient, provide an appreciation for their chance expectations in the general population.

Tritiated Thymidine Labeling of Colonic Crypt Compartments

Details of the methods for investigation of ^{3}HdThD labeling of colonic mucosal crypts have been previously published [Lipkin et al 1984]. These studies detect DNA synthesis in cells at all levels of the colonic crypts, although normally S-phase cells only occur in the lower two-thirds of the glands. These studies have aided our understanding of the neoplastic transformation of colonic epithelial cells in hereditary disorders that may predispose to cancer. In the study of 11 families with the Lynch syndromes, a shift of the major zone for ^{3}HdThd uptake in the distal colonic mucosal crypt compartments were positively associated with cancer risk status in the Lynch syndromes [Lynch et al 1985a].

Oral Calcium Supplementation

Recently, Rozen et al [1989] studied patients at risk for colon cancer and noted that oral calcium supplements significantly suppressed proliferation of the upper crypt compartment in biopsy samples taken from the rectum, as measured by the ^{3}HdThd pattern. Studies of oral calcium supplementation merit investigation in the Lynch syndromes [Lipkin et al 1984; Rozen et al 1989].

Biomolecular Genetics

Biomolecular studies may one day aid in both syndrome classification and clarification of heterogeneity. Recently, two groups [Bodmer et al 1987; Leppert et al 1987] identified a genetic marker on chromosome 5 that was tightly linked to the gene for FAP. In addition, sporadic colorectal carcinomas showed loss of heterozygosity on the long arm of chromosome 5 in 20-30% of cases [Solomon et al 1987; Okamoto et al 1987; Wildrick & Boman 1988].

Three other types of genetic alterations that have been reported in colorectal tumors include: a) point mutations in ras proto-oncogenes [Bos et al 1987; Forrester et al 1987]; b) allelic deletion of chromosome 17 [Vogelstein et al 1988; Monpezat et al 1988; Law et al 1988]; and c) allelic deletion of chromosome 18 [Boman et al 1988; Vogelstein et al 1988; Monpezat et al 1988; Law et al 1988]. Recent studies have also shown that the p53 gene on chromosome 17p is mutated in colorectal carcinoma. This suggests that inactivation of p53 through deletion of chromosome 17p or mutation of the p53 gene is important in colorectal carcinoma [Baker et al 1989].

Vogelstein et al [1988] found that these four molecular alterations accumulated in a fashion that paralleled the clinical progression of tumors. Allelic deletions of chromosome 5 and ras mutations occurred relatively commonly in early stage adenomas, as well as later stage tumors. In contrast, allelic deletions of chromosomes 17 and 18 occurred only occasionally in earlier stage carcinomas, but occurred frequently in advanced adenomas and in carcinomas. A recent study on clinical and pathological associations showed that allelic deletions of chromosomes 17 and 18 identified a subset of colorectal cancer patients with increased predilection for distant metastases and cancer-related death [Kern et al 1989].

In one of our studies, 9 families with Lynch syndrome II and 2 with Lynch syndrome I were assessed with respect to 25 serum and blood group markers [Lynch et al 1985a]. A positive lod score of 3.19 for linkage of the Kidd (JK) blood group and Lynch syndrome II were obtained. JK has been assigned to chromosome 18. This suggests that this chromosome might be the location of the deleterious gene for Lynch syndrome II [Boman et al 1988].

Until the time when advances in molecular biology allow precise genetic classification of colorectal cancer, the diagnosis of the Lynch syndromes will continue to be based on careful clinical observation. The oncologist, cancer geneticist, pathologist, and colonoscopist are in an ideal position to merge phenotypic findings, family history, and knowledge of the natural history of the Lynch syndromes into a powerful tool for cancer control.

Third Party Carriers

Compliance with the rigorous surveillance strategies we have recommended for the Lynch syndromes may be influenced by a variety of factors. Foremost of these are the patient's knowledge of his/her cancer risk, the patient's emotional status (i.e., fear of a colon cancer diagnosis), and the availability, convenience, comfort, and cost of the surveillance procedures(s). The health care team can readily mollify most of these concerns. However, cost may prove to be a significantly limiting variable. More cost-benefit research is therefore needed to establish the efficacy of screening individuals who are at inordinately high risk for the Lynch syndromes. Model studies include those of Eddy et al [1987], Rozen et al [1987], Mecklin [1987b], and Vasen et al [1989], each of which have shown an increased colorectal cancer yield as a result of screening patients at high genetic risk. It would therefore seem logical that third party carriers would show a greater willingness to defray the expenses of surveillance and management of high risk Lynch syndrome patients given the scientific evidence that such screening procedures are cost beneficial.

Cancer-Prone Family Registries

Given the enormous amount of time and effort which goes into the accrual of data for the construction of cancer-prone family pedigrees, it would be ideal to have regional or national registries for the Lynch syndromes. The development of such registries could provide invaluable mechanisms for cancer control through computer-automated systems. Paramount to such registries must be protection of the confidentiality of its informational content, with the assurance of security in the transmission of this valuable knowledge to the family physicians of record. Accompanying this genetic risk information would be a description of those salient aspects of a Lynch syndrome diagnosis, its pertinent natural history, and the melding of this knowledge into highly targeted surveillance and management strategies.

These goals will be fostered through the recent development of an International Hereditary Colon Cancer Collaborative Group which is designed to pool information on the Lynch syndromes. A major commitment of this collaborative effort will be: a) the sharing of expertise in the differing specialty areas dealing with colorectal cancer genetics, particularly pathology and clinical studies with attention to minimal clues for syndrome diagnosis; b) development of registries; c) lay and professional education, with the development of techniques for its worldwide dissemination; and d) sharing of DNA and pedigree information for linkage analysis. Since the Lynch syndromes are known to be ubiquitous throughout the world, we are hoping that clinicians will avail themselves of this planned resource so that recognition of hereditary colorectal cancer problems and their control can be maximal.

In conclusion, we consider knowledge of cancer genetics and the natural history of the cancer phenotype, in concert with a detailed pedigree, to be the Gordian knot for diagnosis, surveillance, and management in the Lynch syndromes.

ACKNOWLEDGEMENTS: Support for this effort was provided by grants from the National Cancer Institute, #1 RO1 CA42705-03, the Nebraska Cancer and Smoking Disease Research Program, #90-04R, and the Health Futures Foundation.

REFERENCES

Bailey-Wilson JE, Elston RC, Schuelke GS, Kimberling WJ, Albano WA, Lynch JF, Lynch HT (1986) Segregation analysis of hereditary nonpolyposis colorectal cancer. Genet Epid 3: 27-38

Baker SJ, Fearon ER, Nigro JM, Hamilton SR, Preisinger AC, Jessup JM, vanTuinen P, Ledbetter DH, Barker DF, Nakamura Y, White R, Vogelstein B (1989) Chromosome 17 deletions and p53 gene mutations in colorectal carcinomas. Science 244:217-221

Bodmer WF, Bailey CJ, Bodmer J, Bussey HJR, Ellis A, Gorman P, Lucibello FC, Murday VA, Rider SH, Scambler P, Sheer D, Solomon E, Spurr NK (1987) Localization of the gene for familial adenomatous polyposis on chromosome 5. Nature 328:614-616

Boman BM, Wildrick DM, Alfaro SR (1988a) Chromosome 18 allele loss at the D18S6 locus in human colorectal carcinomas. Biochem Biophys Res Comm 155: 463-469

Boman BM, Lynch HT, Kimberling WJ, Wildrick DM (1988b) Reassignment of a cancer family syndrome gene to chromosome 18. Ca Genet Cytogenet 34:153-154

Bos JL, Fearon ER, Hamilton SR, Verlaan-deVries M, vanBoom JH, van der Eb AJ, Vogelstein B (1987) Prevalence of ras gene mutations in human colorectal cancers. Nature 327:293-297

Burt RW, Bishop DT, Cannon LA, Dowdle MA, Lee RG, Skolnick MH (1985) Dominant inheritance of adenomatous colonic polyps and colorectal cancer. NEJM 312:1540-1544

Cristofaro G, Lynch HT, Caruso ML, Attolini A, Matteo GI, Giorgio P, Senatore S, Argentieri A, Sbano E, Fusaro R, Giorgio I (1987) New phenotypic aspects in a family with Lynch syndrome II. Cancer 60: 51-58

Eddy DM, Nugent FW, Eddy JF, Coller C, Gilbertsen V, Gottlieb LS, Rice R, Sherlock P, Winawer S (1987) Screening for colorectal cancer in a high risk population: results of a mathematic model. Gastroenterology 92:682-692
Fitzgibbons RJ Jr, Lynch HT, Stanislav GV, Watson P, Lanspa SJ, Marcus JN, Smyrk T, Kriegler MD, Lynch JF (1987) Recognition and treatment of patients with hereditary nonpolyposis colon cancer (Lynch syndromes I and II). Ann Surg 206:289-295
Forrester K, Almoguera C, Han K, Grizzle WE, Perucho M (1987) Detection of high incidence of K-ras oncogenes during human colon tumorigenesis. Nature 327:298-303
Hauser I, Weller CV (1936) A further report on the cancer family of Warthin. Am J Cancer 27:434-449
Kern SE, Fearon ER, Tersmette KWF, Enterline JP, Leppert M, Nakamura Y, White R, Vogelstein B, Hamilton SR (1989) Allelic loss in colorectal carcinomas. JAMA 261:3099-3103
Law DJ, Olschwang S, Monpezat JP, Lefrancois D, Jagelman D, Petrelli NJ, Thomas G, Feinberg AP (1988) Concerted nonsyntenic allelic loss in human colorectal carcinoma. Science 241:961-965
Leppert M, Dobbs M, Scambler P, O'Connell P, Nakamura Y, Stauffer D, Woodward S, Burt RW, Hughes J, Gardner E, Lathrop M, Wasmuth J, Lalouel M, White R (1987) The gene for familial polyposis coli maps to the long arm of chromosome 5. Science 238:1411-1413
Lipkin M, Blattner WA, Gardner EJ, Burt RW, Lynch H, Deschner EE, Winawer S, Fraumeni JF (1984) Classification and risk assessment of individuals with familial polyposis, Gardner's syndrome, and familial nonpolyposis colon cancer from ^{3}[H]thymidine labeling patterns in colonic epithelial cells. Cancer Res 44:4201-4207
Lynch HT, Shaw MW, Magnuson CW, Krush AJ (1966) Hereditary factors in cancer: study of two large midwestern kindreds. Arch Int Med 117:206-212
Lynch HT, Krush AJ (1971) Cancer family G revisited: 1895-1970. Cancer 27:1505-1511
Lynch HT, Kimberling WJ, Albano WA, Lynch JF, Biscone K, Schuelke GS, Sandberg AA, Lipkin M, Deschner EE, Mikol YB, Elston RC, Bailey-Wilson JE, Danes BS (1985a) Hereditary nonpolyposis colorectal cancer (Lynch syndromes I and II), Parts I and II. Cancer 56:934-951
Lynch HT, Voorhees GJ, Lanspa SJ, McGreevy PS, Lynch JF (1985b) Pancreatic carcinoma and hereditary nonpolyposis colorectal cancer: a family study. Br J Cancer 52:271-273
Lynch HT (1986) Frequency of hereditary nonpolyposis colorectal cancer. Gastroenterology 90:486-492
Lynch HT, Kriegler M, Christiansen TA, Smyrk T, Lynch JF, Watson P (1988a) Laryngeal carcinoma in a Lynch syndrome II kindred. Cancer 62:1007-1013
Lynch HT, Watson P, Lanspa SJ, Marcus JN, Smyrk T, Fitzgibbons RJ Jr, Kriegler M, Lynch JF (1988b) Natural history of colorectal cancer in hereditary nonpolyposis colorectal cancer (Lynch syndromes I and II). Dis Colon Rect 31:439-444
Lynch HT, Watson P, Kriegler M, Lynch JF, Lanspa SJ, Marcus J, Smyrk T, Fitzgibbons RJ Jr, Cristofaro G (1988c) Differential diagnosis of hereditary nonpolyposis colorectal cancer (Lynch syndromes I and II). Dis Colon Rect 31:372-377
Lynch HT, Smyrk TC, Lynch PM, Lanspa SJ, Boman BM, Ens JA, Lynch JF, Strayhorn P, Carmody T, Watson P, Cristofaro G (in press-a) Adenocarcinoma of the small bowel in Lynch syndrome II. Cancer
Lynch HT, Ens JA, Lynch JF (in press-b) Lynch syndrome II and urologic manifestations. J Urol
Lynch PM, Lynch HT (1985) Colon cancer genetics. VN Reinhold, New York
Mecklin JP (1987a) Frequency of hereditary colorectal cancer. Gastroenterology 93:1021-1025

Mecklin JP, Jarvinen HJ, Aukee S, Elomaa I, Karjalainen K (1987b) Screening for colorectal carcinoma in Cancer Family Syndrome kindreds. Scan J Gastroent 22:449

Monpezat JP, Delattre O, Bernard A, Grunwald D, Remvikos Y, Muleris M, Salmon RJ, Frelat G, Dutrillaux B, Thomas G (1988) Loss of alleles on chromosome 18 and on the short arm of chromosome 17 in polypoid colon cancer. Int J Cancer 41:404-408

Okamoto M, Sasaki M, Sugio K, Sato C, Iwama T, Ikeuchi T, Tonomura A, Sasazuki T, Miyaki M (1988) Loss of constitutional heterozygosity in colon carcinoma from patients with familial polyposis coli. Nature 331:273-277

Rozen P, Fireman Z, Figer A, Legum C, Ron E, Lynch HT (1987) Family history of colorectal cancer as a marker of potential malignancy within a screening program. Cancer 60:248-254

Rozen P, Fireman Z, Fine N, Wax Y, Ron E (1989) Oral calcium suppresses increased rectal epithelial proliferation of persons at risk of colorectal cancer. Gut 30:650-655

Silverberg E, Lubera JA (1989) Cancer statistics, 1989. Ca 39:3-20

Solomon E, Voss R, Hall V, Bodmer WF, Jass JR, Jeffreys AJ, Lucibello FC, Patel I, Rider SH (1987) Chromosome 5 allele loss in human colorectal carcinomas. Nature 328:616-619

Vogelstein B, Fearon ER, Hamilton SR, Bodmer WF, Jass JR, Jeffreys AJ, Lucibello FC, Patel I, Rider SH (1988) Genetic alterations during colorectal tumor development. NEJM 319:525-532

Warthin AS (1913) Heredity with reference to carcinoma as shown by the study of the cases examined in the pathological laboratory of the University of Michigan, 1895-1913. Arch Int Med 12:546-555

Warthin AS (1925) The further study of a cancer family. J Cancer Res 9:279-286

Wildrick DM, Boman BM (1988) Chromosome 5 allele loss at the glucocorticoid receptor locus in human colorectal carcinoma. Biochem Biophys Res Comm 150:591-598

Eldon Gardner Memorial Lecture: Genetic Mapping and Allelic Heterogeneity of the Familial Polyposis Gene

MARK LEPPERT, YUSUKE NAKAMURA, RANDALL BURT, J.P. HUGHES, WADE SAMOWITZ, SCOTT WOODWARD, ELDON GARDNER, JEAN-MARC LALOUEL, and RAY WHITE

ABSTRACT

The genetic locus that harbors mutation(s) responsible for adenomatous polyposis coli (APC) and for Gardner syndrome has been mapped to chromosome 5 by linkage analysis with DNA markers. New markers have been developed for this region of chromosome 5 in order to refine the location of the gene(s) involved, as an important step toward isolation and characterization of the molecular defects responsible for these two diseases. A third type of polyp syndrome linked to the same locus has been observed in a family originally ascertained by Eldon Gardner. The linkage results in this family suggest that allelic heterogeneity at the APC locus may account for some predispositions to colon cancer even when typical polyposis is absent.

Keywords: adenomatous polyposis coli, genetic linkage, DNA markers, colon cancer

1. INTRODUCTION

Eldon Gardner was among the first to recognize the significance of genetic inheritance in human cancers. His early training and research were in the genetics of Drosophila; the genetics of human cancer came later. As a pioneer of a new field, Eldon had a special opportunity and responsibility to shape and direct the nascent enterprise, and he realized both with superlative style. The pioneers of a field have an orientation and perspective distinct from those of us who enter an established field to train and become professionals. The pioneers are amateurs in the original sense of the word, those who pursue their work out of love. Their role is crucial, for they define the field into which we later come as professionals.

I had the opportunity to work as a colleague with Eldon only during his last years, but these interactions were exemplary in representing the approach of a pioneer. No technology was too new or unapproachable. The important thing, the only important thing, was progress toward understanding the genetic basis of human cancer.

Although driven by an intensity of passion that in many gifted people results in impatience or abruptness, Eldon's civilized and gentle demeanor was never compromised. Despite undoubtable provocation from us then-young technocrats, he remained unruffled and strove to be helpful; to further

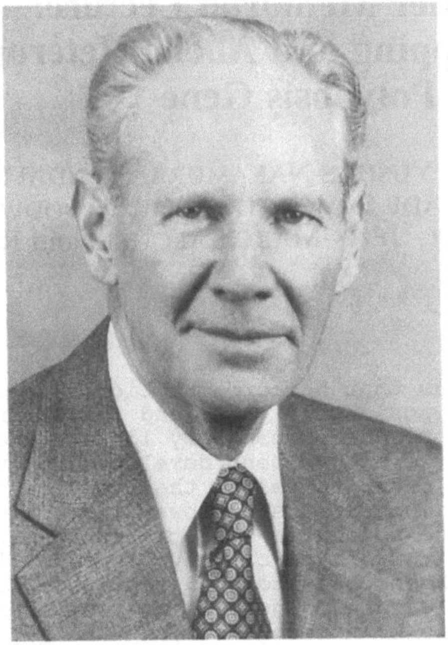

Eldon Gardner

the enterprise, to develop new understandings. Even in his later years, Eldon was remarkably tireless. He spent thousands of hours driving to visit families with unusual clusters of cancer; even to meet with colleagues at the University of Utah required more than an hours' travel.

Eldon Gardner was interested in many forms of inherited cancer, but perhaps his greatest contribution was to the body of knowledge about cancer of the colon, through his recognition and characterization of the intriguing variant form of familial adenomatous polyposis that was subsequently designated Gardner syndrome. In addition to characterizing Gardner syndrome in the classic Kindred 109, Eldon ascertained as well a number of other colon cancer families, in particular the puzzling Kindred 353 which showed a clear inheritance of a polyp syndrome but with a heterogeneous presentation. His personal concern and compassion for these families resulted in enduring relationships and were hallmarks of his approach. As a result these families, ascertained and characterized over several decades, have formed the backbone of our own genetic mapping and characterization of the polyposis gene. We are deeply grateful to Eldon Gardner for his selfless efforts; he was indeed a gentleman and a scholar with a rare insight.

It is an honor and a privilege for me, therefore, to be able to report the progress that has taken place within the last decade in unraveling the genetics of familial polyposis. Much of this work is critically dependent upon the foundation laid by Eldon Gardner in ascertaining and characterizing high-risk colon-cancer families.

This focus on colon cancer partially reflects Dr. Gardner's, and at this meeting our, appreciation that colon carcinoma is a major cause of morbidity and mortality worldwide; in the U.S., it is the second most common cause of death from cancer. Genetic factors may contribute significantly to as much as 10% of colon cancer, and perhaps more. One genetic predisposition, apparently rather rare, is familial adenomatous polyposis coli (APC), a condition that occurs in approximately one in 8000 individuals in all populations. Colon cancer arises in these patients due to the presence of large numbers of adenomatous polyps of the colon (Muto and others, 1975; Burt and Samowitz, 1988). The diagnosis of APC presently depends upon the finding of numerous visible adenomatous polyps --often hundreds or thousands -- in the colon by the end of the second or third decade of life (Bussey, 1975). Many affected individuals also exhibit numerous fundic-gland polyps of the stomach, and/or adenomatous polyps of the duodenum and small bowel.

We became interested some years ago in the effort to map the polyposis gene, with the goal of better characterizing its genetics and in the hope that chromosomal localization would serve as a basis for its cloning and characterization. More than 100 DNA markers had been tested for linkage to APC when we became aware that Herrera *et al*. (1986) had found a deletion in the long arm of chromosome 5 in a polyposis patient. Use of several DNA markers from chromosome 5, especially the C11p11 probe sent to us by Peter Scambler (Leppert and others, 1987), mapped the polyposis gene to chromosome 5q (Leppert and others, 1987; Bodmer and others, 1987) within the region indicated in Figure 1.

In order to improve the precision of the mapping, more markers in the region were needed. We developed a number of these from somatic cell hybrids containing only segments of chromosome 5 as their human component (Cirullo and others, 1983). Our initial DNA markers served to identify the hybrids that contained the region in question, which in turn became a source of new markers for the region through construction of libraries of cloned DNA segments for screening with human DNA.

Maps of the markers developed in normal reference families became the basis for more precise mapping within polyposis families. Figure 2 shows the more highly resolved map location obtained with several new markers (Nakamura and others, 1988). It was somewhat surprising to find that the gene mapped at a distance of approximately 15 cM from the original C11p11 marker, which had been thought to be quite tightly linked. This second round of mapping, however, placed the gene within a 10-cM region, likely reflecting some 10 megabases of genomic DNA. (High-resolution mapping within this region, to serve as a basis for a search for gene transcripts, will be described by Yusuke Nakamura in a separate paper at this conference). These new markers represent powerful new tools for investigating the genetics of familial polyposis.

LOCATION SCORE FOR C11p11 AND GENETIC MAP OF CHROMOSOME 5 (IN MORGANS)

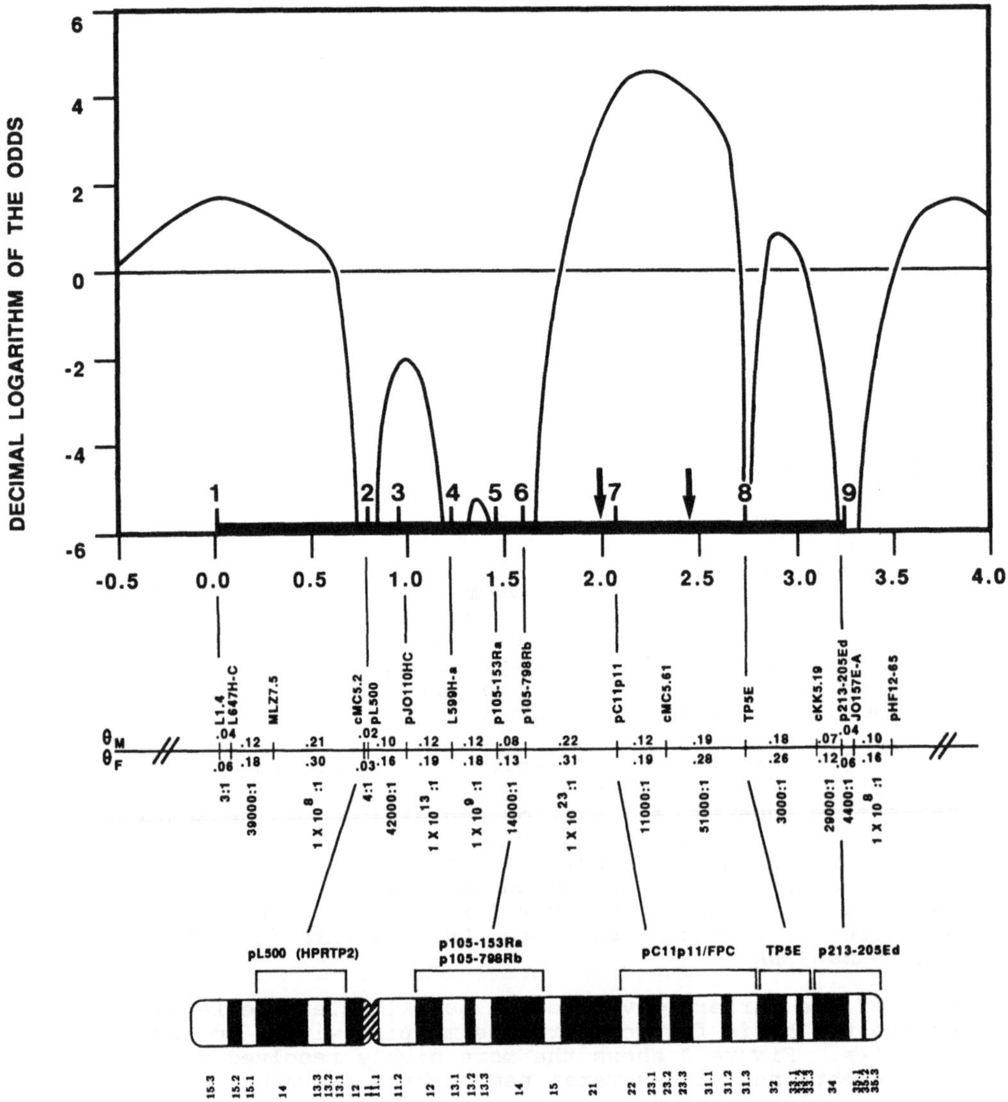

Fig. 1. Genetic linkage map, scaled in Morgans using the Haldane mapping function, of 16 DNA markers on chromosome 5. Logarithmic curve (at top) shows location scores for the APC gene on the relevant portion of the female map, derived from multilocus linkage analysis; the closest marker locus is C11p11. Two arrows on the abscissa indicate the 95% confidence boundaries for the location of APC; the genetic distance between the arrows is approximately 45 centimorgans. The genetic map (center) indicates estimates of recombination distance (theta) between markers for male (above line) and female (below line) meioses, and odds against inversion of adjacent loci are indicated. Physical localizations of selected probes are indicated on the idiogram of chromosome 5. (Reprinted by permission from Leppert and others, 1987. Copyright 1987 by the AAAS).

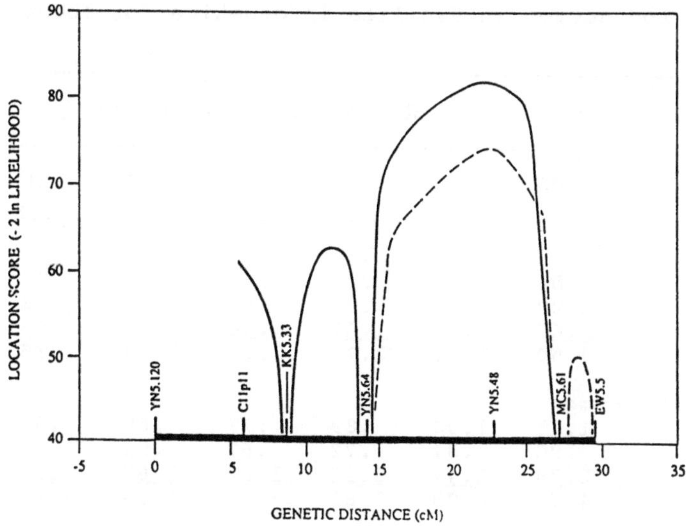

Fig. 2. Location score for the APC gene on the map of a 30-cM region of chromosome 5. The solid line indicates location score with respect to the subset of loci C11p11, KK5.33, YN5.64, and YN5.48; the dashed line indicates location score calculated with respect to the subset YN5.64, YN5.48, MC5.61, and EW5.5. Both curves indicate that the most likely location of APC is very close to the YN5.48 locus. (From Nakamura and others, 1988. Reprinted by permission of the American Society of Human Genetics).

One of the first questions to be addressed in the search for the polyposis gene was the relationship between generic familial polyposis and Gardner syndrome: are the osteomas, fibromas, desmoid tumors, and hyperplastic retinal epithelium -- in addition to adenomatous polyps of the colon -- characteristic of Gardner syndrome, the result of mutations in a gene different from that causing familial polyposis (i.e., locus heterogeneity) or are they the result of a different kind of mutation within the familial polyposis gene (i.e., allelic heterogeneity)? The issue of heterogeneity is fundamental to the genetic description of the phenotype; examples of both locus and allelic heterogeneity are found in human genetics.

The answer came from linkage analysis within both kinds of families. Our expectation was clear; if Gardner syndrome were due to a mutation in a gene distinct from the polyposis gene, then we would expect it to map elsewhere than the location of familial polyposis on chromosome 5. Certainly if we were to find that Gardner syndrome mapped elsewhere, we would have established that two different genes are involved. Therefore, DNA markers expected to be tightly linked to the familial polyposis gene were tested in several Gardner syndrome pedigrees and several familial polyposis pedigrees.

Table 1. Lod scores in families informative for locus YN5.48*

	Recombination Fraction						
Family	.00	.05	.10	.15	.20	.30	.40
APC:							
415	.54	.50	.46	.42	.37	.27	.15
1452	1.29	1.14	.97	.81	.64	.32	.08
1441	1.67	1.48	1.31	1.14	.95	.56	.22
Total	3.50	3.12	2.74	2.37	1.96	1.15	.45
Gardner syndrome:							
1498	1.11	1.00	.89	.77	.65	.38	.13
1507	.90	.81	.72	.62	.51	.30	.09
109	2.74	2.47	2.20	1.92	1.62	.99	.36
Total	4.75	4.28	3.81	3.31	2.78	1.67	.58
Combined lods	8.25	7.40	6.55	5.68	4.74	2.82	1.03

*From Nakamura and others, 1988. Reprinted by permission of the American Society of Human Genetics.

The linkage evidence shown in Table 1 provides strong support for the conclusion that both Gardner syndrome and familial polyposis arise from mutation(s) at the same locus on chromosome 5q (Nakamura and others, 1988). The simplest interpretation is that each form of the disorder represents a different kind of mutation in the polyposis gene. However, at present we cannot rigorously exclude the possibility that two genes, closely colocated, are responsible.

In addition to familial polyposis and Gardner syndrome, we have examined in one kindred a third class of inherited polyp syndrome, one that is characterized by a rather small average number of polyps and by a quite heterogeneous expression of those polyps, ranging in number from hundreds to only a few (one to several). The pedigree, shown in Fig. 3, was ascertained by Eldon Gardner as a kindred (K353) prone to colon cancer. A genetic linkage study with DNA markers in the region of the APC locus has revealed that an inherited defect at or near this locus is responsible for the clinical phenotype in K353.

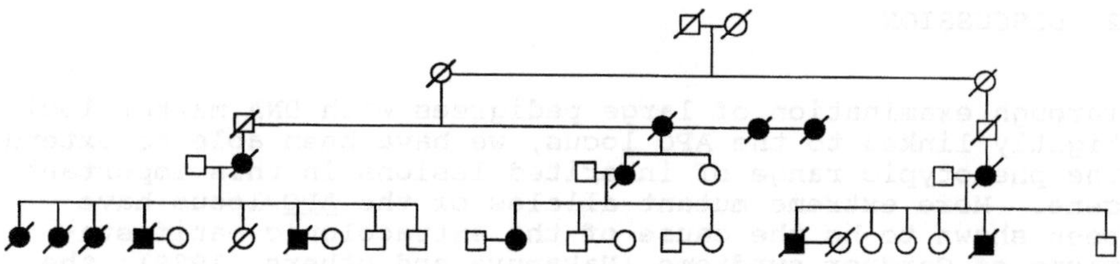

Fig. 3. Historical pedigree K353. Members with colon cancer are indicated by black symbols. Two additional descendant generations were sampled for the linkage analysis.

Endoscopy of more than 100 individuals from several branches of this large kindred indicated the presence of from one or several to as many as hundreds of adenomatous polyps. In order to test for linkage to our DNA markers from the polyposis locus, a clinical phenotype of affection status was defined as the presence of: (1) colon cancer at any age; (2) five or more adenomatous polyps; (3) 2-4 colonic adenomatous polyps plus either multiple gastric fundic gland polyps (Iada and others, 1985) or microadenomas in histologic sections of the colon (Bussey, 1975). Either of the latter two findings, multiple gastric polyps or microadenomas, would be unusual in the general population.

Linkage analysis with two flanking and tightly linked DNA markers that define the polyposis locus provided strong evidence of linkage, independent of our choice of penetrance parameter for the analysis. With penetrance set at 0.5 our LOD score for linkage was 5.5; with the more conservative assumption that unaffected individuals are indeed of unknown phenotype, the LOD score for linkage still reached 4.5. Note that this evidence provides especially significant support for linkage since only a single target locus was hypothesized; only one pairwise test was performed.

The linkage results provided strong support for the hypothesis that the polyp phenotype in K353 is a consequence of the inheritance of a defective allele at or near the <u>APC</u> locus. Therefore, on the basis of genotypes at the flanking marker loci, we were able to identify members of the family who carried the mutant <u>APC</u> allele, specifically those who were deemed "at risk" but originally classified as unaffected, and to examine their phenotypes.

Among the individuals classified as unaffected for the purpose of linkage analysis, four were found to have inherited the mutant <u>APC</u> allele. Two of them, both aged 26, each had only a single adenomatous polyp. The other two individuals also had relatively few polyps; one had two polyps at age 17, and the other had three polyps at age 34. In contrast, 15 of the 16 individuals predicted to be normal on the basis of marker genotypes, had no visible polypoid lesions when screened by endoscopy. The lone individual among the non-carriers in whom a single polyp was identified manifested it at an age (49 years) when polyps are more common in the general population.

2. DISCUSSION

Through examination of large pedigrees with DNA marker loci tightly linked to the APC locus, we have been able to extend the phenotypic range of inherited lesions in this important gene. More extreme mutant alleles of the APC locus have been shown to be the cause of the extracolonic manifestations of Gardner syndrome (Nakamura and others, 1988): the osteomas, desmoid tumors, and retinal hypertrophy that characterize this variant of APC. Furthermore, the variable expression of the inherited polyp syndrome in K353, ranging from colon cancer without colonic polyps, through individuals with only a few polyps, to individuals with hundreds of polyps, is likely to result from less extreme, or less penetrant, mutant alleles at the APC locus.

It is not unreasonable to postulate a diversity of APC alleles, in view of the fact that new mutations are relatively frequent in APC (Bussey, 1975) and because Gardner syndrome, conventional APC, and the variable phenotype in K353 are now known to result from mutations at the same locus. The influence of other genes and/or environmental effects may account for the wide variation of expression at the APC locus in K353.

It is possible that the APC gene may be involved in other, as yet untested, colon-cancer families in which typical polyposis is absent. Furthermore, common colorectal cancer appears to be familial, and Cannon-Albright and others (1988) have suggested that colon cancer in general may often be due to a genetic predisposition to small numbers of polyps. We are led to speculate that some of this hypothesized genetic predisposition may ultimately be explained by alleles at the APC locus that have even lower phenotypic expressivity than the mutation in K353; such alleles would perhaps predispose to an average of 2-5 polyps rather than the 30-40 that are characteristic of K353. For now, this speculative hypothesis is useful only in that it can be tested by linkage analysis with the highly informative set of DNA markers available for the APC locus. The inherited mutation in some colon-cancer families could lie instead at loci involved in tumor progression: the p53 locus on chromosome 17 or loci on chromosome 18q for example (Vogelstein and others, 1988; Baker and others, 1989). It does not seem likely that all colon cancers would be due to inherited predisposition, but somatic mutation of the same gene that is inherited in mutant form in K353 and in APC families could maintain a common etiology. Such a phenomenon has been observed in inherited and sporadic forms of retinoblastoma (Cavenee and others, 1983).

The linkage studies describe here are of immediate interest to persons within K353, however. Those who, on the basis of their genotypes for markers linked to APC, are found to lack the disease allele will be relieved of the need for frequent clinical surveillance, and freed from anxiety concerning risk to their children. Individuals who do carry the disease genotype can be monitored more aggressively. It is possible that individuals who inherit the mutant allele but show only one or a few polyps might be at low risk for the development of colon cancer relative to other family members with many polyps; polypectomy might be an adequate intervention for these individuals, although it is true that a carcinoma was found in one family member who had no visible polyps at all. Refined therapeutic choices for members of K353 will require a more precise description of the prognosis as a function of age and the number of polyps.

A further note, relevant to other families: if the subjects in K353 with only a few adenomatous polyps had been examined outside the context of the large family study, the possibility that they and their relatives might carry an allele conferring a predisposition to polyp formation, and increased risk of colon cancer, might have been missed. Without the statistical power of a large pedigree, it is often difficult to determine for individual patients whether their several polyps are due to an inherited genetic lesion or to somatic mutation. Only when the APC gene is identified, cloned, and sequenced will we have a means of directly determining molecular lesions in the APC alleles of such patients.

REFERENCES

Baker SJ, Fearon ER, Nigro JM, Hamilton SR, Preisinger AC, Jessup JM, vanTuinen, P, Ledbetter D, Barker D, Nakamura Y, White R, Vogelstein B (1989) Chromosome 17 deletions and p53 gene mutations in colorectal carcinomas. Science 244:217-21

Bodmer W, Bailey C, Bodmer J, Bussey HJR, Ellis A, Gorman P, Lucibello FC, Murday VA, Rider SH, Scambler P, Sheer D, Solomon E, Spurr NK (1987) Localization of the gene for familial adenomatous polyposis on chromosome 5. Nature 328:614-16

Burt RW, Samowitz W (1988) The adenomatous polyp and the hereditary polyposis syndromes. Gastro Clin N Amer 17:657 -78

Bussey JJR (1975) Familial Polyposis Coli. Family studies, histopathology, differential diagnosis, and results of treatment. Johns Hopkins University Press, Baltimore, MD

Cannon-Albright LA, Skolnick MH, Bishop DT, Lee RG, Burt RW (1988) Common inheritance of susceptibility to colonic adenomatous polyps and associated colorectal cancers. N Engl J Med 319:533-37

Cavenee WK, Dryja TP, Phillips RA, Benedict WF, Godbout R, Gallie BL, Murphree AL, Strong LC, White R (1983) Expression of recessive alleles by chromosomal mechanisms in retinoblastoma. Nature 305:779-84

Cirullo R, Dana A, Wasmuth J (1983) Efficient procedure for transferring specific human genes into Chinese hamster cell mutants: interspecific transfer of the human genes encoding leucyl- and asparaginyl-tRNA synthetases. Mol Cell Biol 3:892-902

Herrera L, Kakati S, Gibas L, Pietrzak E, Sandberg AA (1986) Brief clinical report: Gardner syndrome in a man with an interstitial deletion of 5q. Amer J Med Genet 25:473-476

Iada M, Yao T, Itoh H (1985) Natural history of fundic gland polyposis in patients with familial adenomatosis coli/Gardner syndrome. Gastroenterology 89: 1021-25

Leppert M, Dobbs M, Scambler P, O'Connell P, Nakamura Y, Stauffer D, Woodward S, Burt R, Hughes J, Gardner E, Lathrop M, Wasmuth J, Lalouel, J-M, White, R (1987) The gene for familial polyposis coli maps to the long arm of chromosome 5. Science 238: 1411-1413

Muto T, Bussey HJR, Morson BC (1975) The evolution of cancer of the colon and rectum. Cancer 36:2251-70.

Nakamura Y, Lathrop M, Leppert M, Dobbs M, Wasmuth J, Wolff E, Carlson M, Fujimoto E, Krapcho K, Sears T, Woodward S, Hughes J, Burt R, Gardner E, Lalouel J-M, White R (1988) Localization of the genetic defect in familial adenomatous polyposis within a small region of chromosome 5. Am J Hum Genet 43: 638-44

Vogelstein B, Fearon ER, Hamilton SR, Kern S, Preisinger AC, Leppert M, Nakamura Y, White R, Smits AMM, Bos JL (1988) Genetic alterations during colorectal-tumor development. N Engl J Med 319:525-32.

Hereditary Colorectal Cancer: A Commentary

WALTER F. BODMER

The human geneticists, unfortunately perhaps and against the advice of the relevant clinicians, have opted for APC as the name for the familial adenomatous polyposis gene because a genetic disease is necessarily familial. However, perhaps FAP can remain the name for the syndrome itself. The uniformity of its distribution worldwide supports its maintenance by mutation-selection balance. Using the frequency of sporadic cases, estimated from complete registers through the frequency of cases with unaffected parents, the mutation rate estimate for the APC gene is from 1:100,000 to 1:125,000 depending on an assumed incidence of 1:10,000 or 1:5,000 and a frequency of sporadic cases of either 40% or 20%. The high mutation rate implies that most families will be new mutants and perhaps suggests the possibility of a large gene. Local drift may give rise to clusters of families in a given area with the same mutation, and this may be the case, for example, for the Mormons and may also explain the apparent association of polyposis with HLA A2 and B44 studied by Terasaki and Lynch and by Julia Bodmer and co-workers (Bodmer et al, 1985).

The rare subsets of isolated constitutional cases of polyposis associated with developmental abnormalities and mental retardation, as in the original case described by Herrera and colleagues, are a source of deletions which are valuable for mapping. The cases described by Chiba are particularly interesting since without a visible chromosomal defect they may represent a micro-deletion and so provide a narrower window on the polyposis gene. The fact that the Chiba cases are severely mentally retarded, as are the two cases described by Solomon and her colleagues from Australia, while their case from Manchester is not, suggests that the mental retardation gene that may be involved maps proximal to, and perhaps close to, the polyposis gene.

There are many approaches to saturating the region around APC with probes, as discussed by Nakamura, Solomon, Frischauf and Tops. Newer approaches, in addition to irradiation hybrids, include chromosome micro-dissection and PCR sampling of relatively small regions using alu probes.

Functional studies may be greatly helped by the availability of many colorectal carcinoma derived cell lines, a number of which can be grown in serum free defined media. These are especially valuable if corresponding normal tissue, preferably from lymphoid lines grown from normal blood samples, is available. The closer to normal the cell lines are, starting from the adenoma lines described by Paraskeva, the better the resolution for finding potential functional effects of inserted sequences from the appropriate region of chromosome 5. In addition to the growth of tumours in nude mice, growth in soft agar and changes in serum requirements as discussed by Sazasuki, changes in the pattern of differentiation should be studied.

The 5q allele loss is so far limited to colorectal carcinomas, in contrast to most of the other chromosome changes which occur in several different types of tumours. The data from Wyllie and colleagues shows most clearly that allele loss focuses on the 5q21 region, with a maximum frequency of over 60%, and implies that APC is the gene which explains the chromosome 5 allele loss. The data of Miyaki and co-workers considerably enlarges the sample of carcinomas from polyposis patients which has been studied, to give an overall estimate of about 40% 5q allele loss, which suggests that a change in the APC gene may in fact occur in most sporadic cases since not all will be detected until the gene itself is identified. Miyaki's data in addition show for the first time that, as expected from family analysis, it is the normal allele which is lost in carcinomas from polyposis cases.

There is uniform agreement that allele loss in polyps from polyposis patients is very low indeed. These data contrast with that in sporadic adenomas, but this may be explained by observational bias, since the sporadic adenomas are likely to be either bigger or nastier, for otherwise they would not be noticed. There is, in my view, no evidence that any additional genetic event is needed to give rise to the APC polyps. This fits in with the threshold model for a focal stochastic event in the development of polyps, as originally discussed by Bodmer and colleagues in 1987. If the polyposis gene is some form of negative regulator which may have wide pleotropic effects, then this could explain the variety of minor differences between APC and normal tissues, such as with respect to TPA responses, repair differences and other phenomena that have been described for fibroblasts and other cell types from polyposis patients. If release from negative growth control is the explanation for polyp formation, this might suggest the switching on of a growth factor and an autocrine mechanism underlying the growth of polyps, including recruitment of neighbouring cells. An approach to prevention may, therefore, be to find agents which will block the activity of such a growth factor.

Why do the polyps in polyposis patients in general only start to appear in the early teens? Is this connected with sexual maturation, which would suggest an effect of steroid hormones that could be investigated? It is surely not likely to be explained by dietary changes. Why is there a preference for the development of polyps in the colon rather than, for example, the upper gastrointestinal tract? Presumably this could be associated with the microenvironment in the colon and an appropriate promotional activity. Miyaki suggested 5q allele loss in desmoids, which would make these analogous to the osteosarcomas found in the retinoblastoma patients which show chromosome 13 allele loss.

Following the threshhold gene dosage model for the effects of the APC gene, mutations which do not completely knock out gene function could give rise to a wide variety of effects, including lesser numbers of polyps developed at later ages, as may be the case for the K353 and other families described by Ray White and colleagues. A gene with half level activity could even give rise to a recessive form of polyposis, since homozygotes for such a gene would be equivalent to heterozygotes for a gene which had completely lost function. Once the functional gene is identified, then transgenic mice with inserted targeted mutations may form the basis for a suitable model for studying the manipulation of the development of polyps.

2. OTHER GENETIC CHANGES IN COLORECTAL CARCINOMAS

There is now little doubt that the majority, if not all, of the 17p allele losses are due to mutations in the p53 gene, as first shown by Bert Vogelstein and colleagues. In our laboratory we have been able to study these changes using a monoclonal antibody from David Lane which has some specificity for the mutant form of p53. We find with this that about 50% of colorectal carcinomas on immunoperoxidase staining show reactivity for, presumably, a mutant form of p53, while none of ten adenomas from both polyposis and sporadic cases showed staining. This, incidentally, indicates that the p53 change, even the first step, is indeed a relatively late event. Elisa assays on cell lines from colorectal carcinomas show greater activity of the mutant than normal anti p53 antibody, with the reverse in lymphoblastoid cell lines with putative normal p53 expression. By this criterion, 17 out of 21 colorectal carcinoma derived cell lines express abnormal p53. It is clear that the first p53 mutation has a dominant effect, most probably through blocking the normal p53 activity, and that this is followed secondarily by further selection against the presence of the remaining allele. (See Bodmer et al. 1989).

The gene described by Vogelstein on chromosome 18, which explains 18q allele loss, is a most exciting development. The fact that it may be a cell adhesion molecule fits in with data suggesting an important role for extracellular matrix receptors in the control of differentiation and for their possible interaction with CEA and other members of the family of adhesion molecules (Pignatelli. In Press). A further and somewhat different example of genetic change in colorectal carcinomas is the comparatively frequent loss of individual HLA alleles as described by Smith et al. (1989) and others. This indicates a relatively high frequency of T cell responses to tumours. Following the discovery by Townsend and colleagues that cytotoxic T cells respond to proteolitically processed proteins which may be intracellular molecules, it is clear that T cells may respond to dominant oncogene mutations such as in p53 and Kras. These immune responses can now be looked for systematically, and suggest the possibility of rational immunomodulation of immune responses for the treatment of tumours and even perhaps of vaccination against dominant oncogene changes. (See Bodmer 1989a).

The overall picture of genetic changes in colorectal carcinomas, now described by many different groups, is remarkably consistant. Apart from Kras, none of the other so far described dominant oncogenes shows any obvious change, and it seems possible that the slight increases in C-myc and Rb products may be secondary to other changes. The extent to which allele loss is being investigated would suggest that there may be no other "recessive" changes to be found, but there could, of course, still be dominant changes that occur in other genes than the presently described oncogenes. Undoubtedly, there are enough genetic changes already described to fit into the multi-step processes analysed by Doll, Armitage and others many years ago. These genetic changes surely describe the pathology of the future. The pathologists will, in future, have to match what they see to the genetic diagnosis, rather than vice versa.

Chromosome 22 allele loss seems to be seen mainly in Japan. This is one example of possible geographic variations in the pattern of genetic change in colorectal carcinomas, which may be paralleled by different patterns of change in different regions of the colon. The geographical variation could be due to an effect of the macroenvironment, most probably the diet, giving rise to different microenvironments within the gut surrounding the potential tumour cells. These may affect differentially the selective advantages of different mutants. Cancer is, after all, an asexual somatic evolutionary process in which one mutational event is selected for and then followed by a second, and so on, to give rise to a series of mutations accumulated sequentially in a clonal fashion. A combination of mutation rates of different genes, influenced by the size of the population in which they occur, and their selective values will determine the expressed genetic changes in a tumour, which must have an inevitable cut off size at a level of say 10^{12} cells at most. There is a case for a new population genetic analysis of this bounded somatic evolutionary process.

Are somatic mutation rates ever really limiting to the development of a tumour? If not, then in general the role of genotoxic carcinogens in giving rise to differential incidences in colorectal cancer would be questionable. The main stage that could be limiting is the first, and for this one needs to know the potential population of stem cells, namely the total number of crypts in the adult colon.

The sequence of genetic changes, as measured by allele loss, only describes the second events for each chromosome and leaves open the possibility that the first event if, for example, it is a mutation such as for p53, occurs at a significantly earlier stage than allele loss. The studies with the antibody to mutant p53 suggest that this is not the case for that particular change and the data of Miyaki on the relatively early loss of alleles in the 5q region suggest that that may be a relatively early event. It seems that most of the events are independent in their effects, and so may occur in different orders in different tumours. The actual observed order in any particular tumour may simply be a function of the chance of when a given mutation arose and the extent of its selective advantage. Karyotype instability may be a concomitant effect of one of the genetic steps selected for, such as the p53 mutations, and may then give rise to a general increase in the rate of allele loss, making second events more likely to occur. Nevertheless, it seems most unlikely that any event will be fixed by random fluctuation in a tumour and so, even with relatively high mutation rates, selection will still be important for fixing those that are found eventually to be expressed.

Positive and negative regulation of growth and differentiation can explain a variety of dominant and recessive effects at the cellular level (Bodmer WF 1989b). It may be efficient for a tumour to select for changes at the transcription or signalling level which may affect several cellular processes at once and so achieve more than one advantageous change through a single mutation event.

3. NON POLYPOSIS INHERITED SYNDROMES

The non polyposis inherited colorectal cancer associated syndromes are a heterogenous collection, including perhaps the Lynch type 2 syndrome itself. This heterogeneity will undoubtedly be sorted out by genetic linkage studies guided by careful clinical descriptions. However, the clinical picture may exaggerate the genetic heterogeneity. For example, it is clear that there is no distinction between polyposis and Gardner's syndromes and therefore that the same gene, though perhaps with different mutations, can be associated with a variety of phenotypic manifestations. Variation could be connected with the genetic background, with environmental effects including diet and sex, with chance variations, and with the consequences of different mutations of the same gene having slightly different effects. All of this can give rise to considerable clinical heterogeneity associated with mutations at a single gene locus.

As discussed by Bishop and his colleagues, there may be an important class of low penetrance relatively common genes influencing the incidence of colorectal cancer. Adenomas may in this case reflect a more penetrant expression of such genes. As in the case of the study of HLA and disease associations, for example with rheumatoid arthritis or Hodgkin's disease, formal linkage analysis is unlikely to be possible and an extension of sib-pair analysis to multiple case family studies should make it possible to locate such a gene or genes provided there is not too much heterogeneity. Such a genetic marker, once found, would of course help in identifying high risk individuals as a focus for screening. If there exists such a common gene, which to be common needs only to have a frequency of, say, more than 1%, it is (a) likely to have a differential population distribution in contrast to polyposis but analogous to cystic fibrosis and PKU and (b) to be explained predominantly by a single allele. This would mean that linkage disequilibrium with closely linked markers would be expected and could help in the search for the gene, though ultimately the mutation itself should be the basis for identification of high risk individuals.

4. REGISTRIES, SCREENING AND DIET

Systematic registries of familial cases of colorectal cancer have proved their value, especially of course for polyposis. These can be selective, as in the St Marks' registry, or population based as in Denmark, Japan and elsewhere. The registries are not only valuable as a resource for investigation, but have been clearly shown to improve survival. Family workers or research nurses, as discussed by Jane Lynch, are an essential resource for such registries. In the United Kingdom we now have a Cancer Family Study Group which brings together all those with an interest in this area throughout the country, in particular those who are running Cancer Family Clinics. Associated with this collaboration there is a network of family workers to help obtain the material and information on families and a specific collaborative project on the genetics of breast cancer and one proposed for ovarian cancers.

There is undoubtedly a need for the development of new screening tests that go beyond endoscopy and fecal occult blood detection. The fecal tests need greater specificity, which may be provided by monoclonal antibodies against novel determinants but including CEA, and even by screening at the DNA level for the genetic alterations themselves. Fecal material contains cellular debris and, in preliminary tests, it is clear that at least some DNA sequences may be detectable in this.

The ultimate goal, not only of the family studies but of overall studies on colorectal cancer, must be prevention. The evidence clearly implicates the diet as underlying the marked differences in incidence, for example in colon and stomach cancer, between Japan and Western societies. And yet it has proved extremely difficult, whether by international comparisons, case control studies or studies on experimental animals, to pinpoint the relevant components in the diet. There seem to be too many clues and it is not clear which really is primary. Increased fibre, decreased fat, increased calcium, prostaglandin synthetase inhibitors, unsaturated fatty acid components, vitamins D, C and A and the retinoids, and even inhibitors of ornithine decarboxylase have all been suggested as a basis for primary prevention. And, in addition, there is the possibility of interactions between two or more of these components. I believe that until the molecular genetics and biology provide convincing clues as to the directions to go, it may be difficult to argue for a systematic prevention trial. Furthermore, there is the question as to whether high-risk situations, and in particular polyposis, provide an appropriate model for testing potential preventative approaches for the majority of sporadic colorectal carcinomas. I believe they may do so, even at the level of preventing the primary development of polyps, but th situation will undoubtedly become clearer once the polyposis gene itself has been identified.

Surely one must hope that by 1991 at the time of the next meeting of the International Symposium on Colorectal Cancer, genetic advances will have identified many of the remaining genes and their functions, and will point to the future directions that need to be taken for screening and prevention of colorectal cancer in both its familial and sporadic forms.

REFERENCES

Bodmer J, Kennedy L, Brennan J,and Bodmer W. HLA and genetic marker studies in adenomatous polyposis. Br.J.Surg. (1985) Vol 72 (September) Sp32-35

Bodmer WF (1989a) Immune attack against cancer - a new look. Cancer Magazine, UICC In press

Bodmer WF (1989b) Genetic Analysis of Tumour Suppression. (Eds. Greg Bock and Joan Marsh). Symposium on Genetic analysis of tumour suppression, held at the Ciba Foundation, London, 19-21 July 1988. Symposium 142. John Wiley & Sons. Page Nos.: 242-244

Bodmer WF, Cottrell S, Frischauf A-M, Jones TA , Kerr IB, Murday VA, Smith MEF, Solomon E, Thomas H, Varesco L, Williams S (1989) Genetics of colorectal cancer. Bristol Myers Symposium on Molecular Mechanisms & new Clinical Applications in Malignancies - Toronto (September 1989)

Pignatelli M, Durbin H, Bodmer WF (1990) Carcinoembryonic antigen functions as an accessory adhesion molecule mediating colon. Proc.Natl.Acad.Sci.USA (in press)

Smith MEF, Marsh SGE, Bodmer JG, Gelsthorpe K, Bodmer WF (1989) Loss of HLA-A,B,C allele products and lymphocyte function-associated antigen-3 in colorectal neoplasia. Proc.Natl.Acad.Sci.USA 86, 5557-5561

Only specific references to work not otherwise discussed in the published papers are given here. The volume itself documents the extensive background on the basis of which this discussion has been written.

Chapter 2

Identification, Surveillance, and Management of Polyposis Syndrome

Summary of Chapter 2: Identification, Surveillance and Management of Polyposis Syndrome

STEFFEN BÜLOW

Bülow S (Denmark):
Surveillance of Danish families with adenomatous polyposis.

The Danish Polyposis Register (DPR) was established in 1971. Probands were ascertained from hospitals, the National Patient Registry and from the Cancer Registry. Their pedigrees were then constructed from genealogical information (from local population registers, parish registers and the Central Population Register) and from medical information (hospitals, specialists in private practice and death certificates). Hitherto unexamined 1. relatives were then offered prophylactic examination with regular proctosigmoidoscopy at regular intervals in the age group 10-60 years and newly diagnosed "call-up cases" referred for prophylactic colectomy. In 1989 the DPR includes 121 families with 381 affected members, of whom 110 are call-up cases. The incidence of colorectal cancer in this group was only 2% versus 67% in probands. The cumulative survival after 10 years was 93% in call-up patients versus only 40% in probands. These differences strongly underline the value of a centralized polyposis register.

Griffioen G, Vasen HFA, den Hartog Jager FCA, Nagengast FM, Verspaget HW, Meera Khan P, Lamers CBHW (Netherlands):
Value of registration in the identification and surveillance of familial adenomatous polyposis in the Netherlands.

The national Dutch Polyposis Registry was set up in 1985 and now includes 107 FAP families of which 82 are fully registered. A total of 230 affected members have been identified: 104 have been referred due to symptoms and 126 were found as a result of screening. At present 204 at risk individuals have not yet been screened. The incidence of colorectal cancer was 47% in probands and 4% in call-up cases. The average age of diagnosis of FAP was 35 years and 24 years, respectively. Gastroduodenal polyps were found in 43% of the patients, one patients died of periampullary carcinoma. The value of a national registration is proved by the identification of many 1. relatives, who are now subjected to regular screening. Furthermore, the early detection of FAP in call-up cases probably will reduce the incidence of colorectal cancer.

Iwama T, Mishima Y, Utsunomiya J (Japan):
Current status of registration at the Polyposis Center, Japan.

The Japanese Center for Polyposis and Intestinal Disease was established in 1985 and includes patients with FAP and other polyposis syndromes. It is based on information from hospital records, autopsy records, death certificates, and family members. The pedigrees have been drawn using the national family registry and family members at risk have been examined prophylactically. In 1989 564 families had been fully surveyed, including 1738 polyposis cases and 4475 living first degree relatives. The frequency of colorectal cancer was 64% among probands and 25% in the call-up group. Ileorectal anastomosis has been performed in 188 patients and ileoanal anastomosis in 263 patients. The number of extracolonic cancers is small, but will probably increase in the future following the improved survival after early colectomy.

Krokowicz P (Poland):
Management of familial polyposis in Poland.

The Familial Polyposis Register in Poland was established in 1979 in Poznan as a regional register, which will include all Poland in the future. Due to lack of archives and parish registers and large emigrations after the second world war the process of constructing the register is difficult. The register now includes 116 FAP cases, of whom 85 have been operated upon. Patients with a limited number of small rectal adenomas had a colectomy and ileorectal anastomosis, those with disseminated small rectal adenomas had a restorative proctocolectomy and an ileoanal pouch, and those with a rectal carcinoma had a total proctocolectomy.

Macrae F, St John DJB, Cuthbertson AC, Muir E (Australia):
Familial adenomatous polyposis: Impact of a hospital-based register on management.

Until recently, there has been no central registration of FAP in Australia. A study was based on 20 families in the Royal Melbourne Hospital including 24 call-up cases, of whom 75% had colorectal cancer. It was demonstrated that surveillance of at risk family members was unsatisfactory due to communication failures, family denial of the hereditary nature of the disease, insufficiency of hospital outpatient surveillance and failure to evaluate the large kindred in all details. The regional Victorian ESSO Familial Polyposis Register was established in 1988 and now 33 call-up cases have been identified, of whom only 6% had colorectal cancer. It is concluded that without the active surveillance of a dedicated register responsible for notifying clinicians and patients about the timing of surveillance procedures lethal delays in diagnosis are likely to occur.

Slack J (England):

The probability of developing familial adenomatous polyposis after combining the diminishing risk with age with negative screening by sigmoidoscopy and linked gene markers.

On the basis of 34 1. relatives who have been followed with regular sigmoidoscopy from negative findings to the diagnosis of FAP the cumulative risk of developing polyps with increasing age was calculated to 20% at age 20 and 8% at age 30. Combining these figures with a negative result from linked gene markers in informative families reduced the risk to 2% at age 15 and 0.5% at age 30. Moreover, if no CHRPE was found the risk of future development of FAP was only 1% at age 10 and 0.1% at age 30. In conclusion, the combination of sigmoidoscopy, gene markers and examination for CHRPE results in excellent opportunities for offering genetic counselling in informative families.

Baba S, Tsuchiya M, Machida H, Yamada M (Japan):

Retinal pigmentations in familial adenomatous polyposis and linkage study on gene probes on chromosome 5q.

A study of 27 families was carried out to evaluate the detection of congenital hypertrophy of the retinal pigment epithelium (CHRPE) as a clinical marker and of linkage analysis by the use of the gene probes C11p11, Pi227 and YN5.48. The study group included 44 FAP patients, 30 1. relatives and 1984 controls. CHRPE was found in 79% of the patients; 43% of 1. relatives and 0.3% of controls. Large pigmentations were found close to the posterior pole and small pigmentations in the periphery; the latter may increase in number with age. The sensitivity was 0.62 for large pigmentations and 0.77 for small and the specificity was 0.999 for large pigmentations. Only one family was informative for Pi227, three for YN5.48 and none for C11p11. It was concluded that CHRPE is an important subclinical marker of FAP, and it should be used until definite DNA diagnosis will be possible.

Ushio K (Japan):

Follow-up study on colonic adenomas and associated tumors in familial polyposis coli and Gardner's syndrome.

In 55 FAP patients from 29 families the incidence of accompanying benign lesions was: Mandibular osteomas 77%, duodenal polyps 64%, gastric polyps 60%, extramandibular skeletal lesions 46%, soft tissue tumors 32%, desmoid tumors 14%, and odontoma 13%. Three patients had malignant tumors: two gastric cancers and one thyroid cancer. Most benign tumors developed during early childhood and increased in size and number at puberty. Malignant tumors very rarely developed from mesodermal or ectodermal tissues, whereas glandular epithelium originating from endodermal elements such as the gastrointestinal tract and the thyroid had a high malignant potential. In conclusion, surveillance of FAP patients primarily should include examination of these organs.

Romania A, Heyen F, Jagelman D, Zakov Z, Lavery I, Fazio V, McGannon E, Church J (U.S.A.):
Congenital hypertrophy of the retinal pigment epithelium: A clinical marker for familial adenomatous polyposis.

In order to determine the predictive value of CHRPE as a marker for FAP 153 members of 56 families were studied with wide-angle fundus photography. All patients also had proctosigmoidoscopy. The presence of four of more bilateral lesions was established as criterion for the presence of FAP. Sixty percent of affected members and 25% of 1. relatives were positive. The families fell into two distinct groups: In group 1 (35 families) all affected members and 40% of 1. relatives were positive. Since then, 5 CHRPE-positive 1. relatives have developed adenomas. In group 2 neither affected members nor 1. relatives were positive, and no 1. relatives have developed adenomas. In conclusion CHRPE is a valuable marker for the presence of FAP in 65% of the families, with a predictive value of 100% during a short follow-up time.

MAJOR CONCLUSIONS

The reports from 5 major national or regional polyposis registries in Denmark, Holland, Japan, Poland and Australia all demonstrate substantial effects of establishing a centralized registration of the disease:

1. A large number of asymptomatic 1. relatives are identified and subjected to regular screening.
2. The frequency of colorectal cancer in newly diagnosed polyposis patients is reduced from 47-67% in probands to 2-25% in call-up cases.
3. The survival of call-up cases is significantly better compared to that of probands.

The conclusions of studies of one or more markers of polyposis are:

1. In 2/3 of families the predictive value of CHRPE is 100% during a short follow-up. CHRPE is a non-invasive and inexpensive subclinical marker of FAP.
   In the future ophthalmoscopy is recommended in all polyposis patients and their 1. relatives.

2. Combining examination for CHRPE, linked gene markers and regular proctosigmoidoscopy (from negative findings) demonstrates that, in DNA-informative families with negative results of all three examinations, the future risk of developing FAP is only 1% at age 10 and 0.1% at age 30.
   This result forms a substantial basis for future genetic counselling.

FUTURE PERSPECTIVES

As stated by Dr. DeCosse in the plenary report from the third Leeds Castle Polyposis Group meeting this summer some of the present major challenges of polyposis are: Progress in molecular genetics toward a precise localization of the FAP gene, improved knowledge of the natural history, control and treatment of duodenal adenomas and desmoid tumors, and long-term evaluation of the functional results and control after restorative proctocolectomy.

These goals can only be achieved on the basis of a continued and even increased international research of this rare disease. The research must be based on data from centralized registries using a common data set. A such data set has now been decided by the Leeds Castle Polyposis Group and we hope that well established polyposis registries as well as new registries will join the cooperation by using this data set.

In Europe a new polyposis research group is now being formed. A proposal of concerted action on genetic studies in cancer families, with primary regard to FAP, has been sent to the Commission of the European Community in Brussels, asking for economic support. The project includes an increased identification and registration of polyposis families by establishing centralized or even national registers and research toward a precise localization and identification of the FAP gene. The cooperation with the Leeds Castle Group is ensured by two members of the European project management group being also members of the council of the Leeds Castle Polyposis Group.

The establishment of similar regional research groups in other continents might further initiate and coordinate future polyposis research in cooperation with the Leeds Castle Polyposis Group.

Familial Adenomatous Polyposis Study: The Report of the Leeds Castle Polyposis Meeting

JEROME J. DECOSSE

ABSTRACT

In June 1989, 52 delegates from 15 nations attended the third Meeting of the Leeds Castle Polyposis Group at Worcestershire, UK. Discussions ranged from basic molecular biology to the importance of collaboration among worldwide registries. A highlight of the meeting was review of worldwide progress in molecular probes of specific genetic aberrations in patients with FAP. The development of registry interchange and central coordination provided a second major focus of the meeting. The fourth meeting will be held in the United States in 1991. Interim goals include development of predictive biomarkers and better control and management of periampullar neoplasia.

Keywords: cancer genetics, desmoid disease, familial adenomatous polyposis, periampullar neoplasia, registries

1. INTRODUCTION

On June 15 to 17, 1989, the third meeting of the Leeds Castle Polyposis Group was held at Worcestershire, UK. At this multidisciplinary meeting, 52 attendees from 15 nations participated in 27 formal presentations and numerous additional free papers, all with the common goal of scientific endeavor and improvement of care for patients with familial adenomatous polyposis (FAP).

Clinicians and scientific investigators interested in this inherited syndrome conducted their first international workshop at Leeds Castle, Kent, UK, in 1985 (Lancet, 1986). Recognizing the need for accurate and comprehensive information, participants developed and distributed questionnaires on demography, surveillance, upper gastrointestinal tumors, desmoid disease, and primary treatment. A number of subsequent studies owe their origins to this meeting, but the questionnaires led directly to a published survey of upper gastrointestinal cancer in patients with FAP (Jagelman et al, 1988).

Acknowledging the unique setting of this first meeting, the participants entitled themselves the Leeds Castle Polyposis Group. Others sharing an interest in the syndrome were invited to join in the group's subsequent studies.

The second meeting of the Leeds Castle Polyposis Group took place in Washington, D.C., April 3-5, 1987. At this meeting, 38 participants from 12 nations addressed the issues of demography, primary management of the large intestine, desmoid disease or fibromatosis, upper gastrointestinal neoplasia, and genetics. A report of this meeting was subsequently published (Thomson, 1988).

2. CLINICAL ISSUES

The first day's session focused on a variety of clinical issues, including desmoid disease, upper gastrointestinal disease, and surgical management of the large bowel in FAP patients. Other topics included histopathology of mucosal tissue in FAP patients, brain tumor associated with FAP (Turcot Syndrome), and anthropomentric measurement for screening purposes. The importance of registries for screening and follow-up of FAP patients was the subject of several papers.

3. GENETICS

The highlight of the meeting was the second morning's session, consisting of a series of reports reviewing the dynamic world-wide progress in molecular studies of the specific genetic aberrations in the polyposis patient. Molecular probes, such as C11, P11, YN5.48, Pi227, and ECB27, are being used to close in on the deletion on chromosome 5q. Additional studies have identified allele losses in colon cancers of FAP patients on chromosomes 17, 18, 22, and less frequently 6 and 12. It is suggested that the inactivation of tumor or growth suppressor genes on these chromosomes, along with the FAP gene on chromosome 5, is associated with malignant transformation in patients with FAP. The relationship of this process with oncogene expression -- in particular the mutation of K-ras-2, which has been found in large adenomatous polyps as well as in cancer -- is slowly emerging. Linkage studies in polyposis families are in progress in the Netherlands as well as the United Kingdom,

4. BIOMARKERS

4.1 Congenital Hypertrophy of the Retinal Pigment Epithelium

Five presentations dealt with congenital hypertrophy of the retinal pigment epithelium (CHRPE). Reports of based on patient populations in England, New Zealand, Japan, and Italy indicated that CHRPE, especially when bilateral, is associated with increased risk in family members not yet diagnosed with FAP. The eye examination is noninvasive and can be performed on children. A number of follow-up studies of patients at risk for FAP who have had negative eye examinations are in progress. Participants discussed techniques for combining results from pedigree, bowel, eye, and DNA examination.

4.2 Sialomucins

Other studies dealt with mucins in the flat mucosa of FAP patients and controls, finding some differences that may be useful for screening at-risk patients in FAP families.

5. INVESTIGATIVE CHALLENGES

From the presentations and free papers, a number of investigative challenges emerged.

5.1 Periampullary Neoplasia

Periampullary neoplasia is much more widespread among FAP patients than is generally known, and needs to be better understood. Regular upper gastro-intestinal endoscopy must become part of the routine surveillance of FAP patients, and appropriate screening policies must be developed for this purpose. What treatment is appropriate when adenomatous change in the ampulla is identified? What management is appropriate for duodenal adenomas too large to be resected endoscopically? Is there a place for conservative operative or endoscopic resection of the ampulla?

Also needed are collaborative trials of nutritional intervention or chemoprevention focusing on benign adenomatous neoplasia in the upper gastrointestinal tract.

5.2 Desmoid Disease

There is need for studies of the imunohistochemistry of desmoid disease. Like upper gastrointestinal cancer, desmoid disease is a more common cause of death in FAP patients who have undergone colectomy than is rectal cancer. Collaborative efforts are necessary to study the inhibition of fibroplasia in FAP patients with desmoid disease. Treatment agents, such as clinoril and tamoxifen, that have shown some promise in small-scale trials should be tried on a larger scale.

5.3 Other Extracolonic Expressions

The pathogenesis and clinical relevance of congenital hypertrophy of the retinal pigment epithelium as well as other nonlife-threatening expressions of FAP, such as osteomata, remain to be resolved. Are extracolonic expressions inversely related to the intensity of colorectal adenomas in FAP patients? Can within-kindred patterns of extracolonic expression or of aggressiveness of the disease be verified? Do rare events, such as hepatoblastoma and medulloblastoma, which are more common in FAP patients and their relatives than in the general population, segregate in particular families or distribute themselves randomly among FAP patients and their relatives worldwide? Is more than one gene involved in these extracolonic expressions?

5.4 Long-term Follow-up

Long-term post-surgical follow-up of the FAP patient is an important area for collaborative study. Among patients who have had a colectomy and ileorectal anastomosis, are there differences between East and West in rectal cancer incidence? Long-term follow-up also is needed for patients who have undergone total excision of the large bowel and ileoanal anastomosis. What methods of reconstruction provide optimal function? How well is anal continence maintained in the patient five, ten, twenty, and more years past ileoanal anastomosis surgery? To what extent do aging, repeated examinations, and length of time since surgery affect continence in this patient population? Given the FAP patient's inherent elevated risk of small bowel cancer, does the introduction of colonic microflora into the small intestinal pouch further increase that risk?

5.5 Other Polyposis Syndromes and Conditions of High Risk for Colorectal Cancer

Other polyposis syndromes, such as Cowden's disease, Cronkhite-Canada syndrome, juvenile polyposis, and Peutz-Jeghers syndrome, as well as other colorectal cancer family syndromes also require investigation. Studies should deal with similarities and differences in molecular genetics. Predictive markers, serological or mucosal, must be identified to promote early detection of cancer risk and permit appropriate preventive measures.

5.6 Registries

The development of FAP registries has proved an effective means of identifying and following-up FAP families. Programs need to be developed to expand registration of FAP families and promote international collaboration and data sharing among registries throughout the world.

At the individual patient level, ascertainment should be timely and accurate. There is a need for much more precision and standardization in counseling, as well as in screening procedures. In at-risk relatives of probands, when should screening start, how often should screening be performed, and by what methods? Finally, at what age may screening stop?

Efforts to facilitate data sharing and coordination among the registries were a major focus of the Leeds Castle meeting. Central coordination of the registries would promote stability, provide a means for sharing registry information and pooling specimens, and permit the development of large-scale clinical trials. In the past few years, the registries have begun trying to standardize their data forms so that information may be shared without prejudice to patient confidentiality. Standardization of data forms also may promote standardization of data collection and surveillance and follow-up procedures.

At the meeting, distinctions between hospital- and population-based registries were noted. Both individual and registry participation in the Leeds Castle Group were encouraged.

6. ACKNOWLEDGEMENTS

Although many individuals have provided active leadership for the meetings of the Leeds Castle Polyposis Group, those who have contributed most to organizing the meetings have come from St. Mark's Hospital in London. These leaders include Sir Ian Todd, Mr. James P. S. Thomson, Mr. John M. A. Northover, Dr. H.J. R. Bussey, Dr. Sheila Ritchie, and Ms. Kay Neale. Outside leaders include, in particular, Dr. Steffen Bulow of Denmark and Dr. David Jagelman of the United States.

7. NEXT MEETING

The fourth meeting of the Leeds Castle Polyposis Group will be held in Fort Lauterdale, Florida, USA, in June 1991.

REFERENCES

Familial adenomatous polyposis. Lancet (1986) 1:1226

Jagelman DG, DeCosse JJ, Bussey HJR, and the Leeds Castle Polyposis Group (1988) Upper gastrointestinal cancer in familial adenomatous polyposis. Lancet 1: 1149-1151.

Thompson JPS (1988) Leeds Castle Polyposis Group Meeting. Dis Colon Rectum 31: 613-616

Surveillance of Danish Families with Adenomatous Polyposis: Results of the Danish Polyposis Register

STEFFEN BÜLOW

ABSTRACT

In Denmark surveillance of patients with familial adenomatous polyposis is coordinated via The Danish Polyposis Register. At present the register includes information about 121 families with 381 patients, of whom 111 have been found as the result of a prophylactic examination. The incidence of colorectal cancer was only 2% in call-up patients versus 67% in patients diagnosed due to bowel symptoms. Since the establishment of the register the survival of polyposis patients has improved significantly.

Keywords: Familial adenomatous polyposis.

AIMS OF THE REGISTER

The Danish Polyposis Register was established in 1971 with the purpose of improving the prognosis of patients with familial adenomatous polyposis (FAP) by: 1) identification and registration of all Danish FAP patients and their family members, 2) coordination of regular prophylactic examination of all first degree members of affected family members, leading to prophylactic colectomy in newly diagnosed call-up cases, 3) information about the disease and 4) research of all aspects of the disease. Via a membership of the "Leeds Castle Polyposis Group" and of a European polyposis group the Danish Polyposis Register cooperates with other centers about international FAP research.

CONSTRUCTION OF THE REGISTER

Probands were ascertained via direct reports from local hospital departments, from the National Patient Resigtry and by examination of medical records of young patients with colorectal cancer reported to the Danish Cancer Registry. The pedigrees of the probands were then constructed following genealogical and medical information about relatives obtained from hospital departments, general practitioners, death certificates, autopsy reports, local population registers and the Central Population Register. Subsequently, hitherto unexamined first-degree relatives were invited to attend prophylactic examination and the result was reported to the Polyposis Register. Affected patients were referred to the regional department of surgery or surgical gastroenterology for further evaluation, prophylactic colectomy and postoperative control.

SCREENING PROGRAM

The Danish screening program in first degree relatives includes rigid proctosigmoidoscopy as the only method. The first examination is carried out at the age of 10 years in order to accustom the children to the examination before puberty. Examination is continued at biannual intervals until the age of 40 years and at intervals of 3-5 years in the age group 40-60 years. After this age the risk of development of adenomas is negligible, provided normal findings at the age of 60 years.

STATUS OF THE REGISTER

At the end of August 1989 the register included information about 121 families, including 381 affected members: 195 probands have been diagnosed due to bowel symptoms, 111 call-up patients have been identified due to a prophylactic examination, and 75 are assumed cases with insufficient information. Furthermore, the register contains information about 453 living first degree relatives of affected patients, who have all been traced. Six have emigrated, and 25 are less than 10 years of age and have not yet been examined. The group aged 10-59 years (341 patients) includes 19, who have refused prophylactic examination despite information about the disease and its consequences, and 322 who are being followed with regular examination and have, as yet, demonstrated normal findings. One hundred first degree relatives are above age 60 and their regular examination program has ended.

CANCER INCIDENCE AND SURVIVAL

Among the call-up patients only 2% had developed colorectal adenocarcinoma at diagnosis of FAP, compared to 67% in probands. The cumulative survival of FAP patients after 10 years was 93% in call-up patients compared to only 40% in probands. The prognosis of all verified Danish FAP patients (probands and call-up patients) increased steadily from a 10-year survival rate of 13% in 1900-49 to 70% in 1970-82. The significant improvement in the prognosis since the establishment of the Danish Polyposis Register strongly underlines the effect of a centralized (regional or national) polyposis register.
The incidence rate of FAP in Denmark (5 mill. inhabitants) is 1.3 per 10^6 inhabitants (Bülow 1987).

FUTURE SCREENING PROGRAM

In the future the recent identification of a specific FAP gene will change the screening program. In families with informative gene markers protosigmoidoscopy probably will be used only in "gene positive" first degree relatives, in order to establish the time of development of adenomas and time of prophylactic colectomy.

COMPUTERIZED REGISTER

The Danish Polyposis Register is now being changed from a manual into a computerized register, which is based on a modified dBase-IV and an IBM personal computer. Details of the computerprogram will be presented.

REFERENCE

Bülow S (1987) Familial polyposis coli. A clinical and epidemiological study. Dan Med Bull 34: 1-15.

Value of Registration in the Identification and Surveillance of Familial Adenomatous Polyposis in the Netherlands

G. GRIFFIOEN, H.F.A. VASEN, F.C.A. DEN HARTOG JAGER, F.M. NAGENGAST, H.W. VERSPAGET, P. MEERA KHAN, C.B.H.W. LAMERS, and E.A. VAN SLOOTEN

ABSTRACT

In order to facilitate the estimation of the risk of familial adenomatous polyposis (FAP) in the first degree relatives of the patients we established the registration of families and the construction of their genealogies. Individuals who are at risk for the disease should be screened at regular intervals and appropriate treatment of the premalignant lesions should be offered. The value of a registry of FAP families is proven by the identification of many fist-degree relatives of FAP patients who were at risk for the disease and had not been screened yet. Moreover it appeared that many individuals were unnecessary under surveillance. Finally it was found that screening could lead to the early detection of FAP patients and eventually to a decrease in the incidence of colorectal cancer in their families.

Keywords: familial adenomatous polyposis, colorectal cancer, registration, surveillance, cancer prevention.

INTRODUCTION

In the Netherlands one out of every six cancer patients (skin cancer excluded) is of colorectal cancer and one out of every thirty deaths is due to colorectal cancer. This disease is the second cause of cancer death in our country (C.B.S. 1987). Most of the patients are beyond cure by the time the diagnosis is made. Moreover its incidence in the Netherlands has been rising by 1.5% annually during the last 30 years (Snel 1988). However, these figures are not unique to the Netherlands but are generally valid to the whole western world in which colorectal cancer has become one of the major oncologic problems.
In the past decades we gained new insights into the pathogenesis, possible precursor lesions and factors predisposing to colorectal cancer. It has now generally been accepted that most, if not all, colorectal adenocarcinomas arise from preexisting adenomas, the adenoma carcinoma sequence (Muto 1975, Day 1978). At present one of the most important prognostic factors for colorectal cancer is the stage of the disease at the time of diagnosis. Because the basis for cancer prevention is the early identification and appropriate treatment of the adenomatous lesions (Gilbertsen 1978) we should consider groups of patients with a more than average risk on the development of colorectal cancer and screen them at regular intervals (Lipkin 1981).
Although not all aetiological factors in the pathogenesis of colorectal cancer are well defined, it is clear that both environmental and genetic factors are involved. The vast majority of the colorectal cancer patients do not have any apparent predisposing genetic factor; it has been estimated, however, that in at least 20% of the patients with colorectal cancer genetic factors may play a significant role (Lynch 1977, Eddy 1987). Less then 6% of the colorectal cancer cases in the western world is due to a single mendelian inherited autosomal dominant gene (Mulvihill 1983). Of these inherited cancers familial adenomatous

polyposis (FAP), formerly called familial polyposis coli is the best characterized premalignant condition. This disease is accompanied by an autosomal dominant mode of inheritance, by a nearly 100% penetrance and by the presence of at least 100, but often thousands of adenomatous polyps in the large bowel (Bussey 1975). Untreated FAP will inevitably lead to colorectal cancer at relatively young age and it represents about 1% of all colorectal cancer deaths (Bussey 1975).
As long as there is no specific gene marker identified, screening of all first degree relatives of a newly diagnosed FAP patient is mandatory because they have, a priori, a 50% risk of carrying the disease gene. This screening requires a complete genealogic inventarisation study of each FAP patient. Most often this was done by the medical specialist. Disadvantages of this procedure are that specialists are not trained in genealogy, this type of work is very time consuming, and the continuity of screening can be endangered for example because the doctor retires or the patient moves to another area.
To ensure the continuation of screening and follow-up in FAP families and because FAP is a relatively rare disorder to many doctors, we came to the establishment of a national registry of heriditary tumors in the Netherlands in 1985.
This chapter deals with the evaluation of registration in the identification and surveillance of FAP families in our country.

THE REGISTRY

After the diagnosis the specialist contacts our registry. A social worker, who is very well trained in genealogy, generally interviews the patients at their homes, prepares a complete pedigree chart of the patient to elicit the family history as complete as possible. Furtheron he/she collects as much information as possible from the patient and from the first and second degree relatives (names, adresses, places of living and birth, dates of birth, as well as names and adresses of their family doctors and medical specialists). We collect in our registry the personal data, the results of the screening and histological examinations, as well as types and results of treatment of the FAP patients and also the personal data and results of screening of family members at risk for the disease.
We are sponsored by the government and one of our responsibilities is to see that the continuity of the investigations by periodic assessment of the screening results is maintained. We send a reminder to the specialists of the family to screen family members who are at risk. Moreover pamphlets are available for patients and their relatives, which contain information about the disease explaining the importance of the continuation of medical surveillance for patients and their first degree relatives.
Written informed consent is obligatory before registration of the data of a person is started. Moreover, each registered person preserves the right to remove his or her data from the registry.
Information about our organisation and the aims of this national registry were disseminated to relevant scientific societies (Gastroenterology, Pathology and Oncology) in the country by talks and lectures as well as by publications in the local media. For that reason and due to the fact that the screening procedures are performed by the patient's own specialists in their local hospitals, a lot of FAP families were referred to the registry.
Flexible endoscopy of at least the rectum and sigmoid colon is advocated at two years intervals as the screening examination of choice for FAP. Endoscopy of the rectum is advocated twice a year for patients in whom an ileorectal anastomosis was performed.

RESULTS

As on January 1st 1989, three years after its establishment, the registry contained data from 107 families. The majority of the members of these families were registered, while only a few of them refused registration mainly for religious reasons. Although the reminder system appeared to function well, several specialists also preferred the help of the registry's social worker for completing the follow-up and screening forms.

Patients

Complete data are available on 82 of the 107 registered families, including 395 patients and 357 first degree relatives. The diagnosis FAP was confirmed after histological examination in 230 patients, 131 males (57%) and 99 females (43%). Unfortunately, in the other 165 patients the diagnosis was based on family history and/or a clinical impression. The group of 230 patients could be divided into a subgroup of patients who had been referred because of symptoms (propositi) and a subgroup of first degree relatives who were asymptomatic in whom FAP was found after screening.

The mean age at diagnosis in the symptomatic group of 104 patients was 35 years (ranging from 13 - 66 years), whereas in the group of 126 asymptomatic relatives the mean age at diagnosis was 24 years (range 8 - 59 years).

In 90% of the asymptomatic patients the diagnosis was made by the age of 40, whereas the diagnosis had been made at the age of 50 in 97% of the patients.

In four of our families the late-onset form of FAP was found.

Colorectal Cancer and FAP

In the subgroup of propositi 49 out of 104 (47%) appeared to have one or more cancerous growth in their colorectum. In the subgroup of asymptomatic patients in whom screening examinations were performed, 5 of 126 patients (4%) had colorectal cancer. The mean age of these 54 patients who developed colorectal cancer was 40 years at the time of diagnosis (range 19 - 64 years).

Surgical Therapy

In the majority of the 230 FAP patients a subtotal colectomy with an ileorectal anastomosis was performed. In 9 of them a carcinoma of the rectum was found during a follow-up period ranging from 2 to 33 years (mean 14 years). In the other patients different types of surgical treatment were performed (total proctocolectomy with or without a continent ileostomy, proctocolectomy, mucosal proctectomy and ileo-anal anastomosis).

Screening

Careful analysis of the families revealed that 49 persons were under unnecessary surveillance, whereas 204 persons who were at risk for the disease had not been screened at all.

De Novo Mutations

In 38 of the 82 families the diagnosis FAP could not be confirmed neither in the parents nor in the brothers or sisters of the propositus. It is possible, but by no means proven, that FAP in these families is the result of a de novo mutation.

FAP and Extra-Colonic Manifestations

Polyps in the Stomach and Duodenum

Screening of the upper GI tract (either radiologically or endoscopically) is not performed routinely in the Netherlands. Therefore we have the results from only 44 of the 230 patients. Nineteen of them (43%) were found to have one or more polyps in the upper GI tract. In some of the patients the stomach polyps appeared to have the typical features of a fundic gland polyposis, whereas most of the small bowel polyps had an adenomatous type of mucosal growth while some of them showed severe dysplasia.

Abdominal Desmoids and Mesenteric Fibromatosis

These serious complications of FAP were found in 11 (5%) of the 230 patients after abdominal surgery at a mean time interval of 8 years (range 1 - 28 years) after the operation. Eight of them were males, 3 females. The mean age at diagnosis was 34 years (range 22 - 51 years).

Periampullary Carcinoma
In our series one patient died due to this complication.

Other Extra-Colonic Manifestations
Because no systematic examination was done in the whole group of patients we are not aware of the prevalence of other extra-colonic manifestations such as osseous, dental, retinal or cutaneous stigmata.

DISCUSSION

The basis of the prevention of colorectal cancer is early identification of the individuals at risk of the disease. They should be recognized at an early age and their premalignant lesions should be treated appropriately.
As familial adenomatous polyposis (FAP) is a well-defined condition with a phenotypic expression that can be recognized easily and because untreated FAP will inevitably lead to colorectal cancer and to death at relatively young age, possible carriers of the FAP gene should identified as soon as possible. Because of the autosomal dominant character of this disease it is important to prepare a complete pedigree chart. However, in the Netherlands most clinicians who deal with FAP patients are not trained in this genealogic type of work. To guarantee the continuation and to promote screening in these families in 1985 we came to the establishment of a national registry of FAP families. Due to the fact that the Netherlands is a relatively small but densely populated country, so far we were able to register 107 families and 82 of them completely. Just a few members of the families refused registration and screening whereas all the attending doctors collaborated and were very enthusiastic. This is probably due to our vision that screening examinations should be performed by the patients own physicians in their local hospitals. The registry just collects the results and sends reminders for follow up examinations when necessary.
During the relatively short period of registration we noticed that many individuals were not screened at all. Also, the genealogic studies showed that many persons who were not at risk were screened at regular intervals.
The incidence of large bowel cancer in the asymptomatic group of patients compared to the propositus group of patients is lower but still considerable. This finding, which is in confirmation with those of other registries (Bussey 1975, Bülow 1986), stresses the necessity and value of registration and screening in the prevention of colorectal cancer in FAP.
The age at which the screening procedures start, depends on the age at which the polyps appear in asymptomatic patients. However, the number of asymptomatic individuals who were found to be free of polyps at the first screening examination(s) and subsequently developed adenomas was small. Moreover, most of the asymptomatic patients already had polyps during the first screening. For those reasons we are not able to decide at what age screening procedures in first degree relatives of a FAP patient should be started, it should obviously be the age the development of colorectal cancer is highly unlikely. Since the youngest patient with a colonic carcinoma in our series of FAP patients was 19 years of age, and because in two other large series (Bussey 1975, Bülow 1986) the youngest colorectal cancer patients were 18 and 17 years of age, we feel that screening should start between the ages of 10 and 15 years. Based on clinical experience we feel that the best compliance is achieved in the early teenages; for these reasons we advocate to start screening investigations in first degree relatives of a FAP patient between the age of 10 and 12 years.
For the advice for how long screening examinations should be continued the following observations are of relevance. At the age of 40 years individuals who are at risk, but without evidence of FAP still have a 9% risk of developing the disease later in live. The chance is only 1% at the age of 50 years. Therefore after the age of 40 the intervals could be longer than 2 years, and they can be stopped after the age of 50. This advice should however be based on the biology of the disease in a given family. It could be, for instance, that a particular family is suffering from an apparently late-onset form of FAP. It is evident that in such

families screening should continue even after the age of 50.
It is well known that patients with FAP are at considerable risk for the development of extra-colonic manifestations of the disease. The best known polyposis syndrome associated with extra-colonic manifestations is Gardner's syndrome (Gardner 1953). The Gardner's syndrome was classically characterized by a triad comprising of adenomatous polyposis in the colorectum, soft tissue abnormalities and bone abnormalities.
This was later expanded with a variety of extra-colonic gastrointestinal manifestations of FAP, such as periampullary carcinomas (Jones 1977), small bowel carcinomas and adenomas (Phillips 1981) and gastric polyps and cancer (Coffey 1985, Sarre 1987). Gardner's syndrome has long been considered as a disorder distinct from FAP, but it appears to be a genetic variant of FAP.
Among those screened for this phenomenon we found a relatively high prevalence of polyps in the proximal part of the gastrointestinal tract. This observation has also been made by others (Bülow 1985). Therefore screening of this part of the GI tract appears to be justified (Järvinen 1986, Kurtz 1987). However, the biology of adenomas in the upper gastrointestinal tract is not known. Prospective studies are needed to elucidate this phenomenon.
In the near future the upcoming knowledge on the FAP linked DNA-markers (Bodmer 1987, Meera Khan 1988) may allow presymptomatic detection (or exclusion) of FAP. Thus the unnecessary anxiety in the group of non-gene carriers can be avoided and we can focus our attention on the cancer prevention in the actual carriers of the FAP-gene.

Acknowledgement

The authors wish to thank Agnes van Es-Isaak and Ilse Vliegenthart-Isaak for typing the manuscript.

REFERENCES

Bodmer WF, Bailey CJ, Bodmer J, Bussey HJR, Ellis A, Gorman P, Lucibello FC, Murday VA, Rider SH, Scambler P, Sheer D, Solomon E, Spurr NK (1987) Localization of the gene for familial adenomatous polyposis on chromosome 5 Nature 328: 614-616

Bülow S, Lauritsen KB, Johansen A, Svendsen LB, Sondergaard JO (1985) Gastroduodenal polyps in familial polyposis coli Dis Colon Rectum 28: 90-93

Bülow S (1986) Familial polyposis coli A clinical and epidemiological study Laegeforeninges Forlag, Copenhagen

Bussey HJR (1975) Familial polyposis coli The Johns Hopkins University Press, Baltimore, London

Centraal bureau voor de statistiek (C.B.S.) (1987) Overledenen naar primaire doodsoorzaak, leeftijd en geslacht in het jaar 1986 Serie Al Voorburg, pp 4-6, 39

Coffey RJ, Knight CD, van Heerden JA, Weiland LH (1985) Gastric adenocarcinoma complicating Gardner's syndrome in a North American woman Gastroenterology 88: 1263-1266

Day DW, Morson BC (1978) The adenoma-carcinoma sequence In: Morson BC (ed) The pathogenesis of colorectal cancer Saunders WB, Philadelphia, pp 58-71

Eddy DM (1987) Screening for colon cancer in a high risk population Gastroenterology 92: 682-692

Gardner EJ, Richards RC (1953) Multiple cutaneous and sub-cutaneous lesions occuring simultaneously with hereditary polyposis and osteomatosis Amer J Human Genet 5: 139-147

Gilbertsen VA, Nelin JM (1978) The prevention of invasive cancer of the rectum Cancer 41: 1137-1139

Järvinen HJ, Sipponen P (1986) Gastroduodenal polyps in familial adenomatous and juvenile polyposis Endoscopy 18: 230-234

Jones TR, Nance FC (1977) Periampullary malignancy in Gardner's syndrome Ann Surg 185: 565-573

Kurtz RC, Sternberg SS, Miller HH, DeCosse JJ (1987) Upper gastrointestinal neoplasia in familial polyposis Dig Dis Scie 32: 459-465

Lipkin M, Winawer SJ, Sherlock P (1981) Early identification of individuals at increased risk for cancer of the large intestine Clinical Bulletin 11: 13-21
Lynch HT, Lynch J, Lynch P (1977) Management and control of familial cancer In: Mulvihill JJ, Miller RW, Fraumeni J (eds) Genetics of human cancer Raven Press, New York, pp 235-255
Meera Khan P, Tops CMJ, vd Broek M, Breukel C, Wijnen JT, Oldenburg M, vd Bos J, van Leeuwen-Cornelisse ISJ, Vasen HFA, Griffioen G, Verspaget HW, den Hartog-Jager FCA, Lamers CBHW (1988) Close linkage of a high polymorphic marker (D5S37) to familial adenomatous polyposis (FAP) and conformation of FAP localization on chromosome 5 q21-q22 Hum Genet 79: 183-185
Morson BC (1976) Genesis of colorectal cancer In: Sherlock P, Zamcheck N (eds) Clinics in Gastroenterology Saunders WB Company Ltd, London Philadelphia Toronto, pp 505-525
Mulvihill JJ (1983) The frequency of hereditary large bowel cancer In: Ingall JRF, Mastromarino AJ (eds) Prevention of hereditary large bowel cancer Alan R Liss, New York, pp 61-75
Muto T, Bussey HJ, Morson BC (1975) The evolution of cancer of the colon and rectum Cancer 36: 2251-2270
Phillips LG (1981) Polyposis and carcinoma of the small bowel and familial colonic polyposis Dis Colon Rectum 24: 478-481
Sarre RG, Frost AG, Jagelman DG, Petras RE, Sivak MV, McGannon E (1987) Gastric and duodenal polyps in familial adenomatous polyposis: a prospective study of the nature and prevalence of upper gastrointestinal polyps Gut 28: 306-314
Snel P, de Wolf AN (1988) Consensus follow-up-onderzoek na poliepectomie Ned Tijdschr Geneesk 132: 489-495

Current Status of the Registration of Familial Adenomatous Polyposis at the Polyposis Center in Japan

TAKEO IWAMA, YOSHIO MISHIMA, and JOJI UTSUNOMIYA

ABSTRACT

The Polyposis Center of Japan had registered 970 cases and 631 families of familial adenomatous polyposis (FAP) up to Oct. 1989. The fusion of families which were registered independently from different institutes was recognized in 104 (16.5%) families. Our survey revealed 1738 affected persons and 4475 persons at risk as carrier of the FAP gene. The frequency of cancer was less in the call-up cases (21%) than the proband cases (60%). Periampullary carcinoma and desmoid tumor were the two most serious extra colonic malignancies. We need to pay attention to the bile duct and to development of desmoid tumor after colo-rectal operation.

OPERATION OF THE POLYPOSIS CENTER

The Center for Analyzing Familial Polyposis (The Polyposis Center) was established at Tokyo Medical and Dental University in 1975 by Utsunomiya. Since 1982, we have been continuing the activity under the name of the Research Center for Polyposis and Intestinal Disease. A part of the activity and purpose of The Polyposis Center is as following. When a doctor diagnoses and treats a hereditary tumor, it is inevitable to inform family members about the disease from the genetic aspects and to explain them the need of screening of FAP before the development of malignant tumor. The detection of persons who are at risk of FAP takes much time and effort which is sometimes impossible for practitioners to perform. When a patient is registered to The Polyposis Center, for each family, an exact family map is made up using the national family register. The information is reported back to the doctor who registered the patient to help him call up and examine the high risk members. The privacy of patients and relatives have been guaranteed. To establish proper strategy based on a scientific evidence for the treatment of familial adenomatous polyposis (FAP) or other hereditary cancer diseases, nation wide collection of data is needed. Information on the patients of familial adenomatous polyposis (FAP) as well as other types of polyposis have been collected from the hospitals through five different sources of information: inquiries to hospitals, autopsy records, published literature, voluntary visits by patients and Japanese Society of Large Bowel Cancer Research. For collection of nation wide data of FAP, The Polyposis Center serves as the information center for the doctors who want to know about the epidemiological details of the disease or the recent development on this disease. At the Department of Cytogenetics of Tokyo Medical and Dental University, fibroblast and lymphocytes of FAP patients and their relatives are stored for chromosome and gene analysis (Fig. 1). Resent development of cellular or molecular biology makes these fundamental efforts more important to clarify the cause of development of cancer in FAP.

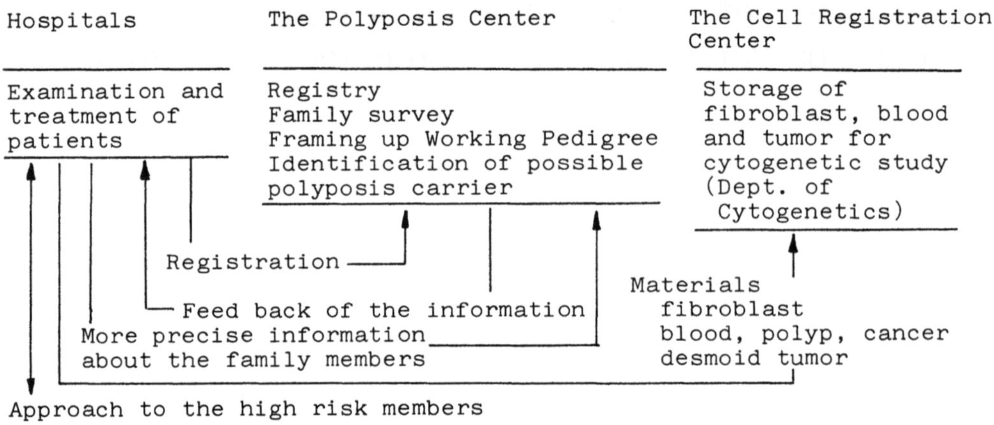

Fig. 1.
Operation of The Polyposis Center of Japan.

RESULTS

Diagnosis of FAP is sometimes difficult. We defined FAP as a case which had more than 100 adenomas in the colon. We had 970 cases of FAP and 631 families registered. Among them, 104 families (16.5%) were composed of two or more families which had been reported independently from different institutes. These fusions have accelerated the ascertainment of the pedigree. A family survey revealed 1738 affected cases and 4475 persons at risk of FAP gene carriers (Table 1).

Table 1.
Registered FAP cases at the Polyposis Center. (Oct. 1989.)

	Number
Cases	970
(call up cases; 230)	
Families	631
Fused families	104
(16.5% of 631 families)	
Completed pedigree maps	564
: members	9604
: affected cases	1738
(alive; 839, dead; 899)	
: living first degree relatives	4475

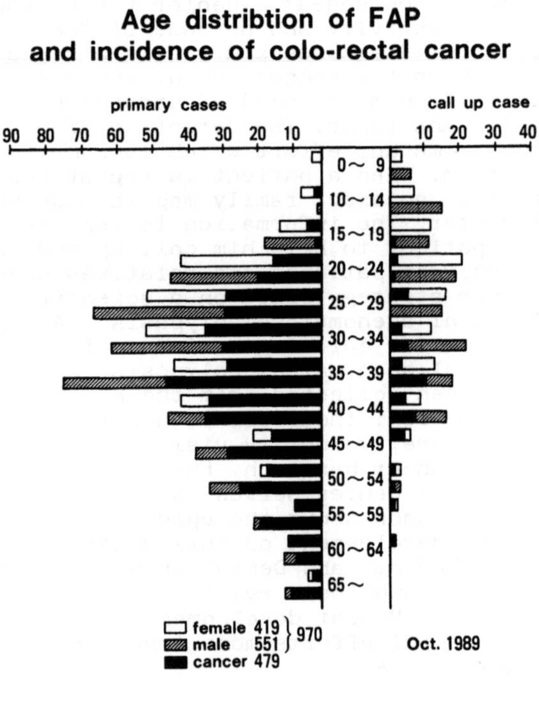

Fig. 2.

The patients which were found by family examination, call up cases, were about 24% of the registered cases after the establishment of our institute (Fig. 2.). Incidence of colon cancer was much less in the call up cases (20%) than in the primary cases (60%). These two

figures were much improved than the frequency of the colo-rectal cancer in both call up and proband cases (29% and 67% respectively) when Utsunomiya (1982) surveyed. But even in the call up cases, the frequency of cancer was very high when they were over 35 years old. Fig. 3. is an example of a family tree in which five independently registered cases were revealed to be the member by our surveillance.
Colonic carcinoma in FAP is frequently multiple. In general population, multiple carcinoma was found only in 4.5% of carcinoma cases but multiple lesions were found in 38% out of 479 FAP carcinoma cases (Table 2).

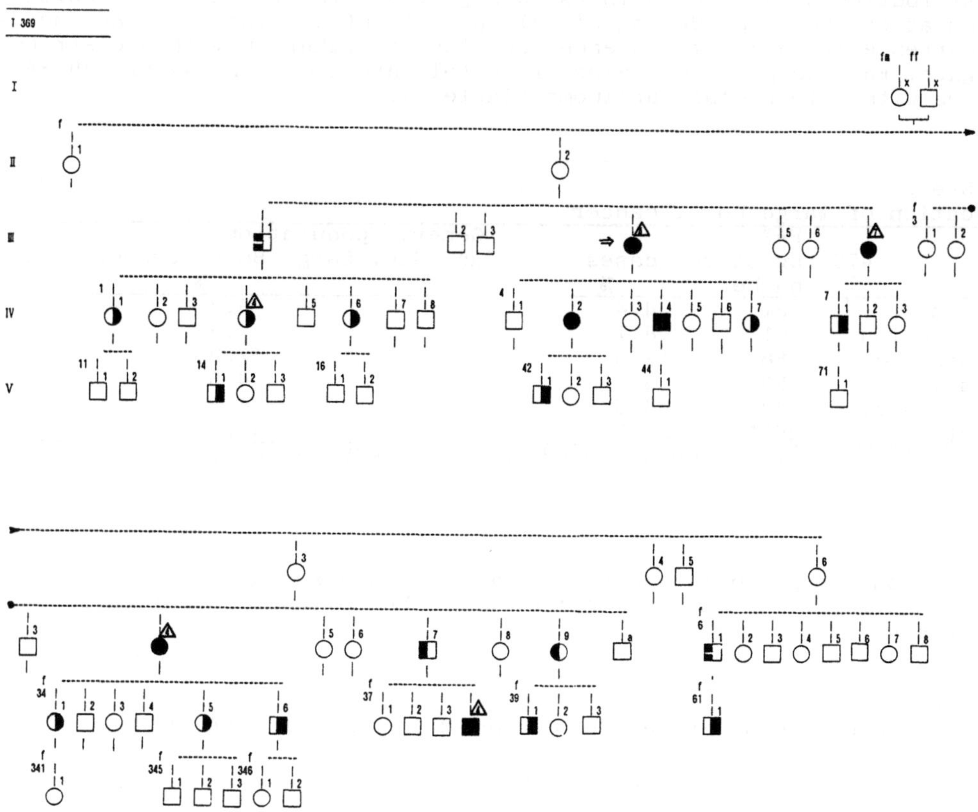

△ ; Cases which fused into the same family.

◧ ; Polyposis, male. ● ; Colo-rectal carcinoma.

◪ ; Colorectal carcinoma + Extra colonic cancer.

Fig. 3

Table .2
Multiplicity of large bowel carcinoma.

No. of Cancer	FAP 479 cases		General population. 24,616 cases *	
Single	398	62.0%	23,504	95.5%
2	106	22.0	895	3.6
3	34	7.0	148	0.6
4	10	2.0	39	0.2
5	31	7.0	30	0.1

* The 16th meeting of Jan. Sac. Large Bowel Cancer Res.

Distribution of carcinoma in FAP was just similar to that of general population. But considering of multiplicity of carcinoma in FAP, actual occurrence of carcinoma at each location is higher than this distribution figure. For example, 261 cases of rectal carcinoma was 54% of 479 FAP cases with colo-rectal carcinoma (Table 3).

Table 3.
Location of large bowel cancer

	FAP 479 registered cases		General population Jan. Sac. Large Bowel Cancer Res.
	number	%	%
Cecum	31	4.4	5.7
Asc. colon	61	8.7	7.6
Transv. c.	88	12.6	7.2
Desc. c.	59	8.4	4.5
Sigmoid c.	199	28.5	24.5
Rectum	261*	37.3	45.1

* : Rectal cancer occurred in 54% of 479 cancer cases of FAP.

Operation was performed on 827 of registered cases and total proctocolectomy or total colectomy were the dominant operation in Japan (Table 4).

Table 4.
Primary operational procedure performed in Japan for FAP (827 cases).

	Cases		Cases
Total procto-colectomy	240	Subtotal colectomy	57
Mucosal proctectomy and ileo-anostomy	78	Miles operation	88
Total colectomy (rectum preserving operation)	247	Others	117

After colonic carcinoma is prevented, then the development of extra colonic malignant tumors becomes important problems, and among them periampullary carcinoma and desmoid tumor are the two big difficulties (Table 5). We reviewed 20 cases (11 males and 9 females) of duodenal or periampullary carcinoma in Japanese literature including three our own cases (Table 6). Their mean age was 44 years. All cases were over 30

Table 5.
Extra colonic malignancies grouped according to primary embryonic layers. (including desmoid tumor)

Endoderm	Case	Mean age	Mesoderm	Case	Mean age	Ectoderm	Case	Mean age
Stomach	23	49	Uterus	5	38	Breast	2	46
Duodenum, papilla	10	46	Ovary	5	40			
Small intestine	3	54	Sarcoma	2	33			
Liver	5	47	Lymphoma	2	31			
Gall bladder	1	77						
Bile duct	1	53	Desmoid tumor	53	31			
Esophagus	1	49	(postoperative	27)				
Thyroid	11	33						
Total	55			67			2	

Table 6.
Duodenal or periampullary carcinoma associated with familial adenomatous polyposis. (References from Japanese literature).

Case	Age	Sex	Site / Operation	Colo-rectal cancer	Interval from colo-rectal ca.	Duodenal polyp	Gastric polyp	Reporter
1	36	M	PA / PD	-		-	-	Kimura '82
2	45	M	PA / PD	+	0	-	-	Takano '82
3	46	M	2nd / PD	+	17 years	256	+	Sugino '82
4	31	F	duodenum / autopsy	-		100	+	Ogawa '83
5	46	M	PA / PD	-		-	+	Yosimi '84
6	47	F	1st / PD	+	22 months	10	-	Iida '84
7	41	M	PA / PD	+	4 years	29	-	Hishiki '84
8	51	M	2nd / PD	+	0	?	?	Kajihara '86
9	43	M	PA / PD	+	- 3 years	?	?	Tada '86
10	44	M	PA / PD	?		+	-	Aioi '87
11	40	F	PA / LE	+	0	+	+	Kuroda '87
12	47	M	PA / LE	+	0	-	-	Shimoda '87
13	48	F	PA / PD	-		-	-	Suzuki '88
14	41	F	PA / PD	+	12 years	5	ca	Yamanaka '88
15	45	M	PA / Autopsy	+	3 years	-	-	Hirokawa '88
16	32	F	PA / PD	-		-	-	Hojo '89
17	49	F	PA / PD	+	25 years	+	ca	Kataoka '89
18	36	M	PA / PD	-		+	+	**
19	43	F	PA / PD	+	12 years	+	+	**
20	63	F	PA / PD	-		-	-	**

PA; Periampullary carcinoma.
PD; Pancreatico-duodenectomy. LE; Local excision. ca; carcinoma.
**; Our experiences.

years and 16 cases (80%) were between 40 and 55 years of age. Although this age distribution of periampullary carcinoma is about 10 years older than that of colo-rectal carcinoma, they are completely overlapped after 30 years of age. Respectable number of cases (8 out of 20 cases) had no polyps in the duodenum, and 80% of the cases developed cancer at the periampullar part. Duodenal adenomas usually small and sometimes too small to detect by X-ray examination. Two cases were treated by partial resection of the ampullar part. These facts indicate that the papilla of Vater in which bile and pancreatic juice are mixed is the point to be paid attention. Periodic fiberscopic observation of the papilla of Vater, ultrasonographic observation of the bile duct or intravenous choledochography may be useful for early detection of the tumor. Early diagnosis of tumor at the papilla of Vater sometimes makes it possible to excise the ampullar part locally. Malignant potential of desmoid tumor varies. Case 1. 30 years old male. He underwent sigmoidectomy in August 1977 because of sigmoid carcinoma with polyposis of the colon. He was referred to our hospital because of huge tumor in the retroperitoneum and this tumor killed the patient in August 1980 (Fig.4). Case 2. 19 years old female. She underwent ileo-anal anastomosis in March 1979. Two big desmoid tumors at the mesentery as well as several tumors in the abdominal wall were found in July 1983. We resected the tumor in the abdominal wall remaining the main tumor in the abdominal cavity. Contrary to our anticipation, the tumor disappeared without any specific medical treatment except theophylline (Waddell 1975) and she married and is working now as a high school teacher. Natural course of desmoid tumor should be more clarified to evaluate several drugs which are considered to be effective for desmoid tumor. We are going to promote the activities of The Polyposis Center of Japan to help doctors and biologists to find the key to open the door through to medical prevention of cancer of FAP.

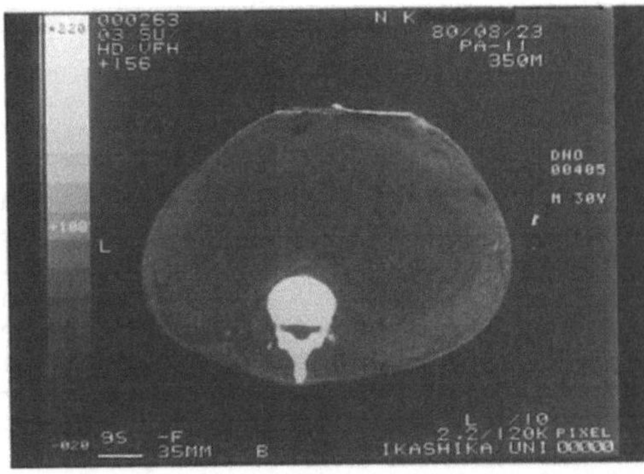

Fig. 4.

REFERENCES

1) Aioi H, Utunomiya J (1987) A follow up study for adenomatosis coli. Gastroent Endoscopy 29(11) 2701-2703. (summary in English)

2) Hirokawa M,Manabe T, Hino K. (1988) Ampullary carcinoma in Gardner's syndrome.Jpn J Clin Oncol. 18(1):43-50.

3) Hishiki S, Baba S, Mitutani K, Morioka S, Nakamura S Sakaguchi S (1985) Cancer of the papilla of Vater associated with familial polyposis coli, report of a case. Ito Cho (Stomach and Intestine) 20(9):1027-1032. (summary in English)

4) Hojo M, Marugami Y, Hashimoto T, Kikuyama N, Takano M, Tomita T, Kojima M (1989) A case of colonic polyposis associated with carcinoma of the papilla Vateri. Nihon Shokaki Geka Gakkai Zasshi (J Jpn Soc Gastroent Surg) 22(8):2126-2129. (in Japanese)

5)Iida M, Yao T, Ito H, Watanabe H, Shigematu H, Iwashita A (1984) Follow up study of Gastroduodenal lesions in familial adenomatosis coli. Ito Cho (Stomach and Intestine) 19(6):621-638. (summary in English)

6) Kajihara S, Kinoshita K, Kimura K, Toda S (1986) A case of intestinal polyposis associated with duodenal carcinoma and colonic carcinoma. Nihonn Shokaki Geka Gakkai Zasshi (J Jpn Soc Gastroent Surg) 19(2):256.

7) Kataoka K, Kitagawa N, Toyoda K, Hashimoto Y, Takano N (1989) A case of adenomatosis coli associated with early periampullary carcinoma and early gastric carcinoma. Gastroent Endoscopy 31(8):2238. (in apanese)

8) Kimura H,Nakamura T, Nakano G, Hoshi H, Nakamura M (1982) Development of early cancer of the ampulla of Vater and Duodenal adenoma as seven years after total colectomy which was performed for familial polyposis coli. Ito Cho (Stomach and Intestine) 17(9):983-987. (summary in English)

9) Kuroda A, Kimura W, Wada Y, Sugihara K, Morioka Y (1987) Periampullary carcinoma. Geka Shinryo (Surgical Clinic) 29(3):323-329. (in Japanese)
10) Ogawa K, Takihara M, Kaji H, Takayasu T, Yamaoka Y, Sugitani A, Hikita J (1983) A case of familial colonic polyposis with duodenal carcinoma. Chubu Gekaigakkai Kiji (Proceeding of the Chubu Surgical Conference) 19:100. (in Japanese)
11) Shimoda T, Suwa T, Hirakata T, Sarashina H Okui K (1987) A case of familial adenomatosis coli associated with carcinoma of the ampulla Vateri. Nihon Shokaki Geka Gakkai Zasshi (J Jpn Soc Gastroent Surg) 20(12):2796-2799. (in Japanese)
12) Sugihara K, Muto T, Sawada T, Konishi F, Kamiya J, Morioka Y. A case of Gardner's syndrome. Ito Cho (Stomach and Intestine) 17(9):977-982. (summary in English)
13) Suzuki N Nabeya K, Hanaoka T, Fukushima H, Kaku C, Kobayashi Y, Oguchi S, Fukuzumi N (1988) A case report of adenomatosis coli associated with carcinoma of the papilla of Vater and fundic gland polyposis. Nihon Shokaki Geka Gakkai Zasshi (J Jpn Soc Gastroent Surg) 21(4);1150-1153. (in Japanese)
14) Tada M, Kato S, Katagiri H, Okamoto K, Tonouchi M (1987) A case of colonic polyposis which was detected after pancreatico-duocenectomy for periampullary carcinoma. Ibarakikenn Rinnsho Igaku Zasshi (J Ibarakikenn Clin Med) 23:70. (in Japanese)
15) Takano N, Akita Y, Karohji S (1982) A case of adenomatosis coli with colonic cancer complicated with carcinoma of the papilla of Vater. Aomorikenritu Byoin Zasshi (J Aomoriken Hosp) 27(4):384-389. (in Japanese)
16) Utsunomiya J. (1982) Hereditary gastrointestinal polyposis. Nihon Iji Shinpoo 3044:126-128. (in Japanese)
17) Waddell WR (1975) Treatment of intra-abdominal and abdominal wall desmoid tumors with drugs that affect the metabolism of cyclic 3',5'-adenosine monophosphate. Ann Surg 181(3):299-302.
18) Yamanaka Y, Morita S, Hayakawa M, Konn M, Ono K (1988) Adenomatosis coli associated with gastric and ampullar cancer; a case report. Nihon Daicho Kohmon Byo Gakkai Zasshi (J Jpn Soc Colo-Proctology) 41:842-848. (summary in English)
19) Yoshimi T, Koizumi S, Muto T, Wada Y, Morioka Y (1984) Gardner's syndrome initially diagnosed as periampullary carcinoma, report of a case. Ito Cho (Stomach and Intestine) 19(12):1373-1378. (summary in English)

(Grant-in-Aid for Cancer Research from The Ministry of Education, Science and Culture, Fund from the Sagawa aid for Cancer Research)

Management of Familial Polyposis in Poland

PIOTR KROKOWICZ

ABSTRACT

In 1979 we have started to organize the Familial Polyposis Register in the Departament of General and Gastroenterological Surgery in Poznań. The Familial Polyposis Register keeps the registry of all the patients operated in our Clinic and their family members. The Registry with 160 cases does not cover the whole Poland yet. In the period 1970-1989, we have operated on 88 patients, among them 28 with ileo-anal pouch anastomosis. Procedure which we have presently applied has an individualized character and consists in a choice of one from three main methods of operation. We make efforts to combine oncological radicality with care for quality of life.

Keywords: familial polyposis in Poland,

The present year is extremely important for the Polish Surgery. One hundred years ago, in October 1989, the I-st Congress of Polish Surgeons was organized and the Polish Society of Surgeons was established.
The I-st Congress of Polish Surgeons was organized by a famous surgeon Ludwik Rydygier, the follower of another famous surgeon, Professor Jan Mikulicz from the University of Cracow.

In spite of widely known economic obstacles and political problems surgery in Poland develops spontaneously and is kept on the modern level. Also in the sphere of the treatment of familial polyposis as well as the management of the Familial Polyposis Register we try to continue the best world patterns.

In 1979 we started to organize the Familial Polyposis Register in the Department of General and Gastroenterological Surgery in the Poznań School of Medicine. The plans of the Register for the future are to cover the whole Poland. The works of the Register were seriously delayed by the introduction of the martial law in Poland in 1981, and also by the economic and political problems, which has made it impossible for us to use the computers for many years (embargo for high-technology) (Krokowicz, 1983).

In the General and Gastroenterological Surgery Clinic in Poznań, the majority of familial polyposis cases from the whole country are operated. It is also the place where the data concerning the patients and their families are kept. At present the population of Poland is about 38 mln. people living on the area of 312.000 square kilometers. The main obstacle in the completion of data is the migration processes after the Second World War, as well as a total destruction of archives and parish church registers kept before the war.
Since last year a computer system has been gradually introduced, but

the process has not been completed yet. So far, all the medical examinations, conducting the family-trees, keeping the records, performing the operations and follow-up examinations - all these activities have been preformed by one man - the author of the present paper. It seems necessary to employ a secretary just to work with documentation of the Register. (Góral, 1987)

MATERIALS AND METHODS

In the years 1970-1989 - 160 patients with the familial polyposis and their family members have been examined in the Departament of General and Gastroenterological Surgery in Poznań. Evident familial polyposis has been stated in 116 patients belonging to 67 families. Eighty eight patients have been operated so far. The patients have been within the range of 15-48 years of age. In the case of 48 patients small polyps showing no malignancy were stated and sphincter-saving operations were performed, out of which 28 operations were performed on ileo-anal anastomosis with creation of pelvic pouch ("J" pouch in 25 cases, and "S" pouch in 3 cases). In every case we created loop ilestomy for the period of 8-12 weeks.

Table 1. Familial polyposis - performed operations

Type of operations	Number of operations
Proctocolectomy with ilestomy.	22
Colectomy with ileo-rectoanastomosis.	20
Restorative proctocolectomy with pouch.	28
Palliative surgery-advanced cancer.	18
Total	88

Out of 88 operated patients we have found 8 cases of evident features of Gardner syndrome (mandibular osteomas, cranial osteomas, numerous fibromas), 1 case of Turcot syndrome with gliosarcoma cerebelli and advanced colon cancer with 5 cancer focuses. Moreover in 2 patients operated for ileus 2 cases of big desmoid tumors of mesenterium were found as well as two advanced cases of retroperitoneal sarcomas. (Krokowicz, 1979)
Since 1987 we have also introduced gastroscopy and retinal pigment examinations in all the patients but the data have not been completed yet.

In the course of the works of the Register we have noticed an interesting phenomenon - the fingers of the patients with confirmed polyposis have features of "clubbed fingers", which was observed in unexpected high frequency compared to the normal population. Simultaneously no constitutional anomalies like cardiac defect have been noticed. The phenomenon seems not to have been described in the literature, but the only explanation for its occurence is the genetic link with the feature of familial polyposis. "Clubbed fingers" have been discovered in 18 patients belonging to 11 families both in man and in women. It is difficult now to draw any definite conclusions at this stage, but the frequency in the occurence of this phenomenon - in the cases above is much higher then in the rest of the population.
I have learned that a similar frequent occurence of the "clubbed fingers" was observed by Professor Fedorov among his familial polyposis patients in the Moscow Institute of Proctology (personal communication). Professor Fedorov is the founder of the Soviet Familial Polyposis Register.

DISCUSSION

At present, in the treatment of the familial polyposis of the colon and rectum we apply "individualized approach", that is choosing one of three operation methods. We try to maintain a full oncological radicality and simultaneously care for the patient's quality of life, that is preservation of sphincters in any possible case. The choice of method depends to a large degree on the size, shape and frequency of the polyps occurence in the rectum.

Table 2. Familial polyposis of the colon. Choosing the method of procedure.

Polyps in rectum	Type of operation
small, nonmalignant, limited number	colectomy, ileo-rectal anastomosis, rectal polypectomy, coagulation,
small, nonmalignant, disseminated,	colectomy, mucosectomy, ileo-anal pouch anastomosis,
cancer focuses in polyps, cancer of rectum,	proctocolectomy and ileostomy,

If the rectum polyps are relatively small and non-malignant and the number of them is limited - we perform colectomy and resection of the upper part of the rectum by means of ileo-rectal end-to-end anastomosis. The polyps in the remaining part of rectum are coagulated during the check-up examinations every 3-6 months. The operation is relatively simple and causes few complications, and the patients avoids permanent ileostomy.
We know from our own experience and from the literature that rectum polyps left in some patients disappeared spontaneously. Unfortunately, they sometimes grow and may become malignant in other patients (Moertel 1970). Another incovenience of the method is the necessesity to conduct regular check-up examinations and periodical coagulations of polyps in rectum. In 17 out of 22 patients operated according to this method the polyps disappeared or stopped their growth after successive coagulations and only in 5 cases the growth of polyps forced us to perform rectum amputation and mucosectomy with ileo-anal anastomosis.

When the polyps are small, non-malignant, but difussed and non-removable, by means of coagulation, because of their multitude, mucosectomy and ileo-anal pouch anastomosis are the opration of choice. The operation was performed in a simplified version by Nissen (1932) and Ravitch (1947) and later in 1975-1980 it was modernized and developed by Parks (1980), Peck (1980), Utsunomiya (1980) and others. Regardless of the shape of the performed pouch, the principle of the operation is to remove mucosa from the rectum and anastomose the pouch with the rectum on the level of dentate line. In any case it is necessary to perform a temporary loop ileostomy, to be closed after 8-12 weeks. We have operated 28 patients in this way-in most of the cases we achieved good results. Nevertheless, the operation is still technically difficult and carries a risk of complications. On the other hand, it assures full radicality and allows for sphincter-saving.

The presence of large, sessile and high-risk-of-malignancy-polyps or fully developed rectum cancer are still according to us the indications for proctocolectomy with permanent ileostomy.

The above remarks support the general rule, that the operations on familial polyposis should be performed the earliest possible prophylactively in the symptom-free period.
Operations performed in this early period assure successful treatment and simultaneously save the sphincters.

The Familial Polyposis Registers and prophylactic examinations of the high risk family's members play enormous role here.
It seems that future belongs to the conducting of the extensive screening examinations based on the genetic knowledge and more and more precise location of the gene responsible for the disease (Bodmer, 1987).

REFERENCES

Berk T., Cohen Z., McLeod R.S., Parker J.A. (1988) Congenital hypertrophy of the retinal pigment epithelium as a marker for familial adenomatous polyposis. Dis. Colon Rectum 31:253-257

Bodmer W.F. at al (1987) Localization of the gene for familial adenomatous polyposis on chromosome 5. Nature 328:614-616

Góral R., Krokowicz P. (1987) Colectomy with mucosectomy and ileoanal anastomosis in the treatment of familial polyposis and ulcerative colitis. Pol. Przegl. Chir. 59:57-65

Krokowicz P. (1979) The Turcot syndrome. Acta Chir Scand 145:113-115

Krokowicz P. (1982) The medical procedure in familial polyposis of the colon and rectum. Poz. Rocz. Med. VI:45-54

Moertel C.C., Hill J.R., Adson M.A. (1970) Surgical treatment of multiple polyposis. The problem of cancer in the retained bowel segment. Arch. Surg. 100:521-524

Parks A.G., Nicholls R.J. (1978) Proctocolectomy without ileostomy for ulcerative colitis. Brit. Med. J. 2:85-88

Peck D.A. (1980) Rectal mucosal replacement. Ann. Surg. 191:294-303

Utsunomiya J., Iwama T., Imajo M., Matsuo S., Sawai S., Yaegashi K., Hirayama R. (1980) Total colectomy, mucosal proctectomy and ileoanal anastomosis. Dis. Colon Rectum 23:459-466.

The Probability of Developing Familial Adenomatous Polyposis: Combining the Diminishing Risks with Age with Negative Screening at Advancing Age and Linked Gene Markers

JOAN SLACK

Familial Adenomatous Polyposis (FAP) is a rare dominantly inherited disorder characterized by multiple premalignant polyposis in the colon and rectum, occasional polyps in the upper gastro-intestinal tract and other extra-intestinal manifestations including osteomas and epidermoid cysts, desmoid formation, congenital hypertrophy of retinal pigment and other malignant changes including in the thyroid gland.

The risk of malignant change in the lower gastro-intestinal tract is so high that elective ileo-rectal anastomosis is usually performed when colorectal polyposis has been identified. For this reason, screening of family members known to be at risk is carried out by regular surveillance of the bowel wall, usually performed by rigid sigmoidoscopy.

As happens in many dominantly inherited conditions, the manifestations of the single mutant gene for FAP are variable even within families and the age of onset of the first symptoms is variable. The question of the ideal age to start screening children at risk and the safe age to stop screening adults who have not manifested the condition has been kept under constant review but consensus opinion of the safe margins for screening has not been established. With the finding of linked gene markers for the mutant gene for FAP there is an opportunity to review the probability that a family member at knownrisk who has no visible polyposis at sigmoidoscopy by a given age is going to be affected, and to combine that probability with information obtained from the family distribution of linked gene markers and the result of ophthalmological examination for congenital hypertrophy of retinal pigment. (CHRPE)

The findings from a study of the experience of screening family members at risk of Familial Adenomatous Polyposis from the Polyposis Register at St. Mark's Hospital, London and the Western Australia Polyposis Register in Perth. (Personal communication Mr. Sol Levitt) are presented. I acknowledge gratefully the work of the clinicians who have kept their patients under surveillance.

In the classical dominant pedigree shown in Fig 1, the risk of A inheriting the single mutant gene is 1 in 2 and while her status remains unknown the risk to B is 1 in 4. These risks are the prior probability which will affect the values of any positive or negative evidence for or against A or B having the disorder.

Careful examination of the records in the St. Mark's Polyposis Register showed that the most consistent screening procedure used was rigid sigmoidoscopy and th ough barium enema or colonoscopy occasionally diagnosed the appearance of polyps earlier than sigmoidoscopy, the diagnosis in the great majority was made by rigid sigmoidoscopy.

I have therefore confined the observations reported in this paper to family members who were screened by rigid sigmoidoscopy because they were known to be at 1 in 2 risk of inheriting the mutant gene for FAP. The results cannot be applied to more remote family members with lower prior probabilities unless they are modified by Baysian calculations.

In the series screened at St. Mark's and Perth, there were 137 affected family members who were screened at a prior prbability of 1 in 2 and whose diagnosis was made by rigid sigmoidoscopy. Fig. 2 shows the percentage chance, that any affected individual will be diagnosed by a given age at first screen.

Table I shows the numerical probabilities of being diagnosed at some relevant ages, read from Fig.2.

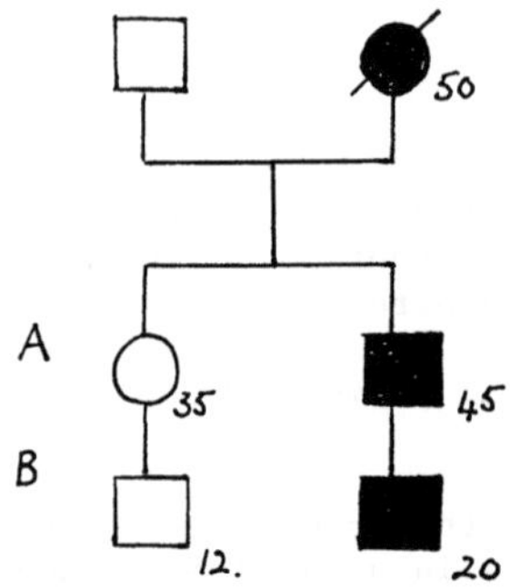

Fig. 1.

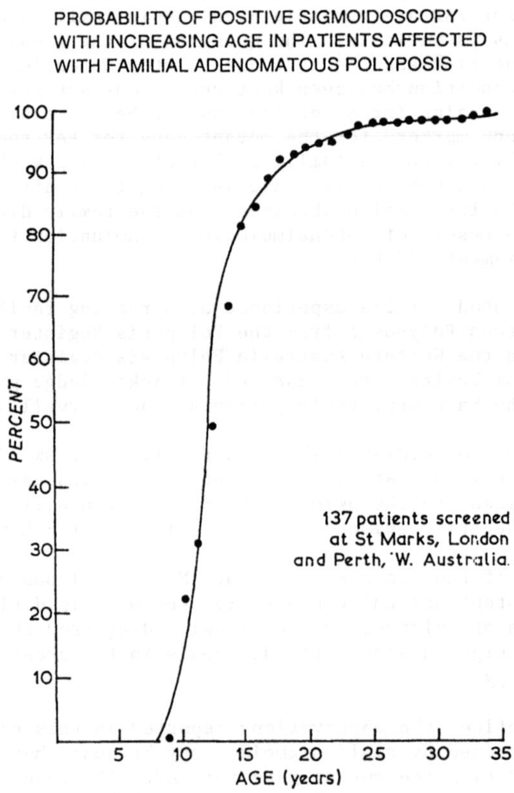

Fig. 2.

Table I. CHANCE OF FINDING POLYPS IN FIRST DEGREE RELATIVES AT 1ST SCREEN BY SIGMOIDOSCOPY IF AFFECTED

AGE	PROBABILITY
10	15%
15	82%
20	94%
30	98%

Of 137 patients picked up by screening in the two centres, 103 were found to be affected at the first screen so it is impossible to know at what age polyps actually developed. It is only amongst those who attended one or more times with negative screening and were subsequently found to have polyps that the age at which polyps developed can be estimated.

These patients will therefore represent a sample biassed towards a late onset of polyposis.

34 patients from the two registers were found to have a negative screen at first examination who subsequently developed polyposis; and from these the mid-point between the first positive and last negative screen was taken as the best estimate of age at which polyps developed. The mean time interval between negative and positive screening was 7.5 years with a range of 1 - 11 years.

Fig. 3 shows the cumulative chance of developing polyps after a negative examination, with increasing age in those affected family members who were screened with 1 in 2 chance of being affected.

The curve gives the practical information which is needed to answer the question likely to be asked by a relative at risk "If I have no polyps now, what is the liklihood that I am a gene carrier and will develop the disease later?"

To answer the question, the prior probability must be combined with the likelihood of showing polyps if affected and this is shown in Fig. 4.

The prior probability starts at 1 in 2, or 50% before any screening. If there are no polyps at age 10, there is a very small diminution in risk, the risk falls rapidly between ages 14 and 20, and in our series all those affected had developed polyps by age 34. In biological terms this curve is more likely to be truely sigmoid and there are reports of affected patients developing polyps after age 34, but there were none who fulfilled the terms of our study in the St. Mark's or Western Australia Registers.

Table II shows the numerical risks read from the curve at a few relevant ages. It is at ages 18 or 20 onwards that the information is most likely to be needed for purposes of genetic counselling. It is now possible to tell a prospective parent that if he or she has not developed polyps by age 20, their risk has dropped from 50% to 20% and the risk to their children of inheriting the gene has dropped from 1 in 4 to 1 in 10. By age 30, a negative screen on sigmoidoscopy will have reduced the risk of having an affected child to 4%.

Since the localization of the mutant gene for Familial Adenomatous Polyposis to the long arm of chromosome 5 and the establishment of linkage to restriction fragment length polymorphisms C11 and Pi 227 and others, it is possible for most families though not all to make use of the linked gene markers to increase the accuracy of a presymptomatic diagnosis. The effect of combining the probability of being affected with age, a negative screen on sigmoidoscopy and a negative result from linked gene markers is shown in Fig. 5.

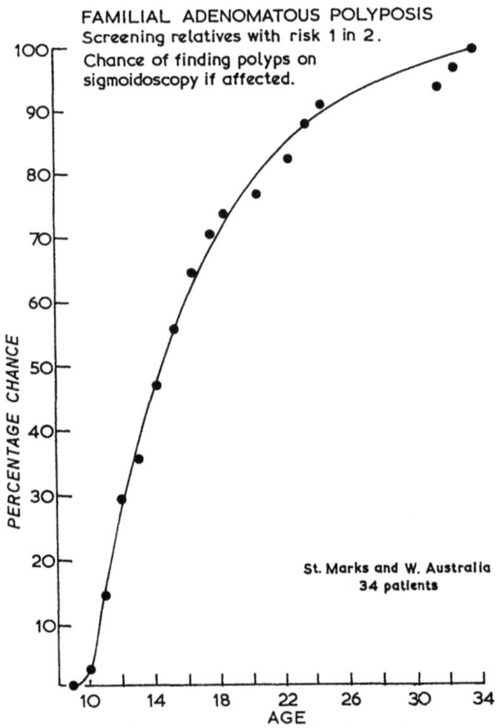
FAMILIAL ADENOMATOUS POLYPOSIS
Screening relatives with risk 1 in 2.
Chance of finding polyps on sigmoidoscopy if affected.
PERCENTAGE CHANCE
100
90
80
70
60
50
40
30
20
10
St. Marks and W. Australia
34 patients
10
14
18
22
26
30
34
AGE

Fig. 3.

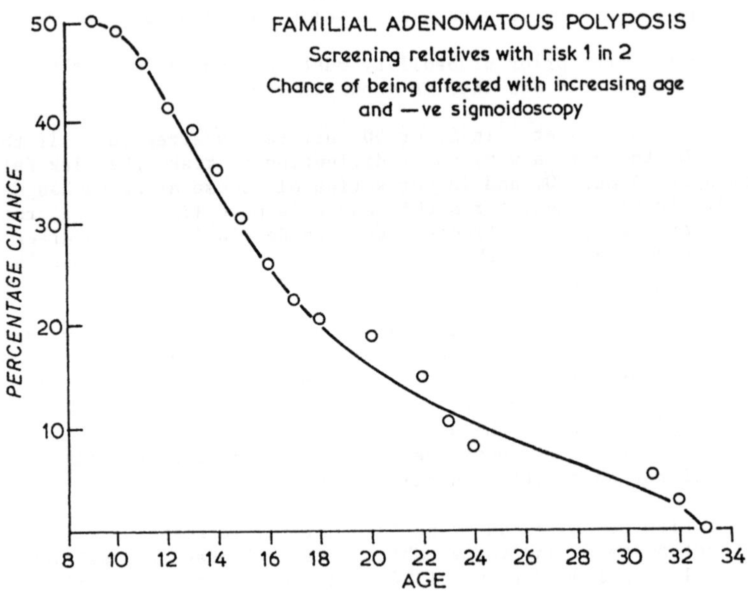
FAMILIAL ADENOMATOUS POLYPOSIS
Screening relatives with risk 1 in 2
Chance of being affected with increasing age and —ve sigmoidoscopy
PERCENTAGE CHANCE
50
40
30
20
10
8
10
12
14
16
18
20
22
24
26
28
30
32
34
AGE

Fig. 4.

Table II.

CHANCE OF FINDING POLYPS AFTER -VE SCREEN BY SIGMOIDOSCOPY AND PRIOR PROBABILITY 1 IN 2

AGE	PROBABILITY
10	49%
15	30%
20	20%
30	8%

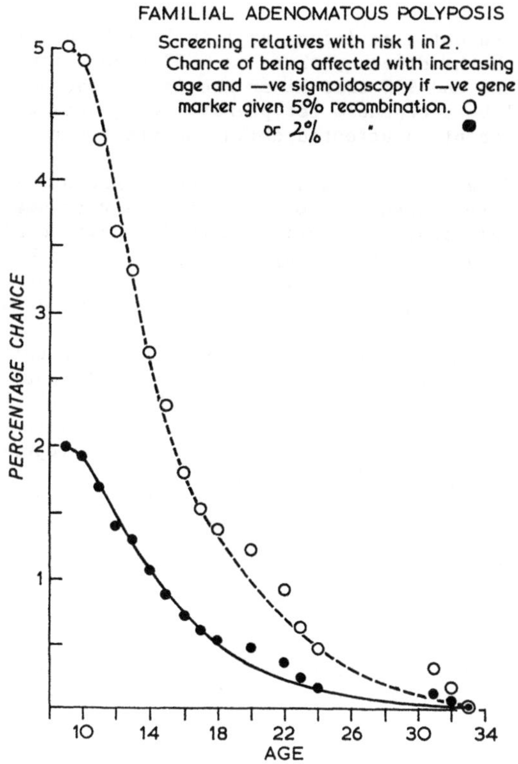

Fig. 5.

At a conservative estimate present available the linked gene markers have a probable 5% recombinant rate so that for informative families a negative gene marker gives a 95% probability that the individual is unaffected. Combining the previous curve of probability with negative sigmoidoscopy with a negative result with C11 P11 gives the probability curve traced through open circles. You will notice that the scale of the vertical axis has changed its upper limits from 100% to 5%, giving an idea of the magnitude of change these markers can make in informative families. The curve traced through closed circles shows the difference made if a linked gene marker with 2% recombination were used - the difference is very little in the older age groups.

Table III.

CHANCE OF FINDING POLYPS AFTER -VE SCREEN BY SIGMOIDOSCOPY AND -VE RESULT FROM LINKED GENE MARKER WITH 5% RECOMBINATION

AGE	PROBABILITY
10	5%
15	1.8%
20	1.2%
30	0.5%

But for now, if an unborn child or infant at 1 in 2 risk inherits markers which are not segretating with the disease, there is a 5% chance that he or she has inherited the mutant gene and 95% that he or she is unaffected. This reduction of probability may well be acceptable for prenatal diagnosis to some parents who would find the 50% chance of an affected child too great a risk to take.

With increasing age and negative sigmoidoscopy the chance of being affected with a satisfactory result with linked gene markers becomes very small indeed so that a comparison with the numerical information shown on previous slides shows that at age 10, the chance is just under 5%, by 15 it is 1.8% and by age age 30 ½% which is only one quarter of the life time risk of a member of the general population developing colorectal cancer. Table III summarizes the numerical effects.

As time goes on more gene markers become available for ante natal and pre-symptomatic diagnosis and recent reports from Japan and Newcastle[3,4] of finding congenital hypertrophy of retinal pigment in families at risk suggest that there is about 80% chance of finding the characteristic pigmentation in affected patients compared with 1% in the general population. If the same proportion of affected children can be shown to exhibit these retinal changes then even at 10 years old a child who is born with a 1 in 2 chance of carrying the gene but who has no hypertrophy of retinal pigment and a satisfactory result from linked gene markers will have only 1 in 100 chance of being affected and by age 30, with negative sigmoidoscopy the probability will have diminished to 1 in 1,000.

REFERENCES:

Bodmer W F, Bailey C J, Bodmer J, Bussey H R J, Ellis A, Gorman P, Lucibello F C, MurdayV A, Rider S H, Scambler P, Sheer D, Soloman E and Spurr N (1987).
Localization of the gene for familial adenomatous polyposis on chromosome 5.
Nature 328 614-616.

Meera Khan P, Tops C M J, v d Broek M, Breukel C, Wijnen J T, Oldenburg M, v d Bos J, Van Leeuwen-Cornellisse I S J, Vasen H F A, Griffioen G, Verspaget H M, den Hartog Jager F C A and Lamers C B H W (1988).
Close linkage of a highly polymorphic marker (D5 S37) to familial adenomatous polyposis (FAP) and confirmation of FAP localisation of chromosome 5q 21-11.
Human Genetics 79 183-185.

Blair N P and Trempe C L (1980).
Hypertrophy of the retinal pigment epithelium associated with Gardner's syndrome.
American Journal of Ophthalmology. 90 661-667.

Chapman P D, Church W, Burn V and Gana A (1989)
Congenital hypertrophy of retinal pigment epithelium: a sign of familial adenomatous polyposis.
British Medical Journal 298 353-354.

Follow-up Study of Associated Tumors in Cases of Familial Adenomatous Polyposis

KYOSUKE USHIO

Abstract

Between 1962 and 1988 we have experienced at the National Cancer Center Hospital 55 cases of familial adenomatous polyposis(FAP) of the colon involving 29 families (43 males, 12 females). The prognosis of the various accompanying FAP tumors were as follows: 1) Benign tumors originated from ectodermal, mesodermal and endodermal tissue had already developed during early childhood and had increased in size and number by puberty, though it was suspected that the tumor growth had generally stopped from that time onwards; 2) Mandibular osteomas developed near the roots of the permanent teeth after the eruption and loss of the deciduous teeth, suggesting that the abnormal repair of the osseous damage plays a great role in mandibular tumorigenesis. 3) Malignant tumors were seen to develop in the glandular epithelium that originated from the endodermal tissue, such as the colon, the small intestine, the stomach, and the thyroid . [Key words : Familial adenomatous polyposis; Associated lesion; Natural history; Mandibular osteoma]

Introduction

Familial adenomatous polyposis (FAP) is characterized by an autosomal dominant mode of inheritance and the presence of at least 100 adenomas in the large intestine. Futher, FAP should be described as being a systemic disease in which a wide variety of accompanying lesions are seen to develop in many regions other than the digestive tract. These tumors are derived from the ecto-, meso-, and endodermal tissue. Thus, the purpose of the present study is to clarify the natural history of these tumors, with especial emphasis placed on the tumorigenesis of FAP mandibular osteomas.

Matreial and Method

Studied were 55 FAP cases involving 29 families (43 males, 12 females) that were treated at the National Cancer Center Hospital between 1962 and 1988. Fourteen patients have since expired. Among the remaining forty-one patients 12 are children less than 15 years old. Whole body systemic examination were conducted, including orthopantomograms and follow-up studies for periods that ranged from 5 to 20 years.

Results

(1) Incidence of associated tumors with FAP

The incidence percentege of accompanying benign lesions that amounted to more than 10 % follows (Table 1) : intramandibular osteomas, 77.3% (34/44); duodenal adenomas, 63.4% (26/41); gastric polyps, 60.0% (30/50); extramandibular skeletal lesions such as osteomas, exostosis, and hypertrophy of the bone, 45.7% (16/35); soft tissue tumors, 31.6% (12/38); mesenteric desmoid tumors, 13.5% (5/37); and, odontomas, 13.2% (5/38). Extracolonic malignant tumors were confirmed in two gastric cancer cases (a 53 year-old male and a 41 year-old female) and one case of a thyroid cancer in a 27 year-old male.

Table 1

Associated Lesions with Familial Polyposis Coli and Gardner's Syndrome

(55 Cases 1962~1988. N.C.C.H)

• Occult osteoma in jaw bone	77.3% (33/44)
• Duodenal adenoma	63.4% (26/41)
• Gastric polyp	60.0% (30/50)
• Bone abnormality	45.7% (16/35)
• Soft tissue tumor of body surface	31.6% (12/38)
• Mesenteric desmoid tumor	13.5% (5/37)
• Odontoma	13.2% (5/38)

(2) Natural history of various tumors

1) Benign tumors originating from ectodermal, mesodermal, and the endodermal tissue had already developed during early childhood and had increased in size and number by puberty, and it was suspected that tumor growth had generally stopped from that time onwards.

2) Mandibular osteomas also were seen to develop near the roots of permanent teeth after the eruption and loss of the deciduous teeth.

3) Malignant tumors were found to have developed only in the glandular epithelium originating from the endodermal tissue, such as the colon, the stomach, and the thyroid .

4) Malignant tumors (sarcomas) originating from the mesodermal tissue were not found.

5) Malignant tumors originating from the ectodermal tissue were not observed.

Discussion

In cases of FAP, a wide variety of tumors that derive from the ecto-, meso-, and endodermal tissue are usually seen to develop, and cases in which "hard tumors", such as osteomas and exostosis, and "soft tumors", such as epidermal cyst and fibrom, are significantly present are classified as Gardner's syndrome (Gardner 1951, Smith 1958) . Recently in Japan it was disclosed that gastric and duodenal tumors are often associated with familial polyposis coli (Utsunomiya et al., 1974, Ushio et al., 1974, 1976; Ohsato et al., 1974, 1977; Yao et al., 1977). This phenomenon has also been observed in foreign countries (Bussey et al., 1978; Pauli et al., 1980; Ranzi et al., 1981; Jarvinen, 1983; Burt,1984). However, the natural history of these lesions is not yet sufficiently known.

(1) Natural history of the mandibular osteoma

Recent investigations (Utsunomiya and Nakamura 1975, Ushio et al. 1976) reported that orthopantomogram and intraoral x-rays revealed multiple osteomatous lesions in 27 of 29 FAP patients (93 percent) and in 13 of 16 patients (81 percent) respectivily. However, the natural history of these lesions remained to be solved.

There seems to be a similiarity in the site and arrangement seen between the unerupted permanent teeth observed in child (Fig.1-a) and multiple osteomas seen in adult FAP patients (Fig.1-b). Figure 2-a is an orthopantomogram of a patient aged 8, and shows a faint abnormal outline indicating osteosclerotic change (arrow) near the root of the permanent tooth. This lesion gradually increased in size and density from age 8 to 16 (Fig.2-b,c) . This same phenomenon as shown in Figure 3 was observed in all 5 cases of chidren that we were able to follow-up for a long period. In contrast, mandibular osteomas that were followed up in 5 adult cases did not change in size and number, as shown in Figure 4. This phenomenon is very important in considering the tumorigenesis of mandibular osteomas and suggests that the abnormal repair of tissue damage after the eruption and loss of deciduous teeth may play a great role in the formation of the tumor.

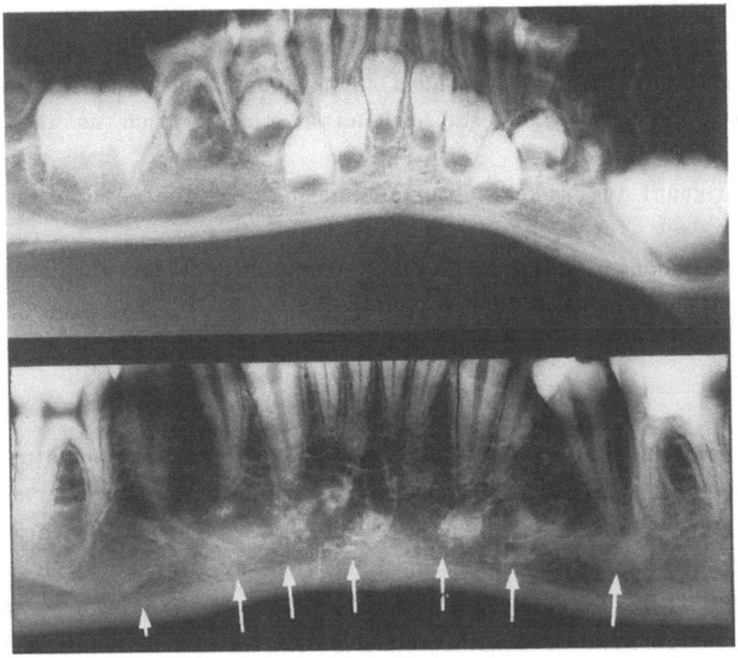

a

b

Fig.1 Panoramic radiographs of the mandibles observed in a 5-year old boy (a) and a 22-year old patient of FAP. There seemes to be a similiarity in the site and arrangement seen between the unerupted permanent teeth observed in child and multiple osteomas seen in adult FAP patient.

Fig. 2 Over eight years' follow-up observation of the osteosclerotic lesion (intramandibular osteoma) of a patient with familial polyposis coli, aged 8. An obscure osteosclerotic change around the root of the tooth was detected in September 1975 (a). Five years and eleven months later (b), this lesion increased in size and density, and after another 2 year and 4 months it formed the well-demarcated osteosclerotic lesion (c).

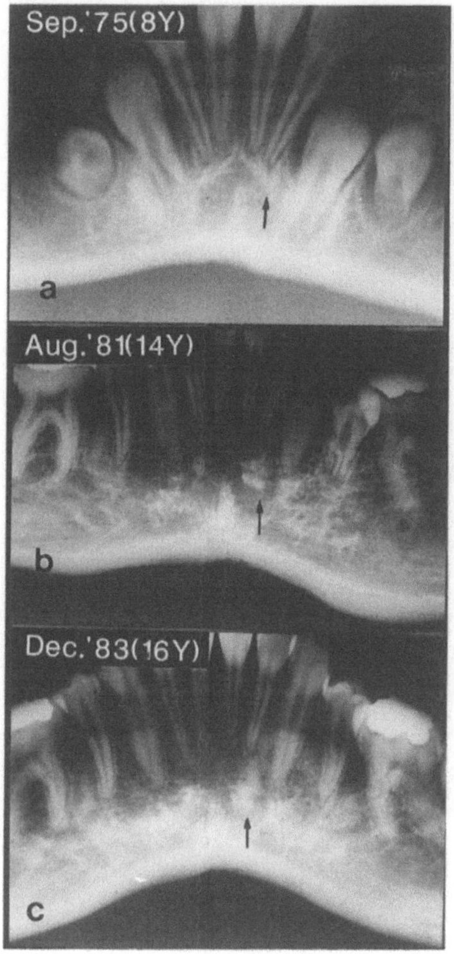

Fig. 2

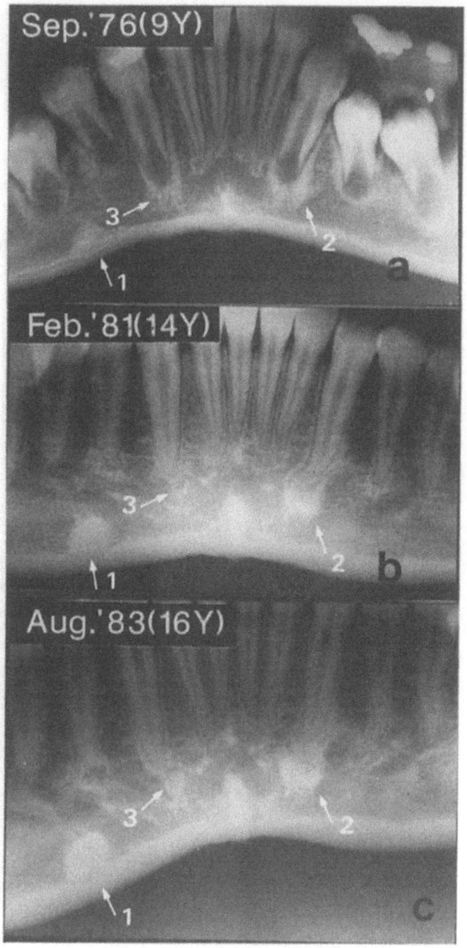

Fig. 3

Fig. 3 Observation by panoramic radiograph of the mandible during 6 years and 11 months of a patient with familial polyposis coli, aged 9. With aging, an osteoma (arrow 1) grew in size, and two ill-defined osteosclerotic shadow (arrow 2, 3) detected in September 1976 (a) became compact (b) and formed well-demarcated lesion (c). It is interesting and important that these osteosclerotic lesions (intramandibular osteoma) were suggested to originate from the area corresponding to the region of the fall-out of the deciduous teeth, and that it became prominent with the development and growth of the permanent teeth.

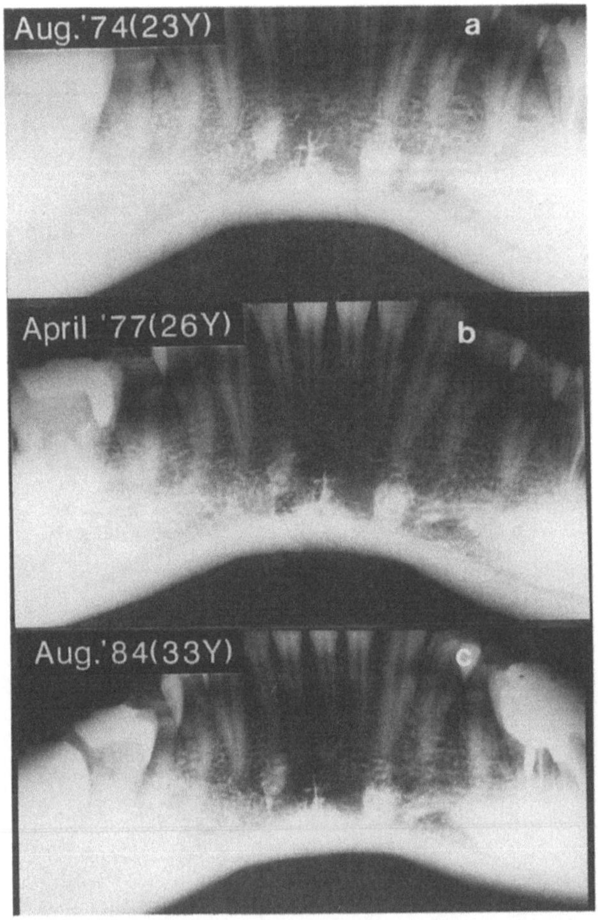

Fig.4

Fig.4 Over 8 years' follow-up observation of the osteosclerotic lesion (intramandibular osteoma) of a patient with familial polyposis coli, aged 23. Note that two osteomas in the body of the mandible, did not change in size and density during 10 years.

(2) Site of the malignant tumor

It is well known that in cases of FAP many and various types of tumors develop throughout the body. These tumors originate from the ectodermal, mesodermal, and endodermal tissue (Table 2). According to our follow-up studies, thus far, no malignant tumor was seen to originate from either the mesodermal or ectodermal tissue. Malignant tumors were confirmed to occur only in the endodermal tissue of the colon, the stomach, and the thyroid. These facts indicate that a tumor of endodermal origin may be more important from a viewpoint of carcinogenesis. Why do malignant tumors develop in the gastrointestinal tract

Table 2

Associated Lesions in Familial Polyposis Coli

Ectodermal

Sebaceous cysts
Epidermoid cysts
Tumours of the central nervous system (Turcot's sy.)

Mesodermal Origin

<Connective tissue>
Fibroma and fibrosarcoma
Desmoid tumours
Diffuse fibrosis : mesenteric, mesocolic, retroperitoneal
Excessive intraabdominal adhesions
<Bone>
Osteoma
Exostosis
Odontomata, Supernumerary teeth

Endodermal Origin

Adenomata of the small intestine, duodenum, stomach
Adenomata of adrenal gland, pancreas, thyroid gland
Carcinoma of ampulla of Vater, stomach, thyroid gland, adrenal gland

and thyroid? The answer may lie in the difference seen in the epithelial tissue of the human body as shown in Table 3. The epithelium of the respiratory and of the lower urinary tract are also derived from the endodermal tissue. However, the epithelium of the gastrointestinal tract and the thyroid are composed of simple, columunal, glandular epithelium. Therefore, in a follow-up stady of FPA patients, it is important to mainly investigate the simple columunal epithelium that originated from the endodermal tissue.

Conclusion

Benign tumors originating from the ectodermal, mesodermal, and endodermal tissue seen to have already developed during early childhood and increase in size and number during puberty, though, it is felt that tumor growth generally stops from this point onwards. Mandibular osteomas also develop near the roots of permanent teeth after the eruption and loss of the deciduous teeth, suggesting that an abnormal repair of the osseous damage plays a great role in mandibular tumorigenesis. Further, malignant tumors tend to develop in the glandular epithelium that originates from the endodermal tissue, such as in the colon, the small intestine, the stomach, and the thyroid.

Table 3

Difference of Tissue and Epithelium in Human Body

A. Origin of Tissue

Ectoderm	Mesoderm	Endoderm
• Epidemis • Sensory and Nervous Tissue	• Connective, Muscle and Bone Tissue • Cardiovascular and Mesenchimal Tissue • Genital and upper Urinary Tissue	• Gastrointestinal Epithelium • Respiratory Epithelium • Lower Urinary Epithelium

B. Epithelium Originated from Endoderm

Gastrointestinal Tract	Respiratory Tract	Lower Urinary Tract
• Esophagus — Stratified Squamous Ep. ► • Stomach, Intestine, • thyroid — Simple Columnar Ep.	• Pseudostratified ciliated Ep.	• Transitional Ep. (stratified)

References

1) Burt W, Berenson MM, Lee RG et al (1984) : Upper gastrointestinal polyps in Gardner's syndrome. Gastroenterology 86 : 295-301

2) Bussey HJR, Veale AMO, Morson BC (1978) : Genetics of gastrointestinal polyposis. Gastroenterology 74 : 1325-1330

3) Gardner EJ (1951) : A genetic and clinical study of intestinal polyposis: A predisposing factor for carcinoma of the colon and rectum. Am J Hum Genet 3 : 167-176

4) Gardner EJ, Plenk HP (1952) : Hereditary pattern for multiple osteoma in a family group. Am J Hum Genet 4 : 31-36

5) Jarvinen H, Nyberg M, Peltokallio P (1983) : Upper gastrointestinal tract polyps in familial adenomatosis coli. Gut 24 : 333-339

6) Ohsato K, Watanabe H , Yao T (1974) : Simultaneous occurrence of multiple gastric carcinoma and familial polyposis of the colon. Jpn J Surg 4 : 165-174

7) Pauli RM, Pauli ME, Hall JG (1980) : Gardner syndrome and periampullary malignancy. Am J Med Genet 6 : 205-219

8) Ranzi T, Castagnone D, Velio P, Bianchi P, Polli EE (1981) : Gastric and duodenal polyps in familial polyposis coli. Gut 22 : 363-367

9) Smith WG (1958) : Multiple polyposis, Gardner's syndrome, and desmoid tumors. Dis Colon Rectum 1 : 323-332

10) Ushio K, Sasagawa M, Doi H, Yamada T, Ichikawa H, Hojo K, Koyama Y, Sano R (1976) : Lesions associated with familial polyposis coli ; Studies of the stomach, duodenum, bones and teeth. Gastrointest Radiol 1 : 67-80

11) Ushio K (1985) : Genetic and familial factors in colorectal cancer. Jpn J Clin Oncol 15 (Suppl 1) : 281-298

12) Utsunomiya J, Maki T, Iwama T, Matsunaga Y, Ichikawa T, Shimomura T, Hamaguchi E, Aoki N (1974) : Gastric lesions of familial polyposis of the large intestine. Cancer 34 : 745-754

13) Utsunomiya J, Nakamura T (1975) : The occult osteomatous changes in the mandible in patient with familial polyposis coli. Br J Surg 62 : 45-51

14) Yao T, Iida M, Ohsato K, Watanabe H, Omae T (1977) : Duodenal lesions in familial polyposis of the colon. Gastroenterology 73 : 1086-1092

Retinal Pigmentations in Familial Adenomatous Polyposis, and Linkage Study on Gene Probes on Chromosome 5q

SHOZO BABA, MASATO TSUCHIYA, HIROYUKI MACHIDA, and MASAO YAMADA

ABSTRACT

Familial adenomatous polyposis (FAP) is a disease of inheritance with autosomal dominant gene, located at chromosome 5 most probably near band 5q21-22. It is important to identify the gene carrier in young age before developing polyposis. In order to assess the importance of retinal pigmentation (Congenital Hypertrophy of the Retinal Pigment Epithelium, CHRPE)[1,2] as a subclinical marker of gene carrier, precise retinal pigmentation and RFLP studies using various 5q DNA probes e.g. C11p11, Pi227 and YN5.48 were carried out. There are no discrepancies between gene carrier and RFLP study.

Keywords: familial adenomatous polyposis, retinal pigmentation, congenital hypertrophy of the retinal pigment epithelium, restriction fragment length polymorphism

1.MATERIALS

Fifty cases of familial adenomatous polyposis in 27 family trees were studied. Sex ratio of patients were 24 to 26. Age of the patient at the time of operation ranges 15 to 66. Association of cancer and extra colonic manifestations in this series were as follows. Early cancer were found 23 lesions in 13 cases. Advanced cancers were found 24 lesions in 15 cases inclusive of the cases with two distant metastasis.

Gastric and duodenal polyps were found 62.5% (25/40) and 71.4% (25/35) respectively. Occult osteoma was found 76.2% (32/42). Soft tissue 70 tumors and desmoid tumors were associated in 35% (14/40) and 11.5% (5/43) respectively. Desmoid tumor was predominantly seen in female in productive age.

The number of the polyps in each individuals were counted at the time of operation. Carpet type polyposis in which the number of polyps were more than 5000 were found in 7 cases, with polyps more than 1000 were 24, more than 500 were 7. The cases with more than 200 and less than 500 were 7 most of which are called up cases and are the second or third generation.

Retinal examination was carried out to 156 eyes in 78 members of 22 Japanese family trees including 34 patients and 44 family members. Among 44 members of FAP family, 28 were possible carriers of the second or third generation. The age distribution of examined cases ranged from 1 to 71.

As for family linkage analysis restriction fragment length polymorphism (RFLP) studies were carried out using various DNA probes such as C11p11, Pi227 and YN5.48 (C11p11 was kindly offered by Sir

W.Bodmer, Pi227 by G.Stewart and YN5.48 by Y.Nakamura). Family linkage analysis were carried out in 9 family trees by the use of Pi227 and YN5.48, and in 20 members in 4 family trees by the use of C11p11.

2.METHODS

2.1 Retinal pigmentation studies

As for retinal pigmentation studies, precise retinal examination were carried out by one ophthalmologist using indirect ophthalmoscope and Goldmann's three mirror contact lens. As a control 1984 retinal examinations were carried out in normal individuals in ophthalmology out patient clinic.

2.2 RFLP studies

For isolation of DNA from peripheral blood lymphocytes blood samples were collected from FAP family members. Lymphocytes were obtained by fraction of peripheral blood. Samples were frozen and stored at -80°C until isolation of DNA.

Samples were treated twice with phenol-chloroform-isoamyl alcohol, and DNA was recovered by ethanol precipitaion. DNA was digested with the restriction enzymes (TaqI, BstXI or MspI) under standard conditions. Samples of about 10 μg of the digest DNA were subjected to electrophoresis on 0.8% agarosegel, and transferred from the gel to filters (Nitrocellulose membrane or Nylon membrane) as described by Southern.[3]

Various DNA probes (C11p11, Pi227 and YN5.48) were labeled with ^{32}P.

The nitrocellulose filters were preincubated for 2hr at 68°C in pre-hybridization solution (6X SSC [1X SSC is 0.15M NaCl / 15mM sodium citrate], 5X Denhardt's solution [1X Denhardt's solution is 0.02% Ficoll / 0.02% polyvinylpyrrolidone / 0.02% bovine serum albumin], sonicated salmon sperm DNA at 0.1 mg/ml and 0.1% SDS). Then filters were incubated for 18hr at 68°C in hybridization solution (6X SSC, 10mM EDTA, 5X Denhardt's solution, sonicated salomon sperm DNA at 0.1mg/ml, 0.1% SDS and 50-100 ng of ^{32}P-labeled DNA probe fragment). The nylon filters were preincubated for 2hr at 42°C in pre-hybridization solution (6X SSC, 5X Denhardt's solution, human placental DNA at 0.1 mg/ml and 0.5% SDS). Then filters were incubated for 18 hr at 42°C in hybridization solution (50% formamide, 5% dextran sulphate, human placental DNA at 0.1 mg/ml, 0.5% SDS and 50-100 ng of ^{32}P-labeled DNA probe fragment). After the hybridization reaction, filters were washed three times. For auto-radiography, the filters were exposed to Kodak X-ray film at -80°C.

3. RESULTS

1) Overall retinal pigmentations of examined patients were calcurated 79.4% (27/34). Pigmentaions of bilateral eyes were found in 23 among 34 FAP patients. Pigmentations in possible carriers were found 12/28 (42.9%). Bilateral pigmentations in possible carriers was found in 8 cases among 12 pigmentation positive children (66.7%).

2) Pigmentation can be classified into two types as Traboulsi reported,[4] namely large pigmentations and small pigmentations (Fig.1,2).

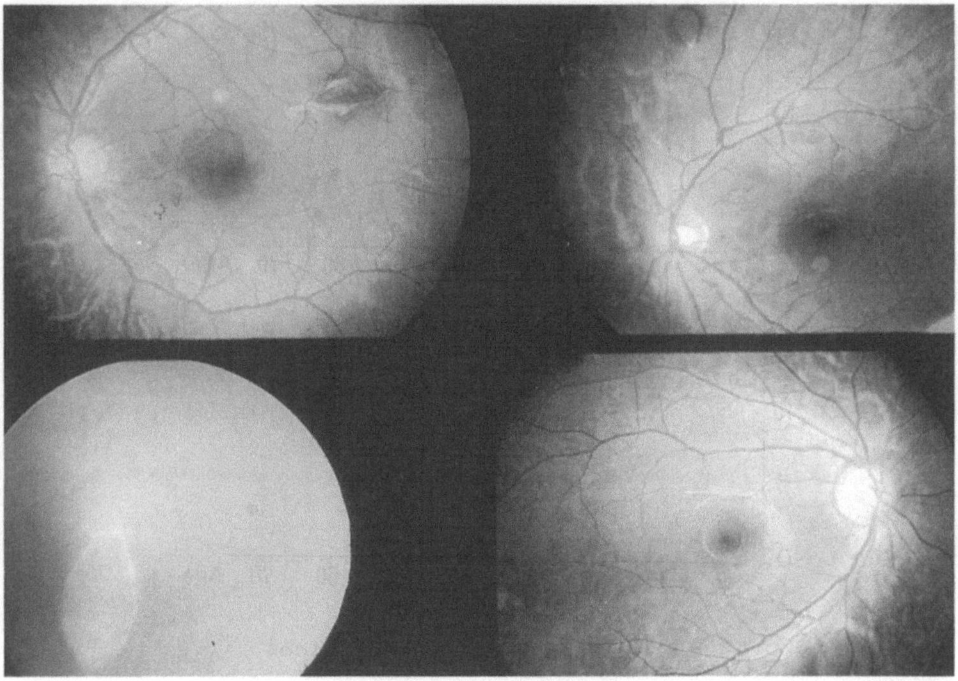

Fig.1. Large pigmentations

Fig.2. Small pigmentations

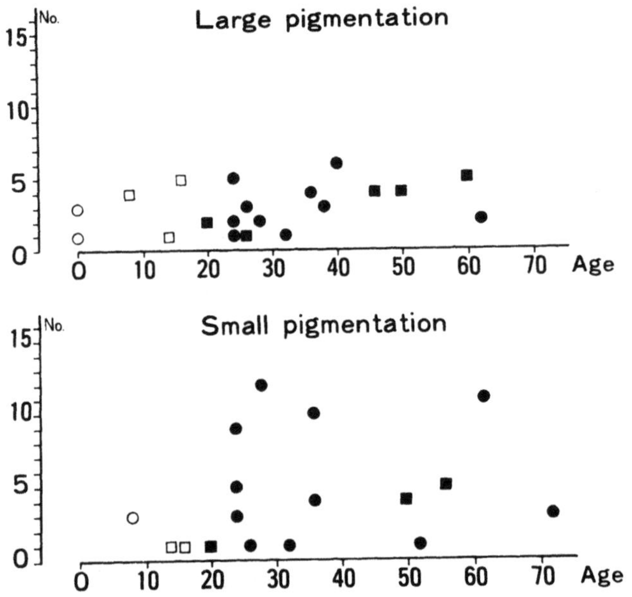

Fig.3. Number of pigmentations

3) The large pigmentation distribute close to the posterior pole and 0.5 to 2 times of papillary diameter in size. Shape of large pigmentation is similar to the seed of water melon or persimon. The small pigmentation distribute in peripheral zone and real black in colour.

4) Between patients and possible carriers of second and third generation, there is no difference in the number of large pigmentation. However, the number of small pigmentation is greater in patients (5.0 on the average in patients and 1.7 in possible carriers). The number of small pigmentation may increase its number or become recognizable at the age when the possible carrier start to develope polyps (Fig.3).

5) In control group only 6 cases with unilateral small pigmentations were recognized. Consequently sensitivity and specificity of large and small pigmentations were calcurated as 0.618, 0.999 in large pigmentation and 0.765, 0.997 in small pigmentation respectively.

6) Two possible carriers with large pigmentations developed polyps during surveillance.

7) So far studied there was no discrepancies between gene carrier and retinal pigmentation.

8) Family linkage study using Pi227 probes was carried out revealing one informative family in 9 family trees (Fig.4). Lod score was calcurated as 0.3 in this study.

9) Family linkage study using YN5.48 probes was also carried out in 9 family trees revealing three informative families.

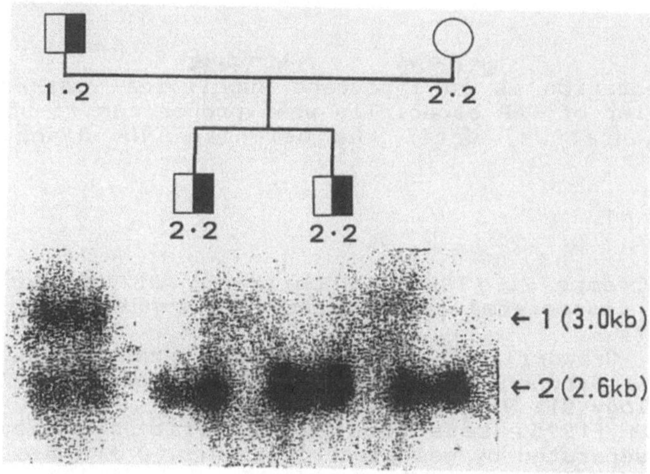

Fig.4. Family linkage analysis of FAP (Family 14) using Pi227

10) There was no informative family in 4 family trees using C11p11 probe so far studied. TaqI polymorphism of C11p11 in Japanese population is different from Caucasian. Frequency of allele 1(4.4kb) is 0.01 and allele 2(3.9kb) is 0.99 (based on 60 Japanese individuals).

4.DISCUSSION

Among the children of FAP patients, possible gene carriers has a 50% risk of manifesting the disease. Therefore, preclinical prediction by reliable marker relieve half of the non-risk persons from anxiety as well as the unnecessary expence and troublesome periodic clinical investigations. To the remaining other half at risk patient, surgeons can plan operative procedures timely to prevent colon cancer. When the parents has large pigmentation there is greater chance to have large pigmentation in gene carrier of second generation. If the children whose parent has pigmentation don't show pigmentation, there is very low risk of developing polyposis.

Bodmer et al[5] reported close linkage between FAP and DNA probe C11p11 among Celtic population, however, we found that C11p11 is not informative among Japanese because of low frequency of the heterozygosity in Japanese population. Khan et al[6] also reported low incidence of heterozygosity in Dutch population. Recently other DNA probe Pi227[6] and YN5.48[7] was also reported to be closely linked to FAP. In our family linkage studies Pi227 reveals one informative family and YN5.48 reveals three informative families. Therefore, among the studied DNA probes YN5.48 is considered to be most useful to predict the possible gene carrier among FAP family in Japanese.

5.CONCLUSION

Retinal pigmentation is an important subclinical marker to identify the gene carrier of FAP especially when propositus of the carrier has typical pigmentation, until the definite DNA diagnosis will be established.

REFERENCES

1)Blair NP, Trempe CL (1980) Hypertrophy of the retinal pigment epithelium associated with Gardner's syndrome. Am J Ophthalmol 90: 661-667
2)Lewis RA, Crowder WE, Eierman RN, Nussbaum RL, Ferrell RE (1984) The Gardner syndrome : Significiance of ocular features. Ophthalomology 91: 916-925
3)Southern EM (1975) Detection of spesific sequences among DNA fragments separated by gel electrophoresis. J Mol Biol 98: 503-517
4)Traboulsi EI, Maumenee IH, Krush AJ, Giardiello FM, Levin LS, Hamilton SR (1988) Pigmented ocular fundus lesion in the inherited gastrointestinal polyposis syndromes and in hereditary nonpolyposis colorectal cancer. Ophthalmology 95: 964-969
5)Bodmer W, Bailey C, Bodmer J, Bussey H, Ellis A, Gorman P, Lucibello FC, Murday VA, Rider SH, Scambler P, Sheer D, Solomon E, Spurr NK (1987) Localization of the gene for familial adenomatous polyposis on chromosome 5. Nature 328: 614-616
6)Khan PM, Tops CM, Broek M, Breukel C, Wijnen JT, Oldenburg M, Bos J, Leeuwen-Cornelisse IS, Vasen HF, Griffioen G, Verspaget HM,Jager H, Lamers W (1988) Close linkage of a highly polymorphic marker (D5S37) to familial adenomatous polylosis (FAP) and confirmation of FAP localization on chromosome 5q21-q22. Hum Genet 79: 183-185
7)Nakamura Y, Lathrop M, Leppert M, Dobbs M, Wasmuth J, Wolff E, Calson M,Fujimoto E, Krapcho K, Sears T, Woodward S, Hughes J, Burt R, Lalouel JM, Gardner E, White R (1988) Localization of the genetic defect in familial adenomatous polyposis within a small region of chromosome 5. Am J Hum Genet 43: 638-644

Congenital Hypertrophy of the Retinal Pigment Epithelium: A Clinical Marker for Familial Adenomatous Polyposis

A. ROMANIA, F. HEYEN, D. JAGELMAN, J. CHURCH, Z. ZAKOV, I. LAVERY, V. FAZIO, E. MCGANNON, and J. OAKLEY

INTRODUCTION

Other than the presence of adenomatous rectal polyps at proctoscopy, there is no satisfactory biomarker available for the early diagnosis of Familial Adenomatous Polyposis (FAP) in at-risk relatives of patients with the disease. Potential markers, such as mandibular osteomas, have not proved helpful as shown by Woods (1989). Recently, several authors' (Berk 1988, Blair 1980, Diaz-Llopis 1988, Lewis 1984, Traboulsi 1987 and 1988) attention has turned to the lesions of congenital hypertrophy of the retinal pigment epithelium (CHRPE), which are present as solitary lesions in a small minority of the normal population but which have been reported as multiple lesions in some families with FAP. The aim of this study was to investigate the incidence of CHRPE in a number of kindreds with FAP, to assess its value as a possible biomarker for polyposis and to evaluate its association with extraintestinal manifestations of the disease.

PATIENTS AND METHODS

Dilated fundus examinations were performed in 148 members of 53 FAP kindreds. Wide-angle fundus photography with multiple (approximately 40) overlapping exposures was performed for each subject and the photographs examined by one author (AR) who did not know the clinical status of the subjects. This had been determined by proctosigmoidoscopy and biopsy of any colorectal polyps found. On the basis of this, patients were classified as either "at risk" or "FAP". Yearly proctosigmoidoscopy is performed in "at risk" family members.

The results of other examinations performed to exclude or diagnose extracolonic manifestations of FAP were recorded. All kindreds were registered with the Cleveland Clinic Familial Adenomatous Polyposis Registry.

Based on the distribution of findings in this study and preliminary work by others (Blair 1980, Lewis 1984, Traboulis 1987), a criterion of at least four lesions of CHRPE, one or more in each eye, was set for a "positive" examination, that is an examination likely to be predictive of inheritance of the FAP gene. Patients and relatives were grouped according to the results of their examination. Data were evaluated using Chi Square, Student's t or the Wilcoxon signed rank tests.

RESULTS

There were 97 patients with FAP and 51 at-risk family members in the study sample. Using the criterion previously described for a positive examination for CHRPE, 61 patients and 13 family members were positive. All of these subjects belonged to a group of 34 kindreds. Clearly distinct from these "positive" kindreds was a second group of 18 kindreds in whom none of the 32 FAP patients nor any of the 34 at-risk relatives had more than four CHRPE lesions.

The only exception from this pattern was family #1002, in whom two mother/daughter pairs from distant branches of the family tree had differing, but homogenous patterns of CHRPE. One pair was positive and one negative. Patients with FAP and a positive eye exam were diagnosed earlier than patients with a negative exam (22.6 years vs 31.2 years, $t=3.9, p<.01$), suggesting a more aggressive form of disease in this group. Follow-up of at least two years has elapsed since the initial eye examinations and during this time 10 of the 13 at-risk family members in the "positive eye kindred" group have been examined proctoscopically. Five have developed polyps, and five have not. Of the 20 at-risk relatives negative for CHRPE in the "positive eye kindreds" 14 have been examined and none have developed polyps.

Extracolonic manifestations of FAP were distributed equally between the two groups of kindreds (positive CHRPE kindreds= 26/34, negative CHRPE kindreds=11/18). Positive kindreds had more extracolonic manifestations per patient, however (.55 vs .30, $t=2.06$, $p<.05$).

There were eight families in who the propositus had no family history of FAP and was deemed a spontaneous mutation. They were present in equal proportions in the two kindred groups.

DISCUSSION

The results obtained in this study suggest that a positive examination for CHRPE in a member of a kindred diagnosed with FAP means that a positive examination in at-risk relative in that kindred has a high predictive value for the development of polyposis. A negative exam in an at-risk relative of the same kindred is a good indication that patient will not develop polyposis. Conversely, a negative examination in a FAP patient means that the examination has no predictive value in at-risk relatives. This type of division of kindreds, based on these criteria, has not been reported previously. The strength of these conclusions is weakened somewhat by the one exception, family #1002. Yet within the two, widely separate parts of this family, the pattern of CHRPE was consistent. Certainly follow-up of at-risk patients over the two years since the initial eye exam was performed has shown no inconsistent results and has confirmed, in a preliminary way, the high predictive value of CHRPE in 65% of FAP kindreds when used according to the criteria presented here.

The results also suggest that in kindreds where CHRPE lesions exist in significant numbers, the FAP phenotype is expressed more strongly: the diagnosis is made earlier and there are more extracolonic manifestations per patient. A more aggressive surveillance program may be justified. There are some difficulties with the widespread application of this technique, however. Further follow-up of our patients is required to establish the true predictive values of the results. Most of the lesions found in this study were small and peripheral, and were documented through the expensive technique of review of many overlapping photographs. A less costly, but less meticulous technique may not detect all these small, peripheral lesions and so the sensitivity and specificity of the method would drop. Offsetting these disadvantages are the relative ease and comfort of the exam and the potential of detection of the FAP trait at an early age. The combination of proctoscopy, eye examination, and gene probes has potential for an accurate determination of the probability of inheritance of the FAP gene at an early age (8). Such an ability, although likely to be superceded by identification of the gene itself, would enable surveillance programs to be pruned, genetic counselling to be given and prophylactic treatment to be more confidently planned.

REFERENCES

Berk T, Cohen Z, McLeod RS, Parker JA (1988) Congenital hypertrophy of the retinal pigment epithelium as a marker for familial adenomatous polyposis. Dis Colon Rectum 31:253-257.

Blair NP, Trempe CL (1980) Hypertrophy of the retinal pigment epithelium associated with Gardner's syndrome. Am J Ophthalmol 90:661-667.

Diaz-Llopis M, Memezo JL (1988) Congenital hypertrophy of the retinal pigment epithelium in familial adenomatous polyposis. Arch Ophthalmol 106:412-3.

Lewis RA, Crowder WE, Eiman LA, et al. (1984) The Gardner's Syndrome: Significance of ocular features. Ophthalmology 91:916-925.

Slack J. (1989) Presented at Fourth International Symposium on Colorectal Cancer, Kobe, Japan.

Traboulsi EI, Krush AJ, Gardner EJ, et al. (1987) Prevalence and importance of pigmented ocular fundus lesions in Gardner's syndrome. N Engl J Med 316:661-667.

Traboulsi EI, Maumenee IH, Krush AJ, et al. (1988) Pigmented ocular fundus lesions in the inherited gastrointestinal polyposis syndromes and hereditary nonpolyposis colorectal cancer. Ophthalmology 95:964-969.

Woods RJ, Sarre RG, Ctercteko GC, Jagelman DJ, Smith JW, Duchesneau PM, McGannon E (1989) Occult radiologic changes in the skull and jaw in familial adenomatous polyposis coli. Dis Colon Rectum 32(4):304-306, 1989.

Chapter 3

Identification, Surveillance, and Management of Hereditary Nonpolyposis Colorectal Cancer

Summary of Chapter 3: Identification, Surveillance and Management of Hereditary Non-polyposis Colorectal Cancer

RANDALL W. BURT

SUMMARIES

The first presentation (#8) of the second section of workshop A2 was given by Hans F.A. Vasen of the Netherlands, and entitled "Screening for hereditary nonpolyposis colorectal cancer in the Netherlands." The investigators compared the stage of colon cancers in 97 patients who belonged to "Lynch" syndrome families and presented with symptoms, to 20 relatives in these families who were screened while asymptomatic. The symptomatic group was found to have more advanced stage tumors than the screened group. Symptomatic group: Dukes A, 6 patients; Dukes B, 43 patients; Dukes C, 24 patients; Dukes D, 11 patients; unclassified, 13 patients. Screened group: adenomas only, 14 patients; Dukes A, 2 patients; Dukes B, 4 patients. The authors noted other features of the Lynch syndromes including early age onset of cancer (mean age 46 years), 60% proximal tumors, 25% metachronous tumors and an excess of endometrial, stomach and urinary-tract tumors. They recommended that periodic colonoscopic screening begin at age 20 years and that subtotal colectomy be performed with the first diagnosis of colon cancer.

The second presentation (#9) was given by Joan Slack, ICRF, London, and entitled "The risks of colorectal cancer and the frequency of recognized family cancer syndromes in 550 sequential referrals for family risks of bowel cancer." A screening clinic for patients with familial risk for bowel cancer was recently established at the St. Marks Hospital in London. The authors described their experience in screening the first 550 patients who have presented to this clinic. They performed screening according to risk calculations based on previous studies at St. Marks: one relative affected with colon cancer, risk 1:17; two relatives affected (first-degree and second-degree relative), risk 1:10; one relative less than 45 years of age affected, risk 1:10; two first-degree relatives affected, risk 1:6; dominant pedigree, risk 1:2. The overall population risk in the U.K. was calculated at 1:50. Colonoscopy was offered if the risk was 1:10 or greater and occult stool blood test if the risk was less. Adenomatous polyps were found in 57 of 316 screened by colonoscopy. Within this high risk group, those with highest risk were consistently more often found to have polyps. In the lower risk categories, two patients with polyps were found by occult stool blood tests, while ten screened in this way were occult blood test negative but were later found to have adenomas. One hundred seventy-three patients from the entire group could be classified into syndromes of colorectal cancer, and 28 of these exhibited adenomatous polyps. The authors concluded that screening could be successfully based on familial risk.

The third presentation (#10) was given by Jens O. Sondergaard, Copenhagen, Denemark, and was entitled "The Incidence of colorectal cancer among first-degree relatives of patients with colorectal cancer." Parents of individuals with colorectal cancer were investigated for the prevalence of cancer. There were 1534 individuals with colorectal cancer from a three year period in the Danish cancer registry. Records were available on 2775 parents (96%). The overall cancer risk among parents was equivalent to that expected by chance, while the colorectal cancer risk was double that expected. The authors stressed the necessity of screening for first-degree relatives of those with colorectal cancer.

The fourth presentation (#11) was given by Randall W. Burt, Salt Lake City, U.S.A., and was entitled "Genetics of adenomas." The authors investigated the hypothesis that inherited susceptibility to adenomatous polyps accounted for the familial clustering of commonly observed colorectal cancers and adenomas. Thirty-four pedigrees selected for a sibling pair with colon cancer (5) or a single individual with an adenomatous polyp (29) were studied. Pedigree members and spouses (studied as controls) were examined by 60-cm flexible proctosigmoidoscopy for the presence of adenomatous polyps. Of pedigree members, 78 of 407 (19%) exhibited adenomas, while 32 of 263 (12%) spouse controls had adenomas. Likelihood analysis demonstrated that a partially penetrant autosomal dominantly inherited gene or genes was much more likely to explain the results than recessive inheritance or sporadic occurrence. The estimated gene frequency in the population examined was 19% (95% confidence limits 14 to 28%). The fraction of polyps observed which occurred from inheritance was estimated to be between 53 and 100%. The authors concluded that a significant fraction of adenomas, possibly the majority, occurred from inherited susceptibility probably interacting with environmental factors.

The fifth presentation (#12) was given by L Bertario of Italy. The title was "Surveillance of individuals at high risk for family history with guaiac test (Hemoccult II)." Occult stool blood screening was applied to 2,629 first-degree relatives of individuals with colorectal cancer. If the test was positive, colonoscopy was performed. If the test was negative, flexible proctosigmoidoscopy was done. Ninety-five persons tested were positive (3.6%). Twenty-one of these had colorectal cancer and 23 had adenomas. Of those with negative stool occult blood tests, 545 (21.5%) agreed to proctosigmoidoscopy. Six of these had cancer and 66 had adenomas. Similar findings were observed during a follow-up period of over five years in a subgroup of the patients. Cancers detected were early stage 75% of the time. The authors concluded that annual stool occult blood screening among first-degree relatives over 40 years of age was justified.

The sixth presentation (#13) was given by James M. Church, Cleveland Clinic, U.S.A., and was entitled "Large bowel neoplasms in patients with and without a family history of rectal cancer---a colonoscopic study." The authors examined the additive risks of family history of colorectal cancer, and personal history of colorectal cancer or adenoma. A total of 448 individuals were examined by colonoscopy. Adenomatous polyps were found in 4 of 27 (15%) of those with family history alone. Adenomas were present in 79 of 313 (25%) of those with a personal history of colonic neoplasm. Of those with both a positive personal history and family history, 77 of 148 (52%) had adenomas. The authors conclude that family and personal history are additive risk factors.

The seventh presentation (#14) was given by Finlay A. Macrae, Melbourne, Australia, and was entitled "Managing surveillance for colorectal cancer: the importance of microcomputers." A software package called "ScreeningMan" (SMan) was developed for categorizing and tracking patients at increased genetic risk or personal risk for colorectal cancer. The program documented cancer risk, organized surveillance, identified non-compliers, notified negative results to participants and their doctors, and documented and analyzed the results of surveillance as scheduled. The authors examined the efficiency of using the software to manage increased risk patients as compared to manual systems. The computerized system proved to be more efficient even with as few as 10 subjects.

CONCLUSIONS

The investigations presented and the discussion which resulted suggested the following conclusions:

1. Screening is justified in those at increased genetic risk for colorectal cancer, because neoplasms are found more often in this group than in the general population, and because the neoplasms are found at an earlier stage than in unscreened groups.
2. Screening may be stratified according to genetic risk, with approximate categories being: a) one affected first-degree relative; b) two affected first-degree relatives; c) hereditary nonpolyposis syndromes; d) hereditary polyposis syndromes.
3. Individual risk should be considered additive to genetic risk.
4. Partially penetrant genetic susceptibilities leading to colonic adenomas and cancers may be very common, and account for a significant fraction of common colonic adenomas and cancers.
5. Computerized data base systems can be effectively utilized to manage screening programs based on personal, familial, and genetic risk.

PROBLEMS REQUIRING SOLUTION AND INVESTIGATION

The presentations and discussion identified the following areas where further investigation is needed:

1. Genetic markers of the various categories of genetic susceptibility are needed to more accurately define risk.
2. Genetic markers will hopefully help to determine whether an adenoma implies affected status in an individual at risk for hereditary nonpolyposis colorectal cancer.
3. A better understanding of the natural history of the hereditary nonpolyposis colorectal cancer syndromes (Lynch syndromes) is needed to more appropriately determine screening intervals.
3. More work should be directed towards defining the genetic-environmental interactions for all levels of genetic risk.

Hereditary Nonpolyposis Colorectal Cancer and Tumorigenesis in the Human Body

KYOSUKE USHIO

ABSTRACT

At the National Cancer Center Hospital in Tokyo, a review has been made of 1,898 case histories, from 1962 through 1986, of colorectal cancer patients who did not exhibit the polyposis syndrome, with particular emphasis placed on identifying cases of familial aggregation and cases involving multiple cancers in the large intestine and/or other organs.

From this total number, found were 141 cases of multiple colorectal cancer (7.4%) and 179 cases of a colorectal cancer associated with an extracolonic cancer (9.4%). Also found were 100 cases (5.3%) of hereditary nonpolyposis colorectal cancer (HNPCC). In the HNPCC cases, several characteristics were found common: an early onset of the cancer (mean: 53.2 years), proximally-sited colonic tumors (38.0% in the right colon), and a high frequency of multiple cancers (31.0%). Among theses HNPCC patients, 7 cases of an associated adenocarcinoma of the uterine body and/or ovaries were identified.

These findings are discussed, along with an overall view of HNPCC clinico-genetic characteristics. [Key words : cancer family syndrome ; colon cancer ; hereditary nonpolyposis colorectal cancer ; endometrial cancer ; hereditary tumor]

INTRODUCTION

A familial history of cancer seems to be the most common verifiable risk factor for determining the liklihood of developing cancer, and the frequency of such a connection when a colorectal carcinoma is involved indicates that the family history is very important. A hereditary nonpolyposis colorectal cancer (HNPCC) is comprised of the following two classifications: 1) a hereditary nonpolyposis site-specific colon cancer, or Lynch Syndrome I, which shows an autosomal dominant inheritance; an onset of the colorectal cancer at an early age; an increase in the synchronous or matachronous colorectal cancer; and a site-specific nonpolyposis colorectal cancer; and, 2) a cancer reflecting the cancer family syndrome (CFS), or Lynch syndrome II, which shows all the characteristics indicated above and associated extracolonic adenocarcinomas as well, particularly an endometrial carcinoma (Table 1).

This paper describes the clinical characteristics of an HNPCC, including seven kindreeds manifesting the CFS. Additionally, the author also presents his views on the relationship that exists among infantile and childhood tumors, hereditary tumors, such as the poplyposis syndrome and the HNPCC, other familial, aggregative tumors often observed in the breast, the thyroid, the stomach, etc., and the usual tumors that are prone to develop during old age.

Table 1

DEFINITION AND CLASSIFICATION OF HERDITARY NONPOLYPOSIS COLORECTAL CANCER (HNPCC)

Hereditary site-specific colorectal cancer (Lynch Syndrome I)
- autosomal dominantly inherited predisposition
- site-specific nonpolyposis colorectal cancer
- early age of onset
- increase in synchronous and metachronous colonic cancers

Cancer family syndrome (Lynch Syndrome II)
- all of the features of Lynch syndrome I
- extracolonic cancer, particularly carcinoma of the endometrium and ovary
  (evidence of tumor heterogeneity has recently been demonstrated by an excess of gastric, small bowel, pancreatic, urologic, and laryngeal cancer in specific extended kindreds.)

SUBJECTS AND METHODS

Reviewed were the case histories of 1,898 patients who had a primary colorectal cancer, confirmed to be an adenocarcinoma, and who underwent surgery at our hospital from 1962 to 1986. As our study was based on investigating the familial medical histories of these patients, primary medical document, consisting of such data surgical and pathological reports as well as autopsy and/or death records, were checked. Patients with a single colorectal cancer, multiple colorectal cancers, and a colorectal cancer with associated malignancies in other organs were especially studied to see whether there had been cases of a colorectal cancer and/or similar malignancies in other organs among relatives within the first degree.

RESULTS

Within the 1,898 cases that were reviewed, identified were 141 cases (7.4%) of multiple colorectal cancer and 179 cases (9.4%) of a colorectal cancer with an associated extracolonic cancer. Further, 100 HNPCC cases were found, which included familial medical histories reflecting a CFS (Lynch syndrome II). 70 cases were excluded because of the insufficient data about the familial medical histories.

A comparison of the clinical date between these HNPCC patients (n=100) and cases that involved sporadic colorectal cancer (n=1,728), as shown in Table 2, has revealed the following characteristics: 1) the average age at the onset of their cancers was 53.3 and 58.2 years, respectively. (Informatively, the youngest HNPCC patient was a 16-year-old male with a history of five colon cancers.); 2) the site of the colorectal cancer in the HNPCC cases was predominantly proximal (38.0%), in comparison with the cases of a sporadic colorectal cancer (14.6%); 3) the average incidence of a multiple primary colorectal cancer in the HNPCC cases and in the sporadic cases was 31.0% and 6.3% respectively; 4) other colonic malignant tumors were seen in 24.0% of all HNPCC patients, a rather high incidence in comparison to the manifestation of such tumors in the sporadic colorectal cancer patients, which only amounted to 9.0%; 5) more associated adenomas were found in the HNPCC patients (28.0%) than in the sporadic patients (15.3%); and, 6) a tendency towards a successively earlier age of cancer onset was seen from one generation to the next in HNPCC cases.

Table 2

Comparsion of Clinical Data Between HNPCC and
Sporadic Colorectal Cancer (N.C.C.H 1989)

	HNPCC (n=100)	Sporadic c.c (n=1728)
Mean age (yr)	53.2	58.2
Multiple colorectal cancer	31.0%	6.3%
Extra colorectal cancer	24.0%	9.0%
Right side colon cancer	38.0%	14.6%
Associated adenoma	28.0%	15.3%

$P<0.01$

Two pedigrees of these kindreds are shown in Fig. 1. Both probands had an adenocarcinoma of the large intestine and the endometrium, and their family histories showed a high incidence of colorectal cancers and associated adenocarcinomas developing at an earlier age than usual, in conformance to the tendency of successive generations to show an even earlier age of cancer onset. Figures 2a and 2b show a colorectal cancer and an endometrial cancer, respectively, in CFS patients.

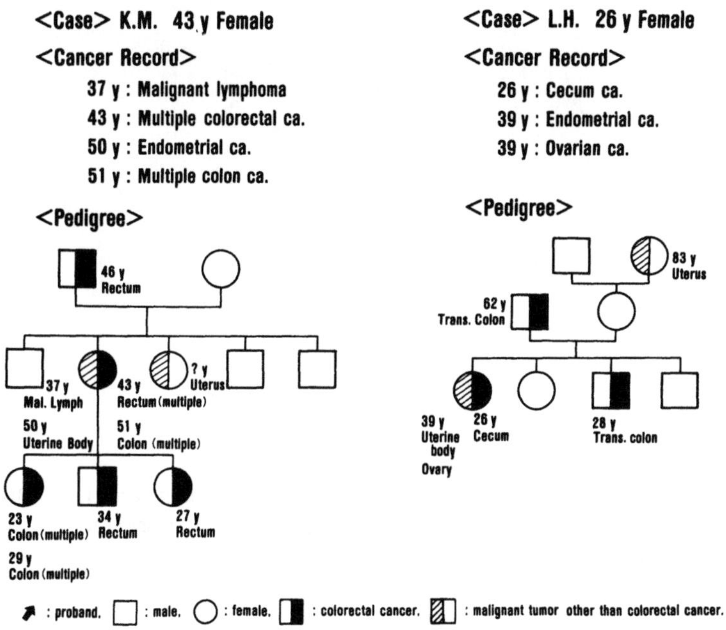

Fig.1: Two pedigrees of cancer family syndrome

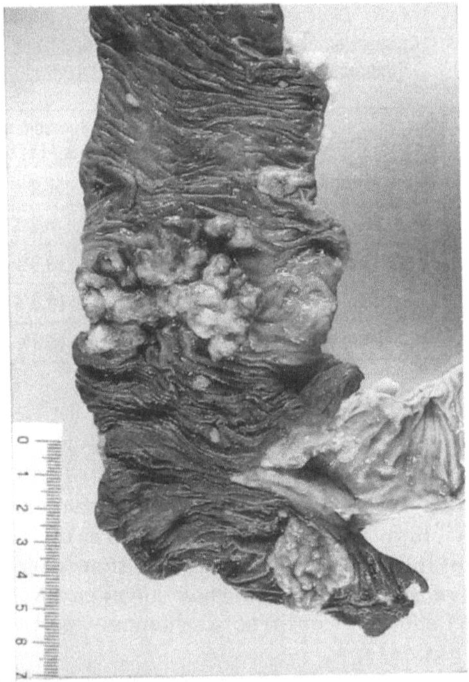

a

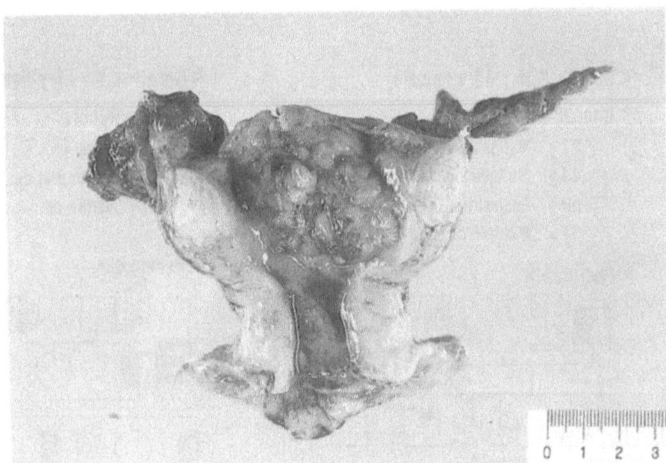

b

Fig.2: Cancer family syndrome. (a) Colectomy specimen revcealing multiple cancers of the cecum and the ascending colon (51-year-old female). (b) An endometrial adenocarcinoma is in the uterin body.

DISCUSSION

(1) Clinico- genetic characteristics of hereditary nonpolyposis colorectal cancer (HNPCC) including cancer family syndrome (CFS)

The CFS was originally proposed as an entity by Lynch and Krush (1971) and its criteria includes the following characteristics: 1) an increase in adenocarcinomas, primarilly of the colon and the endometrium; 2) an increased frequency of multiple primary neoplasms (approximately 20%); 3) an early age of the onset of the cancer; and, 4) a vertical transmission of a cancer with an autosomal dominant inheritance pattern. Several authers (Boland 1978; Aiges 1979; Ushio 1985; Lynch 1985; Mecklin 1985,1987; Abusamra 1987; Li 1988) have been reported in many well- defined kindreds in the world. At present the CFS is included in the HNPCC (Table 1). However in general, its clinical and genetic features are not well known in the medical practice .

As has been stated, our review of the familial medical histories of 1,898 colorectal cancer patients revealed 100 HNPCC cases, representing 5.3% of the total number. However, as it is impossible to identify a HNPCC if there is no familial medical history to check, so that an identification is only possible after a first degree relative also develops a cancerous tumor. Thus this figure -- a 5.3% HNPCC frequency -- is probably underestimated.

In this review of Japanese HNPCC cases, the same characteristics common to caucasian HNPCC patients were observed, e.g., a young age of cancer onset (mean: 53.2 years), a preponderance of proximally-sited colon cancer (38.0%), and a multiplicity of cancers (31.0%). Further, 7 HNPCC cases were found to have a familial medical history confirming a CFS, these cases similarly revealing an early age of cancer onset (mean: 41.4 years), a preponderance of proximally-sited colon cancers (85.7%), and a high frequency of colorectal cancers (71.4%). Thus it appears that orientals and caucasians both share the same CFS manifestations.

These results suggest that special attention must be paid to clues in the patient's familial medical history that might indicate a HNPCC pedigree. At this juncture, it is especially recommended that female colorectal cancer patients belonging to a HNPCC family undergo an annual check of their ovaries and the uterine body.

(2) Considerations regarding the relationship between the human body and various hereditary tumors.

Although complex interactions occurring between the environment and the human body are greatly responsible for the development of certain cancers in man, it also is certainly well established that genetic factors play a great role in tumorigenesis, both malignant and benign. This genetic connection was seen in our review of patients with colorectal cancers, some of whom displayed hereditary disorders such as familial polyposis coli, Gardner's syndrome, Turcot's syndrome, and HNPCC, diseases which evidence a high frequency of colorectal cancers.

Figure 3 is the author's depiction of tumorigenesis in the human body, based on studies of hereditary gastrointestinal polyposis, as seen in such diseases as the familial adenomatous polyposis including Gardner's syndrome, Peutz-Jeghers syndrome, juvenile polyposis, Turcot's syndrome, cases of HNPCC, and other familial aggregative tumors. In this depiction, the X-axis represents the age distribution and the Y-axis shows the frequency or scale of the lesion. The curve above the X-axis indicates tumors or anomalies that have been recognized

Conception of Tumorigenesis in Human Body and Place of Hereditary, Familial Aggregative Tumor.

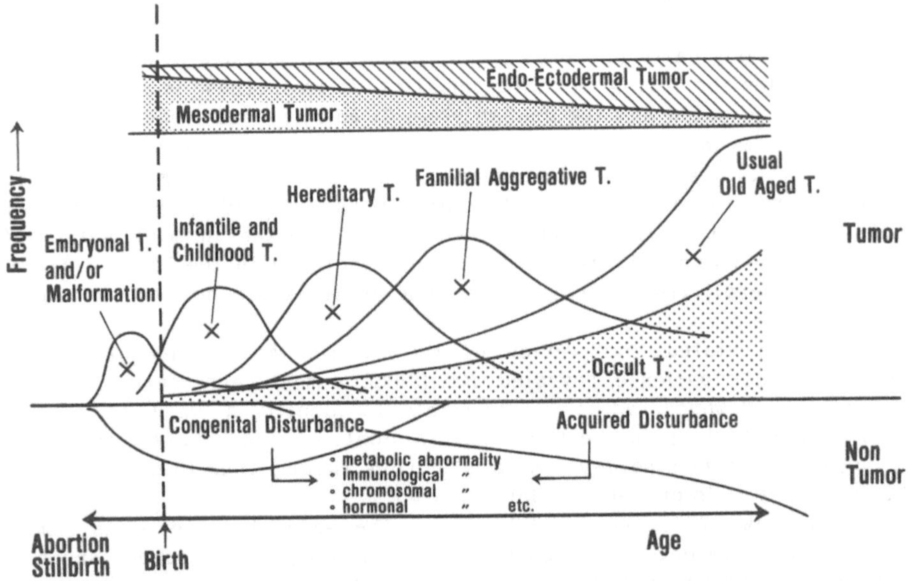

Fig.3

morphologically, while those under the Y-axis are unseen adnormalities of a metabolic, immunological, chromosomal and/or hormonal origin.

In relating tumoral growth to the growth of the body, the neonatal period is especially hazardous to the development of the human since chromosomal abnormalities, as well as congenital metabolic disturbances and anomalies, can occur, culminating in a natural abortion, premature birth or stillbirth.

Following this comes childhood tumors originating from the mesodermal or embryonal tissue. Tumors in the young are often associated with other anomalies, such as phacomatosis, congenital metabolic disturbances, various immunodeficiencies, and DNA and chromosomal abnormalities. Thus it might be said that genetic factors in the young, such as heredity and predisposition, are more greatly related to tumorigenesis than to environmental factors.

Tumors that have a hereditary connection, generally determined by the patient's age at the time of tumoral onset, include some childhood tumors that characteristically originate in two or all three derms. As a consequence, these tumors can later develop in most any tissue and organ, in marked contrast to the majority of non-hereditary tumors seen in the aged, such as carcinomas that most often develop in the ecto-or endoderm.

Thus, multiple primary tumors showing a familial aggregation, including tumors with associated malignancies in other organs, are ranked between the hereditary and childhood tumors and the tumors usually seen in the elderly, suggesting that genetic factors play a greater role than do environmental factors in tumorigenesis.

CONCLUSION

At the National Cancer Center Hospital in Tokyo, 1,898 case histories of colorectal cancers not manifesting the polyposis syndrome have been reviewed, with special emphasis placed on determining cases of familial aggregation and those showing multiple cancers in the large intestine and/or other organs. From this total number, 100 cases of hereditary nonpolyposis coloretal cancer (HNPCC) were found, indicating a frequency of 5.3%.

Common characteristics in these HNPCC patients were an onset of their first colorectal cancer at a relatively early age (mean: 53.2 years), a preponderance of proximally-sited colon cancers (38.0%), and a high frequency of multiple cancers (31.0%). Further, among these HNPCC cases 7 CFS cases were found, each of these CFS patients having an adenocarcinoma of the uterine body and/or of the ovaries, said patients similarly having shown an early age of cancer onset (mean: 41.4 years), a preponderance of proximally-sited colon cancers (85.7%), and a high frequency of multiple cancers (71.4%). Based on these findings, it thus is recommended that female HNPCC patients undergo an annual inspection of their uterine body and ovaries.

REFERENCES

1) Abusamra H, Maximova S, Bar-Meir S, Krispin M, Rotmensch HH (1987) : Cancer family syndrome of Lynch. Am J Med 83 : 981-983

2) Aiges HW, Silverberg KM, Daum F (1979) : Adenocarcinoma of the colon in an adolescent with the family cancer syndrome. J Pediatr 94 : 632- 633

3) Boland CR (1978) : Cancer family syndrome; A case reprot and literature review. Am J Dig Dis 23 (Suppl) : 25-27

4) Li FP, Fraumeni JFJr, Mulvihill JJ, Blattner WA, Dreyfus MG, Tucker MA, Miller RW (1988) : A cancer family syndrome in twenty-four kindreds. Cancer Research 48 : 5358-5362

5) Lynch HT, Krush AJ (1971) : The cancer family syndrome and cancer control. Surg Gynecol Obstet 132 : 247-250

6) Lynch HT, Krush AJ (1973) : Differential diagnosis of the cancer family syndrome. Surg Gynecol Obstet 136 : 221-224

7) Mecklin JP, Jarvinen HJ (1985) : Clinical features of colorectal carcinoma in cancer family syndrome. Dis colon Rectum 29 : 160-164

8) Mecklin JP (1987) : Frequency of hereditary colorectal carcinoma. Gastroenterology 93 : 1021-1025

9) Ushio K (1985) : Genetic and familial factors in colorectal cancer. Jpn J Clin Oncol 15 (Suppl 1) : 281-298

Colonoscopy Findings in a Series of Patients with Hereditary Colorectal Cancer

STEPHEN J. LANSPA, HENRY T. LYNCH, THOMAS C. SMYRK, ROBERT J. FITZGIBBONS JR., PATRICE WATSON, and J.X. JENKINS

ABSTRACT

During a colonoscopy screening program for patients at high risk for hereditary nonpolyposis colorectal cancer (HNPCC), we observed one family which was atypical in that members showed right-sided flat adenomas. The total colonic adenoma counts exceeded those found in HNPCC, but were fewer than that characteristically observed in familial adenomatous polyposis (FAP). There was a high rate of synchronous and metachronous adenomas. These observations highlight the heterogeneity in HNPCC and stress the need for careful delineation of all facets of the colonic phenotype in the interest of etiologic classification of hereditary colorectal cancer syndromes.

Keywords: colonic adenomatous polyps, flat adenomas, genetics, hereditary nonpolyposis colorectal cancer

INTRODUCTION

The clinical characteristics of HNPCC have been presented previously [Lynch et al 1988]. Unlike its counterpart FAP, HNPCC lacks premonitory physical signs which can facilitate diagnosis. This mandates the need for thorough pedigree documentation of cancer and its natural history, since a specific biomarker is lacking.

METHODS

We performed colonoscopy on 44 patients from nine families who were believed to be at high risk for HNPCC. Patients were asymptomatic and had no prior history of colorectal cancer, colonic polyps, or a family history of FAP. Each patient was at 50% risk for HNPCC (Lynch syndromes I and II) by virtue of being in the direct genetic lineage of a Lynch syndrome pedigree.

The reference subject pool consisted of 242 patients undergoing colonoscopy at the Creighton University Gastrointestinal Unit during one calendar year. Patients with inflammatory bowel disease or a previous history of colonic cancer or polyps were excluded. From this reference pool, two patients were age- and sex-matched to each of the Lynch syndrome kindred patients. Comparisons between case and reference patients were made according to the method of Mantel and Haenszel.

RESULTS

Mean age of the 44 Lynch syndrome patients (18 males, 26 females) was 42.2 years. The cecum was reached in all.

As compared to the reference group, the Lynch syndrome group of patients had more frequent right colon adenomas. The Lynch syndrome group had lesions present in 18% of patients vs. 1% of the reference group ($p<.001$; OR = 16). They had more frequent synchronous adenomas with lesions present in 20% of patients vs. 4% of the reference group ($p<.01$; OR = 4.5).

In followup of the patients with excess polyps, it was determined that one family accounted for the statistical difference between the Lynch syndrome patients and the reference group. Members of this family (12 patients, mean age 49.4) differed from the remaining eight families (32 patients, mean age 41.4) in that several family members had multiple adenomas in the right colon, including flat adenomas (utilizing the histologic criteria of Muto et al 1985).

This atypical family will be referred to as "flat adenoma syndrome" and is compared to the remaining eight Lynch syndrome families. None of the adenomas from the other eight Lynch syndrome families were flat adenomas. When this family was excluded from consideration, endoscopic findings of the remaining eight families did not differ from the reference group.

Fifty-eight percent of patients from the flat adenoma syndrome had colonic adenomas (7 of 12); 19% of the Lynch syndrome patients had colonic adenomas (6 of 32). Flat adenoma syndrome patients had a higher prevalence of right-sided colon adenomas, with lesions proximal to the splenic flexure in 42% of the 12 patients screened. In contrast, 9% of the Lynch syndrome group (3 of 32) had right-sided colon adenomas. All patients with adenomas from the flat adenoma syndrome had synchronous adenomas (7 of 7). A third of patients with adenomas from the remaining eight families with Lynch syndrome had multiple adenomas (2 of 6).

Eight members of the flat adenoma syndrome had followup colonoscopy. Of five flat adenoma patients with adenomas at initial exam, all had adenomas at followup. Of three patients from this kindred with negative initial colonoscopy, two had developed adenomas at followup.

DISCUSSION

Of the nine families which originally were considered to be HNPCC, when the single family with flat adenomas was removed, the frequency of colonic adenomas was found to be in accord with our original assessment of adenoma occurrence in HNPCC; namely 19% [Lynch & Lynch 1985].

In a previous report [Lynch et al 1988], we described a colon cancer-prone family with right-sided flat adenomas. At that time, we suggested that the family represented either a variant of the Lynch syndromes or, possibly, a distinct syndrome. An additional family has now been identified with similar characteristics and entered into the colonoscopy screening program. A full report of these two families has been submitted for publication [Lynch et al 1989].

In the flat adenoma kindred, all patients with adenomas had synchronous lesions. In the eight Lynch syndrome families, two patients had multiple adenomas (one patient with 3 adenomas and one patient with 5 adenomas). Of 42 Lynch syndrome patients in Love's series [1986], two of seven patients with adenomas had multiple adenomas at colonoscopy. In Mecklin's study [1986], the percentage of synchronous adenomas in Lynch syndrome patients with cancer was similar to the rate in sporadic colon cancer cases (19% vs. 16%).

We observed that patients from the kindred with multiple flat adenomas who had had adenomas removed at initial colonoscopy continued to show adenomas on subsequent examinations (100%). This is in contrast to colonoscopic followup of adenomas in patients who were from families lacking hereditary colorectal cancer syndromes. In these circumstances, only 3-18% showed metachronous polyps [Grossman et al 1989].

These findings indicate the need for detailed evaluation of the pedigree and family cancer history, along with colonoscopic and histologic information when dealing with patients who are at increased risk for hereditary colorectal cancer. This approach allowed us to redefine a family syndrome previously characterized as HNPCC.

Biomolecular genetic advances will eventually allow hereditary colon cancer syndromes to be grouped according to specific chromosomal defects. Nevertheless, detailed clinicopathologic information will still be necessary so that specific mutations can be correlated with phenotype.

REFERENCES

Grossman S, Milos ML, Tekawa IS, Jewell NP (1989) Colonoscopic screening of persons with suspected risk factors for colon cancer. II. Past history of colorectal neoplasms. Gastroenterology 96:299-306

Love RR, Morrissey JF (1984) Colonoscopy in asympatomatic individuals with a family history of colorectal cancer. Arch Int Med 144:209-211

Lynch HT, Smyrk T,Lanspa SJ, Marcus JN, Kriegler M, Lynch JF, Appelman HD (1988) Flat adenomas in a colon cancer-prone kindred. JNCI 71:278-282

Lynch HT, Smyrk TC, Lanspa SJ, Lynch PM, Watson P, Strayhorn PC (sub mitted) Phenotypic variation in colorectal adenoma/cancer expression in two families: hereditary flat adenoma syndrome. N Eng J Med

Lynch PM, Lynch HT (1985) Colon cancer genetics. VN Reinhold, New York, NY

Mecklin JP, Jarvinen HJ (1986a) Clinical features of colorectal carcinoma in the Cancer Family Syndrome. Dis Colon Rect 29:160-164

Mecklin JP, Sipponen P, Jarvinen HJ (1986b) Histopathology of colorectal carcinomas and adenomas in the Cancer Family Syndrome. Dis Colon Rect 29:840-853

Muto J, Kamiya J, Sawada T, Konishi F, Sugihara K, Kubota Y, Adachi M, Agawa S, Saito Y, Morioka Y, Tanprayoon T (1985) Small "flat adenoma" of the large bowel with special reference to its clinicopathologic features. Dis Colon Rect 28:846-851

Extracolonic Cancer in Hereditary Nonpolyposis Colorectal Cancer

PATRICE WATSON and HENRY T. LYNCH

ABSTRACT

Published studies of families with hereditary nonpolyposis colorectal cancer (HNPCC) frequently report the occurrence of cancers at extra-colonic sites. Our purpose in this study was to compare the observed frequency of cancer at specific sites in members of 18 unrelated HNPCC kindreds with expectations based on general population incidence in order to determine whether there were specific types of cancer for which family members were at elevated risk. We were able to stratify family members according to their risk of carrying the putative HNPCC gene. We found that putative HNPCC gene carriers and their high risk relatives have been diagnosed with cancers other than uterine and colorectal more frequently than expected based on general population incidence figures. Specific sites where elevations are seen include the stomach, small intestine, biliary system (especially the bile ducts), urological system (especially the kidney and ureter), and ovary.

Keywords: hereditary nonpolyposis colorectal cancer, extracolonic cancer, tumor spectrum

INTRODUCTION

Many researchers and physicians studying families with hereditary nonpolyposis colorectal cancer (HNPCC) have noted high frequencies of certain extracolonic malignancies. Most often, endometrial cancer is found to occur cosegregating with colon cancer in the family. A wide variety of other cancers, mostly adenocarcinomas, have been reported to occur at high frequencies in specific families. Families have also been reported which are affected almost exclusively by colon cancer. Reviews of published reports of HNPCC families [Menko et al 1989] indicate the wide variety of cancers reported. These authors compiled a table of 868 tumors in 708 HNPCC patients. Approximately half the tumors were colorectal; uterine and gastric cancers were also quite common. Twenty-five other cancer sites were also mentioned.

Which of these cancer types can be said to occur more frequently in HNPCC than in the general population? This is an issue of clinical importance since management of HNPCC patients might be improved by screening for cancer at extracolonic sites, if we could determine which sites are "high risk." However, compilation and analysis of results in published families could be misleading if there is bias in the choice of families to report, such as bias in favor of families with unusual cancers.

Our purpose in this study was to compare the observed frequency of cancer at specific sites in members of 18 unrelated HNPCC kindreds with expectations based on general population incidence.

METHODS

We studied the frequency of specific types of cancer in members of HNPCC families from the Creighton University/Hereditary Cancer Institute colon cancer family resource. Families in the resource were classified as HNPCC if members were frequently affected by colorectal cancer, if this colon cancer occurred in the family in a pattern consistent with autosomal dominant transmission of a gene conferring susceptibility to colon cancer, and if familial adenomatous polyposis could be ruled out. All HNPCC families in the resource were included as long as the process of cancer verification and data computerization was completed at the time of the study and the family had been classified as HNPCC in our department process of pedigree review. Eighteen unrelated families met these criteria.

The members of these families were classified into risk categories as follows. The pedigrees were reviewed, and the common ancestors of the known affected family members (affected with early onset and/or multiple primary colon cancer) were identified. These two individuals were referred to as the family progenitors. Then, the family data were analyzed by computer to assign risk status by the following rules: all persons not descendant from the progenitors were classifed as "married- in." Of those remaining, all with colorectal cancer or endometrial cancer (including adenocarcinoma of the uterus, or carcinoma of the uterine corpus) were classified as "affected." Of those remaining, those with affected offspring were classified as "unaffected gene carriers;" those with other affected first degree relatives were classified as "high risk;" and all family members descendant from the progenitors but lacking an affected first degree relative were classified as "low risk." For analysis of the occurrence of other cancers, all affected and unaffected gene carriers were combined into a single group, the putative gene carriers; the high risk group was analyzed alone; and the married-in and low risk family members were combined into a single low risk group.

Our aim was to compare the observed numbers of cancer diagnoses in each risk group to the expected numbers, based on general population incidence data. Two methods were used to calculate the expected numbers of cancers among family members.

<u>Method 1: Expected numbers based on year, sex, and age-specific incidence rates:</u> Computation of expected numbers of cancers was done using the calculation of expected numbers on the age and sex-specific incidence rates from the Connecticut Cancer Registry (CCR). Data on cancer incidence is available from 1935; incidence in the years 1925-1934 is estimated based on the 1935 data. Use of year-specific incidence rates allows the adjustment of expected numbers for the secular trends in cancer rates. Estimates produced by Method 1 are designated "CCR" in the Results section.

<u>Method 2. Expected numbers based on sex and age-specific incidence rates:</u> The <u>USDR</u> program does not allow calculation of expected numbers of cancers at all possible sites; rather, it calculates values for organ systems and for some of the commonest sites within those systems. Thus, application of this program might not fully describe the pattern of cancer incidence in the HNPCC families. A second analysis was carried out whenever the results of the USDR analysis indicated that an excess of cancer occurred in a general system which was not fully

accounted for by the specific types of cancer analyzed within that system by USDR. For example, since none of the specific cancer sites within the oral cavity were analyzed by the USDR program, if an excess of buccal cancer was found, we would carry out a secondary analysis of expected and observed numbers of cancers at specific sites within the oral cavity.

Expected numbers of cancers of specific sites were calculated separately for the males and females in each risk group. Age at death or present age was calculated for each of the family members included in the study. These ages were grouped into 5-year intervals for analysis, and the number of males and females in each age group was determined. Incidence data was obtained from Surveillance, Epidemiology, and End Results (SEER) program tables of average annual age and sex-specific incidence rates for malignant neoplasms by primary sites, all races, all areas, 1973-1977 [Young et al 1981]. These data were used to calculate cancer risk up to the end of each 5 year period, using the density methods for calculating risk as described by Kleinbaum et al [1982]. These risks were multiplied by the number of persons in that age category, and summed over all sexes and ages, to compute the expected number of cases of cancer. This procedure was used to calculate expected numbers of specific cancers not obtainable in the USDR program. Estimates produced by Method 2 are designated "SEER" in the Results section.

Determination of observed numbers of cancers: Actual cases of cancer of specific types among the cases in each risk group were counted. Most diagnoses were verified by pathology report and/or by medical records from the hospital at which the diagnosis occurred. However, when such documentation was not available, either because of loss of hospital documents or because no definitive tests had been performed, we were forced to rely upon the diagnoses reported on the death certificate. Finally, in some cases, no verification was available, but we had very reliable family or personal medical history information on the diagnoses. In statistical analyses, diagnoses based on unverified family or self-reports were excluded. We also excluded all cancers of the types used in the risk coding (colorectal and endometrial cancers), all cancers with unknown primary site, and all benign or *in situ* lesions.

Statistical testing: Statistical tests of the hypothesis that the observed number of cancers differed from the expected number were performed using a test attributable to Byar and described by Breslow and Day [1987], which is an accurate approximation of an exact Poisson test. Whenever 2 expected number estimates were available (from Method 1 and 2 above), the one closest to the observed number was relied upon to produce the most conservative test. Standardized incidence ratios (actual/expected numbers of cancers) were also calculated as an approximation of the relative risk.

RESULTS

Putative gene carriers: This group included 298 individuals. There were 257 who were affected by colorectal or endometrial cancer and 41 who were classified as unaffected gene carriers because of their pedigree position. Among the 257 who were classified as affected, 67% had at least one of these carcinomas verified by pathology or autopsy report and 19% had at least one such diagnosis documented by medical records or a death certificate. The remaining 14% of the cases had the diagnosis known only by reliable family reports (usually from multiple close relatives) or self-report. See Table 1 for descriptive characteristics.

Table 1. Characteristics of study groups.

	Males	Females	% Dead	---Mean Age--- Dead	Alive
Putative Gene Carriers					
affected	119	138	63	54.9	58.8
unaffected	18	23	78	58.2	68.3
High Risk	404	387	26	45.6	44.8
Low Risk Group					
low risk relatives	1379	1307	5	27.4	28.7
married in	986	817	18	64.5	48.9

Members of this group had significantly ($p<0.05$) more cancer diagnoses at specific sites than expected. Sites where cancer was found to occur in excess included stomach, small intestine, biliary system, kidney/ ureter, and ovary. No differences were found between males and females in the cohort, except of course, for the excess of ovarian cancer. Details are provided in Table 2.

Table 2. Gastric, small intestine, biliary system, urologic system, and ovarian cancer in putative HNPCC gene carriers.

Cancer Site	Observed (+unverified)	Expected	Observed/Expected Ratio
stomach	12(+2)	1.0 (CCR)	11.6
		1.3 (SEER)	9.6 (p<0.001)
small intestine	4	0.12 (SEER)	32.2 (p<0.001)
biliary system	2(+1)	0.36 (CCR)	5.5 (p<0.10)
biliary system other than liver, gallbladder	2	0.18 (SEER)	11.4 (p<0.04)
urol. system/bladder	4	0.93 (CCR)	4.3
		1.90 (SEER)	2.1 (p<0.25)
urol. system/kidney	6	0.95 (SEER)	6.3 (p<0.002)
urol. system/ureter	2	0.07 (SEER)	29.4 (p<0.001)
ovary	10	0.90 (CCR)	11.0
		1.30 (SEER)	7.7 (p<0.001)

<u>High risk group:</u> This group included 791 individuals who had a first degree relative in the putative gene carrier group. See Table 1 for group characteristics. Two sites were observed to have an excess number of cancers: the ureter, where two diagnoses were observed and 0.14 were expected, and the small intestine, where three diagnoses were observed and 0.23 were expected. Details of these results are provided in Table 3.

Table 3. Small intestine, biliary system, and urinary system cancer in high risk relatives of putative HNPCC gene carriers.

Cancer Site	Observed (+unverified)	Expected	Observed/Expected Ratio
small intestine	3	0.23 (SEER)	12.7 ($p<0.01$)
biliary system	4(+2)	1.05 (CCR)	3.8 ($p<0.05$)
biliary system other than liver, gallbladder	2	0.34 (SEER)	5.9 ($p<0.10$)
urol. system/bladder	1	3.41 (CCR)	0.29
		4.00 (SEER)	0.25
urol. system/kidney	2	1.87 (SEER)	1.1
urol. system/ureter	2	0.14 (SEER)	14.6 ($p<0.025$)

Certain negative findings in the putative gene carrier and high risk group are noteworthy. No excess of pancreatic cancer, lymphatic/hematopoietic cancer, laryngeal cancer, breast cancer, malignant brain tumors, or lung/bronchus cancer was detected (see Table 4). In fact, significantly fewer lung/bronchus cancer cases occurred than were expected ($p<0.02$), regardless of whether the unverified case was included, and whether the CCR or SEER estimate of expected number was used. None of the three reported cases occurred in the putative gene carrier group.

Table 4. Other cancers in putative gene carriers and their high risk relatives.

Cancer Site	Observed (+unverified)	Expected
pancreas	3	2.4 (CCR) or 3.8 (SEER)
lymphatic/hematopoietic	4(+2)	7.1 (CCR)
larynx	1	1.96 (SEER)
breast	17(+5)	14.3 (CCR) or 20.4 (SEER)
brain	3	1.7 (CCR)
lung/bronchus	2(+1)	10.6 (CCR) or 18.9 (SEER)

Low risk group: This group included 4489 individuals in the kindreds who were not classified as putative gene carrier or as high risk (first degree relatives of putative gene carriers). See Table 1 for group characteristics. No significantly excessive numbers of cancer diagnoses were observed in the low risk group, either in any general organ system or in any specific site. Separate analysis of the 2686 low risk family members (excluding the married in family members) also showed no excess of cancer at any site.

DISCUSSION

In the orignal family study of the 'Cancer Family Syndrome,' now known as HNPCC [Lynch et al 1966], the propositus of the family was affected with adrenocortical carcinoma. A wide variety of cancers was reported in family members, with a predominance of carcinoma of the colon and endometrium which appeared to segregate in an autosomal dominant mode of genetic transmission. It is now widely accepted that carcinomas of the colon and endometrium are most characteristic of the disorder. Knowledge of the natural history of the colonic cancer has been refined, with evidence of proximal colon predominance, early age of cancer diagnoseis, and high frequency of multiple primary cancers [Lynch et al 1987]. However, significance of cancers at other sites remains unclear. A variety of other tumors have been associated with HNPCC, including cancers of the ovary, brain, bile duct, small bowel, urologic system, and breasts [Lynch et al 1988a; Lynch et al, in press], larynx [Lynch et al 1988b], stomach [Cristofaro et al 1987], pancreas [Lynch et al 1985], and lymphatic/hematopoietic system [Law et al 1977; Love 1985]. These associations were based on observation of these cancers in HNPCC families, but uncertainty remained about the extent to which the results could be explained by normal cancer incidence rates.

Our results provide good evidence that risk of carcinoma of the small bowel is associated with HNPCC. Putative gene carriers and their high risk relatives had 32 times and 13 times, respectively, the expected number of diagnoses of this rare tumor. These small bowel cancers were adenocarcinomas in all cases where the histological type was known. There was also good evidence that gastric cancer is associated with HNPCC; putative gene carriers had approximately 10 times the expected number of diagnoses of this tumor. Again, these were adenocarcinomas in all cases where histologic type was known. Finally, putative gene carriers had approximately 8 times as many ovarian cancer diagnoses as expected, and these were all adenocarcinomas. With respect to biliary system cancer, the results are more complex. Putative gene carriers had a significant excess of cancers of the common bile duct. Their high risk relatives had a significant excess of the biliary system as a whole; the diagnoses in the high risk group included cancers of the bile ducts and gallbladder. In the urological system, we did not find consistent evidence for an elevated risk of urinary bladder cancer. Putative gene carriers had 6 times as many kidney cancers and almost 30 times as many ureteral cancers as expected. High risk relatives had no significant excess of kidney cancers, but nearly 15 times as many ureteral cancers as expected. Five of the eight kidney cancers observed were transitional cell carcinomas of the renal pelvis; the same histological type was observed in the ureter. It is notable that the renal pelvis is more closely related, histologically, to the ureter than to the rest of the kidney.

One relatively common type of cancer, bronchogenic cancer, occurred very rarely among the putative gene carriers and their high risk relatives. We do not have any plausible explanation for this deficit. We do not believe that lung cancer is under-reported since the questionnaire which we use to gather information about cancer diagnoses asks for reports of cancer at all sites, and lung cancer is specifically mentioned as an example of site specification. We also have no evidence that members of these families avoid exposure to carcinogens. We have limited data on smoking history of family members. In five families where smoking history data had been collected, 497 family members over the age of 19 had provided information on cigarette exposure, and 58% indicated that they were current or former smokers.

On the other hand, cancers of the breast, brain, larynx, pancreas, and lymphatic/hematopoietic system were not observed to occur more frequently than expected in these families. These and other cancer types included in the analysis were found to occur at approximately the expected rate.

The limitations of this study should be noted. Our interest was in the association of extracolonic cancer with HNPCC. The method we have used depends on the assumption that the included families are correctly classified as HNPCC, and that the model of HNPCC as an autosomal dominant trait is correct. We believe that these assumptions are justified. The specific results we have obtained depend also on the correct classification of family members into risk groups. There is no fail-safe rule for doing so which is currently available. For example, we know that sporadic colon cancer may have occurred in family members who were not actually gene carriers. In the present analysis, such a person would have been misclassified as a putative gene carrier. We plan to test several alternative rules for specifying gene carriers to discover how sensitive our results are to such alterations. Finally, it should be pointed out that this analysis does not take into consideration potential heterogeneity among families in extracolonic tumor risk. We have planned future analyses to evaluate the extent of this heterogeneity.

Study of any single collection of families has potential for bias. The inclusion of families in the resource may have been affected by the types of tumors seen in family members. However, the resource we have studied in quite large, and more importantly, the families included are well-documented and extended. Bias related to initial ascertainment would be most related to cancers in the proband and close family members, an effect which will be diluted by inclusion of many distant relatives. Another problem is the relative homogeneity of environments among families from a single resource compared to the marked worldwide variation in exposure to cancer-associated environmental factors. The potentially differing impact of HNPCC on risk for specific cancers in various environments is both a problem (for generalizing the results of the current study) and a tantalizing "experiment of nature" which invites study. We hope that similar studies of other collections of HNPCC families will be carried out so that the generality of our findings can be evaluated and extended.

In summary, we have found that putative HNPCC gene carriers and their high risk relatives have been diagnosed with cancers other than uterine and colorectal more frequently than expected, based on general population incidence figures. Specific sites where elevations are seen include the stomach, small intestine, biliary system (especially the bile ducts), urological system (especially the kidney and ureter), and ovary.

ACKNOWLEDGEMENTS: Support for this effort was provided by a grant from the National Cancer Institute, #1 RO1 CA41371.

REFERENCES

Breslow NE, Day NF (1987) Statistical methods in cancer research. II. The design and analysis of cohort studies. IARC Pub. 82, Lyon, France

Cristofaro G, Lynch HT, Caruso ML, Attolini A, Matteo GI, Giorgio P, Senatore S, Argentieri A, Sbano E, Fusaro RM, Giorgio I (1987) New phenotypic aspects in a family with Lynch syndrome II. Cancer 60:51-58

Kleinbaum DG, Kupper LL, Morgenstern H (1982) Epidemiologic research: principles and quantitative methods. VN Reinhold, New York, NY

Law IP, Hollinshead AC, Whang-Peng J, Dean JH, Oldham RK, Herberman RB, Rhode MC (1977) Familial occurrence of colon and uterine carcinoma and of lymphoproliferative malignancies, II. Cancer 39:1229-1236

Love RR (1985) Small bowel cancers, B-cell lymphatic leukemia, and six primary cancers with metastases and prolonged survival in the Cancer Family Syndrome of Lynch. Cancer 55:499-502

Lynch HT, Shaw MW, Magnuson CW, Larsen AL, Krush AJ (1966) Hereditary factors in cancer: study of two large midwestern kindreds. Arch Int Med 117:206-212

Lynch HT, Voorhees GJ, Lanspa SJ, McGreevy PS, Lynch JF (1985) Pancreatic carcinoma and hereditary nonpolyposis colorectal cancer: a family study. Br J Cancer 52:271-273

Lynch HT, Watson P, Lanspa SJ, Marcus J, Smyrk T, Fitzgibbons RJ Jr, Kriegler M, Lynch JF (1988a) Natural history of colorectal cancer in hereditary nonpolyposis colorectal cancer (Lynch syndromes I and II). Dis Colon Rect 31:439-444

Lynch HT, Ens J, Lynch JF, Watson P (1988b) Tumor variation in three extended Lynch syndomre II kindreds. Am J Gastroent 83:741-747

Lynch HT, Kriegler M, Christiansen TA, Smyrk T, Lynch JF, Watson P (1988c) Laryngeal carcinoma in a Lynch syndrome II kindred. Cancer 62:1007-1013

Lynch HT, Smyrk TC, Lynch PM, Lanspa SJ, Boman BM, Ens J, Lynch JF, Strayhorn P, Carmody T, Watson P, Cristofaro G (in press) Adenocarcinoma of the small bowel in Lynch syndrome II. Cancer

Menko FH, Schakel HJ, vanHuis FG, denHartog Jager FCA, Nagengast FM, Vasen HFA (in press) Cancer Family Syndrome - consideration in diagnosis and management: a case report

Monson RR (1974) Analysis of relative survival and proportional mortality. Comp Biomed Res 7:325-332

Young JL, Percy CL, Asire AJ (1981) Surveillance, epidemiology, and end results: incidence and mortality data, 1973-77. NIH Pub 81-2330, NCI, Bethesda, MD

Endometrial Cancer as Heterogenic Picture of HNPCC: Population-Based Studies in Sweden

STIG KULLANDER

ABSTRACT

The association of neoplasms of female sexual organ and colorectal cancer familial anamnesis has been epidemiologically studied on a population basis in Malmø.

In 51 new diagnosed cases of endometrial adenocarcinoma during a two-year period, cancer was present in a first-degree relative in 17,9 per cent, a significant higher figure than among relatives of controls, 9,4 per cent. There was a higher incidence especially of cancer of the colon and of the sexual organs.

The epidemiological findings suggest the presence of a mutated gene in the population, manifesting itself in several cases of endometrial adenocarcinomas and colon carcinomas.

Keywords: Endometrial cancer, familial aggregation, hereditary non-polyposis colon carcinoma, epidemiological studies.

A number of earlier findings, and confirmatory results from current epidemiological heredity studies at Malmø, justify the assertion that hereditary factors are crucially involved in many cases of endometrial carcinoma.

A high incidence of familial aggregation in cancer may be due either to random clustering of sporadic cases, shared exposure to environmental carcinogens, hereditary factors or a combination of any of these. It is still common to view cancer cases as random or "sporadic" phenomena. Such comments as "No familial aspects of any relevance" used to be standard chlichés in our medical records. A tumour that might at first glance appear to be a "sporadic" case may nonetheless have strong hereditary connotations.

In various hereditary cancer syndromes particulary those with breast cancer, ovarian cancer, or non-polyposis (usually rightsided) colon cancer - the characteristic features have been early tumour onset and a high incidence of multiple primary tumours among family members. A very heterogenous multiple tumour spectrum, with varying expression of the defective gene, sometimes even including malformation, is now considered to be characteristic of cancer families, and to be due to a hereditary cancer-predisposing factor.

Variation in the numbers of relatives and variation in family size and in the interrelations with environment factors may explain differences in individual and pedigree cancer frequency and distribution, even in cases of the same genetic defect.

Population studies are essential, if misleading bias is to be avoided when determining the significance of familial or genetic factors. Endometrial cancer has been shown to be associated with a variety of constitutional entities such as diabetes, obesity, and hypertension.

However, no systematic studies have been made of the occurrence of the same endometrial cancer form, or of other cancer forms, in kindreds. Thus, the approach that seemed to be indicated was that of a controlled epidemiological case-control study of endometrialcancer to be succeded by chromosomal and molecular studies. Malmø is particularly well suited to such studies. Its population of 240,000 is large enough yet manageable, and it is served by a single hospital to wich all tumour cases are remitted and where they are subsequently followed up. The population is fairly static and easily accessible for the purposes of information collection or distribution, and the autopsy frequency is high.

To avoid confusion due to small histological subgroups, detailed analysis was confined to cases of adenocarcinoma - by far the predominant type of malignancy is endometrial cancer.

The series comprised all newly diagnosed cases of endometrial adenocarcinoma treated at Malmø during the two-year period, 1983-84. While attending the clinic patient were interviewed in connection with a review of their answers to as standardised questionnaire on family history. The questionnaire had been distributed in advance to allow patients ample time for contacting and questioning members of their families. Information was collected on malignant disease and malformation for all first degree relatives, both of the patients and their consorts, wich were chosen as controls. As far as possible, all reported instances of cancer were checked with the help of medical record and histopathology and autopsy reports.

At a review two years after the interview study, each case was checked with regard to histopathology, and whether the patient was symtom-free, had suffered recurrence of endometrial cancer, or had died of it. All patients had been given the routine treatment for this cancer, standard at the clinic.

Before starting the study, we examined the families of three index cases. The first family, studied in three generations showed two brothers of the proband, and both had cancer of the ascending colon at an early age. One of them, a survivor manifested a feature typical of cases of hereditary cancer, by subsequently developing an additional primary malignancy, of the prostate. Of the proband's eight sisters, four had endometrial cancer at an early age, and one of their children had a chromosomal abnormality - Turner's syndrome. Another of the proband's sisters and one of her children had cervical cancer.

In a second family both the proband's father and mother had cancer; and of the three sisters, one had breast cancer, ant two had double primary malignancies - colon and endometrial cancer in one case, and ovarian and skin cancer in the other; the proband's brother had rectal cancer.

In the third family the proband's father had early onset colon cancer, and two of the father's sisters had endometrial cancer. Of the proband's four sisters, one died of a congenital heart defect, and two had endometrial cancer; in two cases the endometrial carcinoma was combined with an additional primary malignancy - one in the colon, the other in breast. The sister who remained free of endometrial cancer had a daughter who got cervical cancer. Of the proband's five brothers, one had cancer of the colon - as did his son in turn, at the age of thirty-nine.

In the two-year series of altogether 51 patients investigated at Malmø, additional primary malignancy occurred in nine cases (18%), in one of which there were two additional primary malignancies (one mammary, the other skin cancer). The other additional primary carcinomas had occurred in the breast or cervix, and predated the endometrial cancer and in three cases occurring simultaneously it was ovarian cancer. In these cases of endometrial cancer in combination with additional malignancy, age at onset was significantly lower, a feature typical of hereditary cancer predisposition.

In the series as a whole (n=51), cancer was present in a first degree relative in 26 cases; and of the total of 230 relatives, cancer occurred in 41, or 17,9 per cent - wich is significantly more than corresponding figure of 9,4 per cent for the relatives of controls.

Age at onset was lower among endometrial cancer patients whose cancer predisposition was seemingly inherited from the father, than in those where it was seemingly inherited from the mother.

Not only was the incidence of cancer higher among relatives of endometrial cancer patients than among affected relatives of controls, but age at onset was lower. The difference in inciddence is due to a higher rate of cancer in organs particularly sensitive to hormonal changes - the genital tract, the breast, and the prostate; but it is also due to a high incidence of cancer of the colon.

Endometrial cancer occurred in four mothers or sisters of probands; and where histological findings were reviewed we found identical patterns of poorly differentiated adenocarcinoma in the proband and her sister.

In general, endometrial cancer manifesting multiple malingnancy or familial cancer predisposition was associated with poorly differentiated adenocarcinoma of advanced stage and poorer prognosis.

The epidemiological findings outlined suggest the familial presence of a mutated endometrial gene in around 10 per cent of all cases of adenocarcinoma of the uterine body. No genetic studies with modern recombinant DNA techniques seem to have been done so far in connection with endometrial cancer. Until proper DNA probes are available, such simple and readily performed measures as the taking of a thorough family history are of crucial importance. Familial aggregation of endometrial cancer or suspected genetic cancer predisposition in the patient should alert the physician to the necessity of extra care, also in the surveillance of members of the family.

In addition, it is my personal philosophy that, in such family members, the use of oestrogens for contraceptive or anti-climacteric purposes is to be avoided, as expression of an endometrial oncogene may well be hormon-dependent and oestrogen-associated.

Endometrial cancer is known as a heterogenic picture in women belonging to families exhibiting CFS. This syndrome where HNPCC is characteristic seems more common than has hitherto been assumed. The epidemiological findings in Malmø indicate the occurence of several "fragments" of the syndrome in the population. It is interesting that other cancers in hormone-sensitive genital tissues may be herogenic manifestations in HNPCC as well. Such tumours appeared also both in the pedigrees and as double primaries in the endometrial cancer cases studied. Regarding our findings of ovarian and cervical cancers, it should be noticed that Peutz-Jeghers syndrome, a rare hereditary disorder with gastrointestinal polyposis associated with characteristic skin pigmentation, has an increased risk for the development of cancer of the colon but also of ovarian tumours, sometimes with a rather specific histologic picture with annular tubules, causing hyperestrinisme (Utsunomiya et al 1974, Young et al 1982). A distinctive sex-cord-stromal ovarian tumour also has been described in connexion with Peutz-Jegher (Young et al 1983) as well as mucinous adenocarcinomas of the cervix uteri (Young et al 1982). Accordingly in health surveillance of women belonging to families manifesting more or less obvious HNPCC extra attention should be given to genital organs.

References

Young RH, Welch WR, Dickersin GR and Scully Re Cancer 50 1384, 1982
Utsunomiya J, Gocho H, Miyanaga T, Hamaguchi E, Kashimure A, Aoki N and Komatsu I. The Johns Hopkins Med. J. 136, 71, 1975.
Young RH, Dickersin GR and Scully RE. Am. J.Surg. Pathol. 7,233, 1983.

A Monoclonal Antibody C12 Against Endometrial Carcinoma, Recognize Polyfucosyl Lactosamine-Bearing Glycoprotein

YOSHIYUKI TSUJI

An monoclonal antibody (Mab) termed C12 was established by immunization of BALB/c mouse with endometrial culture cell line (1).
The Mab-C12 was shown strong reactivity to endometrial carcinoma but minimum reaction to normal endometrium.
Therefore Mab-C12 was seemed to recognize tumor associated antigen of endometrial carcinoma.
However, Mab C12 was found to hemagglutinate O type blood erythrocyte, but not to any other blood types erythrocytes.
Normal endometrium was not reacted with Mab-C12, but there were several normal glandular tissues reacted by Mab-C12.
These tissues were salivary, pancreas and stomach glands.
In spite of several reactivities to normal tissues, Mab-C12 showed no reactive to normal endometrium and any other digestive epithelium.
On the other hand, the corresponding antigen was detected in the sera of the patients with carcinoma including endometrial carcinoma using Sandwich radiometric assay.
There were significant high level of C12 antigen in endometrial, ovarial, colon, pancreas carcinoma and hepatoma patients' sera, but no significant increase in normal or benign disease patients' sera except for liver cirrohsis.(figure 1).

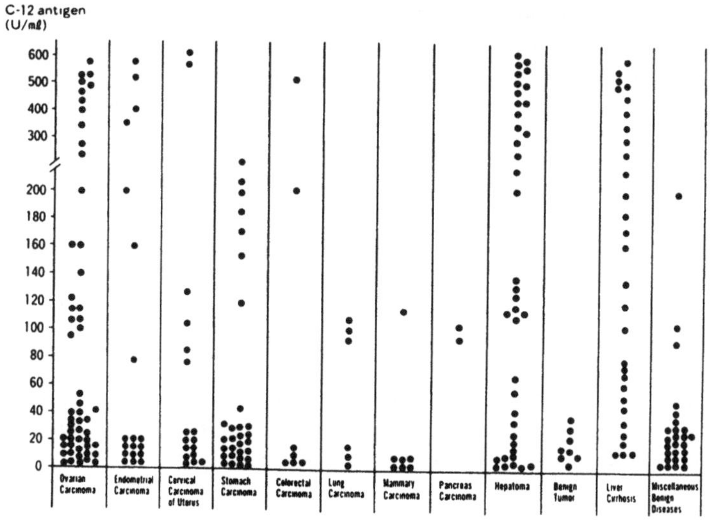

Figure 1.

The biochemical analysis of C12 antigen showed it was high molecular glycoprotein, and possessing periodic acid sensitive, neuraminidase resistance and trypsin sensitive epitope.
These character of glycoprotein is that of mucin type glycoprotein secreted by several glandular tissue, and the epitope of C12 antigen seemed to locate neutral carbohydrate epitope.
The corresponding carbohydrate epitope of C12 was examined by thin layer immuno staining for several standard glycolipids.
Clear TLC-immunostaining bands were detected on terminal fucosil lactosyl ceramide (type II H) and difucosyl lactosyl ceramide (LeY).
This staining result showed the carbohydrate epitopes of Mab-C12 was a common part of type II H and LeY (figure 2).

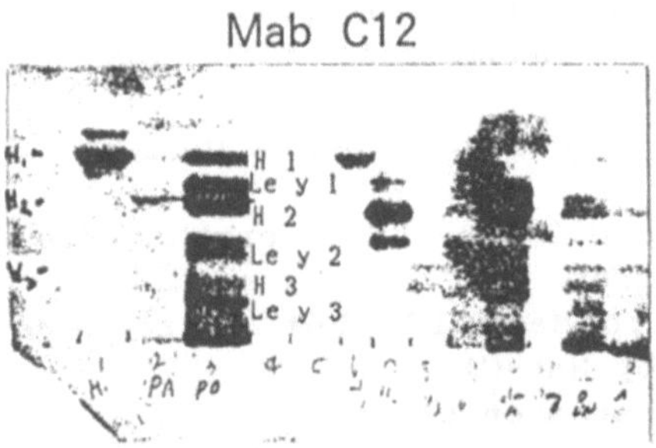

The Carbohydrate Portion Structure of Epitope Recognized by Mab-C12

TypeII H
Galβ1-4GlcNAcβ1-3Galβ1-4GlcNAc-
Fuc

Le y
Galβ1-4GlcNAcβ1-3Galβ1-4GlcNAc-
Fuc Fuc

But Mab-4A4 which had no endometrial carcinoma specificity showed same reactive manner to Le y and typeII H

Figure 2.

We tried to confirm that Mab-C12 recognized H or LeY carbohydrate structure, another monoclonal antibody which reacted LeY or type II H. The endometrial carcinoma were stained with 1B5 or AH6 that reacted to LeY and type II H respectively and the expression of LeY and type II H antigen on endometrial carcinoma was quit similar with C12 staining, but the staining intensity was lower and staining area on carcinoma nests were more limited than that of C12.
In order to elucidate difference C12 antigen and blood group H antigen or LeY antigen cancer serum antigen level was examined by using C12 and Ulex europeas lectin which reacted fucosil mucin.
Several carcinoma sera were examined by radiometric assay using labeled UEA combinated solid phase UEA, or labeled C12 combined by solid phase C12.
As shown in figure 3, UEA radiometric assay detected significance high level in several sera of carcinoma patients, however the level of UEA binding substance in sera were influenced by patients blood group type, especially high level were found in sera of O type group patients.
On the other hand, C12 radiometric assay detected C12 binding substances specifically in carcinoma patients sera and there were relation with patients blood group types.
Thus it can be concluded that the substance which identified by Mab C12 is not merely blood group antigens but it recognized carcinoma specific blood group related antigen.
We studied detail structure of C12 antigenic epitope. The type II H

and LeY glycolipids were reacted by C12, therefore we presumed that the epitope of C12 constituted with combination of peptide and fucose rich lactosamine binding to peptide by O-serine/threonine.
Such conformational epitope is hard to investigate, but first of all we analyzed peptide portion.
On the gel filtration of C12 antigen materials secreted from endometrial culture line, ISHIKAWA was high molecular glycoprotein distributed from 500 k dalton to 2000 k dalton, however we found an associate band of molecular weight 150 k dalton with lesser C12 antigenicity on SDS-PAGE immunoblotting assay.
It was supposed that the smaller substance could be a disassociated materials from major high molecular substance.
We purified the sub materials by immunoaffinity column using Mab-C12 conjugated sepharose 4B.

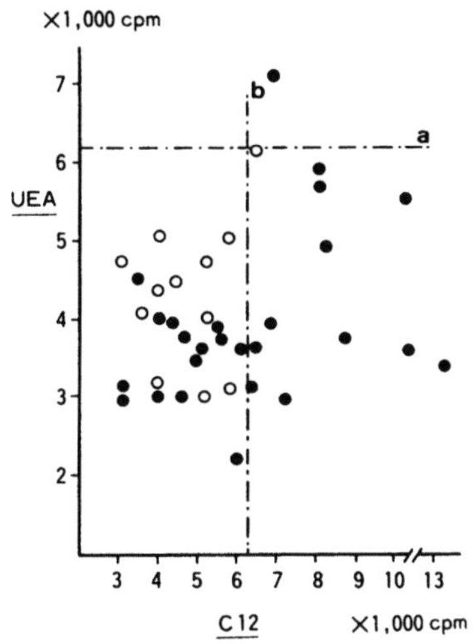

Comparison between UEA RMA and MAb C12 RMA to distinguish carcinoma sera from normal sera. ●, carcinoma sera; ○, normal sera; *broken lines*, man + 2 × SD of cpm level of normal sera measured by MAb C12 RMA (*a*) and that of normal sera measured by UEA RMA, (*b*).

Figure 3.

The semi-purified materials obtained by immunoaffinity column was further purified by FPLC reverse phase chromatography column pro PRC 5, and applied peptide amino sequencer.
The amino acids sequence of the materials were inspected by computer data base, and there were no homological proteins, however interestingly, the presumable corresponding DNA sequences possessed highly homology with pancreatic elastase III.
This data suggested that the gene coding peptide portion of C12 antigen was derived from common ancient gene of pancreatic elastase III. The whole gene cloning of this gene were now under investigation by us.

Refference

1.Tsuji. Y., Yoshioka. M., Ogasawara, T., Takemura, T. and Isojima. S. Identification of an H antigen-like blood group antigen in sera of cancer patients, Using a novel monoclonal antibody raised against endometrial carcinoma. Cancer. Res., 47, 3543-3550, 1987.

A Pedigree of Cancer Family Syndrome with an Aggregation of Transitional Cell Cancer of the Urinary Tract

MITSURO CHIBA, YUKIKO OHYAMA, OSAMU MASAMUNE, TETSURO KATO, KAZUNARI SATO, TOMIO NARISAWA, KENJI SOGA, and RYODO KOIZUMI

ABSTRACT

A pedigree of cancer family syndrome with an aggregation of transitional cell cancer (TCC) of the urinary tract is reported. The proband had left (lt) pelvic cancer at the age of 49, and double cancers of the right (rt) fallopian tube and the uterine body at 50. Various types of cancer, including colon cancer and gastric cancer, were found in four out of her seven siblings. In three siblings, TCC of the urinary tract was found. Although TCC has not been described to be a cancer found in cancer family syndrome, this pedigree clearly demonstrates that TCC is one such cancer.

Key words: cancer family syndrome (Lynch syndrome II), transitional cell cancer, hereditary cancer

INTRODUCTION

The criteria of cancer family syndrome (CFS), otherwise known as Lynch syndrome II, includes: a family tendency to develop adenocarcinomas of numerous organs, but predominantly involving the (proximal) colon and endometrium; a significantly early age of onset of the cancer compared with the same type of cancer in the general population; an extraordinary frequency of multiple, primary malignant neoplasms; and vertical transmission with segregation patterns consistent with an autosomal dominant mode of genetic transmission (Lynch 1979). There have been several pedigrees of CFS in which only a single case with transitional cell cancer (TCC) of the urinary tact was found (Lynch 1983, Igarashi 1986, Tokunaga 1986). To our knowledge, there has been only one report of a pedigree in which multiple cases with TCC were observed (Bender 1988), but the aggregation of TCC was not specifically stated by the authors. We report herein CFS with an aggregation of TCC.

A PEDIGREE

A 49-year-old female had a medical check, together with her eldest sister, in January 1988, because her brothers had had numerous types of cancer. She had a polyp of the uterus excised at the ages of 39, 42 and 45. She had another three polyps of the uterus excised and had posttransfusion hepatitis at 48. The medical check revealed that she had microscopic hematuria, and a further examination revealed a lt pelvic tumor (Figure 1a), which was surgically removed in March 1988. The histology of the tumor was determined to be transitional cell carcinoma. In October, a cystic tumor in the lt abdomen, which was detected by ultrasonography, was surgically removed and histologically confirmed as adenocarcinoma (Figs. 2a, 2b, 2c). She was referred to the First Department of Internal Medicine for further examination of the intestinal tract, because the cystic tumor was adherent to the sigmoid colon in the operation.

Her family history was remarkable (Fig.3). The eldest brother died of rectal cancer at 42. The third eldest brother had multiple, ascending colon cancers (Borrman 2, well-differentiated adenocarcinoma, Dukes C, modified Dukes C1 or C2; Ip, well-differentiated adenocarcinoma, focal cancer "m") at 42, TCC of the lt ureter at 49 (Fig. 1b), and multiple metachronous urinary bladder cancers (pathology report: TCC) at 51. Her youngest brother was found to have a rectal polyp at 37, which was left untreated, and rectal cancer (well-differentiated adenocarcinoma, Dukes B), a rectal polyp, and a gastric polyp (adenoma, group 3) at 40. He also had double cancers of the stomach (IIa + IIc, tubular adenocarcinoma) and the lt pelvis (TCC) (Fig. 1c) with pulmonary metastasis at 45, and then died at 46. The eldest sister, who was 63-year-old, had total hysterectomy about 20 years ago, but the details are unknown. Her mother died of gastric cancer at the age of 52. In all, cancer was found in four out of her seven siblings and, in three of these, TCC was found. There was no skin tumor among these patients, so that the diagnosis of Mure-Torre syndrome was excluded (Rulon 1973, Anderson, 1980). The family members did not live in particular environments in which they were exposed to specific chemical agents, but lived in average surroundings.

Apart from an aggregation of TCC, this family had some features of CFS; an early onset of cancer, cancer of the rt colon, and multiple, primary cancers including gastric cancer. Therefore, She was diagnosed as having CFS, and further examinations were focused on the gastrointestinal tract and female organs.

Her physical examination was unremarkable, except for surgical scars for lt pelvic cancer.

Laboratory data on admission (Table 1) were normal except for a moderate increase of CA-125 (Table 2). The serum levels of CEA and CA 19-9 were normal.

Table 1 Laboratory data on admission

ESR(1°)	18 mm	TP	7.5 g/dl
Hb	11.3 g/dl	Albumin	4.5 g/dl
WBC	6200 /mm³	GOT	17 U/L
Stool: occult blood	-	Bilirubin (T)	0.7 mg/dl
Urine: occult blood	+++	ALP	181 U/L
		LDH	128 U/L

No abnormalities were found in the following examinations; barium enema study, fluoroscopy and endoscopy of the upper gastrointestinal tract, small intestinal fluoroscopy, abdominal ultrasonography and chest X-ray. CT of the abdomen and the pelvis revealed a tumor, 3.5 × 4.0 cm in size, in the rt upper area next to the uterus. Papanicolaou's stain test revealed group 5. Laparotomy on Feb. 14, 1989, revealed double cancers of the rt fallopian tube with intra-abdominal metastasis, and of the uterine body (Ia stage). Subsequently, a semi-radical hysterectomy

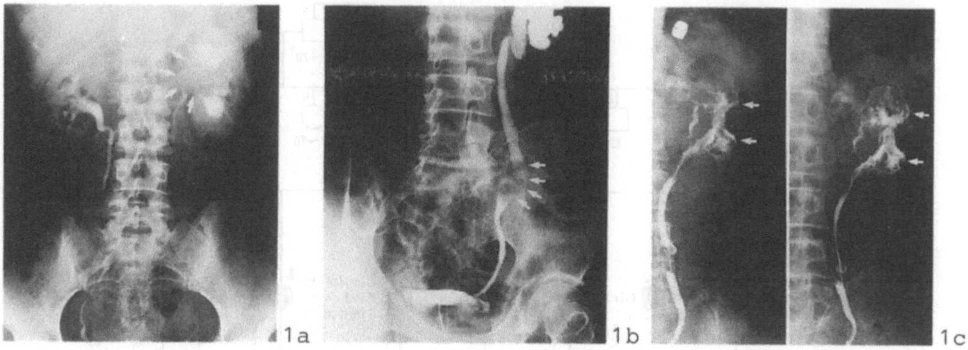

Fig. 1: 1a, lt. pelvic cancer of the proband; 1b, lt. ureteral cancer of III-5; and 1c, lt. pelvic cancer of III-7.

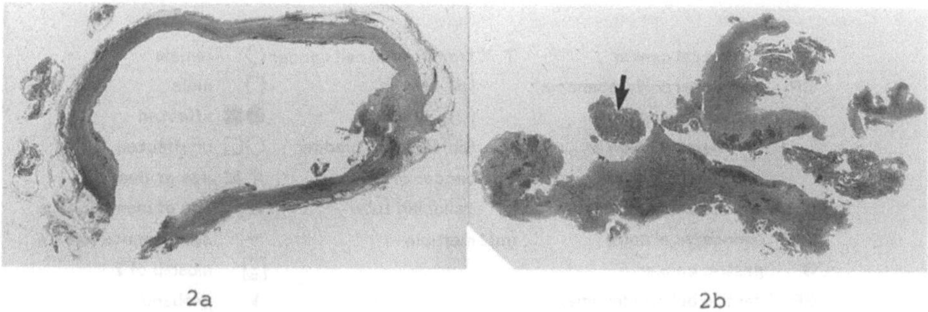

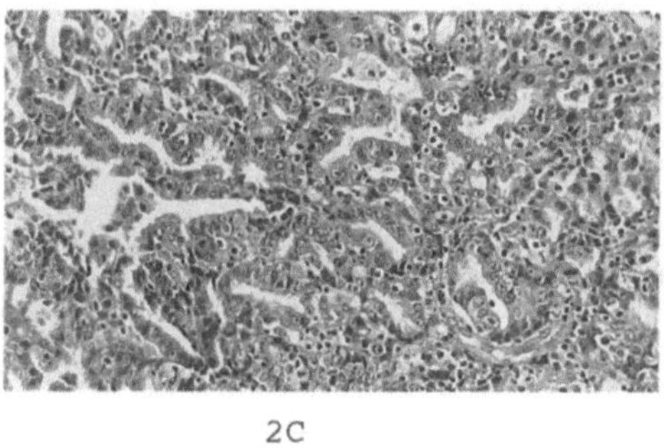

Fig. 2: 2a, the wall of the cystic tumor; 2b, another fragment of the cystic tumor; 2c, high power view (× 64) of a part indicated by an arrow in Fig. 2b.

was performed. Both cancers were found to be adenocarcinomas, and they were histologically confirmed to be primary cancers. Serum levels of CA125 decreased to 50 on Feb. 21, and became normal in April (Table 2). She was discharged on July 8, 1989, after postoperative chemotherapy. The HLA types of the patient and her siblings are presented in Table 3.

A chromosome study of the proband, using peripheral blood lymphocytes with G-banding by the Special Reference Lab. Inc. (Hachiohji, Tokyo), found to be normal.

The eldest sister (III-1) and the second-eldest brother (III-3) underwent a detailed examination of the gastrointestinal tract and the urinary tract, and the former was also checked by a gynecologist. They were both found to be free from cancer.

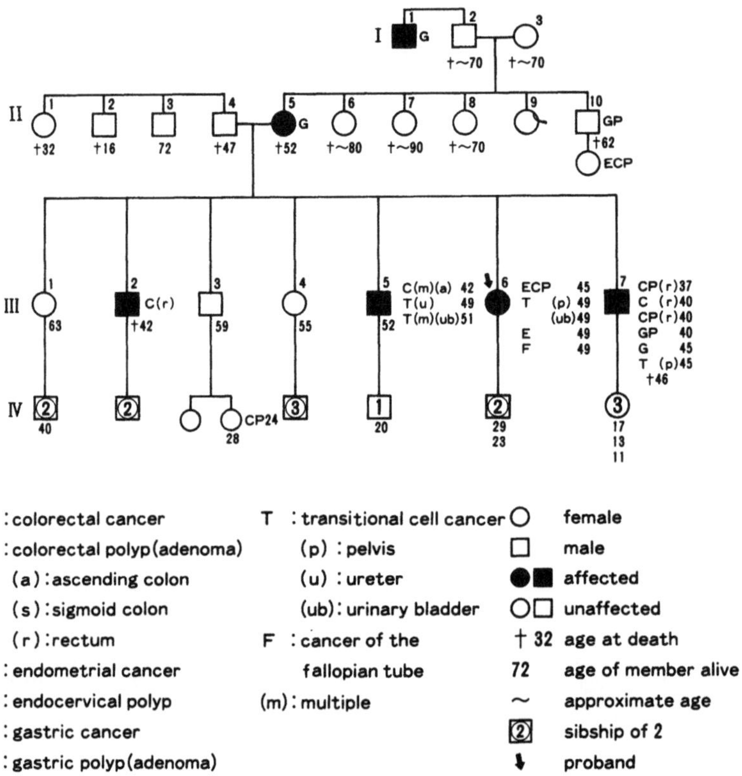

Fig. 3: Pedigree of family

Table 2 Laboratory data of tumor markers

Tumor marker	Date	(normal range)	Value
CEA*	Dec 5, 1988	(<4 ng/ml)	1.7
α-fetoprotein	Mar 3, 1988	(<20 ng/ml)	<20
CA19-9	Dec 5, 1988	(<37 U/ml)	<37
CA125	Mar 3, 1988	(<50 U/ml)	11
	Dec 5, 1988		130
	Jan 11, 1989		130
	Feb 21, 1989#		50
	Apr 19, 1989#		<8
β_2-microglobulin	Oct 26, 1988	(0.8-2.4 μg/ml)	2.0
Ferritin	Mar 14, 1988	(3.4-120 ng/ml)	31
IAP*	Mar 14, 1988	(<500 μg/dl)	851

*CEA: carcinoembryonic antigen
IAP: immunoregulatory acidic protein
#: semi-radical hysterectomy on Feb 14, 1989

Table 3 HLA types

Cases	A locus	B locus	C locus	D locus
III-1 probably unaffected	A2	BW67, BW62(15)	CW3,7	DR2, DRW9
III-3 unaffected	A2	BW67, BW62(15)	CW3,7	DR2, DRW9
III-6 affected	A2, A24(9)	BW52(5), BW67	CW7	DR2
III-7 affected	A2, A10(26)	BW62(15), B35	CW3	DR9

DISCUSSION

There have been about 12 pedigrees of CFS reported in Japan (Sasaki 1984, Nomizu 1986, Igarashi 1986, Tokunaga 1986, Ushio 1987, Matsuyama 1987, Ishibashi 1988, Murakami 1988). Our City, Akita, is located in the northern part of the main island of Honshyu, and has a population of 300,846. We have already reported a pedigree of CFS living in Akita City (Igarashi 1986), and so the pedigree reported here is the second one found in Akita City. Mecklin (1986) found that the minimum frequency of CFS in Finland was 1 in 21,400 to 25,100. We do not have a cancer registry in Akita City, but analysis of such a registry (Mecklin 1986) would certainly find other pedigrees of CFS in Akita City.

The pedigree reported in this paper fulfils the criteria of CFS. The characteristic of the pedigree was an aggregation of TCC of the urinary tract (three out of seven siblings). Since the affected cases had not been exposed to specific substance(s) which might be an initiator or a promotor for TCC of the urinary tract, the aggregation of TCC was thought to have occurred from a hereditary predisposition. Therefore, our cases had to be differentiated from other hereditary TCC of the urinary tract. Muir-Torre syndrome is a hereditary disease characterized by benign and malignant tumors of the genitourinary and gastrointestinal tracts, as well as by multiple skin tumors (Rulon 1973, Fahmy 1982, Lynch 1985). The associated visceral cancers of this syndrome show a low-grade malignancy, resulting in prolonged survival. The cases (III-1, 3, 5, 6, 7) examined in our pedigree had no skin tumors and they died at an early age; at 42 years in III-2, and at 46 years in III-7. These observations thus exclude Muir-Torre syndrome. However, there is issue about the nosology of CFS and Muir-Torre syndrome. Lynch (1980, 1985) proposed that Muir-Torre syndrome is a subtype of CFS, while Anderson (1980) considered them as distinct. The accumulation of Muir-Torre syndrome, together with the advances in molecular genetics, will certainly shed further light on this subject.

Although TCC of the urinary tract is not common in CFS (Lynch 1979, Mecklin 1986), a single case of TCC in CFS has been reported (Lynch 1983, Igarashi 1986, Tokunaga 1986). Recently, while not stated specifically in the text, Bender (1988) presents a pedigree figure (Fig.1) in which three members of family "C" were affected by TCC (father, II -5, bladder; the eldest daughter, III-12, pelvis at 55, ureter at 61; the second son, III -14, pelvis at 51). Frischer (1985) reported the case of a woman with CFS associated with metachronous TCC (lt ureter at 50, rt pelvis at 58), and called attention to the association of TCC in CFS. These reported cases, together with our cases, lead to the

following conclusions; 1) TCC of the urinary tract is rarely associated in CFS; 2) in a certain pedigree of CFS, TCC is commonly associated as colon cancer; 3) histologically, not only adenocarcinoma (Lynch 1979) but also TCC develops in CFS.
TCC of the urinary tract, in our cases, developed in single or in multiple, synchronously or metachronously, in the pelvis, ureter, and urinary bladder. The frequent occurrence of TCC necessitates frequent checks of the urinary tract. Early detection and early excision of TCC are mandatory.

(At the Meeting, Dr. Henry T Lynch mentioned his experience of a pedigree with a similar aggregation of TCC of the urinary tract, which will appear in J. Urology, 1990)

ACKNOWLEDGMENT

The authors thank Miss C. Igarashi for her skilful preparation of the manuscript.

REFERENCES

Anderson DE (1980) An inherited form of large bowel cancer. Muir's syndrome. Cancer 45:1103-1107
Bender MA, Viola MV, Fiore J, Thompson MH, Leonard RC (1988) Normal G2 chromosomal radiosensitivity and cell survival in the cancer family syndrome. Cancer Res 48:2579-2584
Fahmy A, Burgdorf WHC, Schosser RH, Pitha J (1982) Muir-Torre syndrome: Report of a case and reevaluation of the dermatopathologic features. Cancer 49:1898-1903
Frischer Z, Waltzer WC, Gonder MJ (1985) Bilateral transitional cell carcinoma of the renal pelvis in the cancer family syndrome. J Urol 134:1197-1198
Igarashi K, Shima H, Chiba M, Ohtaka M, Ohta H, Yoshida T, Nagasaki A, Arakawa H, Masamune O, Narisawa T, Niwa M, Uesaka Y (1986) A pedigree of cancer family syndrome. Gastroenterol Endosc 28:632-641 (in Jpn)
Ishibashi M, Hirao Y, Nakamura Y, Yoshida A, Kumagai T (1988) A pedigree of cancer family syndrome. Jpn J Gastroenterol 85:15 (abstract)(in Jpn)
Lynch HT, Lynch PM (1979) The cancer family syndrome: a pragmatic basis for syndrome identification. Dis Col Rect 22:106-110
Lynch HT, Lynch PM, Pester J, Fusaro RM (1980) The cancer family syndrome: rare cutaneous phenotypic linkage of Torre's syndrome. Arch Intern Med 141:607-611
Lynch HT, Albano WA, Ruma TA, Douglas Schmitz G, Costello KA, Lynch JF (1983) Surveillance/management of an obligate gene carrier: the cancer family syndrome. Gastroenterology 84:404-408
Lynch HT, Fusaro RM, Roberts L, Voorhees GJ, Lynch JF (1985) Muir-Torre syndrome in several members of a family with a varient of the cancer family syndrome. Br J Dermatol 113:295-301

Matsuyama T, Kawabori K, Matsumura T, Nishimura Y, Maniwa N, Nakagawa Y, Asahara T, Dohi M (1987) Two cases of cancer family syndrome. J Jpn Soc Clin Surg 48:1504 (abstract)(in Jpn)
Mecklin JP, Jarvinen HJ, Peltokallio P (1986) Cancer family syndrome. Genetic analysis of 22 Finnish kindreds. Gastroenterology 90:328-333
Murakami S, Haruma K, Kimura M, Tokumo K, Yoshihara M, Sumii K, Kajiyama G, Kawahori K, Matsuyama T, Okamoto E, Maruhashi A, Kawamoto T (1988) A case of cancer family syndrome. J Hiroshima Med Assoc 41:1886-1889 (in Jpn)
Nomizu T, Watanabe I, Rokkaku G, Sekikawa K, Anndo Y, Tsuchiya A (1986) A pedigree of cancer family syndrome. Gan No Rinsho 32:186-189 (in Jpn)
Rulon DB, Helwig EB (1973) Multiple sebaceous neoplasms of the skin: An association with multiple visceral carcinomas, especially of the colon. AJCP 60:745-752
Sasaki A, Konaga E, Enomoto M, Kawamura T, Haisa M, Hasuoka H, Yagi T, Ide Y (1984) A pedigree of cancer family syndrome. Gan No Rinsho 30:1849-1853 (in Jpn)
Tokunaga A, Matsukura N, Takizawa T, Tanaka N, Moriyama Y, Yamashita K, Onda M, Akimoto S, Asano G (1986) A pedigree of cancer family syndrome. Colorectal cancers in two daughters during follow up of the family of a patient with five metachronous cancers. Gann, Proc J Jpn Cancer Assoc 45th Annual Meeting p585 (abstract)(in Jpn)
Ushio K, Hohjyo K, Hirota E (1987) Cancer family syndrome and familial aggregative colorectal cancer. Gan No Rinsho 33 (supple):527-534 (in Jpn)

Screening for Hereditary Non-polyposis Colorectal Cancer in the Netherlands

H.F.A. VASEN, F.C.A. DEN HARTOG JAGER, F.M. NAGENGAST, F.H. MENKO, G.J.A. OFFERHAUS, and G. GRIFFIOEN

ABSTRACT

Hereditary non-polyposis colorectal cancer (HNPCC) is usually subdivided into two main categories: hereditary site-specific colorectal cancer (Lynch syndrome I) and colorectal cancer in association with other forms of cancer (Lynch syndrome II). Identification of HNPCC is a basis for secondary prevention. The objectives of our study were (1) to assess the value of screening; (2) to investigate the natural history; and (3) the hereditary tumor spectrum in HNPCC. Screening was performed in 24 families (colonoscopy or double-contrast barium enema and sigmoidoscopy). The patients were subdivided into two groups. Group A comprised patients with colorectal cancer who were referred because they were symptomatic. Group B included family members of these patients who were found to have a colorectal lesion by screening. We compared these groups with respect to the stage of tumor growth. Histological examination of the tumors in group A (97 patients) revealed Dukes A carcinomas in six patients, Dukes B carcinomas in 43, Dukes C carcinomas in 24 and Dukes D carcinomas in 11 patients (classification unknown in 13 patients). In group B (20 patients) adenoma was found in 14 and carcinoma in six patients (Dukes A in two and Dukes B in four patients). A total of 103 patients, including those whose tumors were detected by screening, had a colorectal carcinoma. The age at diagnosis ranged from 24 to 81 years (mean age: 46 years). The localization of the colonic tumors was proximal in 60%. Multiple primary tumors were found in 25%. Sixty-five extra-colonic tumors were found : endometrial cancer in 16 patients belonging to 12 families, cancer of the stomach in ten patients representing five families, urinary-tract tumors in eight patients from four families and many other tumors less frequently. The results suggest that screening leads to the early detection of colorectal carcinomas and adenomas in asymptomatic members of HNPCC-families. Screening should be initiated at the age of 20 and continued during the life of the individual. Careful examination of the right colon is indicated because of the frequent occurrence of tumors in the proximal colon. A subtotal colectomy is indicated at the time of diagnosis of the initial colon cancer, because of the risk of multiple primary tumors. Carcinoma of the endometrium, stomach and urinary tract appear to belong to the hereditary tumor spectrum.

Keywords: hereditary non-polyposis colorectal cancer, natural history, screening, tumor spectrum.

INTRODUCTION

The hereditary colonic cancer syndrome without polyposis, also called hereditary non-polyposis colorectal cancer (HNPCC), is an autosomal dominant disease characterized by the development of cancer at an early age, an excess of multiple primary cancers, and a predominance of proximal colonic cancer (Lynch 1981; Mecklin 1986; Vasen 1989). The syndrome can be subdivided into two main categories: hereditary site-specific non-polyposis colorectal cancer (Lynch syndrome I), and colorectal cancer in association with other forms of cancer, particularly endometrial carcinoma (Lynch syndrome II) (Boland 1984, Lynch 1985).

Periodic examination of family members at risk may improve the prognosis, because potentially life-threatening tumors can be detected and treated in an early stage. However, periodic screening may also have disadvantages, which include not only the cost and inconvenience of repeated check-ups, but also violation of privacy and problems with insurance companies. All this makes it essential to know whether large-scale screening of families with hereditary tumors satisfies the criteria maintained in epidemiologic screening programs (Wilson 1968). This means that the natural history must be known; there must be a recognizable latent stage; acceptable tests with a high specificity and sensitivity must be available; the treatment should be generally accepted; and early diagnosis and treatment should improve the prognosis and offer the prospect of prolonged life expectancy. In addition, one must know which types of cancer belong to the hereditary tumor spectrum of HNPCC. To obtain more information on the natural history and the hereditary tumor spectrum of HNPCC and to assess the effect of screening, we reviewed the data of 24 families.

METHODS

A registration center (Foundation for the Detection of Hereditary Tumors) supervised by a multihospital committee was set up in The Netherlands in 1983. The aims of this foundation are: (1) to improve surveillance in families with hereditary tumors; (2) to guarantee the continuity of periodic examination; and (3) to advise general physicians and specialists concerning screening methods. This center records personal and medical data of patients as well as personal data and screening results of all first-degree relatives. The registration center has concentrated its efforts to date on families affected with familial adenomatous polyposis, the multiple endocrine neoplasia syndrome type II (Vasen 1987), and HNPCC families (Vasen 1989).

Kindreds were selected for the study if they had at least three first-degree family members with colorectal cancer and one of the following characteristics: early onset of colon cancer (under 45 years), or multiple primary tumors. These kindreds were detected in four university hospitals in The Netherlands between 1975 and 1987. The average length of follow-up was six years. The family pedigrees were traced backward and laterally as far as possible. The genealogic studies were done by "genetic field workers" connected with the registration center. For each affected patient, the information collected included the age at diagnosis, the surgical and pathological findings, and the results of treatment. The data of deceased patients were obtained from medical records and autopsy reports. The screening program includes either colonoscopy or flexible sigmoidoscopy plus double-contrast barium enema. The intervals between examinations were two to three years.

RESULTS

The data of 24 families of 97 patients referred with signs or symptoms, or both, of colorectal cancer (group A) were collected. No relationship between the families has been established as yet. The total number of first-degree relatives was 264. One hundred and seventy-six (68 percent) of these relatives participated in the screening program. Twenty of them (11 percent) were found to have a colorectal neoplasm (group B). All these patients were asymptomatic and none of them had been screened previously. In 16 of the 20 patients, the colorectal lesions were found at the first screening visit, and in four they were found during follow-up. We compared these groups with respect to the stage of tumor growth. Histological examination of the tumors in group A (97 patients) revealed Dukes A carcinomas in six patients, Dukes B carcinomas in 43, Dukes C carcinomas in 24 and Dukes D carcinomas in 11 patients (classification unknown in 13 patients). In group B (20 patients) adenoma was found in 14 and carcinoma in six patients (Dukes A in two and Dukes B in four patients)(Table 1). A total of 103 patients, including those whose tumors were detected by screening, had a colorectal carcinoma. The age at diagnosis ranged from 24 to 81 years (mean age: 46 years). Fifty-two of the 97 patients from group A died from colorectal cancer. The mean age at death was 51 years (range: 27-81). The localization of the colonic tumors was proximal in 60%. Multiple primary tumors were found in 25% of the patients.

A total of 65 extracolonic tumors were found in the 24 HNPCC families. Endometrial cancer was found in 16 patients belonging to twelve families. The mean age at diagnosis in this group was 52 years (range: 33-79 years). In ten families there was only one relative with endometrial cancer. Twelve of the 16 patients had a second primary as well. Two of the 16 patients eventually died from endometrial cancer; these deaths occurred at the ages of 55 and 56 years. Six of the 16 patients have a child with a colon carcinoma (Table 2). Cancer of the stomach occurred in ten patients belonging to five families. The mean age at diagnosis was 46 years (range: 24-82 years). In four of these ten patients another primary was found. Six of the ten patients have a child with a colon carcinoma (Table 2). Six

Table 1. Pathologic stages of the colorectal tumors in the symptomatic group (A) and the call-up group (B).

		Group A	Group B
Number of patients		97	20
Mean age (years)		46	40
Range (years)		24-81	18-71
Colorectal adenoma only		0	14
Colorectal carcinoma		97	6
Classification	Dukes A	6	2
	Dukes B	43	4
	Dukes C	24	--
	Dukes D	11	--
	Unknown	13	--

Table 2 Relevant characteristics of patients with the most prevalent extra-colonic tumors.

	Number of Families	Number of Patients	Number of patients with second primary tumor	Number of patients with progeny having a tumor
Endometrial cancer	12	16	12	6
Stomach cancer	5	10	4	6
Urinary-tract tumor	4	8	7	3

Table 3. Distribution of location of extracolonic tumors in 24 HNPCC kindreds.

Location	Number	Percentage
Endometrium	16	24
Stomach	10	15
Urinary tract	8	12
Small bowel	5	8
Breast	5	8
Ovary	4	6
Pancreas	4	6
Brain	3	5
Prostate	3	5
Other sites	7	11
Total	65	100

patients died from cancer of the stomach (mean age: 48 years; range: 24-81). Tumors of the urinary tract were found in eight patients belonging to four families. The age at diagnosis ranged from 45 to 73 years (mean age 58 years). Multiple tumors of the urinary tract were found in five of the eight patients. Histologically all tumors were transitional carcinomas. In seven of the eight patients another type of cancer was diagnosed as well. Three of the eight patients had a child with a carcinoma. Two patients died from cancer of the urinary tract at the ages of 45 and 51 years, respectively. Other types of cancer were found as well, but with a lower frequency (Table 3).

DISCUSSION

Problems in Diagnosis

There are many difficulties in diagnosing HNPCC in a particular family under investigation. First, in HNPCC the diagnosis of hereditary cancer can not be made in the individual patient, as opposed to the situation in familial adenomatous polyposis. The latter syndrome can be diagnosed in a single patient by the observation of the characteristic multiple (more than 100) adenomatous colonic polyps, whereas the patient with HNPCC can only be identified as such by a combination of clinical and family data. Various criteria for the diagnosis of the syndrome have been proposed, one of which is the presence of colorectal cancer in three first-degree family members (Mecklin 1986). However, it is recognized that occurrence of a disease in three first-degree family members does nor prove the presence of an autosomal dominant disorder not does an autosomal dominant disorder have to be manifest in three first-degree relatives. Familial aggregation of cancer may be based on so called multifactorial inheritance, in which the action of several genes in combination with exogenous factors are assumed to be the cause of the disease. It can be very difficult or impossible to distinguish an autosomal dominant from a multifactorial pattern of inheritance in a particular family. Second, families are often small and medical data are often difficult to obtain, which further complicated the evaluation of a family history. Our kindreds were selected for the study if they had at least three first-degree relatives with colorectal cancer (sporadic vs hereditary CRC) and either or both of the following characteristics: early onset of colon cancer (under 45 years) and multiple primary colorectal tumors.

Value of screening

Periodic examination of families with HNPCC allows the detection of polyps and cancers at a presymptomatic and still localized stage. It seems almost self-evident that it would be beneficial to screen these families and to diagnose HNPCC before the development of overt symptoms. However, the implications of family investigations are so far-reaching that screening should be well-considered. The best way to prove the benefits of screening would be the demonstration by controlled studies of a prolonged survival rate or a decrease in morbidity. However, there is substantial evidence in the literature indicating a positive effect (Mecklin 1987). In addition, several studies (Albano 1982) have shown that patients in non-screened families had a shorter life expectancy. On the basis of these data, the performance of a randomized controlled trial would seem to be ruled out on ethical grounds. Another way to assess the effect of screening would be to compare the symptomatic (Group A) and the call-up group (Group B) with respect to the stage of the colonic neoplasm. The results of the present study show that in the absence of family screening, colorectal tumors were usually diagnosed clinically in a later stage. We consider this to be an indication of the effectiveness of our screening program.

National history

Knowledge of the natural history of the disease is important for deciding the age at which patients should be screened and for choosing an appropriate screening program. Studies (Mecklin 1987, Fitzgibbons 1987) have shown that the onset of colorectal cancer is usually 20 years earlier in families with HNPCC than in the general population. The highest incidence of colorectal carcinoma in the general population in The Netherlands occurs between 70 and 80 years of age. In this study the age at diagnosis ranged from 24 to 81 years (mean age: 47). The peak age at first manifestation of colorectal cancer was between 30 and 50 years in both men and women (Vasen 1989). These findings are in agreement with those of others (Mecklin 1987, Fitzgibbons 1987). The youngest patient with HNPCC reported in the literature was a 14-year-old girl (Aiges 1979). As far as we know, this is the only report of HNPCC before the age of 20, and this age could therefore be the lower limit for the start of the screening program. The screening protocol should include either colonoscopy or flexible sigmoidoscopy plus double-contrast barium enema. Once kindred members reach age 60, it becomes less likely that they will present with hereditary colorectal cancer (Lynch 1985, Mecklin 1986), and therefore most authors recommend continuation of screening up to the age of 60 years. However, 18 percent of our patients (Vasen 1989) and 14 percent of the patients in the study of Fitzgibbons (1987) were older than 60 when the tumor was diagnosed. On these grounds, we recommend lifelong screening, taking into account, of course, the subject's general physical health. Because of the high frequency of tumors in the proximal colon (60 percent in the present study), careful examination of the right colon is mandatory. On the basis of our data on the occurrence of multiple primary tumors, we recommend a subtotal colectomy with ileorectal anastomosis when a tumor is found.

Hereditary tumor spectrum

Because screening on a lifetime basis is very burdensome, relatives who are at risk should be selected with great care and one must know which types of extracolonic cancer belong to the hereditary tumor spectrum of HNPCC. Any of the following may constitute an indication that a certain type of cancer belongs to the hereditary tumor spectrum: (1) the occurrence of a certain type of cancer in several members of the family (and thus a high incidence of this type of cancer in a series of HNPCC families); (2) the coincidence of these tumors with other primaries, particularly of colorectal cancer, in the same patient; and (3) evidence that a patient with an extracolonic tumor transmits the trait, for example, that some of his children have developed colorectal cancer.

There is strong evidence that endometrial cancer should be considered part of the hereditary tumor spectrum (Mecklin 1986, Fitzgibbons 1987, Vasen 1989). In our series it was the second most common type of carcinoma. In the majority of the patients the endometrial tumor occurred in combination with other types of cancer, particularly colorectal cancer. Six of the 16 patients appeared to transmit the trait, since they had children with colorectal cancer. On such grounds it seems reasonable at first glance to conclude that families in which endometrial cancer occurs should be screened for colorectal cancer and endometrial cancer. However, the value of screening for endometrial cancer in the general population is a matter of discussion (Pritchard 1989). The techniques available for the diagnosis of endometrial cancer are, unfortunately, far from ideal. The routine Papanicolaou smear is inadequate. The techniques used for endometrial biopsy to obtain cells for histological examination are relatively uncomfortable. Cytologic sampling of uterine cells can be done relatively painlessly in an out-patient setting, but has a low positive predictive value. Furthermore, no controlled trials have been performed to evaluate the effectiveness of screening for endometrial cancer. On the other hand, despite its relatively high incidence in Western countries, endometrial cancer is a less important cause of death among women. In view of these considerations, a group of investigators (Pritchard 1989) recently recommended that screening for endometrial cancer be omitted from the periodic examination of postmenopausal women in the general population. Screening of women from certain HNPCC families would be more successful, because the incidence in these families is much higher and the target group is small. Until more specific data become available we recommend screening in HNPCC families with endometrial carcinoma, with the exception of families with a single case of endometrial cancer diagnosed at an advanced age. Our screening protocol includes VABRA curettage once every two years, from the age of 30.

Cancer of the stomach is the third most common tumor reported in HNPCC families (Mecklin 1986). In the first HNPCC family described, i.e., by Warthin (Lynch 1971), stomach cancer had occurred in the earlier generations. Cancer of the stomach had occurred in the previous generation of our families too. Our findings indicate that carcinomas of the stomach should be considered to belong to the tumor spectrum in HNPCC families, and that the offspring of family members with these tumors should be included in the screening program for colorectal cancer. Because almost all of the cases of carcinoma of the stomach occurred in the older generations, screening for these tumors in the present generation does not seem useful. We found regular upper-GI endoscopy justifiable in only one of our families, i.e., one in which the incidence of stomach cancer was very high.

Tumours of the urinary tract also appear to be part of the spectrum in some of our families. Most of these families had more than one case with a urinary-tract tumor; in all but one of these patients, the tumor was concurrent with another type of cancer; and finally, patients with cancer of the urinary tract appear to transmit the gene, because they have children with colorectal cancer. All this means that the progeny should be screened for colorectal cancer and urinary-tract tumors. As far as we know, no data have been published concerning the optimal screening procedures for these tumors. Our screening policy calls for regular cytologic investigation of the urine.

In sum, as a general conclusion drawn from the present study, it may be said that in HNPCC families, carcinoma of the endometrium, stomach, and urinary tract should be considered to belong to the hereditary tumor spectrum. Definite assignment of any given tumor to this spectrum must await the availability of a sensitive and specific biomarker.

REFERENCES

Aiges HW, Kahm E, Silverberg M (1979) Adenocarcinoma of the colon in an adolescent with the family cancer syndrome. J Pediatr 94: 632-633

Albano W, Recabaven JA, Lynch HT, et al (1982) Natural history of hereditary cancer of the breast and colon. Cancer 50: 360-363

Boland CR, Troncale FJ (1984) Familial colonic cancer in the absence of antecedent polyposis. Ann Intern Med 100: 700-701

Fitzgibbons RJ, Lynch HT, Stanislav GV (1987) Recognition and treatments of patient with hereditary nonpolyposis colon cancer (Lynch syndromes I and II) Ann Surg 206: 289-295

Lynch HT, Krush AJ (1971) Cancer family "G" revisited: 1895-1970. Cancer 27: 1505-1511

Lynch HT, Lynch PM, Albano WA, Lynch JF (1981) The cancer syndrome: A status report. Dis Colon Rectum 24: 311-321

Lynch HT, Kimberling N, Albano WA, Lynch JF, Biscomne K, Schuelke GS, Sandberg AA, Lipkin M, Peschner EE, Mikol YB, Elston RC, Bailey-Wilson JE, Danes BS (1985) Hereditary nonpolyposis colorectal cancer (Lynch syndromes I and II) 1. Clinical description of resource. Cancer 56: 934-938

Mecklin J-P, Järvinen HJ (1986) Clinical features of colorectal carcinoma in cancer family syndrome. Dis Colon Rectum 29: 160-164

Mecklin JP, Järvinen HJ, Elomaa J, Karjalainen K. (1987) Screening for colorectal carcinoma in cancer family syndrome kindreds. Scand J Gastroenterol 22: 449-453

Mecklin JP (1987) Cancer Family Syndrome. Studies on the hereditary nonpolyposis colorectal carcinoma syndrome. Thesis. Helsinki.

Pritchard KI (1989) Screening for endometrial cancer: is it effective? Ann Int Med 100: 177-179

Vasen HFA, Nieuwenhuijzen Kruseman AC, Berkel J, Beukers EKM, Delprat CC, van Doorn LG, Geerdink RA, Haak HR, Hackeng WHL, Koppeschaar HPF, Krenning EP, Lamberts SWJ, Lekkerkerker JFF, Michels RPJ, Moers AMJ, Pieters GFFM, Wiersinga WM, Lips CJM (1987) The MEN-2 syndrome: the value of screening and central registration. A study of fifteen kindreds in The Netherlands. Am J Med 83: 847-852

Vasen HFA, den Hartog Jager FCA, Menko FH, Nagengast FM (1989) Screening for hereditary non-polyposis colorectal cancer. A study of twenty-two kindreds in The Netherlands. Am J Med 86: 278-281

Wilson JMG, Junger G. (1968) Principles and practise of screening for disease. Geneva. Switzerland: WHO

The Risks of Colorectal Cancer and the Frequency of Recognised Family Cancer Syndromes in 550 Sequential Referrals for Family Risk of Colorectal Cancer

JOAN SLACK

Key Words: COLORECTAL CANCER FAMILY CANCER SYNDROMES OCCULT BLOOD
ADENOMATOUS POLYPS COLONOSCOPY

Three years ago Dr. Victoria Murday and I opened a clinic at St. Mark's Hospital for family members who were concerned about their risks of colorectal cancer. The clinic was part of a Regional Genetic Service in one of the four Metropolitan London Regions and was supported by the Imperial Cancer Research Fund who provided the genetic nursing sister.

The life time risk of death from colorectal cancer in England and Wales is 1 in 50, increasing rapidly with age.

Surgical treatment for bowel cancer is disappointing with an acknowledged survival rate for patients undergoing surgery with a view to cure of 50%.

Morson (1983) pointed out that the majority of colorectal carcinomas arise in pre-existing adenomas and the hypothesis of the adenoma-carcinoma sequence offers an opportunity for the early diagnosis and treatment if polyps can be identified. Population screening using faecal occult blood tests have generally been found to have a low yield and only moderate compliance. There is therefore a need to explore other approaches to prevention.

In an unselected series of patients attending St. Mark's with colorectal cancer, Lovett (1976) described an increase of deaths from colorectal cancer in 1st degree relatives. She found an overall three-fold increase in 1st degree relatives and noted a high risk in the families of patients under 45. Lovett's pedigrees have been used to examine the risks to relatives by life table methods.

Table I shows the risks of colorectal cancer in 1st degree relatives of index patients under and over 45 years of age, compared to the population risk in England and Wales in 1985.

Table I

LIFETIME RISK OF 1ST DEGREE RELATIVES OF PATIENTS WITH COLORECTAL CANCER
(Calculated from Lovett's series, 1976)

INDEX PATIENTS	RISK TO 1st DEGREE RELATIVE	
45 & under	x 5	1 in 10
Over 45	x 3	1 in 17
Population risk		1 in 50

Table II

EMPIRIC RISKS TO 1ST DEGREE RELATIVES
(Estimated from Lovett's series 1976)

RELATIVES AFFECTED	RISK
One relative affected	1:17
Two relatives (1 + 2)	1:12
One relative < 45 years	1:10
Two relatives 1	1: 6
Dominant pedigree	1: 2

Lovett also drew attention to an increase in risk of breast and stomach cancer in the female relatives and in male relatives a nearly two fold increase in the risk of stomach cancers was found. A two-fold increase in deaths from prostatic cancer failed to reach statistical significance.

Table II shows the estimated risk of colorectal cancer in relatives of patients with colorectal cancer. The empiric risks are based on data from Lovett's pedigrees.

With one affected first degree relative over 45 the risk is 1 in 17, with 2 affected relatives such as a parent and grandparent over 45 the empiric risk is 1 in 12. For 1st degree relatives of young patients of 45 or less the life time risk is just under 1 in 10. When 2 first degree relatives such as a parent and sib are affected, regardless of age, the empiric risk is 1 in 6, and when dominant inheritance is indicated by the family tree the risk of the liability to 1st degree relatives is 1 in 2.

With the risks calculated an arbitary decision was made to offer screening by colonoscopy to look for premalignant polyps in family members whose life time risk was 1 in 10 or more. Since reports from various authors, reviewed by Lynch et al (1988) suggest that the average age at which polyps can be detected in families susceptible to colorectal cancer is between 40 and 45, it was decided to offer screening by colonoscopy 5 yearly between aged 25 and 60, increasing this to 3 yearly if polyps were found. For those with risks between 1 in 10 and 1 in 17, annual screening by faecal occult blood was offered and the Haemoccult test was used.

The Family Cancer Clinic was publicised in the National Press and unusually for a National Health Service Clinic a decision was made to accept patients who referred themselves directly as well as those referred by family doctors and hospital consultants.

Table III shows the source of referrals of patients who came to the clinic. 51% were self referrals. 12% came from general practitioners at the instigation of the patients. Referrals from general practitioners have been increasing over the three years the clinic has been running and direct GP referrals now provide 21% of new patients.

We decided to talk to patients and relatives frankly about their life time risks of cancer, encouraging families to communicate information between themselves and to take responsibility for their screening programmes.

Of the first 550 patients who attended the clinic 356 patients had a life time risk of 1 in 10,167 had a risk between 1 in 10 and 1 in 17, and 26 patients were themselves affected but required further screening. 82% of the patients attending the clinic required screening and 70% at the higher risk required colonoscopy.

Table III

SOURCE OF REFERRALS TO FAMILY CANCER CLINIC		
REFERRAL	NO.	%
SELF	283	51%
PATIENT VIA GP	64	12%
GP	116	21%
HOSPITAL CONSULTANT	81	15%
OTHER (SCREENING PROGRAMS)	6	1%
TOTAL	550	

Table IV

RESULT OF SCREENING BY OCCULT BLOOD TEST		
REFERRAL	1ST SCREEN	2ND SCREEN
NO. OFFERED	130	71
NO RETURNED	121	65
COMPLIANCE	93%	91.5%
TEST +VE	2	1
POLYPS	1	1

Table IV shows the result of screening by occult blood tests. Of the patients offered screening by Haemoccult, 130 have been offered their first screening kit, and 71 have reached the 2nd screen. The compliance for the 1st test was 93% and for the 2nd test 91%. Positive occult blood tests were reported on 3 patients, who went on to colonoscopy. Two were found to have polyps, one with enterocolitis. The third patient had ulcerative colitis.

316 have been examined by colonoscopy.

Table V shows the results of screening patients by colonoscopy. Of the 155 patients whose risk was estimated to be 1 in 2, 31 were found to have adenomatous polyps. Their mean age was 49. Three were found to have colon cancer. In 2 benign colonic polyps were so numerous that colectomy was performed. Of the 119 patients who had colonoscopy because their risk was estimated to be between 1 in 10 and 1 in 2, 14 were found to have polyps. Their mean age was 50. Colonoscopy was performed on 26 patients who were themselves affected with colorectal cancer. Of these 8 were found to have polyps and two metachronous colon cancer. 16 patients were screened by colonoscopy because though their risk was less than 1 in 10 they had symptoms such as rectal bleeding or positive occult blood tests. Of these 3 were found to have polyps.

Haemoccult blood tests were performed by 40 patients prior to colonoscopy. Two tests were positive due to bleeding from ulcerative colitis. Of the 38 negative tests 10 patients had adenomatous polyps, one with carcinoma in situ.

Of the 550 patients seen because of their concern about their family risk of colorectal cancer, 164 showed evidence of dominant inheritance in their family trees and were estimated to have a 1 in 2 risk of inheriting the family liability.

Table V

RESULTS OF SCREENING BY COLONOSCOPY

ADENOMATOUS POLYPS FOUND ON COLONOSCOPY

RISK	NO.	NO. WITH POLYPS	PERCENTAGE
1 in 2	155	31	20
1 in 2-1 in 10	119	14	11.7
AFFECTED	26	8	30.7
1 in 12 with symptoms	16	3	18.7

Table VI

DOMINANTLY INHERITED SYNDROMES IDENTIFIED AMONG 550 FAMILIES SEEN IN CLINIC

SYNDROMES IDENTIFIED	NO. PATIENTS AT RISK	NO WITH POLYPS
SITE SPECIFIC COLON CANCER	58	14
FAMILY CANCER SYNDROME	82	11
FAMILIAL ADENOMATOUS POLYPOSIS	9	2
OTHER SYNDROMES COWDEN'S, MUIRS, GORLIN'S, MULTIPLE LIPOMATA	24	1

Table VI shows the dominantly inherited syndromes identified in the 550 families seen. 58 patients showed evidence of site specific colon cancer and among these 14 were found to have adenomatous polyps. 82 patients showed evidence of Family Cancer Syndrome as described by Lynch. Of these 11 were found to have polyps. 35 women from these families were offered mammography and 4 were found to have breast cancer. 22 women were offered pelvic ultrasound but no pelvic cancer was found.

Nine patients from three families previously undiagnosed were found to be at 1 in 2 risk of Familial Adenomatous Polyposis, and two have been found to have multiple polyps requiring prophylactic colectomy.

24 patients were found to have signs of recognisable syndromes including characteristic features of Cowdens, Torre Muir and Gorlin's syndrome and multiple lipomata. We found that the larger the kindred the greater the probability that signs of these syndromes would overlap within families and are therefore doubtful whether homogeneous groups with named syndromes can be distinguished unless exceptionally large kindreds are available. Genetic markers may eventually identify specific syndromes.

We conclude that a family history can be used to identify patients whose relatives are at increased risk of premalignant polyps. Those at highest risk are first degree relatives of patients who develop colorectal cancer under the age of 45 or whose pedigrees give evidence of dominant inheritance of site specific colon cancer, or one of the Family Cancer Syndromes. For patients at risk of Family Cancer Syndrome there is evidence that breast screening may detect malignant change.

From the onset we have been aware that we might arouse further distress and anxiety amongst a vulnerable population by discussing numerical risks and confronting the possibilities of malignancy.

Our experience has been reassuring. Our genetic sister has been able to assess reactions after consultation while organising appointments for screening, after colonoscopy and during home visits. While no statistical analysis has been attempted, we have been left with a firm impression that this group of patients has been relieved to discuss the family risks of which they have usually been aware, and have derived support by undertaking a screening programme for which they have taken a personal responsibility.

REFERENCES:

Lovett E (1976) Family studies in cancer of the colon and rectum. Br. J. Surg. 63. 13 - 18.

Lynch H H, Watson P, Lanspa S J, et al (1988) Natural history of colerectal cancer in hereditary non polyposis colorectal cancer. (Lynch syndromes I and II). Dis. Colon Rectum. 31 439-444

Morson, B C, Bussey H J R, Daw D W, and Hill M J (1983) Adenomas of large bowel. Cancer Surveys 2. 451 - 477.

The Incidence of Colorectal Cancer Among First Degree Relatives of Patients with Colorectal Cancer

JENS O. SØNDERGAARD, STEFFEN BÜLOW, and ELSEBETH LYNGE

ABSTRACT

During 1982-1984 1524 Danish patients had colorectal cancer at an age of less than 60 years. Their parents were identified and searced in the Danish Cancer Registry. Among these, a significantly increased observed/expected number had colorectal cancer (both sexes) and gastric cancer (males). Our result confirms previous indications of a genetic factor in the pathogenesis of colorectal cancer, and we therefore recommend regular screening of children of colorectal cancer patients.

Keywords: Family History, Colorectal Cancer, Familial Cancer.

Retrospective epidemiological studies have shown that relatives of colorectal cancer patients have an increased risk of developing colorectal cancer. This studies are based upon informations given by the patients, and most series are small.
In order to use a family history of colorectal cancer as a marker to select high risk persons for screening, the results should be based on larger materials and based on verified medical informations.
We therefore decided to examine the cancer incidence among parents of patients with colorectal cancer registered in the Danish Cancer Registry, which was established in 1943.

MATERIAL AND METHODS.

From January 1982 to December 1984, 1528 cancer of the colon or rectum were reported to the Danish Cancer Registry in patients aged less than 60 years. These cancer cases in total represented 1.524 cancer patients = index persons.
The parents of these patients were traced in the administrative registers. First, the parish of birth of each index person was found in the Central Population Register (CPR). Second, the parish registers were asked about name, date of birth, address, and other available information on the parents. Third, identified parents were searched in the CPR and their personal identification number and a possible date of death or emigration was registered. Fourth, the municipality population registers were asked about date of death or emigration of identified parents who could not be found in the CPR. Finally, the National Death Index was searched for date of death of identified parents.
The fully traced parents were searched in the Danish Cancer Registry for incident cancer diagnosed in the period January 1943 to December 1986.

Only parents still living in Denmark on January 1943 were included in the analysis. The individual risk period for parents started on the day of birth of the index person or January 1 1943, which ever came last, and ended on the date of death/emigration, or December 31 1986, which ever came first.

All tumours diagnosed during the individual risk periods were included in the analysis. Expected numbers of cancer were based on cancer incidence rates for the Danish population for sex, 5-year age groups, and the following calendar periods: 1963-67, ... 1983-85. The PYRS program was used for calculation of expected numbers. Standardized incidence ratios (SIR) were calculated by dividing the observed number of cancer cases by the expected number.

The 1524 index persons had a total of 1478 eligible mothers, of whom 1411 (96%) were successfully traced, and a total of 1414 eligible fathers, of whom 1364 (96%) were traced.

RESULTS.

The observed number of all cancer cases 1943-1986 in parents of index patients with colorectal cancer was 783 (28%) versus the expected 721 (26%), SIR = 1.09, (NS).
This number of cancer cases represented 43 different cancer types.
A significantly increased ratio was found in colorectal cancer in both sexes and in males with gastric cancer. (Table 1 and 2).

Table 1. Observed and expected number of cancer cases 1943-86 in fathers of patients with colorectal cancer.

	observed	expected	SIR
Colon	56	28	2.0
Rectum	47	27	1.8
Stomach	56	37	1.5

Table 2. Observed and expected number of cancer cases 1943-86 in mothers of patients with colorectal cancer.

	observed	expected	SIR
Colon	62	32	1.9
Rectum	21	18	1.2
Stomach	22	19	1.2
Corpus uteri	29	20	1.5
Cervix uteri	26	27	0.9
Breast	56	69	0.8

DISCUSSION

The incidence of colorectal cancer among parents of patients with colorectal cancer was nearly twice the expected incidence. This result confirms previous studies and indicates that asymtomatic adult relatives of colorectal cancer patients have an increased risk of developing this tumour.
On this basis we recommend that children above the age of 40 years should be screened by fecal occult blood examination at intervals of 3-5 years and subjected to colonoscopy if woccult bleeding is found.

Genetics of Adenomas

RANDALL W. BURT and D. TIMOTHY BISHOP

ABSTRACT

Current research suggests that inherited susceptibility contributes to the pathogenesis of colonic adenomatous polyps in most individuals with these neoplasms. Highly penetrant inherited factors cause adenomas in adenomatous polyposis and in the hereditary nonpolyposis (Lynch) syndromes. Partially penetrant but more common inherited susceptibilities appear to be a factor in the pathogenesis of common or "sporadic" colonic neoplasms. Molecular genetic research has identified the chromosomal location of the genetic defect in adenomatous polyposis. Further work should elucidate the function of this gene and should likewise define the genetic defects for the nonpolyposis syndromes and the common inherited susceptibilities.

Keywords: adenomatous polyp, colon cancer, inheritance

INTRODUCTION

Inherited factors play an important role in the pathogenesis of adenomatous polyps and colorectal cancer. Recent research indicates that inherited susceptibility may be a factor in a large fraction, and possibly even the majority, of cases of adenomatous polyps. There are three levels or categories of adenomatous polyp inheritance. These are the colonic polyposis syndromes, the "nonpolyposis" inherited conditions of colorectal cancer and the common adenomatous polyps, which are variously referred to as "discrete," "solitary" or "sporadic" adenomas.

SYNDROMES

Hundreds to thousands of colonic adenomatous polyps are observed in the polyposis syndromes, both adenomatous polyposis coli (APC) and Gardner syndrome (GS) (Haggitt 1986). In these conditions multiple adenomas are inherited as a highly penetrant autosomal dominant trait. Polyps develop at a young age and cancer is inevitable if colectomy is not undertaken. APC and GS are rare, however, and together account for less than 1% of individuals with adenomatous polyps or colorectal cancer.

Somewhat more common is the syndrome of hereditary nonpolyposis colorectal cancer (HNPCC) (Lynch 1988). HNPCC is also inherited in an autosomal dominant fashion, although affected individuals express only one or several adenomatous polyps. There is an equally high risk for colon cancer in this syndrome despite the smaller number of polyps. Additional characteristics include early age onset of cancer, a predilection for proximal colonic neoplasms, and a higher than expected rate of synchronous malignancies. HNPCC may account for as many as 5-6% of individuals with adenomatous polyps and colon cancer (Mecklin 1987).

FAMILIAL AGGREGATION OF COLON CANCER AND ADENOMAS

There appear to be familial factors important to the pathogenesis of colonic adenomatous polyps in addition to the well characterized syndromes of APC, GS and HNPCC. Genetic epidemiologic studies have consistently demonstrated that first-degree relatives of those with colon cancer have a three-fold or greater risk of acquiring colon malignancy (Woolf 1958, Macklin 1960, Lovett 1976, Duncan 1982). Recent investigations have demonstrated that first-degree relatives of those with adenomatous polyps have a similar increased risk for colon cancer (Maire 1984, Ponz de Leon 1987, Kune 1987, Rozen 1987, Rozen 1987). Because monogenic inheritance patterns generally have not been apparent in these population studies, it has been suggested that common familial clustering of polyps and cancer might occur on the basis of polygenic inheritance, mendelian inheritance with decreased penetrance, or environmental factors common to family members.

PEDIGREE STUDIES

We recently studied a large kindred to clarify which of the possible mechanisms accounted for familial clustering of colonic neoplasms (Burt 1985). The kindred selected contained a number of cases of colon cancer, but no mendelian patterns of inheritance were present when cancer cases alone were considered. Age of cancer diagnosis and colonic distribution of tumors were typical of the general population. Subjects were screened by 60 cm flexible proctosigmoidoscopy to determine the presence of colonic polyps. Family members exhibited a significant increased prevalence of adenomatous polyps compared to spouse controls. Pedigree analysis was then performed considering adenomas in addition to colon cancer as the positive phenotype. The analysis indicated that autosomal dominant inheritance with partial penetrance was significantly more likely to be the cause of familial clustering of polyps and cancer than recessive inheritance or random clustering.

To determine the frequency of the gene or genes which give susceptibility to adenomatous polyps, 33 additional smaller kindreds were systematically selected and investigated (Cannon-Albright 1988). Kindreds were chosen on the basis of an individual with an adenomatous polyp, or a sibling pair with colon cancer. An excess of adenomas was consistently observed in family members. When all kindreds were considered together, pedigree analysis again indicated that a partially penetrant gene (or genes) was the most likely explanation for the familial clustering of neoplasms. The estimated gene frequency in the population studied was 19%. The most likely model indicated that all observed adenomas arose, at least in part, from inherited susceptibility. The 95% confidence limits for this result, however, ranged from 53 to 100%. Larger sample sizes and other populations are needed to refine the analysis estimates and to verify the findings.

These results suggest that a gene (or genes) which confers susceptibility to colonic adenomatous polyps is common and accounts for a significant fraction of clinically observed adenomas. Given the known association of certain environmental factors to colon cancer, it is likely that environmental factors determine whether polyps and finally cancers are expressed in genetically susceptible individuals.

MOLECULAR GENETICS

Molecular genetic investigations have demonstrated that the genetic defect responsible for both APC and GS is found on the long arm of chromosome 5, now referred to as the APC locus (Nakamura 1988). In a recent study, loss of alleles of APC locus markers correlated with deregulation of c-myc oncogene expression (Erisman 1989). This finding suggests that the normal function of the APC locus may be to regulate expression of the c-myc oncogene. Mutations at the APC locus may also play a role in inherited polyp susceptibility separate from APC and GS. In one large pedigree in which the polyp phenotype linked to the APC locus, only two individuals exhibited polyposis typical of APC. Many others had only a few adenomas or even a single adenoma, but nonetheless demonstrated linkage to the APC locus (see R. White, this volume). Further studies are underway to examine linkage of the APC locus to HNPCC and to familial clusters of common adenomatous polyps.

There is evidence that acquired mutations at the APC locus are often found in "random" adenomatous polyps, especially larger polyps, and in colorectal cancers (Vogelstein 1988). Several additional acquired genetic mutations also are consistently observed in such neoplastic tissues. These include mutations on chromosomes 17p and 18q, as well as mutations of the K-ras oncogene. These loci of acquired mutations are also candidate loci for the investigation of the purported gene or genes which give rise to inherited susceptibility to common adenomatous polyps.

ACKNOWLEDGEMENTS

This research was supported by Public Health Service Awards 28854 and CA-40641.

REFERENCES

Burt RW, Bishop DT, Cannon LA, Dowdell MA, Lee RG, Skolnick MH: Dominant inheritance of adenomatous colonic polyps and colorectal cancer. N Engl J Med 1985; 312:1540-1544.

Cannon-Albright LA, Skolnick MH, Bishop T, Lee RG, Burt RW: Common inheritance of susceptibility to colonic adenomatous polyps and associated colorectal cancers. N Engl J Med 1988; 319:533-537.

Duncan JL, Kyle J: Family incidence of carcinoma of the colon and rectum in north-east Scotland. Gut 1982; 23:169-171.

Erisman MD, Scott JK, Astrin SM: Evidence that the familial adenomatous polyposis gene is involved in a subset of colon cancers with a complementable defect in c-myc regulation. Proc Natl Acad Sci 1989; 86:4264-4268.

Guillem JG, Neugut AI, Forde KA, Waye JD, Treat MR: Colonic neoplasms in asymptomatic first-degree relatives of colon cancer patients. Am J Gastroenterol 1988; 83:271-273.

Haggitt RC, Reid BJ: Hereditary gastrointestinal polyposis syndromes. Am J Surg Pathol 1986; 10:871-887.

Kune GA, Kune S, Watson LF: The Melbourne colorectal cancer study. Characterization of patients with a family history of colorectal cancer. Dis Colon Rectum 1987;30:600-606.

Lovett E: Family studies in cancer of the colon and rectum. Br J Surg 1976; 63:13-18.

Lynch HT, Watson P, Kriegler M, et al: Differential diagnosis of hereditary nonpolyposis colorectal cancer (Lynch syndrome I and Lynch syndrome II). Dis Colon Rectum 1988; 31:372-377.

Macklin MT: Inheritance of cancer of the stomach and large intestine in man. J Nat Cancer Inst 1960; 24:551-571.

Maire P, Morichau-Beauchant M, Drucker J, Barboteau M-A, Barbier J, Matuchansky C. Familiar prevalence of colorectal cancer: A 3 year case-control study. Gastroenterol Clin Biol 1984; 8:22-27.

Mecklin J-P: Frequency of hereditary colorectal carcinoma, Gastroenterology 1987; 93:1021-1025.

Nakamura Y, Lathrop M, Leppert M, et al: Localization of the genetic defect in familial adenomatous polyposis within a small region of chromosome 5. Am J Hum Genet 1988; 43:638-644.

Ponz de Leon M, Antonioli A, Ascari A, Zanghieri G, Sacchetti C: Incidence and familial occurrence of colorectal cancer and polyps in a health-care district of northern Italy. Cancer 1987; 60:2848-2859.

Rozen P, Lynch HT, Figer A, et al: Familial colon cancer in the Tel-Aviv area and the influence of ethnic origin. Cancer 1987; 60:2355-2359.

Rozen P, Fireman Z, Figer A, Legum C, Ron E, Lynch HT: Family history of colorectal cancer as a marker of potential malignancy within a screening program. Cancer 1987; 60:248-254.

Vogelstein B, Fearon ER, Hamilton SR, et al: Genetic alterations during colorectal tumor development. N Engl J Med 1988; 319:525-532.

Woolf CM: A genetic study of carcinoma of the large intestine. Am J Hum Genet 1958; 10:42-47.

Surveillance of High Risk Individuals with Family History using Guaiac Test (Hemoccult II)

L. BERTARIO, P. SALA, P. SPINELLI, L. GENNARI, G. BALLARDINI, and M. VIDALE

ABSTRACT

From 1979 to 1989 at Istituto Nazionale Tumori of Milan, 2,629 individuals at high risk for Family History of Large Bowel Cancer (first degree relatives) were screened by guaiac test combined with endoscopy. The test was positive in 95 patients (3.6%), 88 out of them (92%) and 545 H- (21.5%) accepted the endoscopic examinations. 27 colorectal cancers (21 H+, 6 H-) and 89 patients with adenomas (23 H+, 66 H-), mostly in the left side of bowel, were detected. During the follow-up (median 67 mths) 1,492 individuals (60%) were rescreened: 5 cancers and 50 pts. with adenomas were detected. Instead in the non responders group 3 cancers and 4 adenomas were diagnosed (median interval between cancer, adenoma in H-: 26 mths, 24 mths). The overall prevalence for cancers was 1.3% and 5.5% for adenomas. The sensitivity of the test for cancers and adenomas was calculated in about 77% and 29% with a specificity of 98%. The data confirm the opportunity to screen individuals at high risk for family history suggesting annual rescreening.

KEY WORDS: High risk, Screening, First relative, Family history.

INTRODUCTION

Medical literature provides substantial evidence that family history is a factor likely to cause a three to fourfold increase in Large Bowel Cancer risk (Ponz de Leon 1987; Rozen 1987; Mecklin 1987; Lynch 1986; Lovett 1976). On the other hand, both the high prevalence of the disease and the lack of adequate primary prevention seem to justify the use of early detection methods. For all of these reasons, a long-term program was initiated at I.N.T. of Milan a few years back for screening first degree relatives of patients with colorectal cancers, and a number of screening patterns were developed involving periodical guaiac tests (Hemoccult II +/- rehydration), as well as rectosigmoidoscopy. While the effectiveness of this screening in reducing mortality rate has not been proved so far, it is the aim of this report to assess the latest surveillance results from the above program.

METHODOLOGY

Surveillance involved rescreening of all subjects who - when previously examined with guaiac test (Hemoccult II) - had reported a proved family history with at least one first degree relative suffering from large-bowel cancer. Participants were on a standard high fiber, meat free diet before undergoing the test. All slides were examined within two days of collection of the last stool samples. Results were classified as positive (H+) whenever one of several test samples submitted turned blue. As from March 1983 - based on published data (Macrae 1982) - tests were rehydrated (rH). The subjects found to be positive (H+) underwent the following sequence of examinations to identify the source of bleeding: rectosigmoidoscopy, double contrast barium enema x-ray or colonoscopy and, when appropriate, gastroscopy. Endoscopy (preferably flexible rectosigmoidoscopy) was recommended for H- patients, even when symptom-free. Patients that were found negative on first testing were requested to undergo furher annual examination and specifically summoned if they failed to do so. The carcinoma cases detected were classified according to Duke's criteria. Estimates included only patients with histologically confirmed adenomas exceeding 5 mm. in diameter as measured by the pathologist.

RESULTS

In the period January 1979 to June 1989, a screening program based on guaiac tests (Hemoccult II) was conducted at I.N.T. of Milan, involving some 25,000 subjects. 2,629 individuals (10.5%) reported at least one first-degree relative with large-bowel cancer; 1,987 individuals (75%) reported only one first-degree relative with cancer. The male/female ratio (0.6) as well as distributions according to age and neoplastic prevalence are given in table 1. 3.4% of subjects examined were symptomatic (<6 mths). On initial screening, the rate of positive tests was 3.6% (95 individuals). The result and compliance for diagnostic work-up are shown in table 2. As can be noted, 24% of the patients (21.5% H-, 92% H+) underwent endoscopic examination (colonoscopy in 55% of the H- cases). 27 carcinomas were thus detected (21 H+, 6 H-) - 8 (6 H+, 2 H-) of which symptomatic - as well as 89 adenomas (23 H+, 66 H-). Most neoplastic lesions observed were located below the splenic flexure (table 3). During the follow-up (median 67 mths), as shown in table 4, 1,492 patients (60%) underwent at least a second test with an average of 4 tests per patient, the interval mean between test I and test II being 28 months (table 5). Compliance to repeated tests decreased progressively (12% with 5 or >5 H). 13% of the patients subjected to rescreening underwent endoscopy, resulting in detection of 5 carcinomas (3 H+, 2 "intervals") and 50 adenomas (17 H+, 28 H- and 5 "intervals") 3 cases of carcinoma and 4 of adenomas were detected among nonresponders.

Table 1. Distribution by age and prevalence of neoplastic diseases

Age	Pts	I H		Follow-up		Ca+Ad
		Ca	Ad	Ca	Ad	%
0-39	373	0	1	0	1	0.5
40-49	818	2	27	2	13	5.3
50-59	785	8	31	1	19	7.5
60-69	441	6	20	4	13	9.7
> 70	213	11	10	2	8	14.5
Prev. Ca.		10/1,000		3/1,000		
Ad.		33/1,000		30/1,000		

Table 2. Compliance to the diagnostic work-up for H- and H+ patients

Test	%	No exam.	End. ex.	%	Ca	Ad
rH-		399	161	28.7	2	17
rH+	4.7	4	24	85.7	7	7
H-		1590	384	19.4	4	49
H+	3.2	3	64	95.5	14	16
		1996	633		27	89

Table 3. Site of neoplastic disease

Site	I test				Follow-up			
	Ca	%	Ad	%	Ca	%	Ad	%
<Spl. Flex.	21	77	78	88	8	100	43	80
>Spl. Flex.	6	23	11	12	-	-	11	20
	27		89		8		54	

Table 4. Follow-up of H- patients at the initial screening.

Follow-up: median 67 months

	No rescreening	Rescreening (mean H: 4/pts.)
patients	1,021	1,492
mean age	52 years	51 years
median	54 months	87 months
other npls.	12	21
deaths	30	22
Ca.	3	5 (3 H+, 2 intervals)
Ad.	4	50 (18 H+, 5 intervals)

Median: IH/Ca: 49 mths (3-92); IH/Ad: 34 mths (6-95)
Ca/H-: 27 mths (3-92); Ad/H-: 24 mths (6-59)

Table 5. Results of rescreening in 1,492 patients.

N. Test	rH				H				Total
	-		+		-		+		
II	495	8 Ad	19	1 Ca 4 Ad	960	3 Ad	18	1 Ca 4 Ad	1,492
III	321	5 Ad	22	3 Ad	584	6 Ad	8	1 Ca 4 Ad	935
IV	166		6		379	2 Ad	3	1 Ad	554
V	102	4 Ad	10	1 Ad	220		0		332

Mean I/II H: 28 months (+/- 16 months)

A comparison between neoplastic locations on initial and on subsequent tests is provided in table 3 (85% of the lesions observed were located below the splenic flexure); 75% of the carcinoma cases were classified as Duke's A-B. Validity parameters of the test and for the use of rehydration on initial or subsequent tests are reported in table 6, showing a significant reduction in both the predictive value and specificity in rescreening with rehydrated tests.

DISCUSSION

Our experience seems to confirm that family history is a determinant in age-related risk for large-bowel cancer (table 1): no cancer cases were detected among patients under 40 years. The prevalence observed was consistent with that reported in other published data, specially in reference to the number of patients subjected to endoscopy (carcinomas 4%, adenomas 14%). (Love 1984, Grossman 1988, Roze 1987, Gryska 1987). As family history failed to be investigated in detail, it was not possible to relate the level of risk to the number of relatives with cancer. Screening results (table 6) were similar to those from previous experiences. (Simon 1985, Bertario 1988). However, it should be noted that rehydration was shown to result in drastically lower specificity during rescreening and should therefore be discouraged. No conclusive sensitivity for cancer amounted to 77% (80% rH, 70% H) including the 4 cancer cases diagnosed within 24 months from the Ist test. No significant increase in sensitivity was observed when using rehydrated tests, as a result both of the lower number of carcinomas detected and of the different percent rate of patients actually subjected to negative tests. As only 1 of 4 adenomas versus 3 of 4 carcinomas can be detected using the Hemoccult test, a few authors have suggested that Hemoccult should be combined with endoscopic examination when screening high-risk populations. (Grossman 1988, Winawer 1982, Rozen 1987, Eddy 1987) Since compliance to endoscopy was found to be poor in H- patients, a decisive assessment in this respect can hardly be made even though a fair neoplastic prevalence was observed. The serious cost problem posed by the need for further diagnostic investigations applies essentially to adenomas because of their natural history. (Stryker 1987). The prevalent distribution of both carcinomas and adenomas

Table 6. Validity parameters of Hemoccult with or without rehydration.

		I test	Rescreening	
rH +		4.7%	5.0%	*
H +		3.2%	1.3%	
Pred. value	rH	58.3%	15.7%	*
Ca+Ad	H	46.8%	34.3%	
Specif.	rH	98.0%	95.4%	*
Ca+Ad	H	98.0%	98.9%	
Sensit. Ad	rH	29.0%	32.0%	
	H	24.0%	45.0%	
Sensit. Ca	rH	77.0%	81.0%	overall
	H	77.0%	70.0%	

* p 0.01

in the left colon suggests that patients should be subjected to rectosigmoidoscopy. The median interval (about 24 months) between the occurrence of neoplastic lesions and previous H- findings (table 4) suggests that tests should be repeated within 12 months.

Finally, although no conclusion can be drawn at this stage as to the effectiveness of systematic screening in actually reducing the rate of mortality, emphasis should be placed on the fact that overall survival for cancers was about 85% at 5 years (median follow-up 60 months).

REFERENCES

Bertario L, Spinelli P, Gennari L, Sala P, Pizzetti P, Severini A, Cozzi G, Bellomi M and Berrino F (1988) Sensitivity of Hemoccult test for large bowel cancer in high risk subjects. Dig. Dis. Science 33: 609-613.

Eddy DM, Nugent FW, Eddy JF, Coller J, Gilbersen V, Gottlieb LS, Rice R, Sherlock P, Winawer S (1987) Screening for colorectal cancer in high risk population: results of mathematical model. Gastroenterology 92: 682-692.

Grossman S, Milos ML (1988) Colonoscopic screening of persons with suspected risk factors for colon cancer I: family history. Gastroenterology 94: 395-400.

Gryska P, Cohen AM (1987) Screening of asymptomatic patients at high risk for colon cancer with full colonoscopy. Dis. Col. Rect. 30: 18-20.

Love RR, Morcissey JF (1984) Colonoscopy in asymtomatic individuals with a family history of colorectal cancer. Arch. Intern. Med. 220: 9-11.

Lovett E, (1976) Family studies in cancer of the colon and rectum. Br. J. Surg. 65: 13-18.

Lynch HT (1986) Frequency of hereditary colorectal carcinoma (Lynch syndromes I and II). Gastroenterology 90: 486-489.

Macrae FA, St John DJB (1982) Relationship between patterns of bleeding and Hemoccult sensitivity in patients with colorectal cancers and adenomas. Gastroent. 82: 891-98.

Mecklin JP (1987) Frequency of hereditary colorectal carcinoma. Gastroenterology 93: 1021-1025.

Ponz de Leon M, Antonioli A, Zanghieri G, Sacchetti C (1987) Incidence and familial occurrence of colorectal cancer and polyps in a health-care district of northern Italy. Cancer 60 (11): 2848-2859.

Rozen P, Fireman Z, Figer A, Legum C, Ron E and Lynch HT (1987) Family history of colorectal cancer as a marker of potential malignancy within a screening program. Cancer 60: 248-254.

Simon JB (1985) Occult blood screening for colorectal carcinoma: a critical review. Gastroenterology 88: 820-837.

Stryker SJ, Wolf BC, Culp EC, Libbe SD, Illstrup DM and Maccarty R (1987) Natural history of untreated colonic polyps. Gastroenterology 93: 1009-1013.

Winawer SJ, Sherlock P (1982) Surveillance for colorectal cancer in average risk patients, familial high risk groups and patients with adenomas. Cancer 50: 2609-2614.

Studies on Relatives of Sporadic Colorectal Cancer Patients

PAUL ROZEN, ZVI FIREMAN, and ELAINE RON

ABSTRACT

Epidemiologic studies demonstrate that first degree relatives of sporadic colorectal cancer patients are at increased risk for the same neoplasm. Based on this, a prospective screening study demonstrated a 3-fold risk for neoplasia in relatives aged 40 or more years. The risk rose from 3-fold if there was one affected relative to 5-fold if there were 2 or more such relatives. Calculations of costs demonstrated that it was 4-fold more cost-effective to use colonoscopy as the primary screening exam if there were more than one affected first degree relative, otherwise flexible sigmoidoscopy and fecal occult blood testing were the most economic method. Measuring the rectal epithelial proliferation in a sample of these first degree relatives demonstrated that the probability of it being increased was greatest in the young male relatives. This biomarker may help delineate a high risk subgroup for prospective primary and secondary prevention. Using proliferation as a measure of response we gave 1.25 - 1.5 g calcium ion/day for 3 months to such relatives and significantly suppressed their proliferation only while they took calcium.

Key Words: colorectal cancer, cancer relatives, screening costs, epithelial proliferation, calcium intervention

INTRODUCTION

First degree relatives of colorectal cancer (CRC) patients are at high risk for the same neoplasm. The risk is highest in the uncommon syndrome Familial Adenomatous Polyposis and in the more common (4-fold) Cancer Family Syndrome (Lynch 1986; Mecklin 1987). However, sporadic colorectal cancer is by far more common and thus, it would seem that immediate adult family members of CRC patients could benefit from both primary and secondary prevention. This report summarizes our initial experience in this area.

1. FAMILIAL CRC IN THE TEL AVIV AREA

World-wide epidemiologic studies demonstrate that first degree relatives of colorectal cancer (CRC) patients are at increased risk (3 to 5-fold) for the same neoplasm. We studied this also in Tel Aviv (Rozen, Lynch 1987).

The family history of colon cancer was investigated in 38,823 individuals (2,129 families) who comprised a comparison group and an oncology patient series from Tel Aviv and nearby areas. A significant increased risk for colon cancer was observed among first-degree relatives of colon cancer patients when compared to controls (Table 1). This was more so in the relatives aged less than 65 years. But there was no predilection for right-sided colon cancer or an association with breast cancer, which would have been consistent with a non polyposis hereditary syndrome. When the patient sample was divided into two groups based on country and continent of birth · European and non European - the relatives of the non European subjects showed a reater risk for colon cancer (P<0.05). However, colon cancer was found to be less frequent in non European than in European controls. These findings suggest that although the frequency of CRC in the non European population is lower, the genetic component may be more important than for the European sample. The non European Jews ay represent distinct subgroups that differ with respect to either primary genetic susceptibility to colorectal cancer and, or, they may have been subjected to peculiar, environmental carcinogenic exposures when compared to their European brethren (Table 1). We hypothesise that in populations at low risk for CRC (e.g. non European Jews) genetic risk may play a dominant role, whereas for persons having high CRC rates environmental factors are more important.

Table 1. Comparison of CRC rates by age or ethnic groups

	Comparison group rate 10^3	CRC patients rate 10^3	RR*	P
Age of affected relative				
<65 y	5.8	11.7	2.02	<0.05
≥65 y	20.5	33.8	1.65	>0.05
All	9.0	17.4	1.93	<0.05
Ethnic Group				
European	11.7	13.5	1.15	
Non European	6.5	27.2	4.12	<0.01

* For CRC patients compared to comparison group

2. SECONDARY PREVENTION OF CRC AND EVALUATION OF ITS DIRECT ENDOSCOPIC COSTS.

Because of this small but significant added risk, we encourage relatives of CRC patients to enter our on-going screening program (Rozen, Fireman 1987). Interim analysis of 468 asymptomatic first degree relatives not belonging to a recognized cancer family or polyposis syndrome and 452 asymptomatic volunteers without this family history, demonstrated a 3-fold age-adjusted rate for adenomas or cancer in the relatives older than 40 years. The risk rose from 3-fold with one affected relative to 5-fold if there were 2 or more affected relatives. As the risk for neoplasia becomes significant after age 40 years (Table 2), we now screen these relatives from this age or 5 years younger than the youngest case of CRC in that family.

Table 2. Relative risk of CR neoplasia, by age*, at screening

Age (y)	Comparison group Rate 10^3	CRC relatives Rate 10^3	RR⁺	P
<40	0	36.5	-	
40-49	19.0	65.8	3.0	
50-59	29.3	110.3	3.8	
≥60	52.7	148.8	2.7	
All	29.1	100.3	3.2	<0.001

* Age adjusted for 5 year age intervals
⁺ For CRC relatives compared to comparison group

Because first degree relatives are at increased risk and, in certain families, CRC has a right-sided predilection, some clinicians recommend colonoscopy as the prefered initial screening examination. We used the results from the above screening program to evaluate whether the tumor yield and costs justified this recommendation (Rozen, Ron 1989). Our study groups included 429 patients who had only one relative with colorectal neoplasia and 39 who had two or more such relatives. Persons with one affected relative were screened by fecal occult blood and flexible sigmoidoscopy, followed by colonoscopy if either test was positive, whereas colonoscopy was used as the primary screening test for those having two or more relatives with colorectal neoplasia. The comparison group as screened with fecal occult blood tests and flexible sigmoidoscopy. Estimates were based on a range of US costs, and taking into account the 40% hypothetical increased tumor yield had colonoscopy been used as the primary screening examination for controls and families with only one affected relative. Calculations of costs indicate that screening asymptomatic adults by colonoscopy is markedly more cost-effective if they have 2 or more first degree colon cancer relatives. Otherwise, screening families with only 1 affected relative by flexible sigmoidoscopy together with fecal occult blood tests, would seem the most economic method (Table 3).

Table 3 Actual and hypothetical* costs for detecting neoplasia

		Comparison Group	Family Group One Relative	Family Group >One Relative
Screening test:		FS & FOBT	FS & FOBT	Colonoscopy
Cost⁺:	Low :	$ 2,462	1,730	836
	High :	$ 9,291	6,420	1,950
Screening test:		Colonoscopy*	Colonoscopy*	Colonoscopy
Cost⁺:	Low :	$ 5,697	3,830	836
	High :	$ 13,294	8,938	1,950

* Including an estimated 40% increased number of screenees with neoplasia detected by using colonoscopy as initial screening test
⁺ Range of costs: FOBT - $5-20, FS - $75-300, colonoscopy $300- 700
FS - flexible sigmoidoscopy
FOBT - fecal occult blood test

3. EVALUATION OF RECTAL EPITHELIAL PROLIFERATION IN FIRST DEGREE RELATIVES OF SPORADIC CRC PATIENTS AND THE POSSIBILITY OF PRIMARY PREVENTION

Hyperproliferation of rectal epithelium is characteristic of families at high genetic risk for large bowel neoplasia (Lipkin 1988), but has not been well documented in families of sporadic colorectal cancer patients. This issue was studied in 119 first degree CRC relatives and 44 comparison subjects without this family history. All subjects screened negative for large bowel neoplasia. Within the family group proliferation was significantly higher in the men and those aged less than 45 years, also higher (insignificantly) in non-Europeans and those having more than one first degree colorectal cancer relative. In contrast to the non-family group, the labelling index (LI) of the relatives showed a significant negative correlation with age ($R = -0.20$, $p=0.03$). Within this family group the probability of having an elevated LI (>6.0%) was greatest in the young (<50 years old) men (odds ratio = 2.0). Measurements of rectal epithelial proliferation in these first degree relatives, at a young age, might help delineate a high risk subgroup for prospective primary and secondary intervention (Fireman 1989).

Epidemiological and experimental studies point to a role for dietary calcium in inhibiting colonic carcinogenesis promoted by high fat, phosphate, and low fiber diets. It was reported that, in persons having a familial risk for colon cancer, oral calcium supplements significantly reduced increased rectal epithelial proliferation. We examined this in a cohort of 35 volunteers; 31 first degree relatives of colorectal cancer patients (5 had had adenomas) and 4 persons who only had had colonic adenomas (Rozen, Fireman 1989). Their mean age was 51.6 yrs, 17 (49%) were men and all persons screened negative for large bowel neoplasia. 1.25-1.5g of elemental calcium was given in divided daily doses for 3 months. Rectal pinch biopsies were taken without bowel preparation, before, during (a mean of 8.4 weeks) and 7.2 weeks after therapy and incubated with tritiated thymidine. After autoradiography and hematoxylin and eosin staining the mean number of labelled cells, as a ratio of the total number of crypt cells (labelling index - LI), and their crypt position, were determined (Table 4).

Table 4. Changes in LI during and after calcium treatment

		Treatment		
		Before	During	After
LI% (mean ±SD)		5.3±2.2	3.4±1.3*	4.7±2.3
LI%/compartment+ (mean ±SD)	1.	6.6±4.3	4.4±2.5*	6.3±3.5
	2.	9.7±5.3	6.0±3.3*	8.5±4.1
	3.	7.1±2.8	4.3±2.6*	5.6±3.5
	4.	2.5±1.8	2.1±2.0	2.3±2.1
	5.	0.4±0.6	0.8±2.2	0.3±0.7

* Significantly less than basal values ($P<0.01$)
\+ The crypt was divided into 5 equal compartments.

Compartment 1 being at base of crypt and compartment 5 at surface

The mean number of labelled cells decreased during therapy by 29%, especially in the basal three-fifths of crypts. There was also a significant 10% increase in mean number of crypt cells during therapy. Thus, the mean LI decreased 36% ($p<0.001$) during calcium treatment and almost returned to basal values after cessation. This decrease was independant of risk group (with or without an adenoma), but occurred only in those with an elevated basal LI (>6.0%).

CONCLUSIONS

Accepting that an elevated LI is a marker of potential malignancy a randomized clinical trial should be performed to confirm that calcium suppresses it. Together they may be the basis for dietary intervention in high-risk persons. Such a prospective study should correlate risk for colorectal cancer, dietary habits, large bowel epithelial proliferation and their interactions with calcium supplementation. Such a study has become more feasible following the development of a simplified measure of proliferation using the thymidine analogue bromodeoxyuridine and an immunoperoxidase staining technique for the rapid assessment of proliferation. In the meantime, secondary prevention by fecal occult blood testing, flexible sigmoidoscopy and or colonoscopy, should be recommended to this high risk group.

REFERENCES

Fireman Z, Rozen P, Fine N and Chetrit A (1989) Influence of demographic parameters on rectal epithelial proliferation. Cancer Lett (in press)

Lipkin M (1988) Biomarkers of increased susceptibility to gastrointestinal cancer: New applications to studies of cancer prevention in human studies. Cancer Res 48:235-245

Lynch HT, Schuelke GS and Lynch JF (1986) Hereditary colon cancer syndromes and their surveillance management. In: Rozen P and Winawer SJ (eds) Secondary prevention of colorectal cancer. Karger, Basel, pp 182-194

Mecklin J-P (1987) Frequency of hereditary colorectal carcinoma. Gastroenterology 93: 1021-1025

Rozen P, Fireman Z, Figer A, Legum C, Ron E and Lynch HT (1987) Family history of colorectal cancer as a marker of potential malignancy within a screening program. Cancer 60:248-254

Rozen P, Fireman Z, Fine N, Wax Y and Ron E (1989) Oral calcium uppresses increased rectal epithelial proliferation of persons at risk of colorectal cancer. Gut 30:650-655

Rozen P, Lynch HT, Figer A, Rozen S, Fireman Z, Legum C, Katz L, Moy A, Kimberley W, Lynch J and Watson P (1987) Familial colon cancer in the Tel Aviv area and the influence of ethnic origin. Cancer 60: 2355-2359

Rozen P and Ron E (1989) A cost analysis of screening methodology for family members of colorectal cancer patients. Am J Gastroent (in press)

Managing Surveillance for Colorectal Cancer: The Importance of Microcomputers

F.A. MACRAE, D.J.B. ST. JOHN, E. MUIR, and S. MCPHERSON

ABSTRACT

Large scale screening programmes for colorectal cancer based on genetic risk are difficult to administer because of the need to identify at-risk family members and ensure that surveillance proceeds in an orderly fashion over a lifetime. As at August 1989, 1100 high risk persons have been registered with the Royal Melbourne Hospital Surveillance Programme. Categorisation of risk is done after evaluation of the family's history of cancer. Surveillance protocols are then defined based on the intensity of cancer in the family. Annual occult blood testing is performed in all groups. Colonoscopy is performed every 2 years on at-risk members of families with hereditary non-polyposis colon cancer syndromes (n = 35 families) and 3 to 5 yearly for individuals with two or more first-degree relatives with sporadic colorectal cancer. Flexible sigmoidoscopy is performed every 3 years on some individuals with one affected first-degree relative, particularly where there are other affected relatives more remotely placed in the family. Patients who have had an adenoma/cancer undergo 3-yearly colonoscopy.

ScreeningMan is a menu-driven microcomputer program which documents cancer risk, organises surveillance, identifies non-compliers, notifies negative results to participants and their doctors, and documents and analyses the results of surveillance as scheduled.

In this paper, we compare the efficiency of ScreeningMan with a wordprocessor system and a correctible typewriter system. Personnel time required to administer initial and subsequent surveillance with faecal occult blood testing (FOBT) and colonoscopy was measured for each approach. For ScreeningMan, a database was entered initially and sequential results added directly to the computer; letters were then produced by list-processing. With the Wordprocessing and Typing systems, cards were retrieved and results entered for each contact.

Despite time overheads required for data entry, ScreeningMan handled surveillance administration more rapidly than the manual systems, even with as few as 10 subjects. When 1000 subjects are involved, the computer system was more than twice as quick as either of the other systems. Provided the database is maintained accurately, a computer system offers efficiency, security of follow-up, personalised correspondence and an analysable database for the effective function of a high-risk register.

Key words: colorectal cancer, surveillance, genetics, microcomputer/program

THE PROBLEM

Colorectal cancer is the commonest internal malignancy in Australia (Victorian Cancer Registry 1982). One in twenty people develop the disease in their lifetime. Survival beyond five years after diagnosis is the outcome for only about 40% of people developing the disease (Evans et al 1978). Survival is better (over 60%) for those whose disease is limited to the bowel wall at diagnosis, and is nearly 90% for those whose cancers are detected when no symptoms are present (Hertz REL et al 1960). Given this information, a certain pressure of logic dictates that screening for large bowel cancer should be considered, at least in high-incidence countries like Australia. However the results of controlled trials of screening for faecal occult blood are not yet available (Gilbertsen VA et al 1980; Winawer SJ et al 1980; Hardcastle JD et al 1989). These trials accommodate the epidemiological concerns of lead-time and length-biases which confound the interpretation of uncontrolled field screening studies.

High Risk Groups: High risk groups carry a disproportionate load of the colorectal cancer in the community. Identification and screening of these people for colorectal cancer should be rewarding, offering them some security against the lethal threat of colorectal cancer. In some circumstances, the risk is sufficiently high to warrant the closest of surveillance, using the most sensitive technique available - colonoscopy.

About 6.5% of Australians over 45 years have a first-degree relative with colorectal cancer (Macrae FA et al 1984). First-degree relatives of patients have a 2 to 3 fold increase in their lifetime risk for colorectal cancer in Australia (St John et al 1988). Where two first-degree relatives are affected in a family, the risks may be increased further, approaching the 1-in-2 risk borne by siblings and children of affected family members in familial adenomatous polyposis and the hereditary non-polyposis colon cancer syndromes (Rozen P et al 1987). We consider that the risk of colorectal cancer in first-degree relatives does warrant screening, despite the lack of data from controlled trials to show a mortality benefit. The higher risk implies a greater prevalence of neoplasia in this population compared with an average-risk population. As the predictive value of a test is directly related to the prevalence of the disease in the population (Galen RS, Gambino SR 1975), the yield of colorectal cancer and adenomas from screening should be higher and screening should be more cost-effective.

Logistics: The major difficulty with the plan of introducing surveillance to high risk groups based on family history is logistic. These relatives are well, and may be distant from the index case in the family who is in contact with the health care system - distant in place, distant emotionally, distant in age, and distant in attitude. Genetic-risk pays no account of these variables, so the task of the register is to work its way past these difficulties in the process of recruitment.

Colorectal cancer is a disease which more usually affects older compared with younger people. However, younger relatives often develop an intense concern at the time that their affected relative develops or dies from the disease. As this is when the family is most closely involved with the problem of bowel cancer, relatives can be usefully recruited into screening programmes at thie time. Frequently, this is not their period of maximum risk. Initiation of surveillance may not be appropriate for several decades after registration.

Surveillance: A commitment to, and mechanism for organising, periodic screening over a lifetime is required. This creates an ever-increasing workload on those centres that adopt some responsibility to care for relatives. The number of interested relatives could quickly expand to reach proportions where usual secretarial resources are overwhelmed. Keeping track of relatives who are at risk and encouraging the poorly compliant to participate are large tasks which require a personal and empathetic approach - time that is well spent by the screening team. Risk analysis also is difficult to assign to unsupervised computation, requiring close medical scrutiny.

However, the more mundane tasks of scheduling regular screening, contacting the target population at the correct time, ensuring that the data-base is kept up to date for both disease developments in the family and address changes, documenting and assessing the results of screening, and keeping the participant's family practitioner informed are all tasks that lend themselves to computer assistance.

THE MICROCOMPUTER ANSWER

Our group decided to develop a computer program to carry out these tasks. With the establishment of a database of demographic, contact, referral, risk-factor, compliance and surveillance scheduling information, the tasks of contacting and checking compliance can proceed by microcomputation and subsequent letter/list-processing. The results of screening can be incorporated, with provision for recording results according to genetic (and other) risk determinations. In 1984, we chose to use KnowledgeMan. The volume of data to be recorded for each participant in the program and the number of participants heavily influenced the selection of database package. With 10 tables of information on each participant, including registration, family and medical histories as well as surveillance details, there would be 700 variables of status, history and surveillance information as well as 50 variables recorded for each test the patient performs.

The capacity to cope with a large number of tables, variables, index keys and records as well as fast access times and facilities for ad-hoc queries were required. This eliminated many of the database packages such as DBase and DataFlex which were available at the time.

Systems Analysis: The systems analysis of our manual work highlighted the complexity of what would appear to be a simple task. For example, when dealing with large numbers of people, it is essential to document each step in the participant's surveillance programme. Each contact letter that is sent out must be recorded to avoid omission or unnecessary duplication of correspondence. This is especially important when more than one person is involved in the administration of the surveillance program. It is necessary to update the risk status of individuals when new cancers or adenomas are diagnosed in family members. Results of screening have to be documented and related to risk groups for analysis, and participants and their doctors notified of the results. Where individuals have multiple risks, these records can be difficult to place and cross reference in a manual system.

ScreeningMan

ScreeningMan emerged from many months of discussion and programming. ScreeningMan is a menu-driven program which documents risk, organises surveillance by up to 15 modalities, contacts individuals at due times of surveillance, identifies non-compliers, notifies negative results and documents results of surveillance as scheduled.

The objectives of the microcomputer program are to provide a facility to help with the task of administering colorectal cancer screening based on risk. Results are recorded according to risk group status, allowing ready comparison between different family histories. (How many relatives do you have with bowel cancer? At what age did they develop the cancer?) An average-risk control group is also incorporated in the system.

How KnowledgeMan was used

KnowledgeMan was used to develop the ScreeningMan program. The K-Paint module, an interactive screen editor, was used to create the data entry screens and menus. Reports were written in the KMan command language and used output formats defined by K-Paint. The letters are generated by KMan programs which create intermediate tables for records to be used. The K-Text module, a simple word processor, uses the information in the tables with word processing documents to print customised letters and envelope labels, a process known as "mail-merge".

At a later date the program was upgraded to use KnowledgeMan/2 which significantly improved performance and overcame some memory limitation on the personal computer.

ScreeningMan in Operation

As at August 1989, 1180 high-risk persons have been registered with The Royal Melbourne Hospital Surveillance Programme. Participants have been recruited by referral from surgeons in the hospital, other medical practitioners and from intra-family recruitment. Most attention has been given to recruitment of families with two or more relatives with colorectal cancer, especially those with hereditary non-polyposis colon cancer syndromes. Family members are not contacted without the written consent of the index or a subsequent case, and the details of illness in any particular family member are kept confidential.

Demographic and contact information is recorded for each participant. Each registrant is identified by a unique HASAC code which incorporates elements of the participants' given names, initials and date of birth.

Categorisation: Categorisation of risk is done after evaluation of the family's history of cancer. Risk groupings include the hereditary non-polyposis colon cancer syndromes, two or more first-degree relatives with colorectal cancer and various patterns of one first-degree with other relatives affected with colorectal cancer. Special interest groups are included. Previous adenoma or cancer history is also allocated as a risk group. An average-risk category is provided.

Participants can be recorded in up to three risk groupings. The finding of an adenoma or cancer as end-points for genetic risk surveillance is the starting point for adenoma/colorectal cancer follow-up and surveillance for metachronous tumours.

The family history of colorectal adenomas and cancer and other cancers is recorded for each registrant, acting as a ready check on the categorisation and providing a database for pedigree construction.

Screening Status: A special screening status field is included which aborts the computerized surveillance protocol mechanisms if it is not completed. Particular provision to stop screening is made in this field for participants who have died or who have clearly signalled their wish not to undergo further screening.

Surveillance Protocols: Surveillance protocols are defined by clinicians according to the intensity of cancer in the family. Fifteen screening modalities are listed on the surveillance computation with the number of procedures already done, frequency, date when last done and next due, last request sent, date non-compliance letter sent, date doctor notified of non-compliance, date response sent. With the result of the last surveillance recorded in the results section of the program, the surveillance computation is automatically updated, setting its clock for the next surveillance due. Each of the fifteen modalities functions independently in this respect.

At the beginning of each month, the operator drives the appropriate menu to print out correspondence associated with each of the modalities scheduled for that month. Combined screening modalities due at the same time also are handled by the program. For us, the main screening modalities have been faecal occult blood testing and colonoscopy.

Table 1

Typical Surveillance Protocol

Rec No. 558 Hasac Code 2COSSSAM01JAN1950 UR Number
Surname Initials Entry Status 2

	Respon -sible Agent	Num Done	Freq	Last Done	Next Due	Last Request Sent	Date Non Compl	Date Dr. Notif	Date Response Sent
Registration	R	2	0	1286	0	1286	0	0	1286
Scheduling Notif	R	1	0	285	0	285	0	285	285
FOBT	R	3	12	1088	1089	1188	0	0	1188
Sigmoidoscopy		0	0	0	0	0	0	0	0
Sig. + Biopsy		0	0	0	0	0	0	0	0
Colonoscopy	R	1	24	587	589	789	0	587	587
Col. + Biopsy		0	0	0	0	0	0	0	0
Change Address		0	24	0	589	0	0	0	0
Clinical Exam		0	0	0	0	0	0	0	0
DCBE		0	0	0	0	0	0	0	0
Mammogram		0	0	0	0	0	0	0	0
Breast Examination		0	0	0	0	0	0	0	0
Upper GI Endoscopy		0	0	0	0	0	0	0	0
Ludwig Study		0	0	0	0	0	0	0	0
Other		0	0	0	0	0	0	0	0
Comment									

Software Contracts Group UofM

Results of Screening and Compliance Checks: Results of symptom questionnaires and faecal occult blood testing are fed into the result section and are used to list-process correspondence to the patient and his/her doctor re negative results, as well as updating the clock for next surveillance due, or if not fed in, for non-compliance list-processing routines.

If the test has still not been done after a reminder letter, a letter to the responsible doctor is generated and the participant is flagged as a non-complier for that test. As each letter is generated, the system records the date the letter was sent to ensure that letters are not duplicated and that reminders are only sent a month after the notification-of-test letter. It also provides a history of correspondence for each participant. These results provide an ongoing record of the surveillance programmes performance.

ScreeningMan Outputs

Letters produced by ScreeningMan are listed in Table 2.

Table 2

Standard Letters

1. Registration Letter
2. Registration Letter - Reminder
3. Cancellation Due to Failure to Reply to Registration
4. Notification of Initial Scheduling
5. Notification of Change in Scheduling
6. Notification of Scheduling to Doctor
7. First FOBT Test
8. FOBT Test
9. Reminder for FOBT
10. Cancellation Due to Failure to Comply
11. Notification of FOBT Clear Result
12. Notification to Doctor of FOBT Clear Result
13. Sigmoidoscopy Appointment Due
14. Notification of Sigmoidoscopy/Colonoscopy Clear Result
15. Notification to Dr of Sigmoidoscopy/Colonoscopy Clear Result
16. Colonoscopy Appointment Due
17. Private Patient Sigmoidoscopy/Colonoscopy Due
18. Change of Address Letter
19. Return to Main Menu

Letters generated by the system are thus flagged as "done" by the computer so that each new batch of month's letters produced by the computer exclude all those previously done. A temporary file of letters to be sent that month is generated, in case of printer failure and the need to reprint letters.

ScreeningMan has data input capabilities to import data from other programs, in particular the endoscopy data recording program, Metabase. Data export facilities are also available for detailed statistical analysis.

Multiple reports are generated, mostly sorted by risk group or "time due". These include registrants listings, address listings, scheduled colonoscopies by any time period, results of faecal occult blood testing, participants with adenomas/carcinomas, and various routines to assess work load (see Appendix).

TIME MANAGEMENT STUDY

The overhead in time required to establish a computer database concerning high risk people is substantial and there may be simpler ways to administer the programme, e.g. using standard letters with typewriting used to fill in the gaps. To evaluate this further, we conducted a study to compare the efficiency of ScreeningMan with a wordprocessing system (W/P) and a correctible typewriter system (Typing).

Method

Personnel time required to administer initial and subsequent surveillance with faecal occult blood testing (FOBT) and colonoscopy was measured for each approach. Initial surveillance included registration, communication about policies, first FOBT routines. Subsequent surveillance included FOBT routines only. For ScreeningMan, a database was entered initially and sequential results added directly to the computer; letters were then produced by list-processing. With the W/P and Typing systems, cards were retrieved and results entered for each contact.

The word processing system had standard letters recorded in memory; each new letter-contact required typing the participant's name and "screening due" details into the appropriate blanks on a standard letter.

The time required to administer the programme using these systems was recorded. The time required to collect the family history information (a large task) was not included as this is equivalent for each technique.

Results

Table 3

Personnel Time in Hours

Subjects		Initial			Subsequent	
(n)	SMan	W/P	Typing	SMan	W/P	Typing
1	0.4	0.4	0.4	0.2	0.3	0.3
10	1.7	3.9	3.5	0.5	2.2	2.1
1000	142.4	355.9	320.1	31.6	212.8	204.5

Despite time overheads required for data entry, ScreeningMan handled surveillance administration more rapidly than the manual systems, even with as few as 10 subjects. Provided the database is maintained accurately the computer system offers efficiency, security of follow-up, personalised correspondence and an analysable database for the effective function of a high-risk register.

CONCLUSION

The microcomputer surveillance program which we have had in operation over the last three years has enabled a small research group to handle the demanding task of maintaining an on-going surveillance program for colorectal cancer amongst high-risk groups. The routine tasks of contacting and checking compliance has been competently handled by the microcomputer, saving a large amount of time. The analysis of the findings by the computer program is currently being tested and will lead to some minor modifications in programming to provide ready access to useful data on the overall performance of the screening program. The complexity of the genetic information recorded for each individual may be excessive, at least as far as the straightforward aims of surveillance organisation and recording of results according to risk factor analysis are concerned. However, if the programme is to be used for pedigree construction, this additional information will be required.

References:

Evans JT, Vana J, Aronoff BL, Baker HW, Murphy GP (1978) Management and survival of carcinoma of the colon: results of a national survey by the American College of Surgeons. Ann Surg; 188: 716-720

Galen RS, Gambino SR (1975) Beyond Normality. John Wiley & Sons

Gilbertsen VA, Church TR, Grewe FJ et al (1980) The design of a study to assess occult-blood screening for colon cancer. J Chron Dis; 33: 107-14

Hardcastle JD, Chamberlain J, Sheffield J et al (1989) Randomised, controlled trial of faecal occult blood screening for colorectal cancer. Lancet; I: 1160-64

Hertz REL, Deddish MR, Day E (1960) Value of periodic examinations in detecting cancer of the rectum and colon. Postgrad Med; 27: 290-4

Macrae FA, Hill DJ, StJohn DJB (1984) Predicting colon cancer screening behaviour from health beliefs. Preventive Medicine; 13: 115-26

Rosen P, Fireman Z, Figer A et al (1987) Family history of colorectal cancer as a marker of potential screening program. Cancer; 60: 248-254

StJohn DJB, McDermott FT, Katrivessis H et al (1988) How great is the cancer risk for relatives of colorectal cancer patients? Results of a case control study. Aust NZJ Medicine; 18: 417

Victorian Cancer Registry, Statistical Report (1982)

Winawer SJ, Andrews M, Flehinger B et al (1980) Progress report on controlled trial of faecal occult blood testing for the detection of colorectal neoplasia. Cancer; 45: 2959-64

APPENDIX

Reporting routines in ScreeningMan

PRODUCE REPORTS

1. New Patients by Register
2. Scheduling Information by Procedure
3. Scheduling Information by Procedure - Address List
4. Scheduling Information by Register
5. Scheduling Information by Register - Address List
6. Summary of Letters Sent
7. Summary of Procedures Done
8. FOBT Positive Patients
9. Non Compliance by Procedure - Patient Information
10. Non Compliance by Procedure - Doctor Information
11. Summary of Adenomas/Carcinomas
12. Summary of Rectal Bleeding
13. Summary of Rectal Bleeding - Address List
14. Individual Patient Report
15. Summary of Registers
16. Missing Data Report by Register
17. Families by Register
18. Families by Register - Totals
19. Individual Family Report

Your Choice: __

This menu allows you to select one of the nineteen standard reports that can be produced. The reports may either be output to the printer or viewed on the screen, this is not recommended for the very long reports. Most of these reports are dependent on a time factor, i.e. when did the patient enter the trial or when did they become non-compliers.

When you select a report one of the following forms will be displayed, depending on the type of report, in order to determine the criterion by which the reports are produced.

```
From Date (dd/mm/yy)    __/__/__    (Defaults to 3 Months before Today)
To Date (dd/mm/yy)      __/__/__    (Defaults to Today)

Register __              1 = CFS     2 = CPS     3 = RELS
                         4 = RELC    5 = CAS     6 = CAC
                         7 = ADS     8 = ADC     9 = FAP
                        10 = PJS    11 = JPC    12 = UC
                        13 = URET   14 = SELF   15 = OTHER
                        16 = ALL

View or Print (V/P) __
(Q to Quit)
```

If you select options 1, 4, 5, 8, 12, 13, 16, 17 or 18, this form will be displayed. You enter the appropriate date range and register for the report and either "V" or "P" to view or print.

```
From Date (dd/mm/yy)    __/__/__    (Defaults to 3 Months before Today)
To Date (dd/mm/yy)      __/__/__    (Defaults to Today)

Procedure __ and __      1 = Registration               2 = Scheduling Notif
                         3 = FOBT                       4 = Sigmoidoscopy
                         5 = Sigmoidoscopy + Biop       6 = Colonoscopy
                         7 = Colonoscopy + Biop         8 = Change of Address
                         9 = Clinical Exam             10 = DCBE
                        11 = Mammography               12 = Breast Examination
                        13 = Upper GI Endoscopy        14 = Ludwig Study
                        15 = Other                     16 = ALL

View or Print (V/P) __
(Q to Quit)
```

This form will be displayed if you select options 2 or 3. Here you specify the date range and one or two procedures. If you wish for a report on patients who are scheduled for a combination of the two procedures, i.e. both a FOBT and a Colonoscopy, you would enter "Y" in the Both field. Otherwise just leave the field blank or enter "N", i.e. a FOBT or a Colonoscopy.

```
From Date (dd/mm/yy)    __/__/__    (Defaults to 3 Months before Today)
To Date (dd/mm/yy)      __/__/__    (Defaults to Today)

View or Print (V/P) __
(Q to Quit)
```

This form will be displayed if you select options 6 or 7. Here you simply enter a date range and either "V" to view or "P" to print.

```
From Date (dd/mm/yy)   __/__/__   (Defaults to 3 Months before Today)
To Date (dd/mm/yy)     __/__/__   (Defaults to Today)

Procedure __ and __     1 = Registration             2 = Scheduling Notif
                        3 = FOBT                     4 = Sigmoidoscopy
                        5 = Sigmoidoscopy + Biop     6 = Colonoscopy
                        7 = Colonoscopy + Biop       8 = Change of Address
                        9 = Clinical Exam           10 = DCBE
                       11 = Mammography             12 = Breast Examination
                       13 = Upper GI Endoscopy      14 = Ludwig Study
                       15 = Other                   16 = ALL

View or Print (V/P) __
(Q to Quit)
```

This form will be displayed if you select options 9 or 10. Here you specify a date range, view/print and one or <u>all</u> procedures.

Hereditary Non-polyposis Colorectal Cancer: The University of Texas MD Anderson Cancer Center Experience

Patrick M. LYNCH, RODGER J. WINN, MICHAEL J. WARGOVICH, and BERNARD LEVIN

ABSTRACT

The UT M.D. Anderson Cancer Center recently initiated a registry for Hereditary Non-polyposis Colorectal Cancer (HNPCC). Modelled after the Creighton program, our interests include early detection and clinical management, intermediate laboratory markers, and chemoprevention. Kindreds registered to date have the usual features of HNPCC. Mucosal markers (tritiated thymidine and bromodeoxyuridine labelling) have varied considerable amongst high-risk subjects studied. A multi-centered prospective screening trial, with further evaluation of intermediate markers and chemoprevention strategies is proposed.

KEY WORDS: Hereditary non-polyposis colorectal cancer, intermediate markers, screening, strategies

INTRODUCTION

In 1913 Warthin published a report of a family expressing a high incidence of gastrointestinal cancer, particularly involving the colon (Warthin 1913, Lynch, H & Krush 1971).

Beginning in the 1960's, a flurry of reports described additional families with a similar pattern of expression (Peltokallio & Peltokallio, 1966, Mathis, 1962, H Lynch et al 1988). We will refer to this disorder as Hereditary Non-Polyposis Colorectal Cancer (HNPCC), in order to emphasize that it is a simply inherited disposition toward colorectal cancer (not a vague "familial" phenomenon), and to specify that diffuse polyposis is not a feature.

The criteria for HNPCC that have evolved over the years include:

1. An early age of onset for colorectal adenocarcinoma, with a mean of approximately 45 years, which is only slightly older than the mean for FAP, but many years earlier than in the general population (Mecklin, 1987);
2. An excess of synchronous and metachronous multiple primary colorectal cancers (Lynch H et al, 1977).
3. A tendency toward right sided involvement. In the typical HNPCC family, about two-thirds of all initial colon cancers occur proximal to the splenic flexure, although there is considerable variation from family to family (P Lynch et al, 1977).
4. Extra-colonic carcinoma. In the original reports of the "Cancer Family Syndrome", an association with endometrial carcinoma was emphasized (Lynch & Krush, 1971). As more families were evaluated, an apparent excess of tumors of other sites appeared, including the ovary, breast, upper intestinal tract, and urinary tract (H Lynch et al, 1977)

5. Association with the Muir-Torre syndrome. The coincident occurrence of visceral neoplasms and otherwise rare sebaceous adenomas, carcinomas, and keratoacanthomas has now been seen in multiple members of a subset of families with HNPCC (H Lynch et al 1981).

In this paper we will review the recent UT MD Anderson Cancer Center experience in dealing with HNPCC. The areas to be addressed will include the development of clinical strategies for family evaluation and screening and the role of intermediate "mucosal markers".

METHODS

Development Of A "Special Risk Clinic" and Hereditary Colon Cancer Registry

In 1986, the Community Oncology section (RJW) at the UTMDACC initiated a "Special Risk Clinic", devoted to the clinical assessment of patients with strong family histories of a variety of neoplasms. Assessment consisted of an in-depth interview with affected patients, followed by retrieval of medical records of relatives in selected cases. An attempt was made to determine whether the pedigree of a given family expressed a known or suspected familial cancer syndrome. In positive cases, clinical recommendations were made to patients and to their presumptively high-risk relatives (P Lynch & Winn 1989). Further referrals for specific investigations were made as indicated (indirect ophthalmoscopy for signs of congenital hypertrophy of the retinal pigment epithelium or "CHRPE" (Traboulsi et al, 1987), and bone surveys in the case of FAP/Gardner's Syndrome (Offerhaus et al 1987).

Recently, the registry associated with the Special Risk Clinic adopted as its data base program the software developed at the Creighton School of medicine, with minor modifications to suit local needs. The data base remains poolable with the data base in use at Creighton and has been adopted at several other institutions.

The logistics of family workup and evaluation have been published elsewhere (P Lynch, 1985, P Lynch & Winn, 1989) but basically consists of the following steps:

1. Initial history obtained from an index case or next of kin. A self-administered questionnaire is used for this purpose. The instrument provides for personal medical history and solicits information regarding cancer history in sibs, offspring and parents.
2. Followup. Once the questionnaire is reviewed, the indicated relatives are contacted (often by telephone to expedite the workup) for further details. Documentation is then obtained from hospital or physician records.
3. Pedigree analysis. A fairly brief family workup usually enables a straightforward assessment of the significance of the family history, with classification into one of two categories, "unequivocal" syndrome family or "possible" syndrome family (Bailey-Wilson et al, 1986). Consequently, simple inspection of a pedigree and discussion of the family at our weekly "Special Risk Conference" is usually adequate. At this working conference (modelled after the very successful program at Creighton) further directions for family workup are addressed, as are approaches to screening and management of specific patients or categories of patients. Finally eligibility of subjects for marker studies and chemointervention trials is discussed.

Marker Studies

Several assays are carried out in the laboratory of Dr. M.J. Wargovich, including tritiated thymidine autoradiography and Bromodeoxyuridine immunoperoxidase staining for assessment of proliferative index, as well as Ornithine decarboxylase enzyme activity. Details of these techniques are published elsewhere (Deschner et al, 1966, Risio et al, 1988). See also Dr. Wargovich's manuscript. In the results section below we will limit presentation of data to findings from the high-risk subjects that have been evaluated to date. In certain instances, values for Bromodeoxyuridine only will be presented. Note should be made of the excellent correlation that has been found between this technique and the "gold standard" of tritiated thymidine autoradiography (Isbell, et al., 1989).

RESULTS

To date, eight families with HNPCC have been entered into our registry. The many families that have only equivocal features of the syndrome have not been included. An additional twelve kindreds with at least one FAP affected member are also included in the registry, but are beyond the scope of this discussion.

The following table summarizes the clinical status of the HNPCC families that comprise our registry:

TABLE I

FAMILY	# OF COLO-RECTAL CANCERS (AVG ONSET)	OTHER CA (AVG ONSET)	% MULT PRIMARY	% RIGHT COLON
1.	9 (57)	6 (46)	11	75
2.	3 (35)	1 (36)	33	33
3.	5 (55)	4 (48)	20	unk
4.	11 (44)	12 (50)	unk	64
5.	4 (55)	1 (unk)	25	25
6.	4 (55)	3 (57)	unk	unk
7.	5 (46)	4 (65)	unk	20
8.	18 (49)	6 (41)	11	57

Representative pedigrees are shown in figures 1 & 2.

A modest number of individuals from HNPCC and FAP families have undergone colonic mucosa biopsies for intermediate markers, as noted in methods. Findings are as shown in table II.

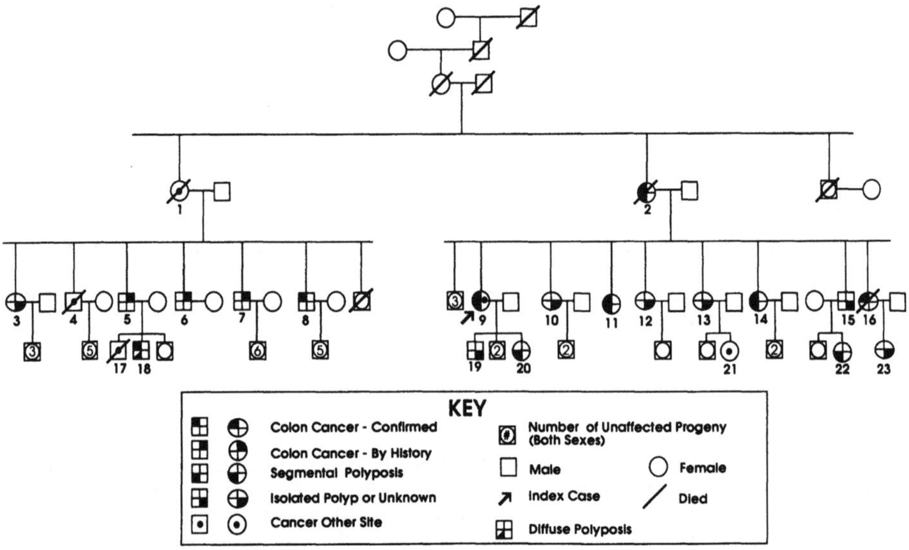
KEY
Colon Cancer - Confirmed
Colon Cancer - By History
Segmental Polyposis
Isolated Polyp or Unknown
Cancer Other Site
Number of Unaffected Progeny (Both Sexes)
Male
Female
Index Case
Died
Diffuse Polyposis

Fig.1

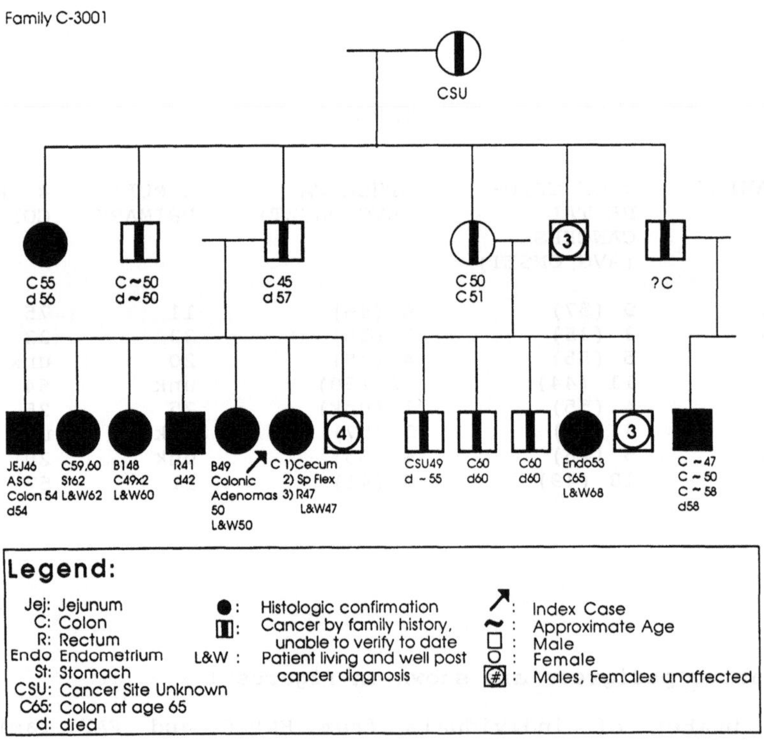
Family C-3001
CSU
C 55
d 56
C ~ 50
d ~ 50
C 45
d 57
C 50
C 51
?C
JEJ46
ASC
Colon 54
d54
C59,60
St62
L&W62
B148
C49x2
L&W60
R41
d42
B49
Colonic
Adenomas
50
L&W50
C 1)Cecum
2) Sp Flex
3) R47
L&W47
CSU49
d ~ 55
C60
d60
C60
d60
Endo53
C65
L&W68
C ~ 47
C ~ 50
C ~ 58
d58
Legend:
Jej: Jejunum
C: Colon
R: Rectum
Endo Endometrium
St: Stomach
CSU: Cancer Site Unknown
C65: Colon at age 65
d: died
Histologic confirmation
Cancer by family history, unable to verify to date
L&W : Patient living and well post cancer diagnosis
Index Case
Approximate Age
Male
Female
Males, Females unaffected
macmscl

Fig.2

TABLE II

INTERMEDIATE MARKERS IN HNPCC PATIENTS

PATIENT	STATUS	3HTDR	BUDR
1.	FPC*	6.56	5.46
2.	HNPCC*	18.11	7.19
3.	HNPCC	5.10	
4.	FPC*		7.0
5.	HNPCC*		7.36
6.	HNPCC^		19.05
7.	FPC^	2.83	3.61
8.	FPC^	10.74	4.07
9.	HNPCC*	3.75	3.27
10.	HNPCC^		5.23
11.	HNPCC*	14.1	14.11P 22.24R, 6.37R
12.	FPC*		6.68R, 6.62 R 6.97 P
13.	HNPCC*	5.04 P	
14.	+Colon Ca*	6.08 R	2.92 R
15.	HNPCC*	9.35 P, 9.1 R	
16.	FPC*		5.82 R 3.82 P
17.	FPC*		

*affected R=rectal
^asymptomatic P=Proximal

DISCUSSION

Our experience and that of a number of other investigators have demonstrated that although HNPCC is not common, neither is it rare (Mecklin 1987). Moreover, the clinical features are sufficiently striking that in many cases recognition of an affected family is relatively straight-forward (H Lynch et al, 1978) . It is in the case of less obviously affected families and asymptomatic members of well-documented kindreds that the role for mucosal markers and molecular genetics studies will be most critical.

Intermediate markers of mucosal proliferation suggest that despite a trend toward increased crypt labelling in cancer and adenoma affected patients, an imperfect correlation exists at the level of the individual subject (Markowitz et al, 1986). Consequently it must be conceded that the predictive value of existing markers is sufficiently weak as to preclude reliance upon such tests in the clinical arena. At the investigational level it is clear that newer markers and combinations of existing markers will need to be evaluated. This is a very active area of study.

Assuming that genetic linkage is eventually established for HNPCC, as it has been for FAP (Bodmer et al, 1987, Leppert et al, 1987), the need will still exist for clinical surveillance, presumably involving a heavy reliance upon colonoscopy (Eddy et al 1987).

Until more definitive characterization of the genotypically affected patient is accomplished, trials devoted to the development of optimal screening strategies will need to be conducted. Such trials will of necessity be multi-centered in order to accrue an adequate series of patients at relatively homogeneous risk.

We propose that a prospective, international, cooperative screening study of HNPCC families be conducted, with primary reliance on colonoscopic evaluation. Its goals would be to determine the optimal age at which surveillance should begin, the appropriate followup interval, and the actual yield of colonoscopic examination. Sub-protocols would include intermediate marker studies and "chemoprevention" trials.

Logically prior to any such large scale project, however, is characterization of the study population of interest. We suggest that contribution of a kindred from any participating institution to a study center data base meet specified eligibility criteria. This is particularly critical given the ongoing controversy as to the significance of any given "familial cluster" of colorectal cancer. We would require that a family have:

1. Aggregation of at least three members with colorectal cancer, with one such affected member being a parent, sib, or child of the other two.

2. At least two affected patients expressing a clinical feature of HNPCC--age at onset below 45 years, right colonic involvement, multiple primary colorectal cancer, "associated" extracolonic malignancy (endometrium, ovary, breast, other GI or genitourinary) if onset is below age 45.

The screening protocol itself would consist of baseline colonoscopy in asymptomatic sibs and offspring of affected patients, starting at age 25 (acceptable alternatives would be to start at age 30 or five years younger than the earliest case in the particular family). Patients with previous colon cancer or adenoma diagnosis would undergo baseline exam at the time the HNPCC diagnosis is made. Exams would be repeated yearly so long as adenomas or carcinomas are found, then every two years following a "clean" exam. Isolated adenomas would be removed endoscopically in the usual fashion, but diagnosis of invasive carcinoma would merit total colectomy.

REFERENCES

Bodmer, WF, Bailey, CJ, Bodmer, J, et al (1987) Localization of the gene for familial adenomatous polyposis on chromosome 5. Nature, 328:614-6.

Bailey-Wilson, JE, Elston, RC, Schuelke, GS, et al. (1986) Segregation analysis of hereditary non-polyposis colon cancer. Genet Epid, 3:27-36.

Deschner, EE, Lipkin, M, Solomon, C (1966) In vitro study of human epithelial cells II: tritiated thymidine incorporation into polyps and adjacent mucosa. JNCI, 36:847-57.

Eddy, DM, Nugent, FW, Eddy, JF, et al. (1987) Screening for colorectal cancer in a high-risk population: results of a mathematical model. Gastro, 92:682-92.

Isbell, GM, Hu, P-J, Lynch, PM et al. (1989) A comparison of tritiated thymidine autoradiography and bromodeoxyuridine immunoperoxidase techniques for measuring epithelial proliferation in the human colon (Abstract) Gastro, 96:875.

Leppert, M, Dobbs, M, Scambler, P, et al. (1987) The gene for familial polyposis coli maps to the long arm of chromosome 5. Science, 238:1411-13.

Luk, GD, Baylin, SB (1984) Ornithine decarboxylase as biologic marker in familial colonic polyposis. NEJM, 311:80-83.

Lynch, HT, Krush, AJ (1971) Cancer family "G" revisited 1895-1970. Cancer, 27:1505-11.

Lynch, HT, Harris, RE, Lynch, PM et al. (1977) The role of heredity in multiple primary cancers. Cancer, 40:1849-54.

Lynch, HT, Lynch, PM, Harris, RE (1978) Minimal genetic findings and their cancer control implications: the cancer family syndrome. JAMA, 240:535-8

Lynch, HT, Lynch, PM, Albano, WA, Lynch, JF (1981) The cancer family syndrome: a status report. Dis Colon & Rect, 24:311-22

Lynch, HT, Lynch, PM, Fusaro, R, Pester, J (1981) The cancer family syndrome: rare cutaneous phenotypic linkage of Torre's syndrome. Arch Int Med, 141:607-11.

Lynch, HT, Lanspa, SJ, Boman, BM, et al. (1988) Hereditary non-polyposis coli-Lynch syndromes I & II. In G Luk Colorectal Cancer, GI Clin of NA, 17(4):679-712.

Lynch, PM, Lynch, HT, Harris, RE (1977) Hereditary proximal colonic cancer. Dis Colon & Rect, 20:661-8.

Lynch, PM, Lynch, HT, Lynch, JF (1985) Hereditary non-polyposis colon cancer: clinical-genetic features In P Lynch & H Lynch (eds) Colon Cancer Genetics, Van Nostrand Reinhold, New York.

Lynch, PM (1985) The process of family registration. In P Lynch & H Lynch (eds) Colon Cancer Genetics, Van Nostrand Reinhold, New York.

Lynch, PM, Winn, RJ (1989) Clinical management of hereditary non-polyposis colorectal cancer: high risk registries and clinics. in B Levin & JE Harris (eds) New Perspectives in Large Bowel Cancer. Hem/Onc Clin of NA, 3(1):75-86.

Markowitz, JF, Aiges, HW, Cunningham-Rundles, S (1986) Cancer family syndrome: marker studies. Gastro, 91:581-9.

Mathis, M (1962) Familiares colonkarzinome. Schweiz Med Wochenschr, 92:1673-8.

Mecklin, J-P (1987) Frequency of hereditary colorectal carcinoma. Gastro, 93:1021-5.

Offerhaus, GJA, Levin, LS, Giardello, FM et al. (1987) Occult radiopaque jaw lesions in familial adenomatous polyposis coli and hereditary non-polyposis colorectal cancer. Gastro, 93:460-7.

Peltokallio, P, Peltokallio, V (1966) Relationship of familial factors to carcinoma of the colon. Dis Colon & Rect, 9:367-70.

Risio, M, Coverlizza, S, Ferrari, A, et al (1988) Immunohistochemical study of epithelial cell proliferation in hyperplastic polyps, adenomas, and adenocarcinomas of the large bowel. Gastro, 94: 899-906.

Traboulsi, EI, Krush, AJ, Gardner, EJ et al (1987) Prevalence and importan.ce of pigmented ocular fundus lesions in Gardner's syndrome. NEJM, 316:661-4

Warthin, AS (1913) Heredity .ith reference to carcinoma as shown by the study of the cases examined in the pathological laboratory of the Univ of Michigan 1895-1913. Arch Int Med, 12:546-55.

Medical/Legal Concerns in the Management of Patients from Lynch Syndromes Kindreds

G. CRISTOFARO, E. DI GIULIO, P.L. MINGAZZINI, P. BUFO, S. SENATORE, P.M. LYNCH, P. WATSON, J.F. LYNCH, and H.T. LYNCH

BACKGROUND

The management of patients affected or at risk for the Lynch Syndromes must focus upon its natural history, early age of onset, predilection for the proximal Colon, excess of synchronous and metachronous Colon cancer, and autosomal dominant mode of inheritance (Lynch Syndrome I). In addition, predisposition to carcinoma of the endometrium, ovary, stomach, pancreas, and other anatomic sites are integral features of the Lynch Syndrome II counterpart [Lynch H.T., 1985, 1988, 1988a]. The absence of biomarkers for the genotype and/or premonitory signs, such as multiple colonic adenomatous polyps, as occurs in the familial adenomatous polyposis (FAP) syndrome, makes the job of the diagnostician a vexing one [Cristofaro G., 1988, 1989].

INTRODUCTION

A physician managing a Lynch Syndrome I or II kindred faces enormous responsibilities which embrace all of these facets of natural history. It is clear that medical/legal implications may abound when the family history is ignored or incompletely compiled. Failure to perform colonoscopy or double contrast barium enema would contribute to failure to examine the area of greatest colonic cancer predilection, namely the proximal Colon. A segmental resection or hemicolectomy, instead of subtotal colectomy, would be surgically insufficient, given the excess of synchronous and methachronous colonic cancer. Failure to evaluate extracolonic cancer target organs, such as the endometrium in Lynch Syndrome II, would render surveillance incomplete. Collectively, inattention to these cardinal features of the Syndrome's natural history could be interpreted as negligence, with malpractice penalties for failure to meet an eventual standard of care for Syndrome at-risk and/or affected patients.

Our attention is focused on a retrospective and longitudinal study of a large Italian Family showing Lynch Syndrome II, composed of 318 subjects over 7 Generations with a relative cancer frequency of 51,2% (range 37%-75%) over the first 5 generations.
The most common cancer localization was the colon, followed by stomach and endometrium/ovary. Respective ages at cancer death were 39, 42 and 50: a specific peculiarity of Lynch Syndromes.
Verification of reported data in clinical records, focused our attention on *five* uncommon cases among which one is well documented by radiology. Cases 3 and 5 were noted during a longitudinal study. All the genealogical tree reported in clinical examples are branches of the *same* large family.

ACKNOWLEDGEMENTS. This Work is partially supported by:
ARNOLDO MONDADORI Editor, MILAN(ITALY)

CLINICAL EXAMPLES

CASE 1: The family history of case 1, a male aged 43 (V-19), is reported in Fig. 1.

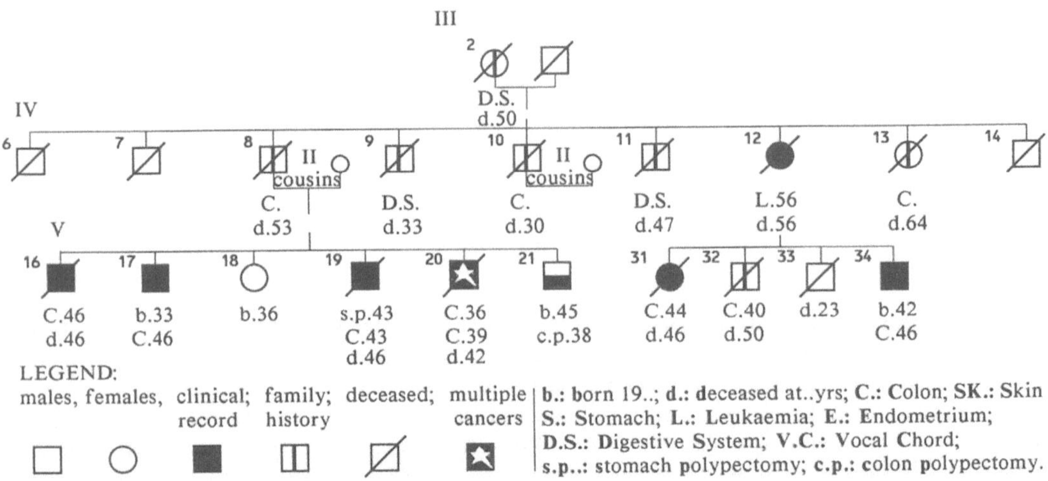

FIG. 1

The subject was hospitalized in February 1980 complaining of occasional abdominal troubles. A double contrast barium enema was performed and, as shown in Fig. 2,3, resulted negative.

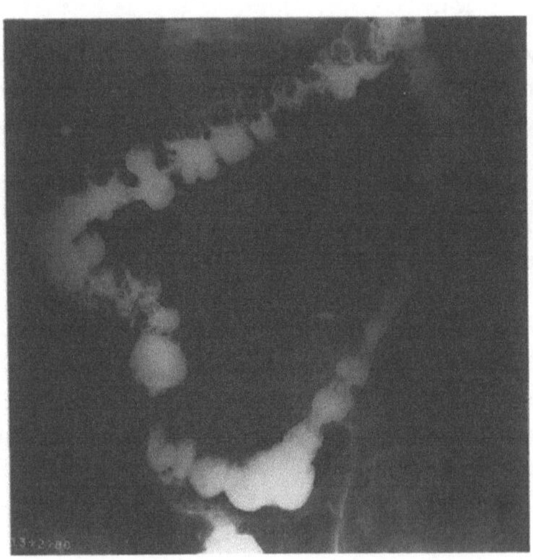

FIG.2

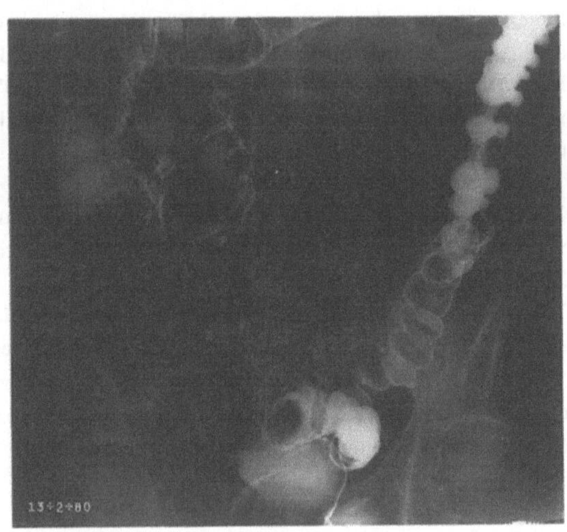

FIG.3

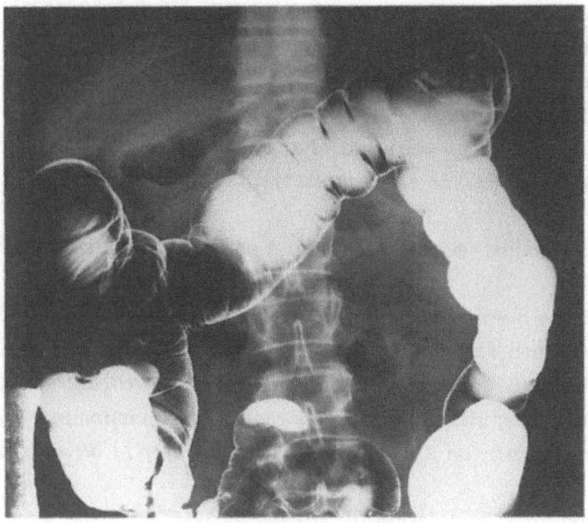

FIG.4

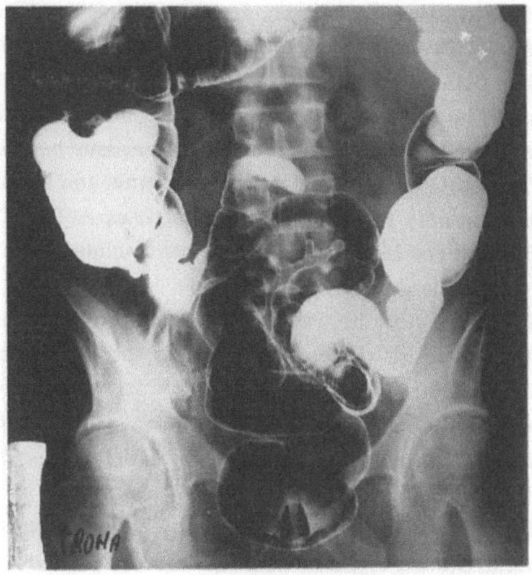

FIG.5

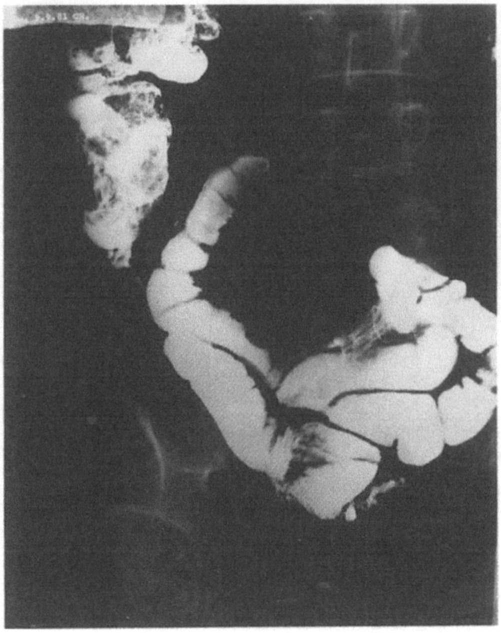

FIG.6

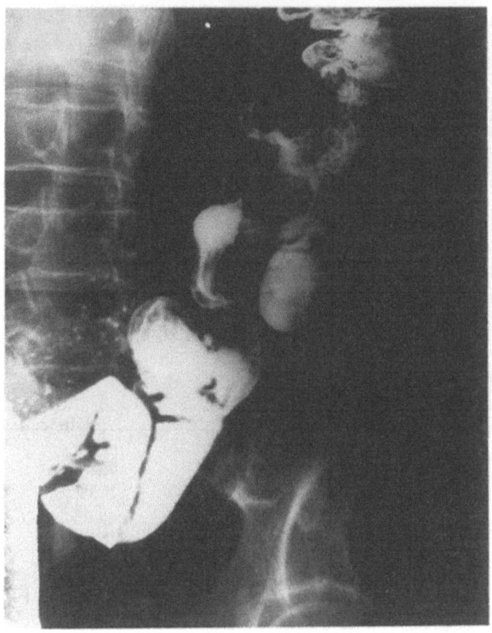

FIG.7

18 months later, due to an epigastric heartburn, he was admitted to another hospital. Standard tests revealed an anaemia, an active duodenal ulcer and a small polyp (histologically hyperplastic) was also removed by diathermic snare during a gastroscopy. Further abdominal troubles necessitated another double contrast barium enema (see Fig. 4, 5.) that was, as documented, negative.

In addition, given a continuous anaemic status and positive FOBT, he underwent a little bowel X-Ray which proved negative (see Fig. 6, 7).

The investigations were completed with a liver profile echotomography (negative) and a routine chest X-ray which the radiologist, searching only for parenchimal lesions, diagnosed as negative.
The patient was discharged a few days later (September 1981) with a diagnosis of "Outcome scar of bulbar ulcer in a patient with hypochromic and hyposideremic anaemia".
43 days later he was readmitted to the same hospital for a peptic ulcer check. The endoscopy showed an ulcer healing. Owing to the persistent anaemia and abdominal troubles, the endoscopist tried to make a colonoscopy but, he only managed the *splenic flexure*. The CEA value was 1,1 ug/ml!
On October 18th, 1981 the Subject discharged himself, against medical advice, not having completed all the examinations.
Four days later he was called by the chief surgeon of the hospital to which he had been originally admitted and where his three other brothers had been admitted earlier.
On the 30th of October 1981 he underwent a new double contrast barium enema which showed a *growing mass on the ascending colon* (clinical record). Nine days later the subject underwent a right hemicolectomy and the histological diagnosis was: *At all wall infiltrating cancer on Ascending Colon with 4 over 11 infiltrated limphnodes: Duke's C2.*
Furthermore a later bone scanning exam demonstrated an accumulation of Tc-99^{m}-Tc-MDP in the V, VI right rib and right clavicle. On the 25th of December the right rib was surgically removed as were the VI right rib and the right clavicle on the 29th of January 1982.
The histology demonstrated: "Metastasis of poorly differentiated adenocarcinoma".
As expected with this Syndrome the subject died after *three years* at the age of 46.

CASE 2: This case was followed-up in a hospital in Northern Italy and, consequently we can only document it with clinical records. Fig. 8 shows the family history of this subject (V-75).

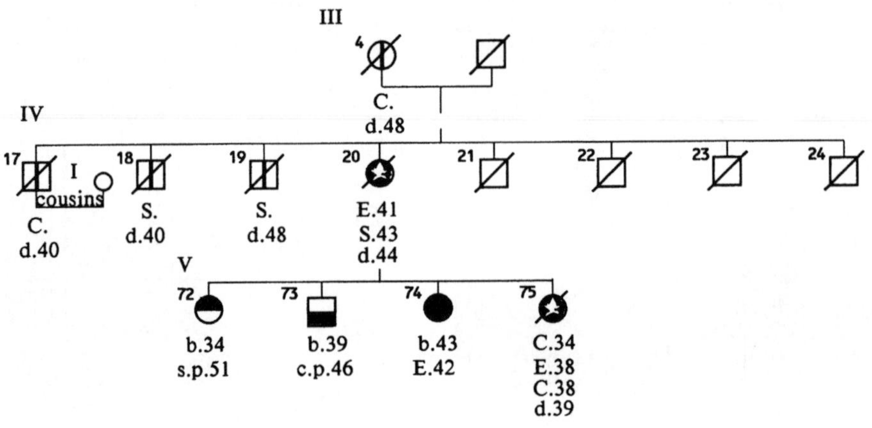

FIG. 8

During 1980 this female, aged 34, developed a rectal tumor. She underwent a surgical anterior rectal resection, a left hemicolectomy and an *appendicectomy.*
Histologically the rectal tumor was a moderately differentiated adenocarcinoma, Duke's B. She subsequently underwent periodical endoscopic controls managing the *splenic flexure only.*
Due to endometrial troubles, at 38 years of age, (1984, October), she was hospitalized and underwent an

histerectomy and bilateral salpingo oophorectomy. The histological diagnosis was: *"poorly differentiated adenocarcinoma with diffuse neoplastic lynphagitis (G3 over 3; IV of Brothers), massive metastasis on the right ovary and lynpho-perilymphatic massive metastasis".*
Her half-brother, a cardiologist who attended the operation assured us that the surgeon had made a thorough manual exploration of all remaining colonic segments which proved *negative.*
23 days later, due to abdominal occlusion, she was urgently admitted to another hospital (Southern Italy). The intraoperative diagnosis was: "Intestinal occlusion due to a growing cancer occluding the *ileo-cecal valve"* (see appendicectomy performed 4 years before). Histologically it was a "Moderately differentiated adenocarcinoma with *aspects of mucinous type:* Duke's B1".
She died a few months later when aged 38.

CASE 3: The family history of this case (VI-111) is reported on Fig. 9.

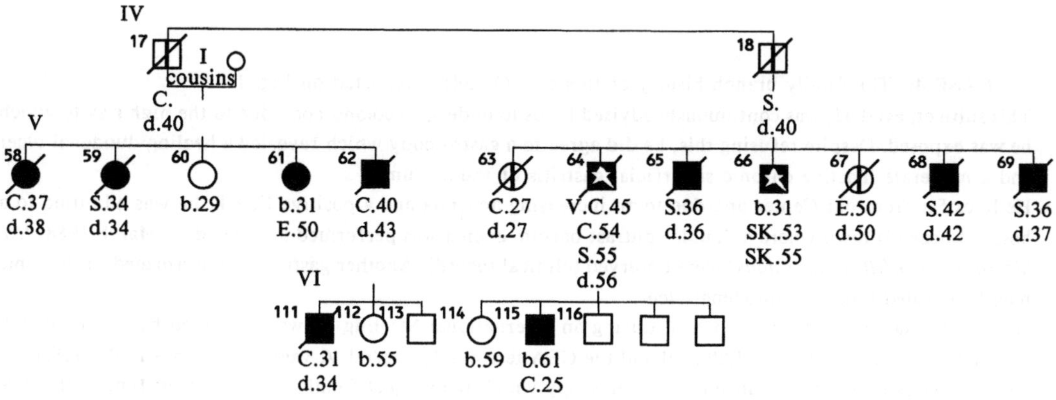

FIG. 9

This young male, aged 31, accepted our Surveillance protocol for asymptomatic subjects showing Lynch Syndrome II. His health and appetite was good and the alvus was perfectly regular.
At the first colonoscopy (January 1985) an infiltrating and growing neoplasia (5 cm.) of the ascending colon was detected. The histology demonstrated a *mucinous adenocarcinoma.*
Due also to the subject's high risk for gastric cancer, and in order to *erroneously* preserve colon segments, an *ileo-transverse-stomy* was performed. The resected colon histology showed 12/27 lynphonodes involved (Duke's C). CEA test was of 5,2 ug/ml.
Six monthly endoscopic control of the remaining colon performing multiple biopsies of the stomy and on other different macroscopically normal segments were made and, until April 1988 proved negative.
There was no weight loss or fever, the alvus was normal and the appetite healthy. Due to a slowly increasing CEA level (December 1987: 7,1; April 1988: 10; May 1988: 11 ug/ml) a TC scan exam was performed in May 1988 which showed liver-right kidney metastasis.
The lower vena cava was infiltrated and a necrotic lymphonodus (Ø=15 mm.) was detected in front of the same vein, thus an attempt of surgical draining of the metastasis was performed 15 days later which also revealed stomach, duodenum and pancreas involvement.
Figs. 10 and 11 show the infiltration removed from the lower vena cava and the remaining Colon including the stomy respectively.
It must be underlined that the metastasis were developed from the stomy, *outside the colonic mucosa.*
Strangely this subject asked us *why* he had to undergo an operation because he said he felt *healthy!*
He died in December 1988.

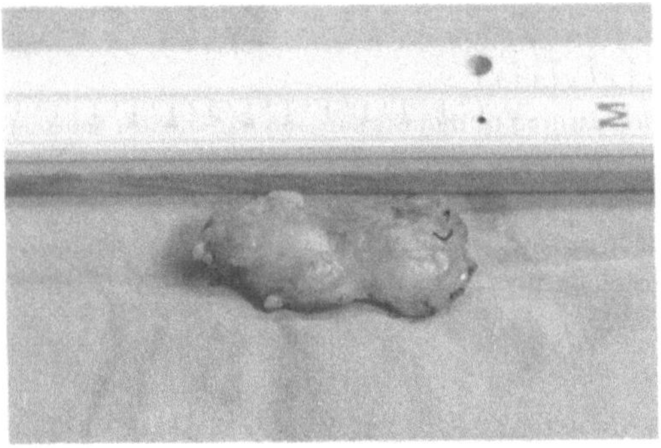

FIG.10

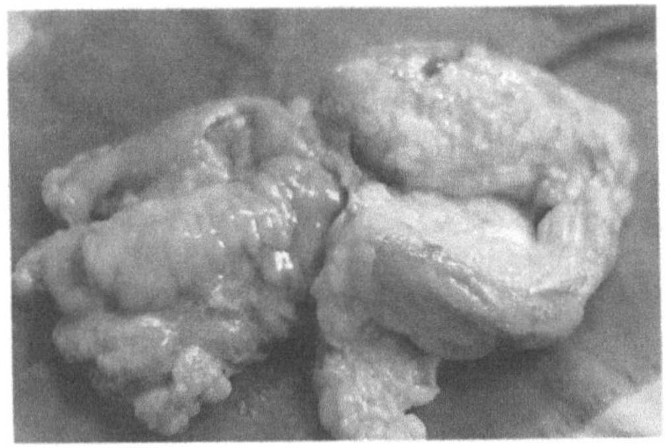

FIG.11

CASE 4: The family branch history of this case (V-34) is reported on Fig. 1.
This subject, aged 43, was continuously advised by us to undergo a colonoscopy due to the high risk to which he was exposed. Despite refusing this, he did agree to a gastroscopy which revealed a healing duodenal ulcer and a moderate inactive chronic superficial gastritis of the antrum.
He lives far from our Center and due to an increasing anaemia and a positive FOBT, he was admitted to a hospital near his town where a double contrast barium enema was performed at the end of March 1988: *"No ulcerative or infiltrating lesions"* were observed (clinical record). Another gastroscopy performed in the same month revealed a healing duodenal ulcer.
He was discharged on May 1st, when, during an International Meeting he was examined by two of us (H. T. L. and G. C.). The Hb was 7,00 g/dl and the CEA test was 1,7 ng/ml. A vague asthenia was also referred. We again stressed the importance of a colonoscopy which the subject finally underwent on June 13th 1988: *"A vegetating and infiltrating mass, 5 cm in length, of the cecum-ascending colon"* was detected. He was operated on a few days later in a hospital near his town but *contrary* to our advice *"a latero-lateral ileotransverse-stomy"* was performed. The histology demonstrated a *"moderately differentiated adenocarcinoma infiltrating at all wall the segment"* no lynphonodes were involved (Duke's B1).

CASE 5: Family history of this young male (VI-115) is shown in Fig. 9.
This asymptomatic subject accepted our instrumental surveillance program started in 1984 and, aged 23, he underwent the first colonoscopy (September 1984) which was macroscopically and histologically negative (biopsies from cecum to rectum). Two years later, at the second exam scheduled and performed in October 1986 a *"flat hyperaemic lesion of ellitic form (cm. 2x0,5)"* was observed and the diagnosis of the bioptic fragments showed a *"severe adenomatous dysplasia of the superficial compartment"*. An ileo descendent stomy was performed with a right colon prophylactic resection. Figs. 12 and 13 show the lesion on the resected segments.
The post surgical histology was *"flat tubular cancerized adenoma with focal aspects of sub-mucosa infilatrations. No metastasis over 31 lynphonodes examined"* Duke's A. This subject, currently in good health, observes a yearly instrumental follow-up.

Lastly we would like to stress that in our experience, over a 5 year instrumental surveillance and follow-up, over the 100 colonoscopies performed on at high risk asymptomatic subjects, apart from three colon cancers described before, we found *6 polyps in 4 Subjects only*, among which two plus two were synchronous and only 4 were true adenomas.
One of these polyps was a "tubular adenoma of the rectum with mild dysplasia" (V-73, Fig. 8); the other two, synchronous (Ø 3 and 1 mm), were rectal pseudopolyps: "diffuse infiltrate of macrophages at basal dislocation"

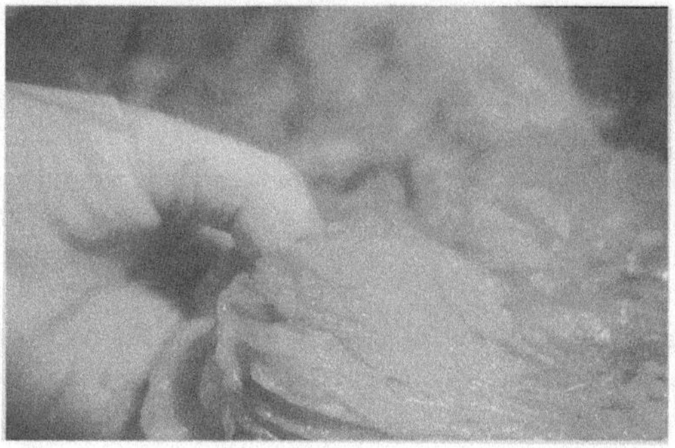

FIG.12

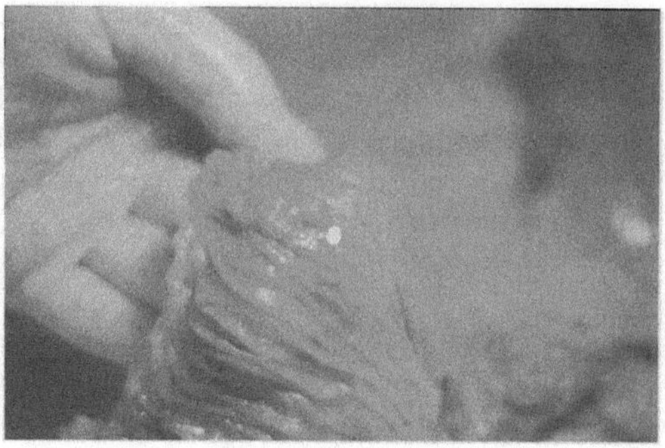

FIG.13

(V-72, Fig.8). Another two synchronous polyps, one of the ascending colon (2 mm., missed) and the other of the rectum (1 cm.) where diathermocoagulated in a 60 year old subject who, 8 years before, had been operated on for a left colectomy due to colon cancer. The rectal polyp was a villous II adenoma (Ø 1,2 cm.) with a moderate dysplasia.
The last resected and unfortunately missed polyp (Ø 3 mm.) was detected on the ascending colon in a 45 year old male (V-21, Fig. 1).

DISCUSSION

CANCER HISTORY: these cases some of which are reconstructed and documented by clinical records and others based on personal experiences, give us the opportunity to discuss the natural history of the adenoma carcinoma sequence and some hypothetical differences in the *cancer history* between *sporadic colon cancer* and *genetic colon cancer.*
In the *sporadic* colon cancer, as reported in the authoritative Literature [Morson B.C., 1979], the Authors on the basis of numerous and well controlled experiences, affirm literally that..."*The adenoma-carcinoma sequence is never less than 5 years (average 10-15 years)*". From research carried out until now, we also know that a polyp of 2 mm. of diameter, to become a polyp of 2 cm. of diameter and therefore potentially dangerous, in terms of cancerous probability, takes an average of *ten* years.
With reference to case 5, we have hypothesized, for example, that it could have been a "missed polyp"; however if the natural history of these lesions is the same as that of "sporadic" lesions, two years before its dimension should have been 1,8xo,4 cm.. We can only assume therefore that the lesion was not existent at the time of the first examination (September 1984).
The discovery of a very low number of polyps in at high risk subjects is in perfect agreement with one of the peculiar characteristics of Lynch Syndromes: a *restricted number of polyps* [Boland C.R., 1984; Lynch H.T. 1988b].
The cases documented lead us to some intriguing hypotheses:
- The *genetic colon cancer history* could reasonably be completely different from that which generally occurs in the *sporadic colon cancer* in terms of *adenomas presence* and *cancer growth.*
- The possibility that a cancer could develop on a colonic mucosa, not preceded by precancerous lesions such as the adenomas, in Lynch Syndrome kindreds *may* unfortunately *exist* especially when some morphological alteration such as *macrophages excess* and *crypt atrophy* are present [Cristofaro G., 1985, 1987].

On the basis of these experiences we can therefore speculate that the assumption that a *colon cancer* is *always preceded by an adenoma* is *not* always ***true***, particularly in subjects showing Lynch Syndromes.
This peculiarity raises enormous medical difficulties in terms of management of these subjects and raises some interesting questions too:

- Are two years sufficient to follow-up those subjects from 25 to 35 years of age? (different cancer growth).
- Is 25 a good age to begin the instrumental exam? (see case 5).
- Is the macrophages excess associated (or not) with crypt atrophy a new and valid biomarker to anticipate endoscopic controls? Would the compliance be the same in this case?
- On the basis of settled and codified acquisition regarding the natural history of adenoma carcinoma sequence, could the physician become legally liable if a carcinoma is detected on a mucosa which two years before was *macroscopically* and *histologically* proved *negative?*

LEGAL CONCERNS. In our own Italian experience and consultation of medical history and physicians, we have heard on several occasions instances of physicians criticising Colleagues or, in other cases, threats of legal action made by relatives to a physician who *apparently* missed a lesion a few months before.
Physicians' insurance against medical mistakes is not common in Italy compared other countries, and particularly the U.S.A.
This constitutes a great difficulty for Insurance Companies both in effecting insurances for medical mistakes and increasingly more in effecting life and medical insurances for subjects showing Lynch Syndromes [Lynch H.T., 1989].
To preserve our professional image and protect ourselves from legal recourse we should advise our subjects that, to date, we know very little about the real and natural history of cancer growth in Lynch Syndromes. Quite frankly the likelihood of finding a carcinoma on a mucosa where nothing was observed earlier is *extremely realistic.*

CONCLUSIONS

This paper, in conclusion, aims at suggesting some guidelines for Preventive Surveillance/Management Strategies:
- A carefully orchestrated family history must be obtained by physicians on all at high risk subjects.
- Genetic counseling with emphasis upon genetic risk, surveillance and management, and a rationale for these preventive strategies must be thoroughly addressed.
- Rigorous surveillance must be performed, even when biomarkers of acceptable sensitivity and specificity to the cancer-prone genotype eventually become known. Instead of double contrast barium enema, when possible, a pancolonoscopy until ileo-cecal valve must be performed. This exam should also include the recognition of flat adenomas, as well as the excess of macrophages and crypt atrophy.
- Surgical prophylaxis by performing a sub-total colectomy may even be indicated in such a setting.
- The peculiar and different cancer history in Lynch Syndromes could be explained and a subscript document about this knowledge should be requested for at high risk subjects, in order to avoid potential litigation.
- More attention and a better knowledge of Lynch Syndromes must be requested by Insurance Companies when they have to draw up a life and medical insurance for at high risk subjects.
- In Countries with a different Health System like Italy, insurance costs both for preventive clinical and instrumental follow-up and medical treatment, could be covered by Governments.

In spite of these *apparently* great difficulties we strongly advise physicians who encounter subjects showing these Syndromes not to succumb to the complexities, both in medical and legal terms, but to persevere with these unlucky patients in an effort to help them and moreover try to do everything they know possible so that we can better our understanding of this particular field.

REFERENCES

BOLAND C.R. and TRONCALE F.J. (1984).
Familial Colonic Cancer Without Antecedent Polyposis. Ann. of Intern. Med. ; 100: 700-701.

CRISTOFARO G., CARUSO M.L., ATTOLINI A. et Al. (1985).
Cancer Family Syndrome (Lynch Syndrome II): Preliminary Report of New Phenotipic Findings.
In: Muller & Weber (Eds.). Familial Cancer; Karger, Basel, Munchen, Paris, London, New York, New Delhi Singapore, Tokyo, Sydney: pp. 85-87.

CRISTOFARO G., LYNCH H.T., CARUSO M.L., ATTOLINI A. et AL. (1987).
New Phenotypic Aspects in a Family With Lynch Syndrome II. Cancer ; 60: 51-58.

CRISTOFARO G., DI GIULIO E., MINGAZZINI P. GUANTI G., BUFO P., MEMEO V., TAURO A., DI GIULIO A. and LYNCH H.T. (1988).
Sindrome II di Lynch: Sorveglianza di un Esteso Gruppo Familiare.
in: CLEUP (Ed.) Padova. Acta of the "II Congresso Nazionale di Coloproctologia".; pp.: 291-301.

CRISTOFARO G., DI GIULIO E., MINGAZZINI P., TIRINDELLI DANESI D., SENATORE S., ME MEO V., TAURO A.V., BUFO P., LYNCH P.M., APPELMAN H.D., SMYRK T.C., WATSON P., LANSPA S.J., BOMAN B.M. and LYNCH H.T. (1989).
"I Tumori del Colon-Retto: le Sindromi di Lynch e Nostre Esperienze. I Fattori Genetici, Recenti Acquisizioni sul loro Ruolo nella Determinazione dell'Alto Rischio"
in: CIC Ed. Internaz. (Ed.) Rome. "Aggiornamenti in Colon-Proctologia".; pp.197-212.

LYNCH H.T., KIMBERLING W., ALBANO W.A., LYNCH J.F., BISCONE K., SCHUELKE G.S., SANDERBERG A.A., LIPKIN M., DESCHNER E.E., MIKOL J.B., ELSTON R.C., BALEY- WIL SON J.E. and SHANNNON DANES B.S. (1985).
Hereditary Nonpolyposis Colorectal Cancer (Lynch Syndrome I and II) p. I and II. Cancer; 56: 934-951.

LYNCH H.T., WATSON P., KRIEGHLER M., LYNCH J.F., MARCUS J., SMYRK T., FITZGIBONS R.J. and CRISTOFARO G. (1988).
Differential Diagnosis of Hereditary Nonpolyposis Colorectal Cancer (Lynch Syndrome I Vs. Lynch Syndrome II). Disease of the Colon and Rectum; 31: 372-377.

LYNCH H.T.,WATSON P.,LANSPA S.J.,MARCUS J.,SMIRK T.,FITZGIBBONS R.Jr., CRISTOFARO G., KRIEGLER M. and LYNCH J.F. (1988a).
Clinical Nuances of Lynch Syndromes I and II.
in: G. Steel, R.W. Burt, S.J. Winawer, J.P. Karr (Eds.): Basic and Clinical Perspectives of Colorectal Polyp and Cancer. Alan Riss, N.Y.; pp.: 177-188.

LYNCH H.T., LANSPA S.J., BOMAN B.M., SMYRK T., WATSON P., LYNCH J.F., CRISTOFARO G., BUFO P., TAURO A.V., MINGAZZINI P. and DI GIULIO E. (1988b).
Hereditary Nonpolyposis Colorectal Cancer-Lynch Syndromes I and II.
in: Gordon Luk (Ed.) Gastroenterology Clinics of North America. Vol.17 N° 4 (Colorectal Cancer) W.B. Saunders Comp. Philadelphia PA; pp.: 679-712.

LYNCH H.T., LANSPA S.J., SMYRK T.C., WATSON P., FITZGIBBONS R.J. Jr, LYNCH J.F., CRISTOFARO G., and ROZEN P. (1989)
Clinicopathologic and Genetic Studies of the Lynch Syndromes: an Update with Screening Recommenda tions. in: Acta of the II International Conference on Gastrointestinal Cancer, Jerusalem (Israel). Karger: Basel, Munchen, Paris, London, New York, New Delhi, Singapore, Tokyo, Sydney (in press).

MORSON B.C., DAWSON M.P., SPRIGGS A.I. and Sir JOHNES F.A. (1979).
The Adenoma Carcinoma Sequence.
In: Gastrointestinal Pathology. Blakwell Scientific Pubblications Onsey Mead, Oxford 2nd Ed. pp.:630-637

The Research Nurse/Family Contact Person and Hereditary Colon Cancer

JANE F. LYNCH

ABSTRACT

A thorough and systematic compilation of the family history of cancer may provide one of the most powerful mechanisms for hereditary cancer syndrome diagnosis. The registered nurse has an ideal background for collecting this family history data. The proband and informative relatives furnish genealogy and cancer history information. Reported cancer occurrences are documented, when possible, by medical and pathology reports, and a working pedigree is compiled. Based on this information, the physician/geneticist provides cancer genetic interpretation and recommends surveillance/management programs. Research protocols into all facets of this process, including a search for biomarkers of cancer susceptibility, are coordinated by the nurse.

Keywords: cancer family history, nurse coordinator

INTRODUCTION

Colorectal cancer is a major health problem in virtually all of the industrialized nations of the world. While a diet that is high in fat and low in fiber has been implicated as a major etiologic factor in colorectal cancer, host factors have also emerged as a major causal concern in this disease. The role of host factors in colorectal cancer's etiology can best be appreciated when one understands the well-defined hereditary colonic cancer-prone syndromes. The most thoroughly accepted hereditary colon cancer syndrome has been familial adenomatous polyposis (FAP) [Bussey 1975]. FAP has the distinct advantage of the presence of myriad adenomatous polyps to aid in its diagnosis. The recognition of its more recently described counterpart, hereditary nonpolyposis colorectal cancer (HNPCC) or Lynch syndromes I and II, is more difficult [Lynch et al 1985]. A well-documented family history is essential in either case.

It is mandatory that the clinician have sufficient pedigree information available for hereditary cancer syndrome diagnosis so that highly targeted surveillance and management programs can be performed. Programs, if they are to be effective for inordinately high genetic risk patients and their at risk relatives, should satisfy one or more of the following criteria: a) the natural history of cancer expression within the given disorder should be known; b) the estimated biologic latent stage of the particular cancer, including its estimated age of onset should be known; c) screening tests employed should have high specificity and sensitivity to the cancer site of concern; and d) effective therapy should be available, with good agreement of who should and who should not be treated. The multiple endocrine neoplasia syndromes (MEN-IIa and IIb) and site-specific medullary thyroid carcinoma are illustrative of this paradigm [Vasen et al 1987]. The calcitonin stimulation test in these disorders is reliable and convenient. The recognition of FAP, with subsequent colectomy, is of course an appropriate model for this discussion. Unfortunately, only a limited number of hereditary cancer syndromes can be managed with this degree of simplicity and efficiency; future biomarker research should ameliorate these important concerns.

NURSE/FAMILY CONTACT PERSON - STUDY COORDINATOR

Until such biomarkers are identified for the nonpolyposis colorectal cancer syndromes, the family history can provide one of the most powerful and potentially cost effective tools for hereditary colorectal cancer diagnosis. It is paradoxical that in this era of extremely expensive, albeit advanced, technologies such as computerized axial tomography, magnetic resonance imaging, and DNA diagnostics, a thorough and systematic compilation of the cancer family history is often either totally ignored or given short shrift. We believe that paramedicals, particularly registered nurses, can readily assist the physician in the compilation of family history from affected and/or genetically high risk colorectal cancer patients. Our purpose therefore is to define the research nurse/family contact person in the clinical practice setting, with appropriate pragmatic implications for management of hereditary colorectal cancer problems.

The most important requirement is that the family contact person be knowledgeable about the significance of the family history and that he/she be highly motivated so that this interest, concern, empathy, and compassion can be effectively understood and appreciated by the family.

Our experience in family history acquisition and its evaluation for hereditary cancer spans a quarter century and involves countless thousands of cancer-prone kindreds. Our Hereditary Cancer Institute at Creighton University is committed to the assessment and management of all varieties of hereditary cancers, including those involving the colorectum. Protocols outlining the logistics for genealogic and medical acquisition have been refined over the years, lending flexibility, so that they can meld with the pursuits of our collaborators from differing institutions throughout the world.

Pedigree Compilation Process

Persons who are concerned about their possible risk for hereditary cancer are either self-referred or they are referred by their physicians to our Consultation Center. The nurse compiles the family history by interviewing the proband, or if the contact was by correspondence, the initiating patient is asked to complete and return a questionnaire. At first, we concentrate on first degree relatives and selected maternal and paternal second degree relatives (grandparents, aunts, uncles). These relatives are more informative than younger individuals because the average age of the syndrome cancers in the kindreds is such as to have made phenotype (cancer) expression more likely in these older relatives than in the more youthful members (progeny, nephews, nieces of probands). Relatives for whom we have been given a specific address are sent a letter explaining the purpose of our contacting them. Included with the letter is a questionnaire which, when completed, will provide us with information on their branch of the family. A lag time of approximately 45 days is allowed before a second questionnaire is sent to nonrespondent individuals.

Telephone calls are often made when there is no response or to clarify information. All family members are given assurances of confidentiality. Family wishes are followed expressly and requests to resign from further study are accommodated. However, cooperation of family members is usually excellent and large, informative pedigrees can be constructed from the questionnaires. As part of our family study protocols, we make a vigorous effort in every circumstance to secure primary medical and pathology documents for cancer verification. Procedures to secure these records are initiated immediately upon return of the questionnaire. A cover letter and the signed release of information form is sent to the appropriate hospital, requesting these documents on the cancer-affected family members. We attempt to verify cancer of all sites, not just those in the gastrointestinal tract. Surviving spouses, children, or closely related individuals are contacted to access decedent records. When records are not available due to destruction or other problems, death certificates are utilized as a means of cancer disclosure.

Unfortunately, the securing of medical and pathology documents and death certificates has become increasingly more difficult due to destruction of the records or a variety of confidentiality requirements. In many cases, the institution responsible for the medical documents may have requirements which create obstacles to their release. For example, the medical record librarian may insist that a permission form be signed within 90 days of the request. In certain circumstances, such an individual may have died since the release form was signed, or they may no longer be traceable. Thus, an exchange of letters and telephone queries may have to take place before the information can be obtained. Occasionally, one may circumvent these problems by requesting that pertinent information such as histologic diagnosis of cancer be read over the telephone from the record. In our experience, this type of approach may be adequate in certain circumstances, while in others, a full medical record (depending on the objectives of the study) may be necesary. Thus, one may have to seek additional legal next of kin, so that release of the document might be possible, given the type of scenario we have described.

Pedigree updating is a dynamic and continuous process which is constantly changing based on the receipt of newly reported family information or medical and pathology documentation. The pedigree is reviewed when new information is received because this may change the risk status of certain family members. Initially, when as much documentation of the cancer family history as possible has been accrued, the pedigree is presented to our weekly pedigree conference, at which time the hereditary status is determined and surveillance recommendations are made.

Regardless of how the family was ascertained, it is essential to identify the high risk patients' family physicians so that all pertinent family history information and surveillance recommendations can be forwarded to them for maximum patient followup, once the pedigree has been compiled and the hereditary cancer syndrome has been diagnosed (figure).

Model for Cancer Genetic Evaluation in HCCC

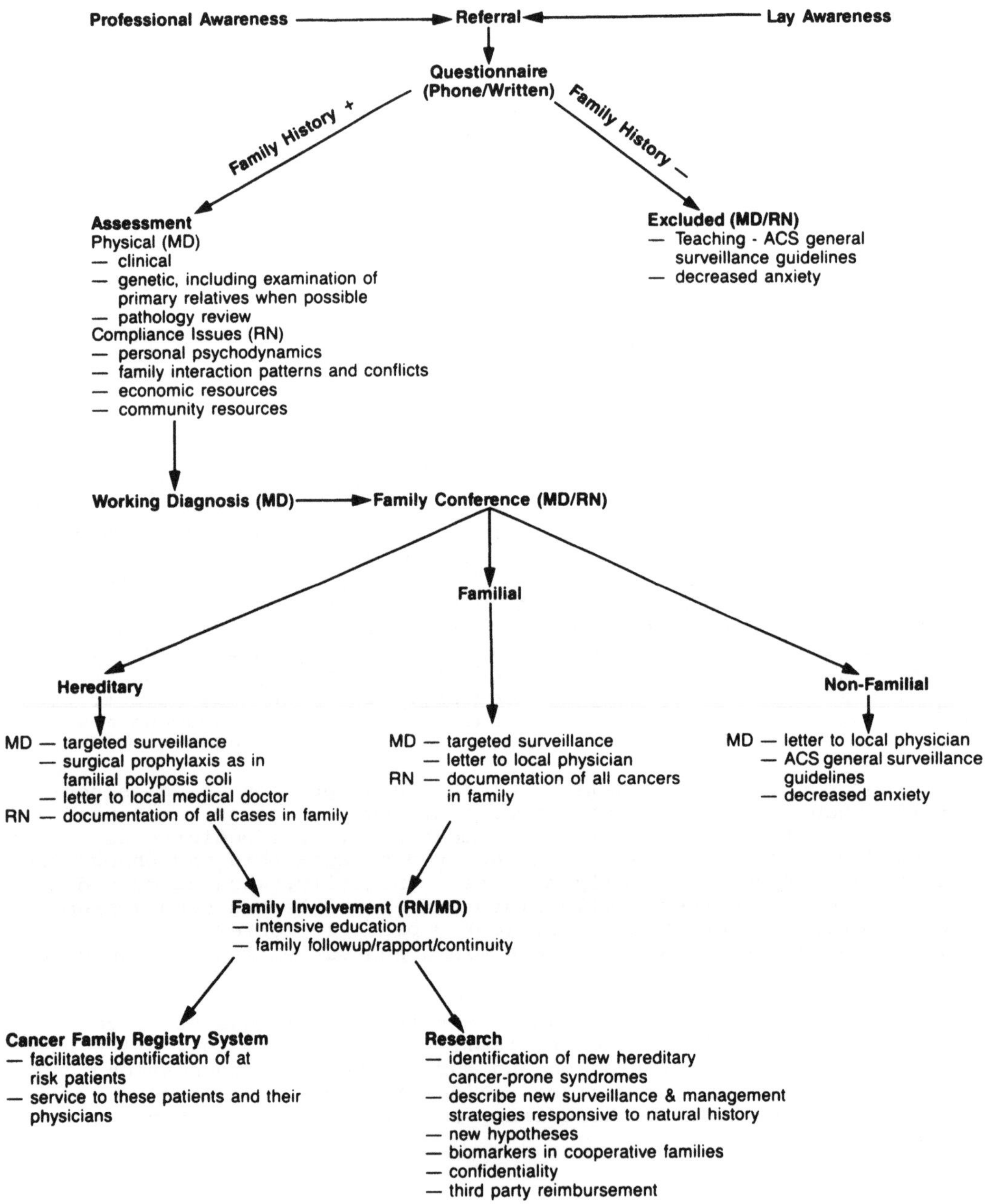

Computerization of Data

We have developed in-house data entry and management systems which facilitate accurate and timely data entry and safe data storage in a central repository, utilizing the dBaseIV (Ashton-Tate) software system. The data recorded includes: family structure information, ascertainment source, family syndrome diagnosis, individual names, addresses, vital statistics, demographic information, personal health and reproductive history, physician contacts, risk status, and details of any cancer diagnosis. We have also computerized a tracking system to record the sending and receipt of questionnaires, requests for medical/pathology records, and pathology blocks and slides. Correspondence appropriate to each situation is generated by the computer, including education/recommendation letters for patient and physician, followup/ requests for screening procedure results, and reminders for repeat procedures. The tracking system can record when items of correspondence were sent by us, when responses were received, and when procedure results were received. The accumulated data is entered into a personal computer by the family contact person, and in the case of routine data entry not requiring interpretation, by the data entry staff.

The analysis programs which use the database files include: a risk code assignment program which allows specification of affection status (e.g., we may define as "affected" any family member with adenocarcinoma of the colon and uterus) and then assigns risk codes (affected, obligate gene carrier, 50% risk, 25% risk, low risk, married-in) to all family members; a program for computing expected numbers of cancer specific to a designated cohort and adjusted for the age and sex of the cohort members based on general population incidence rates, and for comparing these expected numbers to the observed numbers in the cohort; and a program for assessing heterogeneity among families in expression of specific phenotypic traits.

Molecular Genetics and Family Studies

Recent advances in the molecular genetics of colorectal cancer hold promise for precision in colorectal cancer syndrome delineation, with potential for identifying the deleterious gene(s). Ultimately, cloning the cancer-prone gene(s) should provide opportunities for developing antithetic pharmacologic methods for counteracting the carcinogenic expression of these genes. Genetic engineering may even provide methods for primary prevention [Astrin & Costanzi 1989].

The availability of extended colorectal cancer-prone families with highly detailed and accurate genealogic, medical, and pathology corroboration of cancer is essential for biomolecular genetic investigation. This is clearly evident in the case of colorectal cancer wherein linkage research in familial adenomatous polyposis localized the trait on chromosome 5 [Bodmer et al 1987; Leppert et al 1987] and current research has indicated that chromosome 5 deletions (and also deletions on chromosomes 17 and 18) are frequently found in colorectal carcinomas from familial and nonfamilial cases [Solomon et al 1987; Law et al 1988; Vogelstein et al 1988]. Our own findings of linkage in Lynch syndrome II to JK (lod score 3.19) [Lynch et al 1985], with the recent assignment of JK to chromosome 18, suggests that the deleterious gene for Lynch syndrome II may be located on chromosome 18 [Boman et al 1988]. It is therefore clear that the availability of a resource with exceedingly well-defined families prone to the Lynch syndromes could prove to be of invaluable aid to the advancement of biomolecular genetic investigations in the search for clues to carcinogenesis. It is logical to assume that these advances in biomolecular genetics will eventually enable us to determine who is vs. who is not a carrier of the deleterious gene for an increasing number of identifiable hereditary cancer disorders. This would then enable us to target our surveillance strategies to those individuals who are most clearly destined to develop cancer of specific anatomic sites. This would result in a saving of physician and patient time, and would have major economic cost impact.

Field Visits for Biological Sample Collection and Patient Education

Carefully selected families from our resource are utilized for our biomolecular research studies. The family contact person is responsible for coordinating all of the logistics required to collect the biosamples, either on an individual basis or from a large group of assembled family members. For instance, when a family has been selected for linkage studies, a field visit is planned. These trips are conducted by the research team in the geographic areas where the maximum number of cancer-affected and high risk subjects from the family reside. Local medical facilities are made available for our use. Letters and/or phone calls are made to explain to the potential participants the purpose of the study, procedures to be performed, and a proposed date and place for the field visit. Additionally, letters are sent to the patients' physicians explaining the research and eliciting permission to involve their patients in the study. This methodology has in the past provided patients and physicians with sufficient information about our procedures and thereby has assured patient/physician participation.

In addition to the collection of biological material, these field visits provide an opportunity to educate family members, with emphasis on genetic risk status and surveillance recommendations. Education of families is exceedingly important, but is not limited to families involved in field trips. The registered nurse coordinates the construction and distribution of pamphlets and newsletters for all hereitary cancer family members as well as for their physicians. These contain messages about the natural history and genetics of hereditary colorectal cancer, and emphasize the need for surveillance and management which is reflective of the natural history of cancer.

Continued Education of the Family Contact Individual

The nurse continues her own education through participation and presentation at workshops, including visits to the research centers who are collaborating on the particular project, through updating of literature files, and constant collating of data on the families with acquisition of new relatives and new/unrelated families for the particular project. All of this culminates in the preparation of manuscripts. The nurse is an active collaborator on these papers. The sum total of these experiences adds to the professional stature of the nurse/family contact person.

REFERENCES

Astrin SM, Costanzi C (1989) The molecular genetics of colon cancer. Sem Onc 16:138-147

Bodmer WF, Bailey CJ, Bodmer J, Bussey HJR, Ellis A, Gorman P, Lucibello FC, Murday VA, Rider SH, Scambler P, Sheer D, Solomon E, Spurr NK (1987) Localization of the gene for familial adenomatous polyposis on chromosome 5. Nature 328:614-616

Boman BM, Lynch HT, Kimberling WJ, Wildrick DM (1988) Reassignment of a cancer family syndrome gene to chromosome 18. Ca Genet Cytogenet 34:153-154

Bussey HJR (1975) Familial polyposis coli: family study, histopathology, differential diagnosis, and results of treatment. J Hopk Un Press, Baltimore

Law DJ, Olschwang S, Monpezat JP, Lefrancois D, Jagelman D, Petrelli NJ, Thomas G, Feinberg AP (1988) Concerted nonsyntenic allelic loss in human colorectal carcinoma. Science 241:961-965

Leppert M, Dobbs M, Scambler P, O'Connell P, Nakamura Y, Stauffer D, Woodward S, Burt RW, Hughes J, Gardner E, Lathrop M, Wasmuth J, Lalouel M, White R (1987) The gene for familial polyposis coli maps to the long arm of chromosome 5. Science 238:1411-1413

Lynch HT, Kimberling WJ, Albano WA, Lynch JF, Biscone K, Schuelke GS, Sandberg AA, Lipkin M, Deschner EE, Mikol YB, Elston RC, Bailey-Wilson JE, Danes BS (1985) Hereditary nonpolyposis colorectal cancer (Lynch syndromes I and II), Parts I and II. Cancer 56:934-951

Solomon E, Voss R, Hall V, Bodmer WF, Jass JR, Jeffreys AJ, Lucibello FC, Patel I, Rider SH (1987) Chromosome 5 allele loss in human colorectal carcinomas. Nature 328:616-618

Vasen HFA, Kruseman ACN, Berkel H (1987) Multiple endocrine neoplasia syndrome, Type II: the value of screening and central registration. Am J Med 83:847-852

Vogelstein B, Fearon ER, Hamilton SR, Bodmer WF, Jass JR, Jeffreys AJ, Lucibello FC, Patel I, Rider SH (1988) Genetic alterations during colorectal tumor development. N Eng J Med 319:525-532

ACKNOWLEDGEMENTS: Support for this effort was provided by grants from the National Cancer Institute, #1 RO1 CA42705-03, the Nebraska Cancer and Smoking Diseases Research Program, #90-04R, and the Health Futures Foundation.

Surgical Strategies for Management of the Lynch Syndromes

ROBERT J. FITZGIBBONS, HENRY T. LYNCH, STEPHEN J. LANSPA, THOMAS SMYRK, BRUCE BOMAN, JANE LYNCH, and PATRICE WATSON

ABSTRACT

The most important consideration in the treatment of patients with the Lynch Syndromes is recognition. Specific treatment recommendations are based on the natural history of the syndrome. The newly diagnosed colon cancer patient from a Lynch Syndrome family should undergo a subtotal colectomy with low ileorectal anastomosis because of the frequency of synchronous and metachronous colon cancers. Routine sacrifice of the rectum is not justified because of the propensity for the cancers to involve the proximal colon. Lynch Syndrome II patients must have additional recommendations made to address the integrally inherited extracolonic cancer, i.e., total abdominal history and bilateral salpingo-oophorectomy (TAHBSO). For patients who are as yet unaffected by cancer, prophylactic surgery is not felt to be justified because only 50% of first degree relatives of Lynch Syndrome patients are at risk. Finally, for a patient who has been treated for colon cancer before being recognized as a member of a Lynch Syndrome family our current recommendation is aggressive screening. Subtotal colectomy is reserved for the poorly compliant patient.

KEY WORDS:

Lynch Nonpolyposis Hereditary Colon Surgery

INTRODUCTION

Surgeons and the surgical approach to treatment are crucial in the management of patients with either of the Lynch Syndromes of Hereditary Nonpolyposis Colon Cancer (HNPCC). Their importance is in no small part underscored by the fact that in many clinical practice settings the surgeon is the only physician who will see the colon cancer patient. Thus, if the surgeon does not appreciate the presence of the syndrome, there is little chance that the patient will receive appropriate treatment. The key to the surgical management of patients with the Lynch Syndromes is recognition. In contradistinction to Familial Polyposis Coli (FPC), which is recognized by the majority of surgeons because of the distinctive clinical marker of multiple colon polyps, the presence of the Lynch Syndromes is rarely appreciated by the average surgeon because of the absence of a marker lesion. Thus, the real challenge when discussing surgery for the Lynch Syndromes is to promote an educational initiative to the practicing surgeon so that the possibility of the Lynch Syndromes are considered in every patient treated for colon cancer.

Although treatment strategies for the Lynch Syndromes are distinctively different from patients with sporadic colon cancer or other forms of hereditary colon cancer, the average surgeon when cognizant of the existence of the disease process in his patient will have little difficulty in recommending the proper form of treatment. This is because the treatment recommendations flow so logically from the natural history as will be described in this chapter. Our purpose, therefore, will be to discuss first the natural history of the Lynch Syndromes as has been determined by an in-depth review of families from our registry in the Creighton University Hereditary Cancer Institute. Treatment recommendations will then be discussed from the point of view of the way in which patients present to the clinician. Thus, treatment recommendations will be divided into three sections: 1) treatment of patients with a newly diagnosed colon cancer, 2) recommendations for family members as yet unaffected by colon cancer, and 3) recommendations for patients who have had a previous conventional colectomy that is now known to have been inadequate therapy because HNPCC has just been identified.

NATURAL HISTORY OF THE LYNCH SYNDROMES

Lynch Syndrome I and Lynch Syndrome II represents the two subdivisions of the larger group of patients who suffer from hereditary nonpolyposis colon cancer (HNPCC). The natural history of HNPCC has recently been crystallized by review of the past medical histories of ten families currently being followed at the Creighton University Hereditary Cancer Institute.[Fitzgibbons 1987] These families were uniquely suited for study of the family history because very few of the patients had been recognized to be members of a hereditary colon cancer family before the study began. The majority of patients with colon cancers in these families were treated conventionally as if the cancers had occurred sporadically. The ten families represent a mixture of both Lynch Syndrome I and Lynch Syndrome II.

One-hundred and eighty-three histologically confirmed colon cancers were found in 116 individuals in these ten families. There were 64 males and 52 females. The mean age of onset of the first colon cancer was 45.6 years which compares to 63 years of age which was determined by review of several recent reviews in patients considered to have sporadic colon cancer.[Falterman KW 1974; Langevin JM 1984; Reilly JC 1982] In these hereditary colon cancer families, 69.1% of the cancers were located proximal to the splenic flexure with only 23.3% involving the sigmoid colon and rectum. This compares to 28.6% and 66.3%, respectively in the control sporadic colon cancer population. For the purposes of this review, colon cancers occurring within one year's time of the index colon cancer were considered synchronous. This occurred in 18.1% of the HNPCC patients as opposed to 4.8% in the sporadic colon cancer patients. Metachronous colon cancer developed in 24.2% of HNPCC patients with life table analysis disclosing that the risk of metachronous colon cancer in HNPCC patients was 40% by ten years. Finally in all ten families, the inheritance pattern was consistent with an autosomal dominant transmission. The results of this study confirmed the autosomal dominant inheritance pattern in HNPCC patients as well as the importance of the cardinal features of early age of onset, proximal colon involvement, relative sparing of the sigmoid colon and rectum, and increased incidence of synchronous and metachronous colon cancers in confirming the diagnosis.

Review of the data also confirms the importance of dividing the larger population of HNPCC patients into two groups, Lynch Syndrome I and Lynch Syndrome II, as this has important ramifications for treatment and surveillance. Thus, Lynch Syndrome I includes those patients who have colon cancer only being inherited in an autosomal dominant pattern. An increased frequency of cancer in general was noted in some of the Lynch Syndrome I families but not in any clearly definable Mendelian genetic pattern to impact on treatment or surveillance recommendations. This is in contradistinction to the Lynch Syndrome II families in whom extracolonic cancers were inherited in concert with the colon cancer as if the gene(s) for both existed in the same chromosomal location. In these families and in fact in all of the Lynch Syndrome II kindreds in our registry, the extracolonic cancers have been confined to the female genital tract. However, breast, pancreas, and other cancers have been reported by various authors to be inherited in a similar fashion.[Lynch HT 1984]

SURVEILLANCE RECOMMENDATIONS AS THEY RELATE TO TREATMENT

Surgical treatment and surveillance recommendations for patients from Lynch Syndrome families are significantly intertwined and thus it is difficult to discuss them separately. Logistical factors, patient compliance, psychological stability, and other factors may dictate that in similar clinical circumstances, prophylactic surgery might be recommended for one patient while a rigorous surveillance program advised for another. Surveillance recommendations are discussed in depth elsewhere but a brief review would seem to be in order because it must be referred to when discussing treatment and its appropriate follow-up.

The surveillance program currently recommended begins with biannual fecal occult blood testing at age 20. Colonoscopy is initiated on a yearly basis beginning at an age five years before the onset of the earliest colon cancer which has been noted in a particular family. Patients in Lynch Syndrome II families must also have a surveillance program tailored for the extracolonic, integrally inherited cancers. Since all the extracolonic cancers in our experience have been confined to the female genital tract, we recommend biannual pelvic examinations and yearly endometrial suction biopsies. Yearly ovarian ultrasound is occasionally employed if the pedigree indicates that the ovary is the site of the extracolonic cancer. Finally, for the Lynch Syndrome II families whose extracolonic cancers are also extragenital a specific surveillance regimen must be designed to address the organ or organs involved. A summary of the surveillance recommendations for individual organ systems are included as Table 1.

SURGICAL TREATMENT FOR LYNCH SYNDROMES

Treatment considerations are best discussed from the point of view of the way in which patients present to the clinician. These clinical presentations can be divided into three groups: 1) treatment of a Lynch Syndrome patient with a newly diagnosed colon cancer. This will also include those Lynch Syndrome II patients who developed the integrally inherited cancers of the female genital tract before the colon cancer; 2) recommendations for the patient from a Lynch Syndrome kindred as yet unaffected by cancer; 3) recommendations for a patient with a previous conventional colectomy which is now known to have been inadequate because the patient has just been recognized as a member of a Lynch Syndrome family.

TABLE 1

Summary of Surveillance Recommendations

Target Organs	Recommendations
Colon	Education, patient and physician. Genetic Counsuling beginning in mid-teens. Biannual fecal blood testing beginning in at age 20. Yearly colonoscopy beginning at age 25 or five years before the onset of the earliest colon cancer in the family.
Female Genital Tract*	Biannual pelvic examination and yearly endometrial suction biopsy. Ovarian ultrasound if the pedigree indicates it.
Extracolonic, Extragenital Cancer*	Tailored to particular organ involved with cancer as determined by review of the pedigree.
Rectal Remnant After Subtotal Colectomy and Ileorectal Anastomosis	Biannual proctoscopic examination.

*Lynch II Syndrome only

Surveillance Recommendations for Lynch Syndrome Families

The overall management scheme which is employed in our institute when a new patient from an HNPCC kindred presents is shown diagrammatically in Fig. 1. The discussion that follows will begin at column four of the figure after the patient has been categorized as being a member of either a Lynch Syndrome I or Lynch Syndrome II family. Note that both treatment and surveillance recommendations are included because the two disciplines are interrelated when considering the management of Lynch Syndrome patients.

Treatment of The Lynch Syndrome Patient With a Newly Diagnosed Colon Cancer

The natural history of the Lynch Syndromes discloses an inordinately high incidence of synchronous and metachronous colon cancers. The incidence is great enough to justify removal of most of the colonic mucosa at risk. However, it is also important to remember that the natural history also confirms that the majority of colon cancers in Lynch Syndromes are proximal (i.e., 87.4% above the level of the rectum). Thus, routine sacrifice of the rectum with construction of the permanent stoma with the potential morbidity in the form of sexual and urinary tract dysfunction, as a consequence of removal of the rectum, would not appear to be justified. For this reason, we routinely recommend a subtotal colectomy with ileorectal anastomosis. Even the less mutilating mucosal proctectomy, pouch-anal procedures are not believed to be indicated because the incidence of rectal cancer does not justify the added morbidity compared with the ileorectal anastomosis.[Francois Y 1989]

Moertel and his colleagues from the Mayo Clinic in 1970 published a review of their polyposis patients who had been treated by subtotal colectomy. They noted an inordinately high rate of cancer developing in the remaining rectal remnant as patients were followed long-term. This led to skepticism about any procedure less than total colectomy when dealing with familial polyposis coli or for that matter, any form of hereditary colon cancer.[Moertel CG 1970] It should be pointed out that before 1970, subtotal abdominal colectomies included relatively long rectal segments leaving a significant amount of retained colon

FIGURE 1

MANAGEMENT STRATAGIES FOR THE LYNCH SYNDROMES

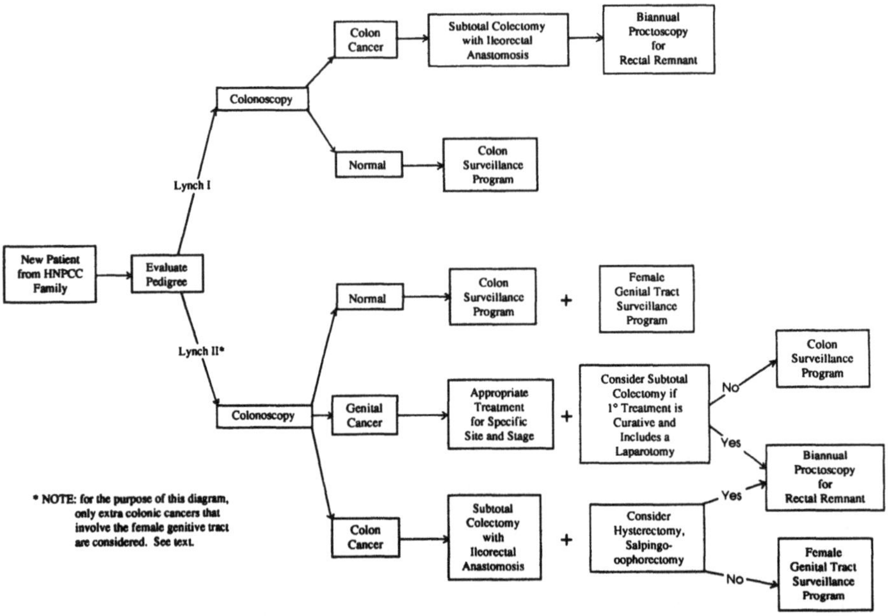

Algorithm From New Patients From HNPCC Kindred

tissue at risk for cancer. With the development of modern stapling devices, a subtotal colectomy can now be performed with a very low ileorectal anastomosis in patients with a premalignant colonic condition. This low rectal anastomosis makes follow-up surveillance straightforward. We perform a rigid proctoscopic examination every six months in our patients, a relatively simple procedure since the rectal segment is invariably less than 15 centimeters and sometimes much shorter. It is our feeling that subtotal abdominal colectomy with a low ileorectal anastomosis is the operation of choice for patients with Lynch Syndromes.

Of some concern however is the concept that by transferring the effluent of the distal ileum and right colon to the rectum, one might establish the same environment in the genetically susceptible mucosa of the rectum which had previously existed in the right colon. This could result in a high incidence of cancer in the retained rectum.[Albano WA] As yet, no data is available to answer this question because so few patients have been treated correctly with a subtotal colectomy when the initial colon cancer is diagnosed. Since the majority of patients we are now following for the Lynch Syndromes are being treated with a subtotal colectomy at diagnosis of the first colon cancer, mature data should be available in several years.[Lynch HT 1983]

Lynch Syndrome II patients must have special consideration for extracolonic cancer. In our registry, all of these extracolonic cancers have been confined to the female genital tract. Thus, for the female patient who presents with a newly diagnosed colon cancer from a Lynch Syndrome II family, we strongly consider prophylactic total abdominal hysterectomy and bilateral salpingo-oophorectomy (TAHBSO). Some of these patients are quite young and therefore childbearing desires and concern about the long-term effects of prolonged estrogen replacement therapy must be considered. If TAHBSO is not performed, a surveillance program consisting of biannual pelvic examinations and yearly endometrial suction curettage as an office procedure is begun. Yearly ovarian ultrasound is also recommended if the individual pedigree suggests that the integrally associated extracolonic cancer involves the ovary.

Another important consideration in Lynch Syndrome II is how best to treat the patient who presents with the integrally associated extracolonic carcinoma first. For example, a female member of a Lynch Syndrome II kindred might present with an endometrial carcinoma and review of the pedigree discloses that this is a particular tumor being inherited integrally with the colon cancer. This, of course, means that the patient almost certainly carries the HNPCC genetic material which puts her at an extremely high risk to ultimately develop colon cancer. Thus, it would be appropriate to combine her therapy for the endometrial malignancy with a prophylactic procedure for the colon. Our approach for these types of patients is to recommend subtotal abdominal colectomy with low ileorectal anastomosis providing that the proposed therapy for the genital malignancy is going to be curative and will include a laparotomy.

Finally, there are Lynch Syndrome II patients whose extracolonic integrally associated cancer is also extragenital. Prophylactic treatment is usually not practical in such patients since the organ involved does not lend itself to prophylactic surgery, i.e., pancreas. An effective surveillance program however must be tailored to meet the needs of these families.

Recommendations For Other Members of The Family as Yet Unaffected by Cancer

A 50% risk to carry the defective genetic material for the Lynch Syndromes exists in any individual member of a kindred because of the autosomal dominant inheritance pattern. Prophylactic therapy, which for the colon would require a major operative procedure, is not justified since 50% of the patients would be treated needlessly. Patients who are members of Lynch Syndrome kindreds who have not yet been affected by cancer are enrolled in a surveillance program as has been previously outlined. For patients from Lynch Syndrome II families, this must include surveillance for the extracolonic cancer also.

Compliance with yearly endoscopic evaluation is sometimes resisted by both the patient and referring physicians in favor of the more liberal regimens employed for sporadic colon cancer patients. Our patients are counselled carefully because it appears that invasive carcinomas can develop quite rapidly in Lynch Syndrome patients without readily detectable precursors. Formerly it was hypothesized that the classic polyp cancer sequence was not active in Lynch Syndrome patients. We now feel that a better explanation is that these patients develop so-called "flat adenomas" which are quite elusive both endoscopically and radiographically. Regardless, the important concept to impress upon the patient is that from a clinical standpoint colon cancers can develop as if they were de novo and therefore frequent surveillance is mandatory.

An exception to our recommendation that surveillance only is indicated in these patients exists for the obligate gene carriers. Thus, if we are making recommendations for a member of a Lynch Syndrome family who gives a history that both a grandparent and an offspring have been affected by cancer, the patient must certainly carry the defective genetic material. In this setting, prophylactic subtotal colectomy is usually recommended as well as prophylactic treatment for the extracolonic organ if the patient is a member of a Lynch Syndrome II family.

Recommendations For a Patient With a Previous Conventional Colectomy Just Recognized As a Member of a Lynch Syndrome Family

Patients who have had a previous conventional partial colectomy and are just now recognized as being members of a Lynch Syndrome kindred represent a particularly perplexing problem. Since the patients have already been affected by colon cancer, they obviously carry the genetic material for the Lynch Syndromes. Our data suggests that their risk for the development of a metachronous colon cancer would be 40% by ten years. Careful patient and family counselling is mandatory. As a rule, we employ surveillance but do not hesitate to recommend a completion subtotal colectomy with ileorectal anastomosis if logistical problems, poor patient compliance, or other factors make adequate surveillance difficult.

CONCLUSION

Treatment recommendations for patients who are members of Lynch Syndrome kindreds are straightforward and based exclusively on the natural history of the condition. The most significant problem with the surgical management of the Lynch Syndromes is that affected patients are difficult to recognize. For this reason, most patients from Lynch Syndrome kindreds who present with a newly diagnosed colon cancer are treated with conventional colectomy and this commonly results in the need for repeated surgeries as they develop metachronous colon cancers. An example is provided in Fig. 2 which is a pedigree of a family currently in our registry. Note the extreme incidence of metachronous colon cancers requiring repeated surgeries. These multiple procedures could have been avoided if the patient would have been treated initially with subtotal colectomy. Thus, the real challenge to improve the surgical treatment of patients from Lynch Syndrome families is to educate surgeons such that the possibility of the existence of the Lynch Syndromes is considered in every patient treated for colon cancer.

FIGURE 2

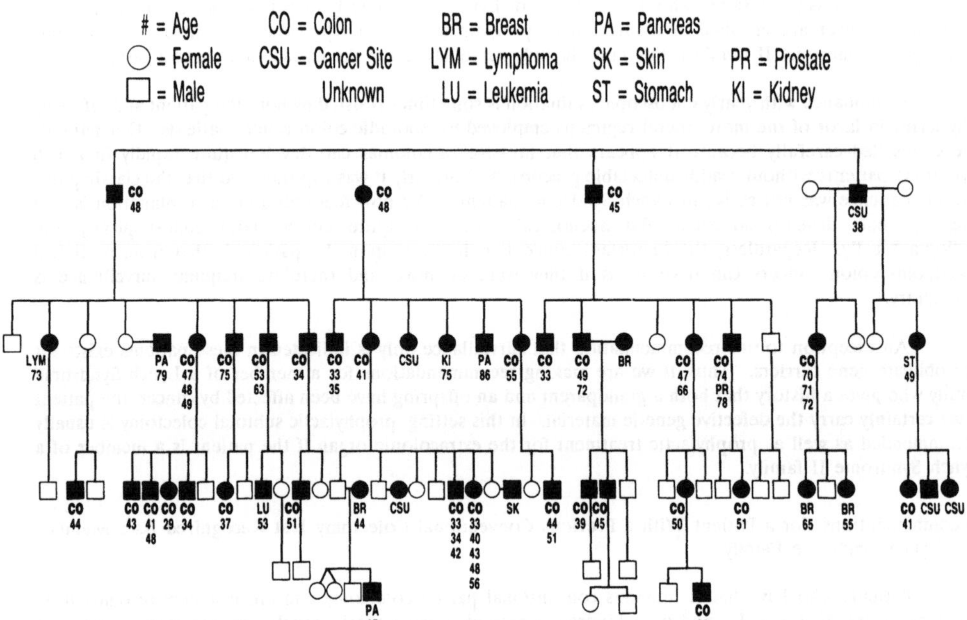

Pedigree for one of the families described. Note the incidence of metachronous colon cancer requiring repeat colectomy.

REFERENCES

1. Albano WA, Lynch HT Clinical management of hereditary colon cancer. Colon Cancer Genetics, New York: VN Reinholt, Co., 99-110.

2. Falterman KW, Hill CB, Markey JC, et al (1974) Cancer of the colon, rectum, and anus: A review of 2313 cases. Cancer 3(suppl):951-959.

3. Fitzgibbons Jr RJ, Lynch HT, Stanislav GV, Watson PA, Lanspa SJ, Marcus JN, Smyrk T, Kriegler MD, Lynch JF (1987) Recognition and treatment of patients with hereditary nonpolyposis colon cancer (Lynch Syndromes I and II). Ann Surg 206(3):289-295.

4. Francois Y, Dozois RR, Kelly KA, Beart RW Jr, Wolff BG, Pemberton JH, Ilstrup DM (1989) Small intestinal obstruction complicating ileal pouch-anal anastomosis. Ann Surg 209(1):46-50.

5. Langevin JM, Nivatvongs S (1984) The true incidence of synchronous cancer of the large bowel. Am J Surg 147:330-333.

6. Lynch HT, Rozen P, Schuelke GS, Lynch JF (1984) Hereditary colorectal cancer review: Colonic polyposis and nonpolyposis colonic cancer (Lynch Syndrome I and II). Surg Dig Dis 2:244-260.

7. Lynch HT, Albano WA, Ruma TA, et al (1983) Surveillance/management of an obligate gene carrier: The cancer family syndrome. Gastroenterology 84:404-408.

8. Moertel CG, Hill RJ, Adson MA (1970) Surgical management of multiple polyposis: The problem of cancer in the retained bowel segment. Arch Surg 100:521-526.

9. Reilly JC, Rusin LC, Theuerkauf FJ Jr (1982) Colonoscopy: Its role in cancer of the colon and rectum. Dis Colon Rectum 25(6):532-538.

An Attempt for Identification of Hereditary Nonpolyposis Colorectal Cancer in Japan

TOORU SAKIYAMA, YOUICHIROU SAKANOUE, YOSHIO MIKI, MASATO KUSUNOKI, and JOJI UTSUNOMIYA

ABSTRACT

In order to identify hereditary non-polyposis colorectal cancer (HNPCC) in Japan, we analyzed clinical characteristics of 10 families of colorectal cancer (CRC) with two or more affected relatives in our department (the personal series) and of 39 families reported as familial CRC or cancer family syndrome in Japanese literatures (the reported series). The characteristics of CRC in the reported series in comparison with general CRC were earlier onset, higher incidence of multiple tumor, predominance in the proximal colon, and excess of multiple primary cancer in the other organs. They were similar to those of USA and Finland except for more frequent association with gastric cancer in the reported series. Gastric cancer patient with onset in age of 60 or younger in family history of CRC may be regarded as a clinical marker suggestive for HNPCC. The reason for failure to demonstrate the characteristics of HNPCC in the personal series is to be further clarified by study with our data based on larger scale.

Key words

Hereditary non-polyposis colorectal cancer, familial colorectal cancer, family history positive colorectal cancer, colorectal index.

Introduction

In Japan adenomatous familial polyposis was first reported in 1925, but HNPCC had been much less appreciated. The first report on a familial occurrence of CRC not associated with polyposis was made by M.Sassa et al. in 1969. They descrived two brothers who underwent surgeries for cancers of the ascending colon in the same year at their age of 53 and 39 respectively. Their mother was known to have cancer of the uterus operated. This was followed by several sporadic case reports on the similar families, but systematic study had not been made until the one by Utsunomiya et al. (1981[a, b]) which was made based on 39 pedigrees of family history positive (fh+) CRC registered at the Polyposis Center. They found that fh+ CRC had an earlier age at onset, more multiple primary cancers and an increased proportion of proximal lesion, compared with fh- cancer as suggested by Lynch et al. and stressed on an importance of familial history positivity to identify HNPCC in general CRC population. In consequence to this study, we are attempting to identify HNPCC in Hyogo area in order to initiate a new field study.

Patients and Method

The proband patients who were known to have CRC in their close blood relatives was extracted by means of reviewing on medical records of CRC patients who underwent surgeries at our department during the last 15 years. A preliminary working pedigree was constructed by reviewing family history. In addition, all the available informations on the cases which were reported as "familial CRC" or "cancer family syndrome" in Japanese literatures published 1969-1989 were also reviewed (references were indicated by * in the list).

RESULTS AND DISCUSSION

There were 44 fh+ cases in 577 CRC patient (7.63%). Ten cases who were found to have two or more blood relatives affected with CRC in their families were subjected to the study following on Mecklin(1987) (the personal series). Cumulative number of CRC patient in the series was 37. Literature review revealed there were 16 relevant reports including 39 well searched families in which 176 members with CRC were identified (the reported series) (Table 1). The data of the two series were compared with that of a large series of general CRC accumulated at Japanese Research Society for Colorectal Cancer. The reported series showed the feature characteristic to HNPCC including much younger one set, more frequent multiple cancer in the colon as well as those in the other organ, increased proportion of right colon lesion, and confirmed the previous study by Utsunomiya et al. (1981[a, b]), but the personal series failed to demonstrate such a marked characteristics. The reason for a discrepancy seen in the personal series and reported series is to be further clarified by study with our data based on a larger scale.

According to the previous study by Utsunomiya et al. 1981, the maximum difference in the age specific prevalence between the fh+ and fh- patients were found in the age of 50-59 (Table 2). Therefore, the age of 60 or younger in CRC patient would be one of clinical indicators for HNPCC.

Regarding to organ spectrum of cancer, gastric cancer which occupied a half (39.6%) of whole extracolonic malignancies Japanese series showed appearently more frequent occurrence compared with USA and Finland's series (Table 3). The colorectal index (CRI), which is expressed by the ratio of frequency of cancer of the other organ to that of CRC was 0.197 while CRI of gastric cancer was 0.071 in USA Series and 0.110

Table 1 Characteristics of colorectal cancer in the familial colorectal cancer in Japan

	Familial colorec. cancer		General Colorec. Cancer (Japan)	Mecklin et al. (Finland)	Fitzgibbons (USA)
	Personal series	Reported series			
No. family	10	39	–	22	10
No. case	37	176	5929*	163	183
Female/male ratio	0.95	0.89	0.75*	–	0.81
Average age (yr.)	55.6	46.3	59.8*	43.2	45.6
Multiple CRC (%)	5.4	14.2	4.5***	23.1	42.3
Multiple primary cancer (%)	10.8	15.3	6.13****	–	–
Right cancer (%)**	26.3 (5/19)	49.3 (66/134)	20.3*	57.4 (66/115)	69.1

* the National Survey Report of Colorectal Cancer in Japan No.4.
** based on number of the lesion which were able to be located.
*** based on 24871 cases of Jap. Res. Soc. Colorect. Cancer (N. Kaibara, et al., 1984)
****based on 53916 cases reported on 31th Meeting of Jap.Res.Soc. for colorect. cancer (1989).

in Finland's series (Table 3). Age of these stomach cancer was much younger than that of the general population suggest the HNPCC gene is also effecting on genesis of this cancer in addition to Japanese specific environmental factor. The evidence suggest that the presense of gastric and other extracolonic cancer with early onset in family history of CRC patient may also be regarded as a clinical member for HNPCC (Utsunomiya et al. 1981[a, b], Cristofaro et al. 1987).

Table 2 Age specific prevalence rate of colorectal cancer with positive and negative family history

	Colorectal cancer with family history				
	positive		negative		
Age	n	prevalence rate (A)	n	prevalence rate (B)	(A) - (B)
10-19	1	2%	5	2%	0%
20-29	6	12%	3	3%	9%
30-39	10	29%	16	10%	19%
40-49	14	52%	38	26%	26%
50-59	15	77%	54	48%	29%
60-69	12	97%	78	81%	16%
70-79	2	100%	42	98%	2%
80-90	0	100%	5	100%	0%

Utsunomiya J, 1981.

Table 3 Organ spectrum of cancer in HNPCC in different countries

Reporter	Personal series				Reported series			
No. family	10				39			
	No.	%	CRI*	age	No.	%	CRI	age
Total no organ	52	100.0			267	100.0		
Colorect.	37	71.2	1.00	55.6	176	65.9	1.00	46.3
Stomach	6	11.5	0.16	52.5	36	13.5	0.20	52.3
Uterus**	2	3.8	} 0.05	54.0	16	6.0	} 0.15	53.5
Endometr.	0	0.0			10	3.8		
Breast	3	5.8	0.08	58.5	7	2.6	0.04	55.0
Urinary	0	0.0			1	0.4		
Lung	1	1.9			2	0.8		
Others	3	5.8			19	7.1		

Reporter	Mecklin et al. (Finland)				Fitzgibbons (USA)			
No. family	—				10			
	No.	%	CRI	age	No.	%	CRI	age
Total no organ	276	100.0			334	100.0		
Colorect.	163	59.1	1.00	43.2	183	54.8	1.00	45.6
Stomach	18	6.4	0.11	50.2	13	3.9	0.07	
Uterus** / Endometr.	25	9.1	0.15	50.8	45	13.5***	0.25	
Breast	4	1.4	0.02	46.3	17	5.1		
Urinary					17	5.1		
Lung	4	1.5			1	0.3		
Others	62	22.5			58	17.4		

* colorectal cancer index explained in text.

** cancer of the uterus including the cervical and unknown site.

*** female genital tracts.

A family (FC55) in the personal series is worthwhile for special presentation (Fig.1). In Tokyo, 1981, Utsunomiya experienced a female patient who underwent two surgeries at her age of 45 for rectal cancer and at the age of 52 for colon cancer (case 1). Since her family history revealed an appearent cancer aggregation suggesting rather typical cancer family syndrome, her four children were called up and as a result, an advanced diffusely infiltrating cancer of the sigmoid colon was found and radically removed in her son of 31 years old at that time (case 2). Other three children were negative for cancer nor polyp (Ichikawa et al. 1982). In 1989, after discontact for many years, he (case 2) visited us in Hyogo with a cancer of ascending colon to undergo surgery. Revisiting on his family history revealed that her mother (case 1) already died of cancer of the urinary bledder at her age of 62 and three member of his family were found to undergo surgeries for colon cancers. This particular family suggested an effective result of family examination and an appearent necessity of continuous surveillance on HNPCC family members.

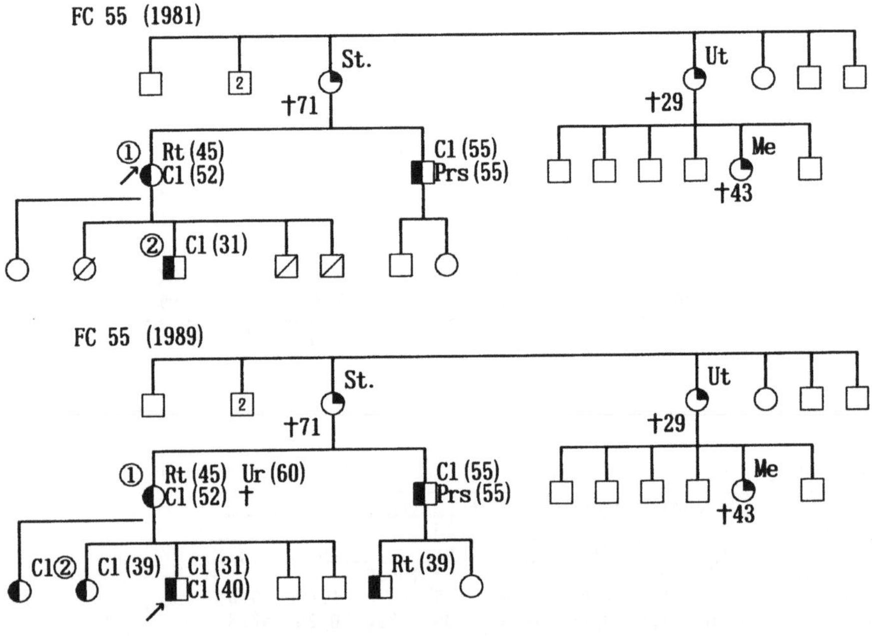

Cl: colon, Rt: rectum, Ut: uterus, St: stomach, Ur: urinary tract
Prs: prostate, Me: mesenterium

Fig.1 A Family with HNPCC suggesting the necessity of family surveillance

REFERENCES * indicates the Japaneses literatures submitted for the present study

Cristofaro G, Lynch HT, Caruso ML, Attolini A, Dimatteo G, Giorgio P, Senatore S, Argentieri A, Sbano E, Guanti G, Fusaro R, Giorgio I (1987) New Phenotypic Aspects in a Family with Lynch Syndrome II. Cancer 60: 51-58

Fitzgibbons RJ, Lynch HT, Stanislav GV, Watson PA, Lanspa SJ, Marcus JN, Smyrk T, Kriegler MD, Lynch JF (1987) Recognition and Treatment of Patients with Hereditary Nonpolyposis Colon Cancer. (Lynch Syndromes I and II) Ann.Surg 206: 289-295.

* Ichikawa T, Utsunomiya J, Iwama T, Yaegashi K, Nagai K, Saito K, Suzuki H, Maeda M, Matsubara O, Kamiyama R (1982) A case of linitis plastica type rectal cancer detected by family study. J Jpn Soc Colo-Proct 35(1):35-41 (In Japanese).

Kaibara N, Koga S, Jinnai D (1984) Synchronous and Metachronous Malignancies of the Colon and Rectum in Japan With Special Reference to a Coexisting Early Cancer. Cancer 54: 1870-1874

* Katano M, Fujiwara H, Toyoda K, Torisu M (1980) Immunogenetic studies of familial large bowel cancer. Gann 71(5): 538-588.

* Kawamura K, Harikane M, Oohara H, Sato H, Oda M, Kojima M, Watanabe H (1988) A case of cancer family syndrome- Associated with four synchronous colorectal cancers. Jpn J Cancer Clin 34(7): 932-937 (In Japanese).

* Koike Y, Adachi W, Ishizaka K, Ohashi M, Nakafuji H (1982) Experience of 2 cases with double cancer observed in cancer family. Jpn J Gastroenterol Surg 15(4): 666-670 (In Japanese).

Lynch HT, Kimberling W, Albano WA, Lynch JF, Biscone K, Schuelke GS, Sandberg AA, Lipkin M, Deschner EE, Mikol YB, Elston RC, Bailey-Willson JE, Danes BS (1985) Hereditary Nonpolyposis Colorectal Cancer (Lynch syndrome I and II). Cancer 56: 934-951.

Lynch HT, Watson P, Kriegler M, Lynch JF, Lanspa SJ, Marcus T, Smyrk T, Fitzgibbons RJ, Cristofaro G (1988) Differential Diagnosis of Hereditary Nonpolyposis Colorectal Cancer (Lynch Syndrome I and Lynch Syndrome II). Dis.Col.Rect. 31: 372-377

Mecklin JP, Jarvinen HJ (1986) Clinical Features of colorectal carcinoma in Cancer Family Syndrome. Dis Col Rect 29: 160-164

* Mikawa K, Narabayashi T, Nishigami T, Ohno T, Satomi M, Tamura K, Shimoyama T (1977) A case of familial colorectal cancer. Clinic All-Round 26(9): 2510-2516 (In Japanese).

* Noji N, Yamagiwa H (1973) Familial Solitary Carcinoma of the Large Intestine. Jpn J Cancer Clin 19(11): 1115-1120 (In Japanese).

* Nomizu T, Watanabe I, Suzuki S, Urazumi K, Endo S, Nihei M, Rokkaku Y, Tsuchiya A, Abe R, Endo S (1986) Clinical investigation on familial clustering of cancer of alimentary tract. Jpn J Gastroenterol Surg 19 (11): 2320-2323 (In Japanese).

* Ochi T, Asai T, Okamura S, Yamaguchi H, Oohashi S, Mitake M (1987) Clinicopathological study on CRC in young adult including a case with cancer family syndrome Jpn J Cancer Clin 33(4): 386-391 (In Japanese).

* Ohara T, Ihara O (1981) Non-polyposis colorectal cancer. Jpn J Clin Med 39(5): 2061-2066 (In Japanese).

* Oshima S, Kawai S, Maruyama T, Kanai M, Tominaga H, Hamada S, Utsunomiya J, Mishima Y, Hirokawa K, Yanagida T, Kurosu Y (1984) A case of familial large bowel cancer. Surg Therapy 51(3): 683-685 (In Japanese).

* Sassa M, Watanabe A, Kurotaki Y, Sakai H, Tori K, Kubo A (1969) Two cases of carcinoma of ascending colon successively seen in a short period of time in brothers. Jpn J Cancer Clin 15(11): 1010-1014 (In Japanese).

* Sasaki A, Konaga E, Enomoto M, Kawamura T, Haisa M, Hasuoka H, Yagi T, Ide A (1984) A case of cancer family syndrome. Jpn J Cancer Clin 30(14):1849-1953 (In Japanese).

* Tarao K, Kamishiro A, Matsuzaki M, Endo O, Shindoh K, Sugimasa T, Funayama M, Hiroi M, Watanabe T (1975) A Family with Six Members Affected by Colorectal Cancer. J Kanagawa Med Ass 2(2): 151-152 (In Japanese).

* Tomoda H, Furusawa M (1988) Familial CRC. Jpn J Clin Experrim Med 65(9): 2865-2868 (In Japanese).

* Ushio K (1989) Practice of diagnosis on colorectal disease vol.2 Colorectal tumor, gastrointestinal polyposis. Igaku-Shoin, Tokyo (In Japanese).

* Utsunomiya J, Iwama T, Matsumura T, Ichikawa T, Tanimura M, Nishiura M (1981[a]) A study on non-polyposis family large bowel cancer. Surgery 43(9): 881-889 (In Japanese).

Utsunomiya J, Iwama T, Hirayama R (1981[b]) Familial large bowel cancer. In: DeCosse JJ (ed) Large bowel cancer. Churchill Livingstone New York pp.16-33

* Utsunomiya J (1981[c]) Cancer family syndrome in colorectal cancer. Clin Adult Dis 11 (12): 1875-1882 (In Japanese).

Utsunomiya J (1990) The concept of hereditary CRC and an implication of the study. In this issue.

* Yagita A, Abe O, Baba S, Sekiguchi S (1977) HLA typing in patients with colon and rectum cancer, and ulcerative colitis with special reference to cancer susceptability. Jpn J Cancer Chemother 4(5): 939-945 (In Japanese).

Chapter 4

Chemoprevention of Colorectal Cancer

Summary of Chapter 4: Chemoprevention of Colorectal Cancer

MARTIN LIPKIN and PAUL ROZEN

In recent years increasing interest has developed in human studies in the field of chemoprevention. Several factors have contributed to this interest. They include preclinical studies showing tumor-inhibitory activity in many classes of naturally occurring nutrients; and studies demonstrating that biochemical changes within cells (intermediate biomarkers) might identify tumor inhibition in humans at an early stage. Recent reviews of this topic include Wattenberg (1985), Bertram (1987), Lipkin (1988).

Thus, it has been pointed out that compounds belonging to over 20 different classes of chemicals have potential capability for chemoprevention in human populations; some of these are naturally occurring constituents of food. The chemopreventive agents have been classified into two broad categories: inhibitors effective against the formation or activation of tumor initiating agents (i.e., genotoxic agents), or against tumor promoters.

Within the first group are compounds that prevent the formation of carcinogens from precursor substances, i.e., ascorbic acid, -tocopherol and certain plant phenols: caffeic and ferulic acids; compounds that prevent carcinogenic substances from reaching or reacting with critical target sites in the tissues, i.e., phenols, and certain plant flavonoids, flavones, coumarins and isothiocyanates; and compounds that act after exposure to carcinogenic agents by inhibiting the expression of neoplasia, i.e., retinoids and carotenoids, selenium salts, protease inhibitors, inhibitors of arachadonic acid metabolism, sterols and a steroid hormone.

Compounds that inhibit tumor promotion include retinoids, protease inhibitors, inhibitors of arachadonic acid metabolism, phenols, agents that increase intracellular cyclic AMP, and modulators of calcium metabolism.

Thus, new rationales for dietary intervention have emerged from epidemiological studies, and from studies of animal models, that might lead to further evaluation in human populations for possible tumor inhibition. In human subjects, however, it is difficult to determine whether dietary modifications or chemopreventive agents will actually inhibit tumor development; when neoplasia itself is used as an endpoint in studies of this type, very large numbers of subjects tested for long durations are often required. However, intermediate endpoints or biomarkers that are directly associated with the evolution of neoplasia, and that develop with much higher frequency in abnormal cells of susceptible individuals than do the actual tumors, now make it possible to carry out many studies on fewer subjects for shorter durations. If such biomarkers were found to be modified by a particular intervention regimen in short-term studies, leading to the regrowth of gastrointestinal cells having more normal and mature properties, a rationale would be provided for carrying out longer-term studies that could attempt to modify the later evolution of human tumors.

At this Workshop new studies related to the two major areas referred to above were presented: studies involving dietary and pharmacologic interventions, and others beginning to evaluate the utility of various biomarkers in this field.

The studies are briefly described below and are enumerated in Tables 1-3.

Table 1. Epidemiology and Animal Model Studies

Epidemiology review	T. Hirayama
Animal model studies	S. Hamilton
Indomethacin	T. Narisawa
Sarcophytol A	
Eicosapentaenoic Acid	H. Takada

Table 1 lists an epidemiologic study, and several studies carried out in animal models. Dr. T. Hirayana presented recent findings on the epidemiology of colorectal cancer in Japan. He referred to earlier work indicating an inverse relationship between green and yellow vegetable consumption and the incidence of large bowel cancer. He further described the fact that the incidence of colorectal cancer is increasing in Japan, and the possibility that by the year 2000 A.D. this disease may be more prevalent in Japan than gastric cancer. A recent study by Dr. Hirayama and his groups led to the finding of an association of carcinoma of the sigmoid colon and alcohol (beer) intake.

Potential chemopreventive agents have previously been studied in animal models. Dr. S. Hamilton reviewed characteristics of the various models. He pointed out the influence of genetic differences in rodent species; how some of these can resemble human populations; and how the differences might influence the outcome of chemoprevention trials. The important concept of genetic-environmental interactions in chemoprevention should be further expored. Types of carcinogens used in these experiments include direct (local) acting carcinogens that cause dysplasias and carcinomas as seen in humans, and indirect acting carcinogens that act via hepatic metabolism and produce derivatives inducing these cellular changes.

T. Narisawa described studies with inhibitors of prostaglandin synthesis, e.g., indomethacin, which inhibited the development of colorectal cancer in a hemicolectomy model, and which reduced the activity of ornithine decarboxylase. Newer measurements using sarcophytol A also inhibited carcinogenesis. In human subjects, indomethacin reduced ornithine decarboxylase activity in flat colonic mucosa of colonic cancer patients. A. Takada further described antitumor effects of a prostaglandin synthesis inhibitor, eicosapentaenoic acid (EPA). Administration of this compound reduced AOM-induced experimental colorectal cancer. This was associated with inhibition of prostaglandin E synthesis, reduction of bile acid output, and decreased ornithine decarboxylase activity.

Table 2. Biomarkers Involved in Intervention Studies

Tritiated thymidine	M. Wargovich D. Ernest H. Stern P. Rozen
Bromodeoxyuridine	M. Wargovich P. Rozen
Proliferating cell nuclear antigen (PCNA)	M. Wargovich
Ornithine decarboxylase	T. Narisawa M. Wargovich L. Herrera

Table 2 enumerates studies involving the further application of intermediate biomarkers to chemoprevention studies, mainly involving human subjects. The general subject of application of biomarkers to human studies was reviewed by M. Lipkin. M. Wargovich further described the development and application of several biomarkers to chemoprevention studies. Newer biomarkers of cell proliferation include bromdeoxyuridine (BUdR). Cell proliferation measurements with BUdR correlated well with tritiated thymidine, and specimen preparation time was more rapid with the former. Cell proliferation is also being studied with proliferating cell nuclear antigen (PCNA) which also labels proliferating cells outside of S-phase. Chromatographic patterns of ODC may be of further interest in measurement of this enzyme. Tritiated thymidine was used in clinical studies described below, by D. Ernest, H. Stern and P. Rozen; BUdR was used by M. Wargovich; PCNA by M. Wargovich; and ODC by T. Narisawa, M. Wargovich and L. Herrera.

Table 3. Adenoma Trials in Human Subjects

Calcium	B. Levin
Calcium	P. Rozen
Calcium, DFMO	L. Herrera
Fiber	D. Ernest
Fiber	J. DeCosse
Fiber, beta carotene, low fat diet	R. Macrae

In Table 3, further studies were described using the biomarker of advanced benign neoplastic disease, the colonic adenoma. It is important to note that when colonic cells become transformed and develop into adenomas, their responses to growth factors and growth inhibitors become modified, and some of these differ when compared to normal colonic epithelial cells. Therefore, chemopreventive agents that inhibit the growth of colonic adenomas could have no effect on inhibiting the neoplastic transformation of normal cells, and chemopreventive modalities inhibiting tumor initiation might have no effect on adenoma development. Therefore, in assaying the possible utility of a wide variety of chemopreventive agents in human subjects, it appears that it will be necessary to analyze many types of biomarkers to identify cell growth and development in many stages.

As noted in Table 3, B. Levin described a randomized controlled study in which patients received 2000 mg of elemental calcium or placebo for 30 days, with treatment crossover for an additional 30 days. A significant reduction in colonic epithelial cell proliferation was observed in subject who first consumed the placebo control, and then crossed over to calcium. When subjects began on calcium, they did not significantly increase cell proliferation when crossed over to the placebo. Increased cell proliferation has generally been found in the upper and lower gi tract in diseases predisposing to gi cancer, and following chemical carcinogens in rodent models.

P. Rozen reported that first-degree relatives of colorectal cancer patients with hyperproliferating colonic mucosa, consuming supplementary dietary calcium (1.25 - 1.5 gms daily), had reduced colonic cell proliferation while taking the calcium supplements. He further reported first degree relatives of sporadic colorectal cancer patients have increased colonic cell proliferation at a young age. BUdR also was successfully used to assay cell proliferation in the colon. In a further experiment with the carcinogen MNNG, a significant reduction of cell proliferation was found in rats when supplemental dietary calcium was given; diets were high or low in calcium, low in fat, calcium and Vitamin D content, and high in residue.

In contrast to the above studies on normal colonic epithelial cells, H. Stern reported no decrease in cell proliferation in familial polyposis mucosa after ileorectal anastomosis. L. Herrera reported a further randomized controlled trial of calcium in familial polyposis which is underway, using long-term adenoma recurrance as well as a series of biochemical markers to evaluate the effect of calcium in familial polyposis. He further described studies utilizing the biomarker ornithine decarboxylase together with studies of gene regulation of ODC.

Several studies involving the administration of supplemental dietary fiber to human subjects were described. D. Ernest reported a study in which wheat bran was given to patients following partial colonic resection for colorectal cancer. Patients whose colonic mucosa was hyperproliferating had significant reductions in cell proliferation after fiber supplementation. Additional measurements following piroxicam administration, given to patients whose adenomas had been removed, demonstrated decreased prostaglandin E2 and cell proliferation.

J. DeCosse reported that high fiber and vitamins C and E supplementation led to decreased numbers of rectal adenomas after-partial colectomy in familial polyposis, although compliance to the regimen was poor. A large multicenter trial of recurrent adenoma formation currently underway, was further reported by F. Macrae in which diets supplemented by betacarotene, low dietary fat content, and high fiber are being evaluated. Patients for the study have been recruited and two years of intervention have been completed.

References

Wattenberg LW. (1985) Chemoprevention of cancer. Cancer Res 45: 1-8.

Bertram JS, Kolonel LN. and Meyskens FL,Jr. (1987) Rationale and strategies for chemoprevention of cancer in humans. Cancer Res. 47: 3012-3031.

Lipkin M. (1988) Biomarkers of increased susceptibility to gastrointestinal cancer: New application to studies of cancer prevention in human subjects. Perspectives in cancer research, Cancer Research, 48: 235-245.

Primary and Secondary Chemoprevention of Colorectal Cancer

S. PHILIP BRALOW

ABSTRACT

Chemoprevention of colorectal cancer is defined as the use of pharmacological, chemical, or specific dietary agents that are capable of interrupting the carcinogenic process; progression or frank malignancy. Primary chemoprevention occurs when these agents are made available to the population at large. Secondary chemoprevention is used for individuals at high risk. Review of multiple studies in both animal models treated with chemical carcinogens and in small groups of patients at high risk with familial polyposis, sporadic polyps, and ulcerative colitis suggest that secondary chemoprevention is feasible. The most likely candidate agents appear to be supplemental calcium, prostaglandin inhibitors and possibly vitamins C and E when coupled with wheat bran. As yet none of these agents have been sufficiently tested to warrant their use in primary chemoprevention. A prudent diet of low animal fat, high fiber and controlled total calories does not require any additional supplements for the average or low risk population.

Keywords: colorectal cancer, chemoprevention

INTRODUCTION

The potential control of colorectal cancer is of universal concern. In Western societies, it is the second most frequent site of cancer. In the USA, it is estimated that more than 145,000 new cases of colorectal cancer will be diagnosed and more than 66,000 deaths will occur in 1989 (Silverberg 1988). Earlier diagnoses and treatment are not likely to decrease these figures significantly. The most effective control measure, both in lives saved and cost, will be in prevention.

The National Cancer Institute in the U.S. has announced its goal of reducing the mortality from cancer by 50 percent before the year 2000 (Lerman 1989). It is believed that this goal can be accomplished by modifying diet, initiating smoking cessation programs and avoidance of known occupational hazards. Types of prevention have been divided into two major groups, primary and secondary (Higgenson 1966, Winawer 1984). Primary prevention would be ideal as it would prevent the initiation phase of cancer by eliminating carcinogens from the lifestyle of the population. Secondary prevention would utilize screening techniques to identify high risk individuals and to detect neoplastic changes at an early stage when the cancer is amenable to available therapy. The rationale for primary prevention is based on epidemiologic data which has shown a relationship of colorectal cancer with diets of high animal fat and low intake of fiber. Doll and Preto (1981) have estimated that these dietary factors may account for at least 30 percent of the incidence of this type of cancer. Despite these data, it is exceedingly difficult to incriminate any dietary factor specifically (Mogadam 1988). The human diet contains many components; some are mutagenic, promoters, or frankly carcinogenic, while others are anti-promoters or anti-carcinogenic. However, the epidemiologic and animal data regarding various fats and fibers are highly suggestive and cannot be ignored.

A more direct method to control colorectal cancer may be by chemoprevention (Bertram 1987). The use of defined pharmacological or chemical agents may be capable of interrupting the carcinogenic process at various phases; initiation, promotion, progression or malignancy. We define primary chemoprevention of colorectal cancer as the incorporation of known anti-carcinogens into our diet that prevent the initiation phase or the promotional stage. Secondary chemopreventional agents act at either the promotional or progression stage of neoplasia. Consequently, primary chemoprevention would be of benefit to the entire population at risk and secondary chemoprevention would benefit high risk individuals for colorectal cancer because of genetic factors or pre-malignant lesions such as adenomas. Interventional studies of potential chemoprevention agents should show a decrease in actual cancer incidence or mortality, but such studies would require large populations, long follow-up periods and obviously are not feasible (Zelen 1988). Currently, it is necessary to test these agents using known intermediate markers such as cellular proliferation, modified gene expression, blood group antigens, and cytokeratin expression (Lipkin 1988). Much work has been reported using calcium, retinoids, carotenoids, vitamins A, D, E, and C and other anti-oxidants with mixed results. Prostaglandin inhibitors, such as sulindac and piroxicam have been reported to inhibit adenoma formation in high risk individuals (Waddell 1989).

This review will attempt to summarize the present state-of-the-art knowledge in chemoprevention for colorectal cancer. Much of the work is ongoing and the data is far from complete. Many of the participants in this symposium are currently involved in these studies and will present new information that should help clarify some of the confusion. At present, the most likely candidates for active chemoprevention in colorectal cancer appears to be calcium supplementation, prostaglandin inhibitors and possibly wheat bran coupled with high doses of ascorbic acid (4 gm per day) and *a* tocopherol (400 mg per day) using cellular proliferation or inhibition of polyp formation as intermediate markers. This review may be biased by the need of the clinical gastroenterologist to learn his future role in the eventual control of colorectal cancer.

INTERMEDIATE TUMOR MARKERS

The regulation of epithelial cellular growth in the gastrointestinal tract is complex and controlled by many factors both luminal, such as food, and systemic by trophic hormones such as gastrin, growth hormones, thyroxin and glucocorticoids (Bertram 1987). Extensive studies by Lipkin (1988) have demonstrated that the proliferative compartment of epithelial colonic cells can be used as a marker of abnormal cellular growth and differentiation early in the carcinogenic evolution. This increased cellular proliferation is measured by tritiated thymidine labelling of active DNA synthesizing cells using radioautography of biopsy material. Abnormal activity has been demonstrated in patients with familial polyposis, hereditary non-polyposis syndromes as well as ulcerative colitis and sporadic polyps (Lipkin 1988, 1989). It has also been noted early in the carcinogenic process in rodent models using various chemical carcinogens.

During abnormal cellular proliferation, cells migrate from the basal crypts of the colonic gland up to the luminal surface. Terminal differentiation of the mature cells is delayed and other cellular events take place which also can serve as intermediate markers. Blood group antigen of the ABH phenotypes as well as the Lewis antigens appear in the pre-neoplastic cells. Le Y expression has been found to correlate with the degree of dysplasia in adenomatous tissue but are not found in normal mucosa (Sakamoto 1986, Kim 1986). These haptens may be highly specific markers for premalignancy. Alterations in gene structure occur together with the delay in cell maturation and differentiation. Deletions of chromosomal sequences have been noted in high risk individuals with familial polyposis and sporadic polyps. C-myc oncogens are expressed in the mid-zone region of the crypt in dysplastic adenomatous polyps while ras genes can be found in the upper region of the crypt as a marker for differentiation of the carcinomatous cell (Augenlicht 1987). Endogenous growth modifiers, TGFa and TGFb are secreted by colonic cancer cells and may lead to aberrant pre-neoplastic cells.

Currently, the estimation of changes in the proliferative compartment of the colonic epithelial cell appears to be the most feasible intermediate tumor marker for interventional studies in both animal models and humans. "Non-prep" biopsies of rectal mucosa can be used for these measurements and are virtually non-invasive (Lipkin 1987). Patients with familial polyposis and with sporadic polyps can be followed by flexible sigmoidoscopy or total colonoscopy to estimate polyp recurrence (DeCosse 1989). If such pilot studies show the effectiveness of a candidate chemopreventive agent, expanded studies in high risk populations may be planned (Lipkin 1988). Such studies would require four to five year follow-up with sufficient subjects to achieve statistical significance. The agent must be safe, available, and receptive to the patient. Efforts to control patient compliance must be built into the program. Even if the agent is successful for this limited high risk population, careful analysis would be necessary before recommending its use for the general population (Bertram 1987).

DIETARY FACTORS IN PRIMARY CHEMOPREVENTION

Epidemiological studies have implicated animal fat intake as a major factor in colorectal carcinogensis. A direct relationship between fat consumption and colorectal cancer incidence has been shown for certain populations but not others. Prospective and case control studies have been equivocal (Vogel 1989). Total calorie intake and dietary fiber content helps to confound these epidemiologic data. Animal studies do implicate the role of fat in chemically induced colonic carcinogenesis. Chemical carcinogenesis is enhanced when rodents are fed high fat diets regardless of the degree of saturation. Several mechanisms have been postulated but not proven as yet. Fat intake influences bile acid production and the composition of the colonic microflora. Excessive fat may increase fecal mutagens as well.

Unsaturated fat in the diet enhances carcinogenesis in animal models to a greater degree than saturated fats. It is theorized that unsaturated fats activate a lipid-dependent protein on the cell membrane that plays a major role in cellular proliferation. The amount of dietary fat in the lumen of the gut may increase bile acid metabolites which are injurious to the epithelial cells and thereby promote cellular proliferation and carcinogenesis. Total fat appears to act as a promoter in both dimethylhydrazine (DMH) (Reddy 1976) and azoxymethane (AOM) protocols (Nigro 1975). Linoleic acid is a precursor for prostaglandin synthesis and these agents also promote cellular proliferation (Carrell 1986). Several studies suggest that prostaglandin inhibitors can block polyp formation in high risk individuals as well as in animal models (Table 1). Several studies suggest that prostaglandin inhibitors can block polyp formation in high risk individuals as well as in animal models.

Table 1: Prostaglandin inhibitors in chemoprevention.

Pollard (1981)	rats (DMH)	indomethacin	↓concurrent
Moorghan (1988)	mice (DMH)	sulindac	↓concurrent 0 later
Reddy (1987)	rats (AOM)	piroxicam	↓concurrent ↓later
Metzger (1984)	rats (DMH)	indomethacin piroxicam	↓concurrent ↓concurrent
Waddell (1989)	Gardner's (4 pts) polyps (7 pts)	sulindac indometacin	↓polyps

↓ - decrease in number, 0 - no effect.

Retrospective studies have reported mixed results in correlating the incidence or mortality of colorectal cancer to the dietary intake of animal fats. Four prospective studies have failed to show any relationship between fat consumptions and colorectal cancer (Vogel 1989). The prospective autopsy study of Hawaiian-Japanese men failed to show any relationship of animal protein or fat with the prevalence of colonic adenamatous polyps (Stemmerman 1987). The dietary intake of fiber has been shown to be protective against colorectal carcinogenesis but these effects are difficult to analyze. Countries with a high fiber diet generally have a low incidence of colorectal cancer (Burkitt 1980). Animal studies have demonstrated some protection for insoluble fiber against chemically induced carcinogenesis in rodents but this protective effects could be eliminated when high fat, high energy diets were administered (Nauss 1987, Nigro 1975). High fiber diets may act by reducing colonic pH, the reduction of secondary bile salts, and dilutional effects on intraluminal carcinogens. Fecal mutagenicity may also be reduced by high fiber diets (Reddy 1989). When dietary insoluble fiber is fermented by colonic bacteria, butyric acid is released which is preferentially used by colonic epithelial cells and promotes cellular proliferation.

Several problems confound the role of dietary fiber in colon cancer. Dietary fiber has many components, both soluble and insoluble, which may exert different influences in the carcinogenic process. Total fiber is positively correlated with total caloric and energy intake (Potter 1986), but this characteristic may vary among vegetables or fruits obtained from different geographic regions; from one part of the plant from another, and even from one season of the year to the next. Animal models indicate that wheat bran and cellulose protect against chemical carcinogenesis while dietary oat fiber enhances the process (Reddy 1981).

Various micronutrients have been identified as possibly related to colonic carcinogenesis in rodents as well as humans (Mogadam 1988). Among the potential inhibitors are vitamins A, C, E, carotenoids, and selenium. Other possible food factors include saponins, phytates, lectins, phytoestrogens and lignans. Calcium in the diet has been shown to suppress chronic epithelial cellular proliferation and tie up intraluminal fatty acids and secondary bile salts as calcium soaps (Lipkin 1984). Intraluminal calcium may inhibit mucosal protein kinase C which is an active stimulator of epithelial cellular proliferation. Supplemental calcium given to rodents has been shown to decrease hyperproliferation induced by deoxycholic acid, fatty acids (Wargovich 1983), cholic acid (Bird 1986), and partial enteric resection (Appleton 1966). The action of calcium may be through calmodulin regulated pathways. Wargovich (1983) hypothesizes that the cellular regulatory mechanism of calmodulin is by stimulating protein kinases in the initiation of DNA synthesis. This integration of molecular events may be of fundamental importance in maintaining cellular homeostasis and the hyperproliferation seen in colorectal neoplasia.

Table 2: Chemoprevention in animal models

Model	Agent	Result	Reference
DMH/rats	ascorbic acid	↓	Collachio, et al, 1986
	a tocopheral	↓	
	B carotene	0	
	canthozanthin	0	
DMH/rats	0.5% cagluconate	↓	Pence et al, 1988
H.F. - 20% corn oil	1.0% cagluconate	↓	
L.F. - 5% corn oil	Vitamin D_3	0	
AOM/rats	0.04% Ca. lactate	control	Wargovich et al, 1989
20% corn oil	0.32% Ca. lactate	↓↓	
AOM/rats	Ca lactate	↓	Appleton, 1987
post enterrectomy	same	↓	
AOM/rats	50% calcium	↓	Pence, 1988
23.5% fat	300% calcium	↓↓↓	Skypec, 1988

H.F. - high fat, 20% corn oil in diet
L.F. - low fat, 5% corn oil
- relative decrease in cancers per rat
DMH - Dimethylhydrazine administration
AOM - Azoxymethane administration

Current evidence indicates that dietary factors do play some role in the primary prevention of colorectal cancer. Since dietary histories in humans are subject to major discrepancies and animal data is controversial, the dietary role cannot be ignored. The suggested "prudent diet" of low fat, low calorie, high fiber with cruciferous vegetable should be adequate to supply enough macro- and micro-nutrients to play a protective role in primary prevention. Primary chemoprevention will still require the addition of some chemical agent that can be added to the "prudent diet" and directly inhibit the initiation phase of colorectal carcinogenesis. At present, the most likely candidates for this role are supplemental calcium and vitamin D.

SECONDARY CHEMOPREVENTION STUDIES

Potential chemopreventative agents should be classified by site of action in the carcinogenic process. Wattenberg (1981) listed the sites of progression in the carcinogeneic process for a great number of potential chemopreventive agents. The sequence of events from initiation of the process to the eventual development of the malignant cell may take many years in the human (Bertram 1987). The period from exposure to initiation may take only 1-2 days. The initial damage may be reversible or converted into a fixed state within the DNA structure during replication. Agents that can prevent initiation must be given immediately prior or shortly after exposure. The initiated cell is then converted to a pre-malignant cell by various promoters. The promotion phase may take as long as 10 years and chemoprevention during this period can be given after exposure and can delay the development of malignancy but may require continuous administration. No agent has been found to prevent further invasion by the malignant cell to surrounding structures.

Rodent models have been particularly useful in defining these stages of colorectal cancer progression. Chemical carcinogens; 1,2-dimethylhydrazine and it metabolites, N-methyl-N-nitro-N-nitroso guanidine, and N-methyl-N-nitroso urea can initiate an expansion of the proliferative compartment in rodents, as well as lead to the development of adenomatous polyps and eventually invasive adenocarcinoma (Lipkin 1988). The chemically induced carcinogenic process can be blocked at various levels. Ascorbic acid and *a* tocopheral act at the initiation phase and by its anti-oxidant action may block the production of mutagens as well as preventing the conversion of various chemical pre-carcinogens into their more active metabolites (Colacchio 1989). High dose calcium supplements is especially effective in blocking the effect of high fat diets in these animal models (Skrypec 1988).

Chemoprevention in the control of human colorectal carcinogenesis has its greatest potential during the promotion or pre-neoplastic phase. Intervention can be started long after the initiation stage and its effectiveness can be judged in a few years by known intermediate end points. Several prospective studies have been completed in small series of patients with familial polyposis, sporadic polyps and in normal average risk individuals (Table 3). Ascorbic acid and *a* tocopheral have been reported to decrease fecal mutagens in humans (Dion 1983). McKeown-Eyssen et al (1988) studied 200 patients who were polyp-free after successful colonoscopic polypectomy. A slight decrease in the number of new polyps was found in the group of 100 patients given ascorbic acid (400 mg) and *a* tocopheral on repeat colonoscopy 2 years later. DeCosse (1975) treated five patients with familial polyposis with a previous ileoproctostomy by adding ascorbic acid (3 gm) to their diet. He noted a decrease in the number of size of polyps recurring in the rectal area. This study was repeated in 49 patients by Bussey (1982) and again there was a decrease in the number of polyps but this difference was not significant. A recent double-blind, randomized study on 58 patients with familial polyposis and previous ileoproctostomy was carefully carried out by DeCosse et al. Their results indicate a high fiber diet in excess off 11 gms per day coupled with ascorbic acid (4 gm per day) and *a* tocopheral (400 mg per day) significantly inhibited the polyp formation in the rectal stump over a four year period but more so during the middle two years of the study. The data was adjusted to account for patient compliance, spontaneous regression of polyps and other environmental variables. Ascorbic acid and *a* tocopherol supplements may have had weak independent effects. Total fat intake was positively correlated with polyp formation but total caloric intake (energy) or percentage of polyunsaturated fat had no independent effect.

Table 3: Completed chemoprevention trials in humans using new polyp formation as a marker

Disease	Treatment	Patients	Remarks
Familial Polyposis	Ascorbic Acid	5	Decrease in number and size of polyps (DeCosse 1975).
		49	Reduction in polyp areas. (Bussey 1982).
	Ascorbic Acid *a* tocopherol wheat bran	58	(DeCosse 1989)
Normal	Ascorbic Acid *a* tocopheral	20	Reduction fecal mutagens. (Bruce 1981).
Sporadic Polyps	Ascorbic Acid *a* tocopheral	100	Small but not significant reduction in new polyp formation. (McKeown-Eyssen 1988)

Prospective dietary studies over a 19-year period at Western Electric demonstrated that the risk of colorectal cancer was inversely correlated with the dietary intake of vitamin D and calcium (Garland 1985). A population study conducted in Utah compared the calcium intake in the diets of 231 patients with recently diagnosed colorectal cancer with 391 matched controls. A protective effect was found for males (Slattery 1988). Calcium supplementation (1200 - 1500 mg) has been shown to be effective in suppressing cellular proliferation in high risk populations such as familial polyposis in 10 such subjects (Lipkin 1985). The increased proliferative compartment in these high risk individuals return towards normal proliferation but once polyp formation has occurred additional calcium does not reverse the hyperproliferative activity. Several longitudinal studies are still in progress using calcium carbonate in familial polyposis, *B* carotene in sporadic polyps; *B* carotene plus vitamins C and E in patients with polyps, and vitamins C and E in normal low risk individuals (Table 4).

Table 4: Current controlled long-term studies now in progress (not complete)

Familial polyposis	Calcium carbonate	Lipkin
Adenomatous polyps	*B* carotene	Bowen
Adenomatous polyps	*B* carotene Vitamins C & E	Greenberg
Normal	Vitamins C & E	Colacchio

Increased prostaglandin synthesis has been found to be associated with chemical carcinogenesis in rodents (Pollard 1981). The calcium phospholipid dependent protein kinase is a receptor for TPA and is activated by cellular membrane degradation and leads to prostaglandin synthesis. Prostaglandin inhibitors such as sulindac, indomethacin, aspirin, and piroxicam have been shown to inhibit polyp formation in rodents as well as patients with familial polyposis (Table 1). Moorghan (1988) reported that sulindac can inhibit colonic tumors in mice when given concurrently with DMH but when given after cancer has developed, the drug is ineffective. Reddy (1987) found that piroxicam was effective in rats even 23 weeks after the administration of azoxymethane and tumors were inhibited in a dose dependent manner. Waddell (1989) administered sulindac to 4 patients with Gardner's Syndrome after an ileoproctostomy. Residual polyps in the rectal mucosa disappeared within one year after the drug was given. Four patients had intact colons with diffuse polyposis but surgery was not done. They were followed from 12 to 24 months on sulindac with an almost complete reduction of existing polyps.

CONCLUSION

Primary chemoprevention by the addition of specific micro- or macro-nutrient to the diet has not been proven to be effective in clinical practice. It is reasonable from current information to recommend a "prudent diet" consisting of a total fat intake of less than 30 percent of total calories and increased fiber up to 30 gm per day. The total calories should not exceed normal body needs. These changes in lifestyle may influence the cancer sequence at the pre-initiation phase and offers the greatest potential for primary prevention in the general population.

Secondary chemoprevention, on the other hand, appears to be feasible. Several candidate agents are available that may interrupt the promotional phase of carcinogenesis. Long term prospective studies in large populations are needed to confirm the effectiveness of these agents in both high risk and low risk population studies. Since it is not practical to follow large populations for many years to determine the effectiveness of candidate chemoprevention agents, intermediate markers can be used in high risk patients. An effective agent should be able to return an exaggerated proliferative cellular compartment to normal activity. The agent should be able to inhibit polyp formation over a short period of two to four years. The most promising agents that can easily be added to the diet for long term usage are calcium supplementation at doses between 1.0 and 2.0 gm per day; anti-prostaglandins (sulindac and piroxicam) and possibly ascorbic acid at doses of 4.0 gm per day coupled with wheat bran and *a* tocopherol.

Lipkin (1988) has proposed a three phase program to study these agents using intermediate markers in an interventional study. Pilot studies using high risk populations can be used to measure short term effects on cell proliferation, differentiation and possible gene expression. If these agents prove promising, expanded studies on a larger survey population such as patients with sporadic polyps may be undertaken. Finally, if candidate chemoprevention agents prove safe and effective, they can be added to the diet of the general population and the incidence of colorectal cancer monitored.

Before a long term study can be undertaken, many questions remain to be answered. The choice and dosage of the agent must be confirmed in short term studies. A comparison of decreased risk using the agent with alternative therapy must be demonstrated. The interventional trials must be designed to allow adequate recruitment, subject compliance, clear measurement of outcome and sufficient statistical power to permit a definitive result. As yet, no such study has been developed. In the meantime, the gastroenterologist and surgeon might prescribe supplemental calcium, prostaglandin inhibitors or additional ascorbic acid and wheat fiber to selected cases at high risk.

BIBLIOGRAPHY

Appleton, C.V.N., Davies, P.W., Bristol, J.B. et al. (1987) Inhibition of intestinal carcinogenesis by dietary supplementation with calcium. Brit. J. Surg. 74: 523-525

Augenlicht, L.H., Augeron, C., Yander, G. and Laboisse, C. (1987) Overexpression of ras in mucus-secreting human colon carcinoma cells of low tumorigenicity. Cancer Res. 47: 3763-3765

Bertram, J.S., Kolonel, L.N., and Meyskens, F.L. (1987) Rationale and strategies for chemoprevention of cancer in humans. Cancer Res. 47: 3012-3031

Burkitt, D.P. (1980) Colon cancer: emergence of a concept. In: Spiller, G.A., Kay, R.M. (eds.) Medical Aspects of Dietary Fiber Plenum Publishing Corp. New York, N.Y. pp 75-81

Buset, M., Lipkin, M., Winawer, S. Swaroop, S. and Friedman, E. (1986) Inhibition of human colonic epithelial cell proliferation in vivo and in vitro by calcium. Cancer Res. 46: 5426-5430

Bussey, H.B.J., DeCosse, J.J., Deschner, E.E. et al. (1982) A randomized trial of ascorbic acid in polyposis coli. Cancer 50: 1434-1439

Carrol, K.K., Braden, L.M., Bell, J.A. et al. (1986) Fat and cancer. Cancer 56: 1818-1825

Colacchio, T.A., Memoli, V.A. (1986) Chemoprevention of colorectal neoplasms. Arch. Surg. 121: 1421-1424.

DeCosse, J.J., Adams, M.B., Kuzma, J.F. et al. (1975) Effect of ascorbic acid on rectal polyps of patients with familial polyposis. Surgery 78: 608-612

DeCosse, J.J., Miller, H.H., and Lesser, M.L. (1989) Effect of wheat fiber and vitamin C and E on rectal polyps in patients with familial adenomatous polyposis. JNCI 81: 1290-1297

Dion, P.W., Bright-See, E.B., Smith, C.C. and Bruce, W.R. (1983) The effect of dietary ascorbic acid and *a* tocopheral on fecal mutagenicity. Mutat. Res. 102: 27-37

Doll, R., Peto, R. (1981) The causes for cancer: quantitative estimates of avoidable risks of cancer in the United States today. JNCI 66: 1191-1308

Garland, C., Shekelle, R.B., Barrett-Conner, E. et al. (1985) Dietary vitamin D and calcium and risk of colorectal cancer: a 19-year prospective study in men. Lancet 1: 307-309

Higgenson, J. (1966) Etiological factors in gastrointestinal cancer in man. JNCI 37: 527-545

Kim, Y.S., Yuan, M. Itzkowitz, S.H. et al. (1986) Expression of Le Y and extended Le Y blood group related antigens in human malignant, premalignant, and non-malignant colonic tissues. Cancer Res. 46: 5985-5992

Lerman, C., Rimer, B. and Engstrom, P. (1989) Reducing avoidable cancer mortality through prevention and early detection regimens. Cancer Res. 49: 4955-4962

Lipkin, M. (1988) Biomarkers of increased susceptibility to gastrointestinal cancer: new applications to studies of cancer prevention in human subjects. Cancer Res. 48: 235-245

Lipkin, M., Enker, W.F., and Winawer, S.J. (1987) Tritiated-thymidine labeling of rectal epithelial cells in "non-prep" biopsies of individuals at increased risk for colonic neoplasia. Cancer Lett. 37: 153-161

Lipkin, M., Friedman, E. Winawer, S.J., and Newmark, H. (1989) Colonic epithelial cell proliferation in responders and non responders to supplemental dietary calcium. Cancer Res. 49: 248-254

Lipkin, M. and Newmark, H. (1985) Effect of added dietary calcium on colonic epithelial cell proliferation in subjects at high risk for familial colonic cancer. New Engl. J. Med. 313: 1381-1384

McKeown-Eyssen, G., Holloway, C. Jazmaji, V. et al. (1988) A randomized trial of vitamins C & E in the prevention or recurrence of colorectal polyps. Cancer Res. 48: 4701-4705

Metzger, U., Meier, J., Unischmid, G., Weine, H. (1984) Influence of various prostaglandin synthesis inhibitors on DMH-induced rat colon cancer. Dis. Colon Rectum 27: 366-369

Mogadam, M. (1988) Cancer and nutritional misconceptions: a perspective. Am. J. Gastro. 88: 1346-1351

Moorghen, M., Ince, P., Finney, K.J., Sunter, J.P. et al (1988) A protective effect of sulindac against chemically-induced primary colonic tumors in mice. J. Path. (Eng.) 156: 341-347

Nauss, K.M., Jacobs, L.R., Newberne, DVM. (1987) Dietary fat and fiber: relationship to caloric intake, body growth, and colon carcinogenesis. Am. J. Clin. Nutr. 45: 243-251

Nigro, N.D., Singh, D.V., Campbell, R.I. et al. (1975) Effect of dietary beef fat on intestinal tumor formation by azoxymethane in rats. JNCI 54: 439-442

Pence, B.C. and Buddingh, F. (1988) Inhibition of dietary fat promoted colon carcinogenesis in rats by supplemental calcium or vitamin D. Carcinogenesis 9: 187-190

Pollard, M. Luckert, P.H. (1981) Effect of indomethacin on intestinal tumors induced in rats by the acetate derivative of dimethylnitrosamine. Science 214: 558-559

Potter, J.D., and McMichael, A.J. (1986) Diet and cancer of the colon and rectum: a case-control study. JNCI 76: 557-569

Reddy, B., Engle, A. Katsifis, S., Simi, B. et al. (1989) Biochemical epidemiology of colon cancer: effect of types of dietary fiber on fecal mutagens, acid, and neutral sterals in healthy subjects. Cancer Res. 49: 4629-4635

Reddy, B.S., Maruyama, H., Kelloff, G. (1987) Dose related inhibition of colon carcinogenesis by dietary piroxicam, a nonsteroidal anti-inflammatory drug, during different stages of rat colon tumor development. Cancer Res. 47: 5340-5346

Reddy, B.S., Mori, H. and Nicolais, M. (1981) Effect of dietary wheat bran and dehydrated citrus fiber on azoxymethane-induced intestinal carcinogenesis in Fisher 344 rats. JNCI 66: 553-557

Reddy, B.S., Narisawa, Vukusich, D. et al. (1976) Effect of quality and quantity of dietary fat and dimethylhydrazine in colon carcinogenesis in rats. Proc. Soc. Exper. Biol. Med. 151: 237-239

Rozen, P., Fireman, Z., Fine, N., Wax, Y. and Ron, E. (1989) Oral calcium suppresses increased rectal proliferation of persons at risk for colorectal cancer. Gut 301: 650-655

Sakamoto, J., Furukawa, K., Cordon-Cardo, C. et al. (1986) Expression of Lewis^{a}, Lewis^{b}, X and Y blood group antigens in human colonic tumors and normal tissue and in human tumor-derived cell lines. Cancer Res. 46: 1553-1561

Silverberg, E. (1988) Cancer facts and figures. American Cancer Society, New York, N.Y.

Skrypec, D.J., and Bursey, R.G. (1988) Effect of dietary calcium on azoxymethane-induced intestinal carcinogenesis in male F344 rats fed high fat diets FASEB Journal 2: AB57

Slattery, M.L., Sorenson, A.W., and Ford, M.H. (1988) Dietary calcium intake as a mitigating factor in colon cancer. Am. J. Epidemiol 128: 504-514

Stemmerman, G.N., Heilbrun, L.K., and Nomura, A.M.Y. (1988) Association of diet and other factors with adenomatous polyps in the large bowel: a prospective autopsy study. Am. J. Clin. Nutr. 47: 312-317

Vogel, V.G. and McPherson (1989) Dietary epidemiology of colon cancer. Hemat./Oncology Clinics of N. America 3: 35-63

Waddell, W.R., Ganser, G.F., Cerise, E.J., Loughry, R.W. (1989) Sulindac for polyposis of the colon. Am. J. Surg. 157: 175-179

Wattenberg, L. (1981) Inhibitors of chemical carcinogens. In: J.D. Burchenal (ed) Cancer Achievements, Challenges, and Prospects for the 1980s Grune and Stratton, New York pp 517-539

Wargovich, M.J. (1988) Calcium and colon cancer. J. Am. Coll. Nutrition. 7: 295-300

Winawer, S.J. (1984) Introduction to position papers from the Third International Symposium on Colorectal Cancer. CA- A Cancer Journal for Clinicians. 34 :130

Zelen, M. (1988) Are primary cancer prevention trials feasible? JNCI 80: 2-4

Chemoprevention of Large Bowel Cancer in Animal Models and Its Possibility in Humans

TOMIO NARISAWA, MASAHIRO TAKAHASHI, NAOSHI KUSAKA, YOSHIHIKO YAMAZAKI, HIROFUMI KOYAMA, HITOSHI KOTANAGI, and YOKO FUKAURA

ABSTRACT

Indomethacin (prostaglandin synthesis inhibitor), sarcophytol A (product from marine soft coral) and perilla oil (rich in α-linolenic acid) suppressed large bowel mucosal ornithine decarboxylase induction as a biomarker of tumor promotion and inhibited methylnitrosourea-induced large bowel tumor development in rats. The elevated level of this enzyme activity in large bowel cancer patients lowered by indomethacin treatment. Thus, it was expected that those agents may prevent large bowel carcinogenesis in individuals at high risk, probably through the mechanism involving in changes of biologic property of the large bowel mucosa.

Keywords: large bowel cancer, cancer prevention, indomethacin, sarcophytol A, perilla oil

Introduction

Various epidemiologic, clinical and laboratory investigations have suggested to be detectable the populations at high risk for large bowel cancer. In addition to genetic predisposition (Utsunomiya and Iwama 1980; Burt et al. 1985; Lynch et al. 1985, 1985), the environmental factors, particularly dietary habits, have an important role in large bowel carcinogenesis (Weisburger and Wynder 1987). A significant correlation between high fat and low fiber diet and large bowel cancer incidence has been indicated in many epidemiologic studies. It was supported by animal studies, in which high fat diet enhances the development of carcinogen-induced large bowel tumors. Thus, it has been postulated that large bowel cancer can prevent by a change of dietary habits with decreased fat intake and increased fiber intake, which reduces tumor promoting substances such as bile acids and fatty acids in the feces. Furthermore, a supplement of peroral dose of calcium seems to be effective for prevention of large bowel carcinogenesis through inactivation of those substances, which conjugate with calcium in the large bowel (Wargovich et al. 1983, 1984; Lipkin and Newmark 1985). In this paper, the results in our studies conducted for another means to prevent large bowel cancer are presented.

Anti-promoting Effect of Indomethacin

An anti-tumor activity of a non-steroid anti-inflammatory drug indomethacin has been investigated with transplantable tumors and primary tumors in rodents (Powles et al. 1982; Fisher and Slaga 1985). A primary pharmacologic activity of this drug is to inhibit endogenous prostaglandin (PG) synthesis, which plays a role in control of differentiation and proliferation of neoplastic and non-neoplastic cells, and of immune function. A number of tumors of animals and humans, including large bowel cancer, produce a large amount of PGs. PGE_2 may promote the neoplastic transformation of carcinogen-induced or initiated-tumor cells. We observed firstly an anti-tumor activity of indomethacin against methylazoxymethanol-induced large bowel tumors in rats (Kudo et al. 1980). Thereafter, we confirmed an anti-promoting effect of this drug on large bowel carcinogenesis of rats in repeated experiments (Narisawa et al. 1981, 1982, 1983). In these experiments, rats received varieties of dose schedules of a potent direct-acting carcinogen N-methylnitrosourea (MNU) for one or a few weeks as a tumor initiation procedure. After completion of the carcinogen doses, the rats started to have the treatment with 0.001% or 0.002% water solution of indomethacin as drinking water until termination of the experiment. A significant reduction of large bowel tumor development in treated groups of rats, compared to respective untreated controls, was observed at autopsy at weeks 25 to 35 in all the experiments. The inhibition rate of tumor development was 41% to 79%. However, the cessation of the treatment permitted the tumor development at the same incidence as untreated control. It suggests that a number of initiated cells may escape from the activity of tumor promoters in the large bowel during indomethacin administration, but may not be eliminated. The body weight gains of rats were identical in treated and untreated groups, and the toxicity of this drug was not observed grossly. The same effectiveness of other non-steroid anti-inflammatory drugs were reported in studies using rats and other large bowel carcinogens such as 1,2-dimethylhydrazine (Pollard and Luckert 1980, 1983, 1984; Metzger et al. 1984; Reddy et al. 1987). Also the inhibition by indomethacin of carcinogen-induced tumor development in other organs such as mammary gland (Carter et al. 1983; McCormick and Moon 1983), esophagus (Rubio 1984) and skin (Furstenberger and Marks 1978; Verma et al. 1980) in rodents were demonstrated. Thus, it seems likely that PG synthesis inhibitors can prevent cancer development in many organs through a probable mechanism involving in endogenous PGs.

The next study was done in a combination treatment with large bowel resection and peroral indomethacin in rats (Narisawa et al. 1985). After the completion of carcinogen administration with intrarectal doses of MNU, the rats received right hemicolectomy operation with anastomosis of the terminal ileum and the left colon, and started to have a water solution of indomethacin as drinking water. The inhibition rate of tumor development in the left side of large bowel was 88%, compared to untreated control without colectomy and indomethacin. The treatment with colectomy alone or indomethacin alone resulted also a significant inhibition of tumor development. The inhibition rate was 55% and 41%, respectively (Table 1). The analysis of fecal bile acids in colectomized rats showed a much lower concentration of total bile acids with a significant increase of primary bile acids and a significant decrease of secondary bile acids, compared to unoperated control. The intestinal transit time shortened significantly in colectomized rats. The results suggest that in addition to the suppression of endogenous PG production by indomethacin the changes of fecal bile acid composition and of intestinal transit time after right hemicolectomy affected further the promotion phase of large bowel carcinogenesis.

Table 1. Inhibition of methylnitrosourea-induced large bowel tumor development in CD-Fischer rats treated with peroral indomethacin and right hemicolectomy

Treatments[a]	Tumor incidence	% inhibition[b]
Untreated	25/34 (74%)	–
Indomethacin	15/34 (44%)[c]	41%
Rt. hemicolectomy	8/24 (33%)[c]	55%
Indomethacin and rt. hemicolectomy	2/23 (9%)[c,d]	88%

a. All rats received intrarectal dose of 2 mg methylnitrosourea thrice weekly for weeks 1-5. Then, treated rats had right hemicolectomy and/or 0.001% water solution of indomethacin as drinking water. All rats were autopsied at week 36.
b. (1 - tumor incidence of treated group/tumor incidence of untreated group) x 100 (%).
c. Significantly different from untreated group: $p < 0.01$.
d. Significantly different from indomethacin group and rt. hemicolectomy group: $p < 0.05$.

Large Bowel Mucosal Ornithine Decarboxylase Activity as a Biomarker of Promotion

A significantly increased induction of ornithine decarboxylase (ODC), the first rate-limiting enzyme of polyamine biosynthesis, by tumor promoters can be demonstrated in mouse skin epidermis (O'Brien 1976; Verma et al. 1980) and in rat large bowel mucosa (Takano et al. 1981). Thus, the enzyme may provide a good biological signal for tumor promotion. On the other hand, it was demonstrated that a specific irreversible inhibitor of ODC, α-difluoromethylornithine, inhibited the development of large bowel tumors in rats and mice (Kingsnorth et al. 1983; Razhin et al. 1984). We examined the enzyme activity in the large bowel mucosa for investigating the mechanism of anti-promoting effect of indomethacin (Narisawa et al. 1985, 1987). Rats received the peroral treatment with indomethacin in drinking water, and then a single intrarectal dose of a potent tumor promoter deoxycholic acid. Indomethacin treatment significantly lowered the level of ODC activity in the large bowel mucosa, compared to untreated controls (Table 2). It was confirmed also that indomethacin treatment significantly reduced PGE_2 production in the large bowel mucosa. A single subcutaneous injection of PGE_2 to indomethacin-treated rats restored deoxycholic acid-augmented ODC activity as well as PGE_2 level in the large bowel mucosa. The results indicate that PGE_2, of which the production in the large bowel mucosa is stimulated by intrarectal deoxycholic acid, is involved in the induction of ODC in the large bowel mucosa. This is probably why PG synthesis inhibitors may inhibit the tumor promotion and prevent the tumor development in the large bowel

Table 2. Suppression by peroral indomethacin and its restoration by subcutaneous prostaglandin E_2 of intrarectal deoxycholic acid-augmented ornithine decarboxylase activity in rat large bowel mucosa

		Prostaglandin E_2		
Treatments[a]	0 μg	40 μg	200 μg	1,000 μg
Deoxycholic acid and:				
Non-Indomethacin	0.36 ± 0.07[b]	0.40 ± 0.11[c]	0.81 ± 0.22[c]	0.87 ± 0.15[c,d]
Indomethacin	0.10 ± 0.02	0.23 ± 0.07[c]	1.04 ± 0.24[c,d]	1.11 ± 0.11[c,d]
No deoxycholic acid and:				
Non-indomethacin	0.01 ± 0.002	0.004 ± 0.002	0.02 ± 0.01	0.05 ± 0.01[d]
Indomethacin	0	–	–	–

a. Rats had 0.002% water solution of indomethacin as drinking water for 3 days. Then, they received a subcutaneous dose of prostaglandin E_2 and an intrarectal dose of 12 μmol deoxycholic acid, and were killed 4 hours later for measuring ornithine decarboxylase activity.
b. Mean ± SEM in 6 rats each, nmol CO_2/60 min/mg protein.
c. Value in vertical row that do not share a common superscript were significantly different each other: $p < 0.01$ or 0.001.
d. Significantly different from 0 μg and 40 μg prostaglandin E_2 groups in horizontal row: $p < 0.02$ or 0.01.

Large Bowel Mucosal Ornithine Decarboxylase Activity in Humans

We examined the ODC activity of normal-appearing mucosa obtained from large bowel specimens surgically resected in 67 patients with large bowel cancer and 6 control patients with cancer in other organs (Narisawa et al. 1989). The level of the enzyme activity of multiple tumor cases with carcinoma(s) and adenoma(s) was noted to be significantly higher than that of solitary tumor cases with one carcinoma alone (Table 3). Both groups of the cases significantly increased the enzyme activity, compared to control cases. It appears to be the larger the number of tumors the greater the enzyme activity. The result agrees with the observations by others (Razhin et al. 1984; LaMuraglia et al. 1986; Porter et al. 1987). Furthermore, it was clearly demonstrated that the enzyme activity remarkably increased in the normal-appearing mucosa of familial polyposis coli patients and of half of their first-degree relatives (Luk and Baylin 1984). Our findings seem to suggest that the large bowel with carcinoma and/or adenoma, particularly multiple tumors, has been exposed to a large amount of tumor promoters such as bile acids or has been susceptible to such substances. Also in humans, thus, the mucosal ODC can be a useful biomarker to detect individuals at high risk for large bowel cancer. Importantly, pre-operative treatment with indomethacin resulted in a marked low level of the enzyme activity in multiple tumor cases, compared to indomethacin-untreated cases (Table 3). Recently it was reported that the most of polyps in familial polyposis coli patients disappeared after the long term treatment with non-steroid anti-inflammatory drug sulindac (Waddell et al. 1989). Our results and reported observations suggest that non-steroid anti-inflammatory drugs may demonstrate an anti-promoting activity against large bowel cancer development also in humans as observed in animal models.

Table 3. Ornithine decarboxylase activity in large bowel mucosa obtained from large bowel cancer patients with or without indomethacin treatment

	Untreated cases		Treated cases	
Non-tumor cases	9.7 ± 3.9[b]	(6)[c]	–	
Solitary tumor cases	28.0 ± 4.9[d]	(31)	25.5 ± 4.3	(13)
Multiple tumor cases	82.8 ± 21.0[d]	(17)	18.0 ± 4.5[d,e]	(6)

a. Treated cases were given peroral dose of 75 mg indomethacin daily for 7 days before operation.
b. Mean ± SEM, pmol CO_2/60 min/mg protein.
c. Number of examined cases.
d. Significantly different from other groups: $p < 0.01$.
e. Significantly different from untreated cases: $p < 0.05$.

Anti-promoting Effect of Sarcophytol A

Recently, we found a new compound, a simple monohydroxycembraene sarcophytol A (SaA) isolated from a marine soft coral _Sarcophyton glaucum_, effective in anti-promoting action against large bowel carcinogenesis and less in toxicity in animal models (Narisawa et al. 1989). A potent anti-promoting effect of this compound had been demonstrated in mouse skin tumorigenesis study (Fujiki et al. 1989). CD-Fischer rats received intrarectal doses of MNU and the treatment with SaA mixed in chow. The inhibition rate of large bowel tumor develoment was 41% or 32%, compared to control fed chow without SaA (Table 4). The same result was obtained the repreated experiment (unpublished data). Body weight gain and consumed chow were the same between rats with and without SaA. The large bowel mucosal ODC activity augmented with intrarectal deoxycholic acid in rats fed SaA chow for one week was measured (Narisawa et al. 1989). The enzyme activity was significantly lower than that in rats fed control chow without SaA. Thus, it was proposed that SaA is another agent to be capable of inhibition of large bowel carcinogenesis, probably through an anti-promoting mechanism. We are interested in this agent in view of its less toxicity even in the range of grams per kg body weight at a single intragastric dose. A large amount of SaA was found in the liver and in the feces without decomposition. It is hypothesized that ingested SaA acts directly on the large bowel mucosa as same as painted SaA does on the mouse skin.

Table 4. Inhibition of methylnitrosourea-induced large bowel tumor development in CD-Fischer rats treated with peroral sarcophytol A

Treatments[a]	Tumor incidence	% Inhibition
Untreated	22/26 (85%)	–
Sarcophytol A from week 1	13/26 (50%)[b]	41%
Sarcophytol A from week 4	15/26 (58%)[b]	32%

a. All rats received intrarectal dose of 2 mg methylnitrosourea thrice weekly for weeks 1-3, and autopsied at week 26. Sarcophytol A-treated rats fed 0.01% sarcophytol A containing chow.
b. Significantly different from untreated group: $p < 0.01$ or 0.05.

Anti-promoting Effect of Dietary Perilla Oil

Studies in animal models made clear that diet high in fat from both animal and vegetable sources enhances the development of carcinogen-induced large bowel tumors as well as mammary tumors. However, some kinds of fats such as olive oil did not demonstrate such an effect (Reddy and Maeura 1984). Thus, the quality or fatty acid composition of fats may be a significant determining factor of large bowel carcinogenesis. Following such a hypothesis, it was demonstrated that high fish oil diet did not enhance, but rather suppressed, the development of large bowel tumors in rats (Reddy and Maruyama 1986) as well as mammary tumors (Carroll and Braden 1985; Jurkowski and Cave 1985) and pancreatic preneoplastic lesions (O'Connor et al. 1989). Fish oil has a unique fatty acid composition containing an appreciable amount of eicosapentaenoic acid and docosahexaenoic acid, n-3 family polyunsaturated fatty acids. On the other hand, most vegetable oils contain a large amount of n-6 family polyunsaturated fatty acid linoleic acid, which appears to promote potentially large bowel carcinogenesis in rats. We tested an anti-promoting effect of perilla oil, which consists of a large quantity of n-3 fatty acid α-linolenic acid but a less quantity of linoleic acid. CD-Fischer rats received intrarectal doses of MNU and were fed with high perilla oil diet. The large bowel tumor development significantly reduced, compared to rats fed with high safflower oil diet, which is rich in linoleic acid, and even though compared to rats fed with low safflower oil diet (Table 5). The inhibition rate was 66%. It was observed that perilla oil feeding resulted in significant low levels of plasma PGE_2 and serum lipids. Our results indicate that the large bowel tumor development can be inhibited also with terrestrial n-3 fatty acids at the same extent as with marine n-3 fatty acids. It might be supposed that the mechanisms are involving in changes of fecal bile acids with decreased total bile acids and secondary bile acids (Minoura et al. 1988), and in the altered cell membrane fatty acid composition followed by changes of the cell membrane function and by changes of the endogenous PG production (Stubbs and Smith 1984; Hagve 1988).

Table 5. Methylnitrosourea-induced large bowel tumors in CD-Fischer rats fed with diet high in safflower oil rich in n-6 fatty acid or perilla oil rich in n-3 fatty acid

Groups by diets[a]	Tumor incidence	% Inhibition
5% safflower oil	12/26 (46%)	–
12% safflower oil	14/25 (56%)	–
12% perilla oil	5/26 (19%)[b]	66%

a. All rats received intrarectal dose of 2 mg methylnitrosourea thrice weekly for weeks 1-2, and were autopsied at week 36.
b. Significantly different from other groups: $p < 0.05$ or 0.01.

Conclusion

The results from investigations described above indicate that the changes in function or biologic property of the large bowel mucosa (biologic means) as shown in altered ODC activity by the treatments with indomethacin, SaA and perhaps n-3 fatty acid suppressed promotion phase of large bowel carcinogenesis and led to inhibit the development of large bowel tumors in rats. Thus, it is expected that the development of large bowel cancer can prevent also in individuals at high risk, since the same changes of the mucosal ODC activity by indomethacin treatment was observed in large bowel cancer patients, markedly in the patients with multiple tumors. There is another means for prevention of this cancer. It may succeed with a decrease of promoting substances in the feces by decreased fat intake and increased fiber intake (physical means) or by an inactivation of such substances by peroral administration of calcium (chemical means). It is needed to test further effective treatments, e.g. the combination of those treatments.

REFERENCES

Burt RW, Bishop DT, Cannon LA, Dowdle MA, Lee RG, Skolnick MH (1985) Dominant inheritance of adenomatous colonic polyps and colorectal cancer. New Engl J med 312: 1540-1544

Carroll KK, Braden LM (1985) Dietary fat and mammary carcinogenesis. Nutr Cancer 6: 254-259

Carter CA, Milholland RJ, Shea W, Ip MM (1983) Effect of prostaglandin synthesis inhibitor indomethacin on 7,12-dimethylbenz(a)anthracene-induced mammary tumorigenesis in rats fed different levels of fat. Cancer Res 43: 3559-3562

Fischer SM, Slaga TJ (ed) (1985) Arachidonic acid metabolism and tumor promotion. Martinus Nijhoff, Boston

Fujiki H, Suganuma M, Suguri H, Yoshizawa S, Takagi K, Kobayasi M (1989) Sarcophytols A and B inhibit tumor promotion by teleocidin in two-stage carcinogenesis in mouse skin. J Cancer Res Clin Oncol 115: 25-28

Furstenberger G, Marks F (1978) Indomethacin inhibition of cell proliferation induced by the phorbol ester TPA is reversed by prostaglandin E_2 in mouse epidermis in vivo. Biochem Biophys Res Comm 84: 1103-1111
Hagve TA (1988) Effects of unsaturated fatty acids on cell membrane functions. Scand J Clin Lab Invest 48: 381-388
Jurkowski JJ, Cave WT Jr (1985) Dietary effects of menhaden oil on the growth and membrane lipid composition of rat mammary tumors. J Natl Cancer Inst 74: 1145-1150
Kingsnorth AK, King WWK, Diekema KA, McCann PP, Ross JS, Malt RA (1983) Inhibition of ornithine decarboxylase with 2-difluoromethylornithine; reduced incidence of dimethylhydrazine-induced colon tumors in mice. Cancer Res 43: 2545-2549
Kudo T, Narisawa T, Abo S (1980) Antitumor activity of indomethacin on methylazoxymethanol-induced large bowel tumors in rats. Gann 71: 260-264
LaMuraglia GM, Lacaine F, Malt RA (1986) High ornithine decarboxylase activity and polyamine levels in human colorectal neoplasia. Ann Surg 204: 89-93
Lipkin M, Newmark H (1985) Effect of added dietary calcium on colonic epithelial-cell proliferation in subjects at high risk for familial colonic cancer. New Engl J Med 313: 1381-1384
Luk GD, Baylin SB (1984) Ornithine decarboxylase as a biological marker in familial colonic polyposis. New Engl J Med 311:80-83
Lynch HT, Kimberling W, Albano WA, Lynch JF, Biscone K, Schuelke GS, Sandberg AA, Lipkin M, Deschner EE, Mikol YB, Elston RC, Bailey-Wilson JE, Danes BS (1985) Hereditary nonpolyposis colorectal cancer (Lynch syndromes I and II), I. clinical description of resource. Cancer 56: 934-938
Lynch HT, Schuelke GS, Kimberling WJ, Albano WA, Lynch JF, Biscone KA, Lipkin M, Deschner EE, Mikol YB, Sandberg AA, Elston RC, Bailey-Eilson JE, Danes BS (1985) Hereditary nonpolyposis colorectal cancer (Lynch syndrome I and II), II. biomarker studies. Cancer 56: 939-951
McCormick DL, Moon RC (1983) Inhibition of mammary carcinogenesis by flurbiprofen, a non-steroid anti-inflammatory agent. Brit J Cancer 48: 859-861
Metzger U, Meier J, Uhlschnid G, Weihe H (1984) Influence of various prostaglandin synthesis inhibitors on DMH-induced rat colon cancer. Dis colon rectum 27: 366-369
Minoura T, Takada T, Sakaguchi M, Takada H, Yamaura M, Hioki K, Yamamoto M (1988) Effect of dietary eicosapentaenoic acid on azoxymethane-induced colon carcinogenesis in rats. Cancer Res 48: 4790-4794
Narisawa T, Sato M, Tani M, Kudo T, Takahashi T, Goto A (1981) Inhibition of development of methylnitrosourea-induced rat colon tumors by indomethacin treatment. Cancer Res 41: 1954-1957
Narisawa T, Sato M, Sano M, Takahashi T (1982) Inhibition of development of methylnitrosourea-induced rat colonic tumors by peroral administration of indomethacin. Gann 73: 377-381
Narisawa T, Satoh M, Sano M, Takahashi T (1983) Inhibition of initiation and promotion on N-methylnitrosourea-induced colon carcinogenesis in rats by non-steroid anti-inflammatory agent indomethacin. Carcinogenesis 4: 1225-1227
Narisawa T, Hosaka S, Niwa M (1985) Prostaglandin E_2 counteracts the inhibition by indomethacin of rat colonic ornithine decarboxylase induction by deoxycholic acid. Jpn J Cancer Res (Gann) 76: 338-344
Narisawa T, Sato M, Sano M, Niwa M, Takahashi M, Ito T, Tanida N, Shimoyama T (1985) Prevention of colon polyposis and carcinomas by right hemicolectomy and indomethacin in animal model. Cancer 56: 1719-1724
Narisawa T, Takahashi M, Niwa M, Fukaura Y, Wakizaka A (1987) Involvement of prostaglandin E_2 in bile acid-caused promotion of colon carcinogenesis and anti-promotion by cyclooxygenase inhibitor indomethacin. Jpn J Cancer Res (Gann) 78: 791-798

Narisawa T, Takahashi M, Niwa M, Koyama H, Kotanagi H, Kusaka N, Yamazaki Y, Nagasawa O, Koyama K, Wakizaka A, Fukaura Y (1989) Increased mucosal ornithine decarboxylase activity in large bowel with multiple tumors, adenocarcinoma, and adenoma. Cancer 63: 1572-1576

Narisawa T, Takahashi M, Niwa M, Fukaura Y, Fujiki H (1989) Inhibition of methylnitrosourea-induced large bowel cancer development in rats by sarcophytol A, a product from a marine soft coral Sarcophyton glaucum. Cancer Res 49: 3287-3289

O'Brien TG (1976) The induction of ornithine decarboxylase as an early, possibly obligatory event in mouse skin carcinogenesis. Cancer Res 36: 2644-2653

O'Connor TP, Roebuck BD, Peterson FJ, Lokesh B, Kinsella JE, Campbell TC (1989) Effect of dietary omega-3 and omega-6 fatty acids on development of azaserine-induced preneoplastic lesions in rat pancreas. J Natl Cancer Inst 81: 858-863

Pollard M, Luckert PH (1980) Indomethacin treatment of rats with dimethylhydrazine-induced intestinal tumors. Cancer Treat Rep 64: 1323-1327

Pollard M, Luckert PH (1983) Prolonged antitumor effect of indomethacin on autochthonous intestinal tumors in rats. J Natl Cancer Inst 70:1103-1105

Pollard M, Luckert PH (1984) Effect of piroxicam on primary intestinal tumors induced in rats by N-methylnitrosourea. Cancer Lett 25: 117-121

Porter CW, Herrera-Ornelas L, Pere O, Petrelli NF, Mittelman A (1987) Polyamine synthetic activity in normal and neoplastic human colorectal tissues. Cancer 60: 1275-1281

Powles TJ, Bockman RB, Honn KV, Ramwell P (ed) (1982) Prostaglandin and cancer. Alan R Liss, New York

Razhin J, Wilson RS, Bull AW, Nigro ND (1984) Ornithine decarboxylase activity in the rat and human colon. Cancer Res 44: 3226-3230

Reddy BS, Maeura Y (1984) Tumor promotion by dietary fat in azoxymethane-induced colon carcinogenesis in female F344 rats; influence of amount and source of dietary fat. J Natl Cancer Inst 72: 745-750

Reddy BS, Maruyama H (1986) Effect of dietary fish oil on azoxymethane-induced colon carcinogenesis in male F344 rats. Cancer Res 46:3367-3370

Reddy BS, Maruyama H, Kelloff G (1987) Dose-related inhibition of colon carcinogenesis by dietary piroxicam, a nonsteroid anti-inflammatory drug, during different stages of rat colon tumor development. Cancer Res 47: 5340-5346

Rubio CA (1984) Antitumor activity of indomethacin on experimental esophageal tumors. J Natl Cancer Inst 72: 705-707

Stubbs CD, Smith AD, (1984) The modification of mammalian membrane polyunsaturated fatty acid composition in relation to membrane fluidity and function. Biochem Biophys Acta 779: 89-137

Takano S, Matsushima M, Erturk E, Bryan GT (1981) Early induction of rat colonic epithelial ornithine and S-adenosyl-L-methionine decarboxylase activities by N-methyl-N'-nitro-N-nitrosoguanidine or bile salts. Cancer Res 41: 624-628

Utsunomiya J, Iwama T (1980) Adenomatosis coli in Japan. In: Winawer SJ, Schattenfeld D, Sherlock P (ed) Colorectal cancer: prevention, epidemiology, and screening. Raven Press, New York, pp 83-96

Verma AK, Ashendel CL, Boutwell RK (1980) Inhibition by prostaglandin synthesis inhibitors of the induction of epidermal ornithine decarboxylase activity, the accumulation of prostaglandins, and tumor promotion caused by 12-O-tetradecanoylphorbol-13-acetate. Cancer Res 40: 308-315

Waddell WR, Ganser GF, Cerise EJ (1989) Sulindac for polyposis of the colon. Amer J Surg 157: 175-179

Weisburger JH, Wynder EL (1987) Etiology of colorectal cancer with emphasis on mechanism of action and prevention. In: DeVita VT Jr, Hellman S, Rosenberg SA (ed) Important advances on oncology 1987. JB Lippincott, Philadelphia, pp 197-220

Wargovich MJ, Eng VWS, Newmark HL, Bruce WR (1983) Calcium ameliorates the toxic effect of deoxycholic acid on colonic epithelium. Carcinogenesis 4: 1205-1207
Wargovich MJ, Eng VWS, Newmark HL (1984) Calcium inhibits the damaging compensatory proliferative effects of fatty acids on mouse colon epithelium. Cancer Lett 23: 253-258

Inhibitory Effect of Eicosapentaenoic Acid on Colon Carcinogenesis

HIDEHO TAKADA, TOSHIYUKI MINOURA, TOSHIYUKI TAKATA, MICHITOMO SAKAGUCHI, KAZUHIKO YOSHIOKA, MANABU YAMAMURA, KOSHIRO HIOKI, and MASAKATSU YAMAMOTO

ABSTRACT

The effect of purified eicosapentaenoic acid (EPA, n-3 polyunsaturated fatty acid) on azoxymethane(AOM)-induced colon carcinogenesis, the alteration of fatty acid composition, and prostaglandin E_2 in colon tumors and normal colon mucosa were studied, in comparison to linoleic acid(n-6 polyunsaturated fatty acid). The tumor incidence and tumor multiplicity(tumors per rat) in the colon were significantly lower in rats on an EPA diet than in those on a linoleic acid diet. The results suggest that EPA has an inhibitory effect on colon carcinogenesis by modulating prostaglandin synthesis and bile acid metabolism.

KEY WORDS

Colon Carcinogenesis, EPA, Linoleic Acid, Prostaglandin E_2

INTRODUCTION

Epidemiological and biochemical epidemiologic studies (Reddy 1980; Jain 1980; Carroll 1986) have shown that dietary factors, especially diets high in total fat and animal fat, are closely associated with the risk of colon cancer . Alaskan and Greenland Eskimos, however, characteristically have had low incidences of cancer, considering their total fat intake which has always been comparable with high-risk Danish levels, and an upward shift of their cancer risk has been associated with increased westernization (Lanier 1976; Nielsen 1980). Compared with Danish food, the fatty acid pattern of consumed lipids, essentially of mammalian marine origin, showed a higher content of n-3 polyunsaturated fatty acid, especially EPA(C 22:6) and docosahexaenoic acid(DHA; C 22:6), and lower contents of linoleic and linolenic acid (Bang 1972). Furthermore, low plasma lipid concentrations in spite of a high dietary intake of fat were reported (Bang 1972; Dyerberg 1975). This attributes to the low incidence of ischemic heart disease (Dyerberg 1978) which well correlates with the incidence of colon cancer (Wynder 1975).

Several laboratory animal model studies (Bull 1981; Sakaguchi 1984; Reddy 1984, 1985; Minoura 1988) suggest that the fatty acid composition and the amount of dietary fat are determining factors in colon carcinogenesis. Recently, Reddy (1986 1988) demonstrated that Menhaden oil(rich in n-3 polyunsaturated fatty acids) produced significant inhibition of AOM-induced colon tumors in rats, compared to a corn oil (rich in n-6 polyunsaturated fatty acid) diet.

The question has been raised as to which component of fish oil exerts this inhibitory effect. Moreover, commercial fish oil contains other fatty acids besides EPA and DHA at various levels. In this study, the effects of purified EPA on AOM-induced colon carcinogenesis were compared with those of purified linoleic acid (n-6 polyunsaturated fatty acid). To shed light on the underlying mechanism, the effects of these diets on mucosal and tumor fatty acid composition and prostaglandin(PG) E_2 were also studied.

MATERIALS AND METHODS

Fatty Acids

EPA ethyl ester refined from fish oil was kindly supplied by Nisshin Flour Milling Co., Ltd., Tokyo, Japan, and linoleic acid ethyl ester was kindly supplied by Ono Pharmaceutical Co., Osaka, Japan. The purity of these fatty acids determined in our laboratory was as follows; EPA: 91.1% and linoleic acid: 91.5%.

Animals and Diet

Weanling male Donryu rats (5 weeks old) were obtained from Laboric Service Co., Shiga, Japan. Semipurified fat-free diets were prepared at Oriental Yeast Co., Tokyo, Japan and the compositions of the experimental diets are shown in Table 1. Two types of 5% fat diets were prepared in our laboratory every other day and stored in the dark at 4°C. 0.3%(v/v) linoleic acid was added to 4.7%(v/v) EPA diet to alleviate any essential fatty acid deficiency. The peroxide content of freshly prepared diets and those stored for 2 days in a cold room was analyzed and the values were very small and similar for both EPA and linoleic acid diets. The rats were given fresh food every night and water *ad libitum* throughout the experiment.

Table 1 Composition of experimental diet

Casein vitamin-free	25%
Corn starch	39
α-Wheat starch	10
Sucrose	5
Cellulose	8
Mineral mixture	6
Vitamin mixture	2
Fat	5

EPA diet (EPA 4.7+Linoleic acid 0.3)
Linoleic acid diet (Linoleic acid 5)

Experimental Procedure

Beginning at 5 weeks of age, all animals were divided into two groups and given two types of diets containing 4.7% EPA plus 0.3% linoleic acid or 5% linoleic acid until the termination of the experiment. At 6 weeks of age, animals intended for carcinogen treatment were administered AOM s.c. at a dose rate of 7.4 mg/Kg body weight once a week for 11 weeks. Animals intended for vehicle treatment were given an equal volume of normal saline s.c. All animals were weighed once a week. Fifteen weeks after the last injection of AOM, 30 rats treated with AOM in both dietary groups were sacrificed and the number, size and location of all intestinal tumors were examined. Tumors and major organs were fixed in 10% formalin, embedded in paraffin and the sections were stained with hematoxylin and eosin for histological evaluation. The remaining rats, including vehicle treatment groups, were sacrificed at 20 weeks after the last injection of AOM and used for analysis of fatty acid and PG E_2.

Biochemical Analyses

The fatty acid composition of tumors and mucosa was determined as described previously (Sakaguchi 1984; Minoura 1988). Tissue protein content was measured by the method of Lowry(1951).

The PG E_2 concentration in colon tumor and mucosa was determined by radioimmunoassay as described previously (Minoura 1988). The content of PG E_2 was quantified with a commercially available radioimmunoassay kit(New England Nuclear, Boston, MA, USA). Radioactivity in the precipitate was counted in a gamma counter. The cross-reactivity of PG E_2 antibody to PG E_1 was less than 4%.

Statistical Analysis

Tumor incidence was analyzed with the X^2 method, and other data were analyzed with Student's t-test.

RESULTS

All animals survived until termination of the experiment except for one rat treated with AOM in the linoleic acid diet group, which died 3 weeks into the experiment due to pneumonia. There was no evidence of essential fatty acid deficiency in the EPA group. On the other hand, the rats of the EPA group were 10-15% smaller than those of the linoleic acid group from 1 week after the start of experimental diet, although food consumption was not significantly different between two diet groups. The lung, liver, spleen and kidneys were examined histologically at autopsy, but there were no specific changes associated with the diet.

Tumor Incidence

Table 2 summarizes the AOM-induced colon tumor incidence and tumor multiplicity(number of tumors/rat) in animals fed diets containing EPA or linoleic acid. The rats fed the EPA diet had a significantly lower tumor incidence and tumor multiplicity than those fed the linoleic acid diet. Histological examination showed that rats in the EPA diet group had fewer well differentiated adenocarcinomas and more mucinous adenocarcinomas than those of the linoleic acid group. Tumors of the small intestine were observed in two rats on linoleic acid diets, but not in those on EPA diets. No tumors developed in the rats treated with vehicle in both diet groups.

Table 2 AOM-induced intestinal tumors in rats fed the diet containing EPA or linoleic acid

	No.of rats	Colon tumor incidence (rat with colon tumor)	Colon tumors/rat (tumor multiplicity)	Small intestinal tumors (rat with intestinal tumor)
EPA diet	30	10[a] (33)[b]	0.41 ± 0.61[a,c]	0
Linoleic acid diet	29	20 (69)	1.66 ± 1.69	2

[a] Significantly different from linoleic acid group ($p < 0.01$)

[b] Number in parentheses, percentage of rats with colon tumors

[c] Mean ± SD

Biochemical Observation

Table 3 shows phospholipid fatty acid composition of colon tumors and normal colon mucosa in both diet groups. The monounsaturated and saturated fatty acids were unaffected in colonic mucosa by the fatty acids ingested except for the increase of the proportion of C18:0 in the EPA diet group. But, the polyunsaturated fatty acids were modified by dietary fatty acid. On the other hand, in colon tumors, the proportion of C16:0 and C20:4 was higher, and the proportion of C18:0 and C18:2 was lower than that of each paired colon mucosa. Furthermore, the contents of C18:2 and C20:4 in colon tumors were significantly lower in the EPA group than in the linoleic acid group.

Table 3 Phospholipids fatty acid composition (mol %) of colon tumors and colon mucosa in rats fed EPA or linoleic acid diets

Fatty acids		Colon tumor		Normal colon mucosa	
		EPA diet	Linoleic acid diet	EPA diet	Linoleic acid diet
Palmitic acid	C16:0	22.5 ± 0.9[a,b]	20.7 ± 1.9[b]	11.8 ± 0.8	12.9 ± 1.5
Palmitoleic acid	C16:1	3.7 ± 0.2	3.0 ± 0.3	5.2 ± 0.8	3.9 ± 0.4
Stearic acid	C18:0	13.6 ± 2.1[b]	13.5 ± 0.4	40.7 ± 2.9[c]	23.1 ± 3.7
Oleic acid	C18:1	29.5 ± 3.8[b]	20.7 ± 2.9	13.5 ± 3.2	8.1 ± 2.5
Linoleic acid	C18:2	2.4 ± 1.7[b,c]	12.6 ± 2.9[b]	10.7 ± 0.6	26.9 ± 7.1
Arachidonic acid	C20:4	10.3 ± 3.1[b,c]	18.5 ± 2.8[b]	4.1 ± 1.4	6.3 ± 3.1
EPA	C20:5	6.4 ± 1.7	Trace	3.6 ± 0.3	Trace
DHA	C22:6	1.9 ± 0.7	Trace	1.4 ± 0.5	Trace

[a] Mean ± SD

[b] Significantly different from paired control ($p < 0.05$)

[c] Significantly different from linoleic acid group ($p < 0.05$)

Table 4 shows the content of PG E_2 in colon tumors and mucosa. In the linoleic acid group, the content of PG E_2 in colon tumors was markedly higher than that of paired colon mucosa. The content of PG E_2, however, was almost the same between colon tumor and mucosa in the EPA diet group.

Table 4 PG E_2 contents of colon tumor and normal colon mucosa in rats fed EPA or linoleic acid diet

	Colon tumor		Normal colon mucosa	
	EPA diet	Linoleic acid diet	EPA diet	Linoleic acid diet
PG E_2 (ng/g wet tissue)	$8.91 \pm 3.17^{a,b}$	45.76 ± 12.09^{c}	9.78 ± 3.50	13.80 ± 4.01

[a] Mean ± SD

[b] Significantly different from linoleic acid diet group ($p < 0.01$)

[c] Significantly different from paired control ($p < 0.01$)

DISCUSSION

Diets rich in fat are known to enhance the development of tumors in several rodent colon cancer models. In addition to the quantity of fat, the type of fat has also been considered to be important (Sakaguchi 1984, 1986; Wargovich 1985; Reddy 1985, 1988; Minoura 1988). Our previous study (Sakaguchi 1984) showed that an n-6 polyunsaturated fatty acid (linoleic acid) had a promoting effect on AOM-induced colon carcinogenesis rather than saturated fatty acid (stearic acid) at low levels of dietary fat (5%). The results of our present study show that EPA, an n-3 polyunsaturated fatty acid, had an inhibitory effect on colon carcinogenesis compared to linoleic acid in the same experimental model, confirming the finding of Reddy (1986, 1988). These results indicate that the fatty acid composition of dietary fat is one of the determining factors in colon carcinogenesis.

Reddy (1988) demonstrated that feeding Menhaden oil, rich in n-3 polyunsaturated fatty acids, altered the incorporation of fatty acids into the microsomes of colonic mucosa cells and tumors. In the present study, the linoleic acid diet markedly increased the proportion of linoleic acid in the phospholipid fraction of colon tumors and mucosa, whereas the EPA diet only increased the chain-shortened fatty acids. The phospholipid composition in biological membranes determines the functional specificity and membrane structure which influences fluidity and lipid-protein interactions (Brenner 1984). The differences in the composition of colon mucosa and tumor fatty acids between the rats given EPA or linoleic acid suggest that fatty acid changes could play a role in colon carcinogenesis.
The linoleic acid group showed a marked decrease in linoleic acid and an increase in arachidonic acid in the phospholipid fatty acid composition of colon tumors compared to colon mucosa. However, EPA may in part displace n-6 fatty acids in colon tumors because the ratio

of n-3 fatty acids to n-6 fatty acids in colon tumors was greater compared to that in colon mucosa. EPA has been reported to inhibit the conversion of linoleic acid to arachidonic acid (Brenner 1967) and also to inhibit the lipoxygenase and cyclooxygenase pathways involved in prostaglandin synthesis (Culp 1979; Meydani 1988). Bennett (1977) observed excessive amounts of PG in human colon cancer and Narisawa (1981) showed that indomethacin, cyclooxygenase inhibitor, inhibited colon carcinogenesis in rats. Our present study showed that excessive production of PG E_2 in colon tumors was inhibited by EPA. And it is therefore possible that the inhibitory effect of EPA on colon carcinogenesis might be due to its inhibitory effect on PG synthesis.

Several studies (Pegg 1982; Slaga 1983) have indicated that ornithine decarboxylase (ODC), a rate-limiting enzyme in polyamine biosynthesis, is required for tumor promotion and cell proliferation in various organs. Reddy (1988) showed an increase in the colonic mucosal ODC activity in rats fed a 23.5% corn oil diet (rich in linoleic acid) compared to those fed a 5% corn oil diet, and the inhibition of ODC activity in colonic mucosa by dietary fish oil (rich in n-3 polyunsaturated fatty acid). Our recent study (unpublished data) confirmed Reddy's observation and the ODC activity in colonic mucosa of rats treated with AOM in the EPA group was lower than that of the linoleic acid group. Furthermore, the ODC activity of colonic tumors in the EPA diet group was lower than that in the linoleic acid group.

Another mechanism may involve bile acid metabolism. The important role of fecal bile acids, particularly secondary bile acids, in colon carcinogenesis has been demonstrated in animal models (Narisawa 1974, 1987; Hiramatsu 1983; Sakaguchi 1986) and biochemical epidemiological studies (Hill 1975; Owen 1987). Our previous studies (Hiramatsu 1983; Sakaguchi 1986) showed that cholesterol and linoleic acid increase the excretion of fecal secondary bile acids, resulting in the promotion of colon carcinogenesis in rats. Fish oil has been suggested to reduce the plasma cholesterol level in rats by increasing the transfer of cholesterol into bile without an increase in bile acid secretion (Balasubramaniam 1985). Our recent study (unpublished data) showed that EPA diet significantly decreased the level of serum cholesterol compared to linoleic acid or stearic acid diets. And, dietary EPA was associated with a decrease in biliary bile acid secretion compared to the linoleic acid group, but the biliary bile acid composition was similar in the two diet groups. Furthermore, fecal excretion of total and secondary bile acids was significantly decreased in rats fed an EPA diet compared to the linoleic acid group.

These dietary effects may be involved in the change of the intestinal bacterial flora which could affect colon carcinogenesis (Hill 1975; Takada 1982). Further studies are required to elucidate the complex involvement of EPA on colon carcinogenesis.

In conclusion, the present study demonstrated that EPA has an inhibitory effect on colon carcinogenesis by modulating prostaglandin synthesis and bile acid metabolism.

ACKNOWLEDGMENT

This study was supported in part by Grant-in-Aid (61570626,01570727) for Scientific Research from the Japanese Ministry of Education, Science and Culture .

We wish to thank Nisshin Flour Milling Co., LTD., Tokyo, Japan, for kindly providing EPA.

REFERENCES

Balasubramaniam S, Simons LA, Chang S, Hickie JB (1985) Reduction in plasma cholesterol and increase in biliary cholesterol by a diet rich in n-3 fatty acids in rats. J.Lipid Res. 26: 684-689
Bang HO, Dyerberg J (1972) Plasma lipids and lipoproteins in Greenlandic west coast Eskimos. Acta Med.Scand. 192: 85-94
Bang HO, Dyerberg J, NjØrne N (1976) The composition of food consumed by Greenland Eskimos. Acta Med.Scand. 200: 69-73
Bennett A, Tacca MD, Stamford IF, Zebro T (1977) Prostaglandins from tumors of human large bowel. Br.J.Cancer 35: 881-884
Brenner RR, Peluffo RO (1967) Inhibitory effect of docosa-4,7,10,13,16,19-hexaenoic acid upon the oxidative desaturation of linoleic into γ-linoleic acid and α-linoleic acid into octadeca-6,9,12,15-tetraenoic acid. Biochim.Biophys.Acta 137: 184-186
Brenner RR (1984) Effect of unsaturated acids on membrane structure and enzyme kinetics. Proc.Lipid Res. 23: 69-96
Bull AW, Soullier BK, Wilson PS, Hayden MT, Nigro ND (1981) Promotion of azoxymethane-induced intestinal cancer by high fat diet in rats. Cancer Res.41: 3700-3705
Carroll KK, Braden LM, Bell JA, Kalamegham R (1986) Fat and cancer. Cancer(Phila) 58: 1818-1825
Culp BR, Titus BG, Land WEM (1979) Inhibition of prostaglandin biosynthesis by eicosapentaenoic acid. Prostaglandins Med. 3: 269-278
Dyerberg J, Bang HO, NjØrne N (1975) Fatty acid composition of the plasma lipids in Greenland Eskimos. Am.J.Clin.Nutr. 28: 958-966
Dyerberg J, Bang HO, Stoffersen E, Moncada S, Uane JR (1978) Eicosapentaenoic acid and prevention of thrombosis and atherosclerosis ? Lancet 2: 117-119
Hill MJ, Drasar BS, Williams REO, Maeda TW, Cox AG, Simpson JEP, Morson BC (1975) Faecal bile-acids and clostridia in patients with cancer of the large bowel. Lancet 1: 535-539
Hiramatsu Y, Takada H, Yamamura M, Hioki K, Saito K, Yamamoto M (1983) Effect of dietary cholesterol on azoxymethane-induced colon carcinogenesis in rats. Carcinogenesis 4: 553-558
Jain M, Cook GM, Davis FG, Grace MG, Home GP, Miller AB (1980) A case-control study of diet and colo-rectal cancer. Int.J.Cancer 26: 757-768
Lanier AP, Bender TR, Blot WJ, Fraumeri Jr JF, Hurlburt WB (1976) Cancer incidence in Alaska natives. Int.J.Cancer 18: 409-412
Lowry OH, Rosebrough NJ, Farr AL, Randall RJ (1951) Protein measurement with the folin phenol reagent. J.Biol.Chem. 193: 265-275
Meydani SN, Stocking LM, Shapiro AC, Meydani M, Blumberg JB (1988) Fish oil and tocopherol induced changes in *ex vivo* synthesis of spleen and lung leukotrien B_4. Ann.N.Y.Acad.Sci. 524: 395-398
Minoura T, Takata T, Sakaguchi M, Takada H, Yamamura M, Hioki K, Yamamoto M (1988) Effect of dietary eicosapentaenoic acid on azoxymethane-induced colon carcinogenesis in rats. Cancer Res. 48: 4790-4794
Narisawa T, Magadia NE, Weisburger JH, Wynder EL (1974) Promoting effect of bile acids on colon carcinogenesis after intrarectal instillation of N-methyl-N'-nitro-N-nitrosoguanidine in rats. J.Natl.Cancer Inst. 53: 1093-1097
Narisawa T, Sato M, Tani M, Kudo T, Takahashi T, Goto A (1981) Inhibition of development of methylnitrosourea-induced rat colon tumors by indomethacin treatment. Cancer Res. 41:1954-1957
Narisawa T, Takahashi M, Niwa M, Fukaura Y, Wakizaka A (1987) Involvement of prostaglandin E_2 in bile acid-caused promotion of colon carcinogenesis and antipromotion by the cyclooxygenase inhibitor indomethacin. Jpn.J.Cancer Res.(Gann) 78: 791-798

Nielsen NH, Hansen JPH (1980) Breast cancer in Greenland-selected epidemiological, clinical and histological features. J. Cancer Res.Clin.Oncol. 98: 287-299
Owen RW, Tompson MH, Hill MJ, Wilpart M, Mainguet P, Roberfroid M (1987) The importance of ratio of lithocholic to deoxycholic acid in large bowel carcinogenesis. Nutr. and Cancer 9: 67-71
Owen RW, Dodo M, Thompson MH, Hill MJ (1987) Fecal steroids and colorectal cancer. Nutr. and Cancer 9: 73-80
Pegg AE, McCann PP (1982) Polyamine metabolism and function. Am.J.Physiol. 243: 212-221
Reddy BS, Cohen LA, McCoy GD, Hill P, Weisburger JH, Wynder EL (1980) Nutrition and its relationship to cancer. Adv.Cancer Res. 32: 237-345
Reddy BS, Maeura Y (1984) Tumor promotion by dietary fat in azoxymethane-induced colon carcinogenesis in female F344 rats: influence of amount and sources of dietary fat. J.Natl.Cancer Inst. 72: 745-750
Reddy BS, Tanaka T, Simi B (1985) Effect of different levels of dietary trans fat or corn oil on azoxymethane-induced colon carcinogenesis in F344 rats. J.Natl.Cancer Inst. 75: 791-798
Reddy BS, Maruyama H (1986) Effect of dietary fish oil on azoxymethane-induced colon carcinogenesis in male F344 rats. Cancer Res. 46: 3367-3370
Reddy BS, Sugie S (1988) Effect of different levels of omega-3 and omega-6 fatty acids on azoxymethane-induced colon carcinogenesis in F344 rats. Cancer Res. 48: 6642-6647
Sakaguchi M, Hiramatsu Y, Takada H, Yamamura M, Hioki K, Saito K, Yamamoto M (1984) Effect of dietary unsaturated and saturated fats on azoxymethane-induced colon carcinogenesis in rats. Cancer Res. 44: 1472-1477
Sakaguchi M, Minoura T, Hiramatsu Y, Takada H, Yamamura M, Hioki K, Yamamoto M (1986) Effect of dietary saturated and unsaturated fatty acids on fecal bile acids and colon carcinogenesis induced by azoxymethane in rats. Cancer Res. 46: 61-65
Slaga TJ (1983) Overview of tumor promotion in animals. Environ.Health Perspect. 50: 3-14
Takada H, Hirooka T, Hiramatsu Y, Yamamoto M (1982) Effect of β-glucuronidase inhibitor on azoxymethane-induced colonic carcinogenesis in rats. Cancer Res. 42: 331-334
Wargovich MJ, Felkner IC (1985) Metabolic activation of DMH by colonic microsomes : a process influenced by types of dietary fat. Nutr.Cancer 4:146-153
Wynder EL (1975) The epidemiology of large bowel cancer. Cancer Res. 35: 3388-3394

Life Styles and Cancer of the Sigmoid Colon with Special Reference to the Role of Alcohol Consumption

TAKESHI HIRAYAMA

ABSTRACTS

A 17-year follow up of 265,118 Japanese adults aged 40 years and above revealed a close association between cancer of the sigmoid colon (n=91) and alcohol consumption: relative risk (RR) for drinkers verses non drinkers was 4.38 (90% CI 1.75-10.97) in men and 1.92 (1.13-3.26) in women. In men, attributable risk was 74% and RRs in non, infrequent, occasional, and daily drinkers were 1.00, 2.03, 3.83, and 5.42, respectively. Both alcohol drinking and fat-rich-fibre-deficient diet were observed to be mutually independent risk factors of cancer of the sigmoid colon.
Key Words : cancer of the sigmoid colon, alcohol, beer, diet, cohort study.

INTRODUCTION

The number of deaths from cancer of the sigmoid colon has been increasing sharply in Japan. In 1987 there were 2,709 such deaths, compared with 1,665 in 1978 - ratio of increase 1.65. The rise has been much steeper than that for other colon cancers and is almost as high as those for cancers of lung (1.71), liver (1.70), and pancreas (1.77)(Fig. 1). Among cancers of each anatomical site of colon, ratio of increase was most striking for sigmoid colon (Fig. 2). To clarify the reason of such sharp increase data from a large cohort study (1966 -1982) were examined and major risk factors were identified.

MATERIALS AND METHODS

From October to December, 1965, a questionnaire survey of all the residents aged 40 or older in 29 health districts in six selected Japanese prefectures was conducted by trained public health nurses and mid-wives. The prefectures (Miyagi, Aichi, Osaka, Hyogo, Okayama, and Kagoshima) were selected because they geographically represent the entire country and all but one (Kagoshima) had cancer registration systems. Respondents numbered 122,261 men and 142,857 women and the proportion of the respondents, as judged from the 1965 National Census population, was 94.8%. A one-page questionnaire was used in the survey to obtain information on smoking, drinking and dietary habits, occupation, marital status, and reproductive history. 98% of the men and 95% of the women responded to questions about consumption of alcoholic beverages: 32.8% of these men were daily drinkers, 27.9% occasional drinkers (once or twice a week), 14.1% infrequent drinkers (once or twice a month), and 23.1% non-drinkers; the corresponding percentages for women were 1.2, 5.5, 10.2 and 78.5. 92% of the male drinkers answered questions about their usual drink - it was sake in 65%, beer in 22%, shochu (local hard liquor) in 10%, whisky in 2%, and other in 1%.

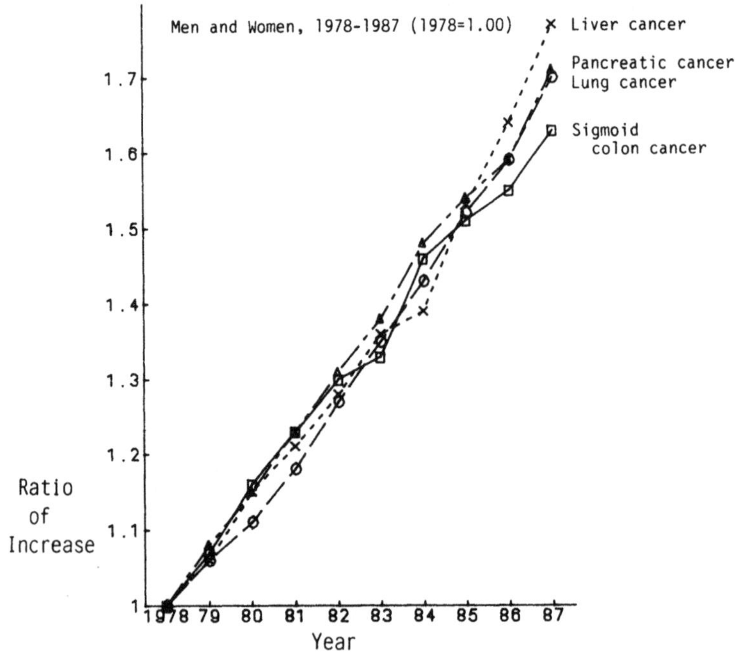

"Fig. 1" Ratio of increase in number of death from cancer of selected sites during past 10 years in Japan.

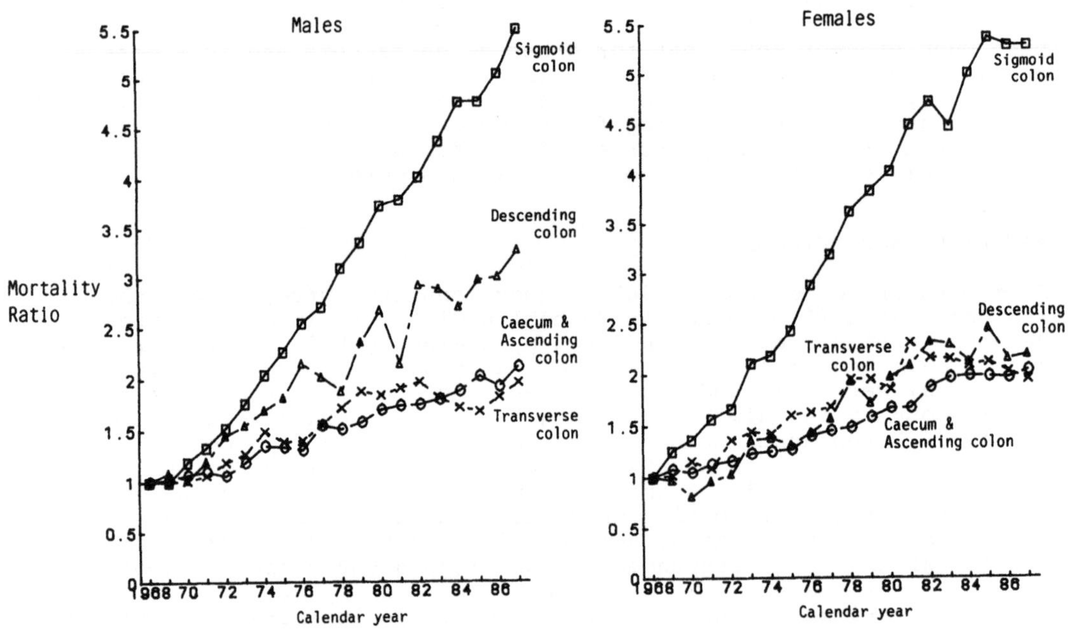

"Fig. 2" Mortality ratio of colon cancer by anatomical sites, 1968-1987, Japan (number of death in 1968=1.00).

At the beginning of each follow-up year, a migration survey was conducted, by reference to the local residence registration, and those who were found to have migrated from the residential public health districts during the previous year were tabulated separately.

During 17 years of follow-up (1966-1982), 14,740 (8,794 M, 5,946 F) died of cancer; 574 died of cancer of the colon (256 M, 318 F) and 91 of these (43 M, 48F) were identified as having died of cancer of the sigmoid colon.

RESULTS

Diet

The age-standardized mortality ratio or relative risk (RR) of daily and occasional consumers versus infrequent and non consumers of selected foods was studied for cancer of the sigmoid colon and other parts of the colon. For proximal colon no significant association with any of the foods was observed: RRs (90% confidence interval) were 1.04 (0.83-1.32) for milk, 1.04 (0.79-1.37) for meat, 1.29 (0.74-2.26) for fish, 1.42 (0.62-3.24) for green-yellow vegetables, 0.96 (0.72-1.28) for rice/wheat, and 1.23 (0.68-2.33) for soybean paste soup. For cancer of the sigmoid colon, age-adjusted RRs of daily or occasional versus infrequent or never for consumption of milk and meat were 2.59 (1.52-4.42) and 1.79 (0.87-3.66), respectively, suggesting a possible risk-rising effect of animal fats; no increase in risk was associated with fish, RR 0.76 (0.29-2.02). The RRs for consumption of green-yellow vegetables, rice/wheat, and soybean paste soup - 0.36 (0.14-0.92), 0.44 (0.26-0.73), and 0.30 (0.15-0.58), respectively - suggested a possible risk lowering effect of dietary fibre (Fig. 3).

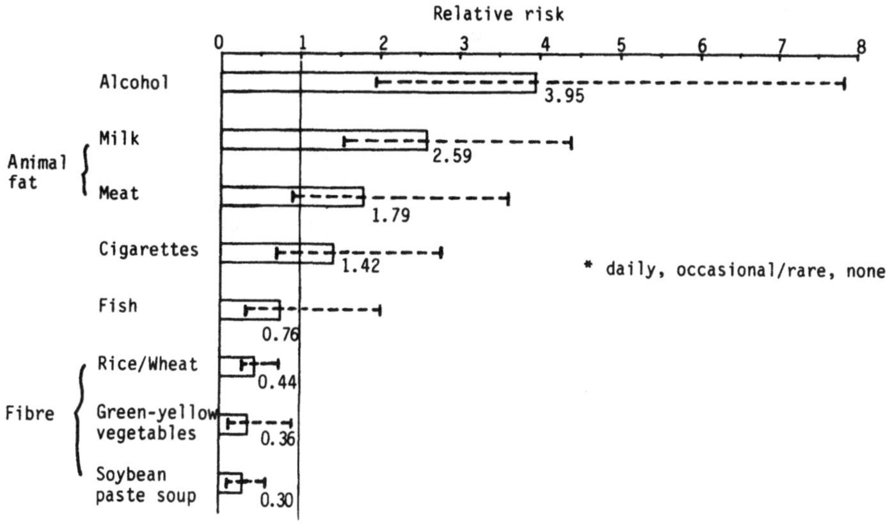

"Fig. 3" Age standardized relative risk* for cancer of the sigmoid colon by selected life styles (Cohort study, 1966-1982, Japan, Males).

Cigarette Smoking

No significant association was observed with the habit of cigarette smoking: the age-adjusted RRs for daily smokers were 1.21 (0.90-1.62) for proximal colon and 1.42 (0.72-2.79) for sigmoid colon.

Alcohol

a. Relative Risk
A striking association was observed between alcohol consumption and cancer of the sigmoid colon (Fig. 3). The age-standardized mortality ratio or RR of daily and occasional consumers versus infrequent and non consumers was 3.95 (1.98-7.86) for sigmoid colon, compared with a non-significant 1.07 (0.85-1.35) for proximal colon. The association between alcohol drinking and cancer of the sigmoid colon was seen in both sexes: RR of alcohol drinkers versus non-drinkers was 4.38 (1.75-10.97) in men and 1.92 (1.13-3.26) in women.

b. Attributable Risk
The age standardized mortality rates per 100,000 for cancer of the sigmoid colon in men are 2.52 for all groups and 0.66 for non alcohol drinkers. From these rates the population attributable risk of alcohol drinking is 74% ([2.52-0.66]÷2.52x100).

c. Type of Alcoholic Beverage
The highest risk for cancer of the sigmoid colon was observed in daily beer drinkers, RR versus non-drinkers 12.57 (3.62-43.66). However, the importance of daily drinking of other types of alcoholic beverages cannot be neglected - daily drinkers of sake had an RR of 4.56 (1.63-12.19) and of shochu 5.90 (2.00-17.42).

d. Frequency-Response Relation
There was a clear-cut frequency-response relation: the RRs for cancer of the sigmoid in non, infrequent, occasional, and daily alcohol consumers were 1.00, 2.03 (0.54-7.32), 3.83 (1.55-12.10), and 5.42 (2.24-13.99), respectively.

e. Comparison with known Alcohol-related Disease
The strength of the association with alcohol consumption was much higher for cancer of the sigmoid colon than that for known alcohol-related diseases. RRs in non, infrequent, occasional, and daily drinkers were 1.00, 0.69, 0.85, and 1.66 for liver cirrhosis, 1.00, 0.70, 0.88, and 2.44 for cancer of the pharynx, and 1.00, 0.87, 1.04, and 2.29 for cancer of the oesophagus.

f. Alcohol plus Cigarette Smoking
For known alcohol-related diseases there was a clear increase in risk with cigarette smoking: RRs in those neither drinking nor smoking daily, in those drinking daily but not smoking daily, and in those both drinking and smoking daily were 1.00, 1.91, and 3.19 for cancer of mouth; 1.00, unassessable, and 4.54 for cancer of pharynx; and 1.00, 1.07, and 3.55 for cancer of the oesophagus. However, for cancer of the sigmoid colon no such tendency was observed and individuals who both smoked and drank even showed a slightly lower risk - RRs 1.00, 2.72, and 2.21. A similar pattern of association was seen with cancer of the rectum - RRs 1.00, 1.92, and 1.75.

g. Alcohol Consumption and Other Cancers of Digestive Tract
Alcohol drinking was closely associated with certain cancers of both upper and lower digestive tract, RRs of daily versus non-daily drinkers being 2.82 for cancer of the mouth, 2.87 for cancer of the

pharynx, 2.28 for cancer of the oesophagus, 2.12 for cancer of the sigmoid colon, and 1.32 for cancer of the rectum; almost no association, however, was seen with cancer of the stomach (1.01), duodenum and small intestine (1.20), caecum (1.05), upper and transverse colon (0.95), or descending colon (1.0). A more impressive pattern was observed when RRs of daily drinkers were compared with those of non-drinkers - mouth 2.27, pharynx 2.44, oesophagus 2.29, stomach 0.92, proximal colon 0.98, sigmoid colon 5.42, and rectum 1.39 (Fig. 4).

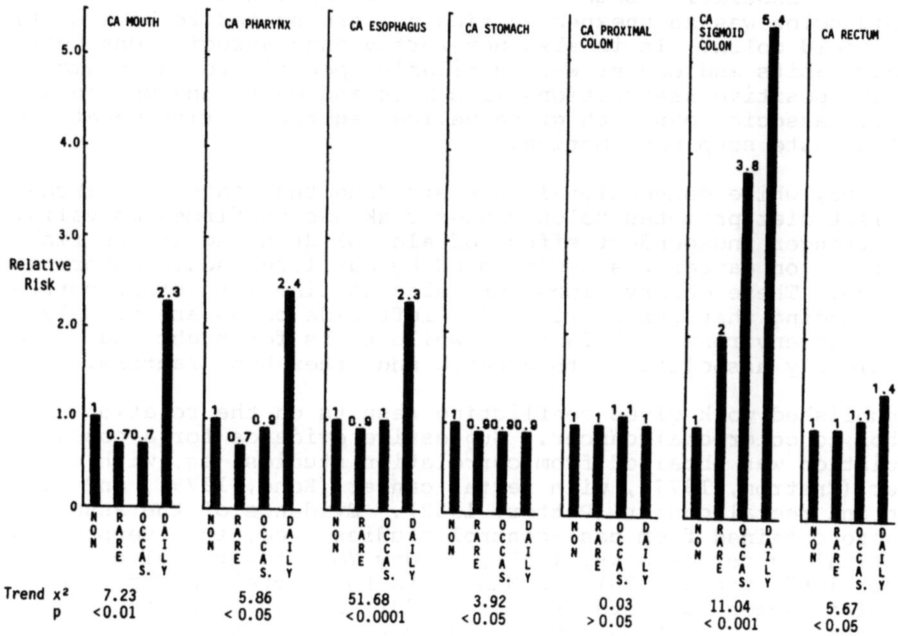

"Fig. 4" Age standardized relative risk for cancers of digestive tracts by frequency of alcohol consumption. Cohort study, 1966-1982, Japan.

h. RR for Cancer of Sigmoid Colon adjusted for Cigarette Smoking and Diet

The RR of daily versus non-daily alcohol consumption was adjusted, by the Mantel-Haenszel method, for smoking and consumption of meat and green-yellow vegetables: it was 2.138 (90% CI 1.316-3.471; x^2=6.65, $p<0.05$), while RRs for daily smoking, daily consumption of meat, and daily consumption of green-yellow vegetables were 1.177 (0.611-2.267; X^2=0.17, $p>0.05$), 0.561 (0.176-1.782; X^2=0.68, $p > 0.05$), and 0.684 (0.410-1.139; X^2=1.50, $p > 0.05$) when other factors were adjusted. RR was essentially unchanged when alcohol consumption was examined by frequency of milk consumption: RR for daily and occasional versus infrequent and non drinkers was 3.61 (1.48-3.81) in daily and occasional milk drinkers, 3.45 (1.01-11.79) in infrequent and non milk drinkers, and 3.53 (1.73-7.31; $X^2=8.33$, $p < 0.01$) when frequency of milk consumption was adjusted. The association with milk consumption persisted when adjusted for frequency of alcohol drinking, the RR for daily and occasional versus infrequent and non consumption being 2.21 (1.16-4.21) in daily and occasional alcohol drinkers, 2.11 (0.50-8.87) in infrequent and non alcohol drinkers, and 2.20 (1.22-3.95; $X^2=4.86$, $p < 0.05$) when frequency of alcohol drinking was adjusted. Thus these two factors were associated almost independently with the disease.

DISCUSSION

The close association between alcohol consumption and cancer of the sigmoid colon was an unexpected finding, and seemed to be specific to the sigmoid colon. It is also noteworthy that associations between dietary habits and cancer were similarly specific to the sigmoid colon -eg, the positive associations with milk and meat consumption and the negative associations with green-yellow vegetable, rice/wheat, and soybean paste soup consumption.

Therefore, while conventional understanding that fat-rich-fibre-deficient diet promotes colon cancer risk was confirmed as valid, an even stronger independent effect of alcohol drinking on the risk of sigmoid colon cancer was newly found by our large scale cohort study in Japan. These observations were also in line with other current understanding that cancer risks for left side colon are closely related to environmental factors, while risks for right side colon are more closely associated with genetic and other host factors.

The published work gives conflicting results on the relation of alcohol to colorectal cancer. Suggestive evidence for a possible association was obtained from correlation studies -eg, with colorectal cancer (Enstrom, 1977), with rectal cancer (Kono, 1979), and with both colon and rectal cancer (Potter, 1982). Evidence of the association was also obtained from case-control studies - eg, in Liverpool for intestinal cancer (Stocks, 1957), in New York for rectal cancer (beer) (Wynder 1967; Kabat 1986), in Minnesota for rectal cancer (beer) and for colon cancer (spirits)(Bjelke, 1973), in a patient interview as part of the third National Cancer Survey in USA for colon cancer, in men but not in women, and for rectal cancer in women but not in men (Williams, 1977), in Toronto, for rectal cancer (beer) but not for colon cancer (Miller, 1983), in Adelaide for colon and rectal cancer (Potter, 1986), and in Melbourne for rectal cancer (beer) but not for colon cancer (Kune, 1987). However some case-control studies did not show any association (Bjelke 1973, Higginson 1966; Tuyns 1982). The issue was also examined in cohort studies. Findings for alcoholics were mostly negative (Sundby 1967; Hakulinen 1974, Adelstein 1976; Monson 1975; Schmidt 1981). Danish brewery workers had no excess of colorectal cancer (Jensen, 1979) whereas Irish brewery workers had twice the expected rate (Dean, 1979). Alcohol use was not significantly associated with colon cancer in the Framingham study (Gordon, 1984). In Hawaiian Japanese there was a positive relation for rectal cancer but not for colon cancer after adjustment for age and smoking (Pollack, 1984). A study in Japanese doctors showed no relation for colorectal cancer (Kono, 1986). In a cohort study conducted in California (Wu, 1987) the RR for colorectal cancer was 2.2 (90% CI 1.2-3.8) after multivariate adjustment. Essentially the same results were obtained when the cases of rectal cancer were omitted.

None of these reports dealt specifically with cancer of the sigmoid colon. The mechanism of the close association between alcohol consumption and sigmoid cancer must be different from that of other known alcohol-related cancers (mouth, pharynx, and oesophagus) where alcohol is synergic with cigarette smoking. If cancer of the sigmoid colon is confirmed to be a purely alcohol-related disease what could be the mechanism? There may be a parallel with cancer of the rectum. It is noteworthy that in our current study the highest risk was observed in daily beer drinkers. Possible mechanisms are: a direct effect of alcohol on the motor system (eg, slowing down or causing irregularity of bowel movement) and on blood vessels (eg, congestion); effects of contaminants of alcoholic beverages such as mycotoxin, polycyclic hydrocarbons, N-nitrosamines, and asbestos fibres; induction of microsomal enzymes and activation of procarcinogens; effects of alcohol on hormonal balance and on the chemical composition of bile acids through liver damage by long-term heavy drinking; prevention of first-pass clearance by the liver of selected carcinogens (Anderson 1986; IARC 1988), effects of alcohol on the intestinal flora; dietary habits peculiar to alcohol drinkers (eg, highly salted food and low fibre diet); and effects of various nutritional deficiencies characteristic of alcohol drinkers, some of which may be associated with immunosuppression.

REFERENCES

Adelstein A, White G (1976) Alcoholism and mortality. Popul Trends 6: 7-13

Anderson LM, Harrington GW, Pylypiw HM Jr, Hagiwara A, Magee PN (1986) Tissue levels and biological effects on N-nitrosodimethylamine in mice during chronic low or high dose exposure with or without ethanol. Drug Metab Disposition 14: 733-739

Bjelke E (1973) Epidemiologic studies of cancer of the stomach, colon, and rectum: with special emphasis on the role of diet. Thesis, Univ of Minnesota

Dean G, MacLennan R, McLoughlin H, Shelley B (1979) Causes of death of blue-collar workers at a Dublin brewery, 1954-73. Br J Cancer 40: 581-589

Enstrom JE (1977) Colorectal cancer and beer dirnking. Br J Cancer 35: 674-683

Gordon T, Kannel WB (1984) Drinking and mortality : the Framingham study. Am J Epidemiol 120: 97-107

Hakulinen T, Lehtimäki L, Lehtonen M, Teppo L (1974) Cancer morbidity among two male cohorts with increased alcohol consumption in Finland. J Natl Cancer Inst 52: 1711-1714

Higginson J (1966) Etiological factors in gastrointestinal cancer in man. J Natl Cancer Inst 37: 527-545

IARC (1988) Alcohol drinking. In: IARC Monogr Eval Carcinogenic Risks Hum. IARC, Lyon, pp 120-121

Jensen OM (1979) Cancer morbidity and causes of death among Danish brewery workers. Int J Cancer 23: 454-463

Kabat CG, Howson CP, Wynder EL (1986) Beer consumption and rectal cancer. Int J Epidemiol 15: 454-501

Kono S, Ikeda M (1979) Correlation between cancer mortality and alcoholic beverage in Japan. Br J Cancer 40: 449-455

Kono S, Ikeda M, Tokumode S, Nishizumi M, Kuratsune M (1986) Alcohol and mortality : a cohort study of male Japanese physicians. Int J Epidemiol 15: 527-532

Kune S, June GA, Watson LF (1987) Case-control study on alcoholic beverages as etiological factor: The Melbourne Colorectal Cancer Study. Nutr Cancer 9: 43-51

Miller AB, Howe GR, Jain M, Craib KJP, Harrison L (1983) Food items and food groups as risk factors in a case-control study of diet and colo-rectal cancer. Int J Cancer 32: 155-161

Monson RR, Lyon JL, (1975) Proportional mortality among alcoholics. Cancer 36: 1077-1079

Pollack ES, Nomura AMY, Heibrun Lk, Stemmermann GN, Green SB (1984) Prospective study of alcohol consumption and cancer. N Engl J Med 310: 617-621

Potter JD, McMichael AJ (1986) Diet and cancer of the colon and rectum: a case-control study. J Natl Cancer Inst 76; 557-569

Potter JD, McMichael AJ, Hartshome JM (1982) Alcohol and beer consumption in relation to cancers of bowel and lung; an extended correlation analysis. J Chron Dis 35: 833-842

Schmidt W, Popham RE (1981) The role of drinking and smoking in mortality from cancer and other causes in male alcoholics. Cancer 47: 1031-1041

Stocks P (1957) Cancer incidence in North Wales and Liverpool region in relation to habits and environment. In: British Empire Cancer Campaign 35th Annual Report, part II (suppl), London

Sundby P (1967) Alcoholism and mortality. Universitetsforlaget, Oslo

Tuyns AJ, Péquignot G, Gignoux M, Valla A (1982) Cancers of the digestive tract, alcohol and tobacco. Int J Cancer 30: 9-11

Williams RR, Horm JW (1977) Association of cancer sites with tobacco and alcohol consumption and socio-economic status of patients: Interview study from the Third National Cancer Survey. J Natl Cancer Inst 58: 525-547

Wu AH, Paganini-Hill A, Ross RK, Henderson BE (1987) Alcohol, physical activity and other risk factors for colorectal cancer: a prospective study. Br J Cancer 55: 687-694

Wynder EL, Shigematsu T (1967) Environmental factors of cancer of the colon and rectum. Cancer 20: 1520-1561

Calcium Regulation of Colon Epithelial Cytokinetics in High Risk Subjects for Colon Cancer: Application of New Proliferation Markers

MICHAEL J. WARGOVICH, BERNARD LEVIN, PATRICK LYNCH, HIROMICHI SUMIYOSHI, ALLAN BAER, GERALD ISBELL, PIN-JIN HU, LEOR ROUBEIN, and RODGER WINN

ABSTRACT

A disorder of the rate in which colonic epithelial cells reproduce seems to underlay the process of colon carcinogenesis. As well, dysregulation of proliferation appears to be common to several cancers of the gastrointestinal tract appearing well in advance of cancer. Calcium is vital to the proliferative process. A number of animal and human studies have shown that calcium modulates proliferative control in the colon. To clinically test the hypothesis that calcium may reduce the risk of colon cancer new immunohistochemical techniques that permit rapid evaluation of colonic proliferation rates have been developed.

Keywords: Calcium, proliferation markers, colorectal cancer prevention

DYSREGULATION OF EPITHELIAL CELL PROLIFERATION IN COLON CANCER

Cytokinetic studies of colonic cell renewal have clearly demonstrated a relatively well regulated pattern of epithelial cell production in the normal bowel (Lipkin 1987). In rodents, where much exploratory work has been done, the kinetics of mucosal cell growth have been shown to be governed by a constellation of factors including innate diurnal rhythm, availability of certain nutrients, trophic hormones, and exogenous tumor promoters (Simanoski, et al., 1989). In spite of these forces the colon, in general, exhibits a steady state kinetic pattern where the exfoliated cells are roughly replaced by those borne from the primordial stem cells located in the base of each colonic crypt. Disorders in the normal rate of colonic proliferation seems to be constantly associated with the process of colonic carcinogenesis (Lipkin 1974). How the epithelium becomes dysregulated is a matter for speculation but probably in the precancerous cell involves the loss of cellular suppressors to uncontrolled cell division.

Evidence for dysregulation of proliferation can be found both in animal models for colon cancer and in human investigations. In the dimethylhydrazine-induced colon cancer model rodents typically develop hyperplastic crypts coincident with increases in the size of the proliferative compartment within a few weeks of carcinogen treatment (Wargovich 1983). From areas of hyperplastic epithelium foci of dysplasia evolve into microadenona, then into the adenoma-adenocarcinoma sequence (Rogers, et al., 1985). When tumors are detectable gross aberrations in colonic cell division are apparent. In the rodent tritiated thymidine kinetics, ornithine decarboxylase activity, and other markers of cellular proliferation are substantially elevated prior to the appearance of colonic tumors (Deschner, et al., 1983, Luk, et al., 1982).

In man, hyperproliferative disorders of the normal appearing epithelial mucosa have been identified in premalignant conditions of the esophagus, and stomach as well as the colon. (Lipkin 1988). In the undiseased colon replication of the entire mucosal epithelium is completed in approximately 7-10 days (Wright 1989). For diseases that lead to an increased risk for colon cancer defects in the proliferative behavior of the mucosa have been reported in patients afflicted with familial polyposis, non-familial colon cancer syndrome, and adenomas (Lipkin 1988). In ulcerative colitis an expansion of the proliferative zone has also been reported. Aberrant proliferative rates are well-documented in the normal appearing mucosa in the presence of colonic tumors (Romagnoli, et al., 1986).

What factors are responsible for the creation of a dysregulated epithelium? At the level of the gene, increasing evidence points to the loss of genomic material as an important feature of tumorigenesis (Bodmer, et al., 1987). If critical regulatory genes that govern homeostatic control of cellular proliferation are lost or deleted it becomes conceivable that uncurbed expansion of cells would occur. Clonal expansion of cells containing mutational lesions in the DNA that confer additional growth advantages to the incipient tumor seems to be a plausible sequence initiating colon tumorigenesis. At the cellular level a number of environmental hazards could afflict colon cell survival. Any toxic component from the diet that reached the colon could have locally deleterious effects on colonic crypts, affecting cell viability, and ultimately influencing the rate of cell replacement. Indeed the concept of "differential necrosis with regeneration" has been put forth by Farber (1982) to account for the role of hepatotoxins in the evolution of liver cancer.

The digestion of dietary lipid infuses the colon with unabsorbed fatty acids and biles acids (released from the liver) which in a basic pH environment cause disruption of the surface of the crypt cells resulting in epitheliolysis (Vahouny, et al., 1984). Secondary to cell loss by the exfoliative action of these lipids the colon responds by hyperproliferation. A number of animal studies have confirmed the "tumor promoting" effects of fatty and bile acids on colonic proliferation and an even greater number of studies have clearly shown that differing types and amounts of dietary fat act as tumor promoters for colon cancer in rodents (Wargovich 1984). Further, limited studies in man have tended to implicate the lipid portion of the diet as a risk factor for colon cancer (Kolonel, et al., 1986).

If the colonic epithelium suffers a persistent loss of regulation over proliferation it is important to demonstrate that the hyperproliferative phenotype persists over time in spite of factors stated above that could modulate the rate of cell division in the short term. To this end a number of ongoing and proposed colon cancer prevention trials propose to investigate the persistence of dysregulated epithelium over time. Validation of markers of epithelial cell proliferation as bona fide forerunners of colon cancer is essential for their proposed use in clinical intervention trials. Properly validated proliferative markers could be used as an early signal of impending risk for colon cancer.

CALCIUM REGULATION OF COLONIC PROLIFERATION

Loss of epithelial cells due to the toxic effect of secondary lipids has been considered one of the cardinal features of the tumor promoting aspects of dietary fat. Interest has been kindled in the use of calcium as an avenue of colon cancer protection since it was first recognized by Newmark and colleagues (1984) that calcium could abrogate the toxicity of dietary lipids to the colonic mucosa. In a number of relatively recent experiments the potential benefit of calcium on the epithelium has become recognized. Historically, however, one of the first clinical investigations of the effect of calcium on colonic function was conducted by LeVeen et al.(1967) who found that $CaCO_3$ administration to human volunteers blocked the action of ricinoleic acid-induced diarrhea of the intestine. Lipkin and Newmark (1985) observed that supplemental $CaCO_3$ decreased the epithelial proliferation rate in patients at high risk for colon cancer. The abnormally high rate of colonic epithelial proliferation characteristic of familial cancer patients was found to be significantly reduced after consumption of approximately 1250 mg of calcium daily for 3-4 months. Rozen et al. (1989) treated 30 first degree relatives of colon cancer patients and eight persons with colonic polyps with 1250 mg of $CaCO_3$ or calcium gluconate-lactate. Colonic proliferation was reduced by 30% during calcium treatment but rebounded to high levels after cessation of the supplementation. Buset et al. (1986) demonstrated that, although calcium chloride caused a decrease in epithelial proliferation in vitro, adenomas and carcinomas failed to respond to calcium added to the medium and proliferated independently of the concentrations tested. Several case-control studies of the effect of calcium supplementation (mostly as $CaCO_3$) on adenomas are under way in the United States and abroad.

UT MD ANDERSON CANCER CENTER PILOT COLON CANCER PREVENTION STUDIES: EFFECT OF CALCIUM OF EPITHELIAL CYTOKINETICS IN SUBJECTS WITH RESECTED ADENOMA

The recognition from animal studies (Wargovich 1988) that calcium could protect the bowel from tumor promoting aspects of dietary fat has led to several pilot studies to determine the effect of calcium supplementation on the epithelial cell kinetics of the human colon. We have investigated the effect of calcium on colonic proliferation markers in three small scale clinical studies. In the first study four patients with resected adenoma and two with resected colon cancer were given 1500 mg of calcium (as $CaCO_3$) daily for 3 months. Sigmoidoscopy provided biopsies for an initial baseline measures of colonic cytokinetics via short-term culture with tritiated thymidine. After 90 days we noted a 21% average suppression of the number of proliferating cells. While not statistically significant this study encouraged us to recruit 6 further adenoma subjects. These individuals consumed 2000 mg of calcium daily for 4 weeks. Proliferation analysis of initial and final biopsies revealed a significant ($p<.001$) 31% reduction in crypt proliferation rates (Isbell et al., 1989). Our final study features a crossover design placebo-controlled single blinded study of 2000 mg of calcium in 20 subjects with adenoma treated for 4 weeks on either calcium or placebo alternating with the opposite treatment arm in the second 4 weeks. Thymidine uptake studies are performed initially, at cross-over, and at the end of the trial. The results of these 3 pilot studies (Wargovich et al, in preparation) suggest that the kinetics of colon cell renewal are modulated by dietary calcium. Whether this modulation predicts a favorable outcome in terms of prevention of adenoma recurrence is the focus of ongoing and proposed clinical trials.

DEVELOPMENTAL MARKERS OF COLONIC CELL PROLIFERATION

Bromodeoxyuridine (BUdR) Incorporation

The development of immunohistochemistry technology has enlarged the repertoire of investigational proliferation markers that may be highly useful in colon cancer prevention trials in man. While historically very informative, cytokinetic studies using tritiated thymidine suffer from delays in the time required to perform autoradiography. This limitation has been circumvented by the use of a monoclonal antibody to bromodeoxyuridine (BUdR), a nucleoside analogue of thymidine (Gratzner 1982). BUdR substantially reduces the time required to calculate labeling indices on histologic sections of colonic tissue. Visualized by immunoperoxidase staining, the detection of S phase cells can be achieved within 1 or 2 days of a biopsy procedure. Risio et al. (1988) have recently demonstrated that an expansion of the proliferative compartment in subjects with hyperplastic polyps, adenomas, or adenocarcinomas is detectable, complementing early work by Lipkin and colleagues using traditional thymidine technology. Our ongoing studies at the M.D. Anderson Cancer Center confirm that BUdR and thymidine give essentially the same information from adjacent biopsies taken in the same subjects (Isbell, et al., 1989) with a substantial increase in assay performance time.

Cyclin (Proliferating Cell Nuclear Antigen) - Immunohistochemistry

Proliferating cell nuclear antigen (PCNA or cyclin) is a 36 kd protein also termed the auxiliary protein of mammalian polymerase δ (Takasaki et al., 1984). PCNA is expressed on most proliferating mammalian cells and has been shown to be maximally expressed in S phase and declines in later parts of the cell cycle (Celis, et al., 1984). Monoclonal antibodies to PCNA therefore are able to provide information about the <u>entire</u> proliferative fraction of normal and neoplastic tissue. Recent studies from the University of Colorado (Ahnen et al., 1988) have shown that PCNA positive cells increase in the normal epithelium of the rat colon in response to the colonic carcinogen, dimethylhydrazine. Our laboratory has worked to optimize the requirements for PCNA immunoperoxidase staining in fixed specimens of human colon. Numerically PCNA labels a higher fraction of proliferating cells and labeling indices reflect this increase. We are currently comparing this technique with other S-phase specific markers. Amongst the advantages of PCNA is the obviation for incubation of colon mucosa with an isotope or biochemical precursor of DNA.

Ornithine Decarboxylase Physio-Chemical Behavior

Polyamines are small, cationic molecules which have been implicated as essential biochemical elements of a proliferating cell (Pegg 1986). Ornithine decarboxylase (ODC), which catalyzes the conversion of ornithine to putrescine, is detectably higher in the colon mucosa than in other tissue (Ball et al., 1976). In animal studies, infusion of the colon with bile salts or fatty acids or colon carcinogens administered parenterally elicits an elevation in ODC (Luk, et al., 1982). In carcinogenicity experiments a persistence in elevated ODC levels in normal epithelium has been shown. Levels of the enzyme have been reported to be higher in subjects with adenomas or colon cancer when compared to subjects with an endoscopically normal colon (Herrera-Ornelas, et al., 1987).

We have found that at least two forms of ODC exist in the colon separable by charge. In the normal mouse colon a more acidic form of

ODC predominates over a second minor peak detected by DEAE Sepharose gtcolumn chromatography. The peak pattern is exactly reversed in colon tumors (Sumiyoshi et al, in preparation). In limited studies using human tissue, we have detected an identical pattern in ODC separation comparable to the normal and tumor patterns in the mouse. Whether these separate forms of ODC imply a unique biochemical evolution for the colon tumor or whether it represents a devolution of a dysregulated colonocytes remains to be determined.

SUMMARY

Abnormalities in colonic cell renewal rates have been clearly shown in animal models for colon cancer and in studies of the colon mucosa from high risk individuals for the disease. Because proliferation is a normal process for the colon markers of neoplastic risk should measure marked and persistent increases in the proliferative compartment. Short-term studies utilizing calcium have shown a benefit by surpressing colonic hyperproliferation in the high risk individual. The final link will be to conclusively show that proliferation markers are not only prognosticative for malignancy but that modulation of the marker response indicates a re-regulation of colonic epithelial proliferation, a step in the direction of cancer prevention.

REFERENCES

Ball WJ, Salser JS, Balis ME (1976) Biochemical changes in preneoplastic rodent intestines. Cancer Res 36:2686-2689.

Bodmer WF, Bailey CJ, Bodmer J, Bussey HJR, Ellis A, Gorman P, Lucibello FC, Murday VA, Rider SH, Scrambler P, Sheer P, Solomon E, Spurr NK (1987) Localization of the gene for familial adenomatous polyposis on chromosome 5. Nature 328:614-616.

Bravo R, Frank R, Blundell PA, MacDonald-Bravo H (1987) Cyclin /PCNA is the auxiliary protein of DNA polymerase. Nature 326-515-517.

Buset M, Lipkin M, Winawer S, Swaroop S, Friedman E (1986) Inhibition of human colonic epithelial cell proliferation in vivo and in vitro by calcium. Cancer Res 46:5426-5429.

Celis J, Bravo R (1984) Synthesis of the nuclear protein cyclin in growing, senescent, and morphologically transformed skin fibroblasts. FEBS Lett 165:21-25.

Deschner EE, Long FC, Hakissan M, Hormann SL (1983) Differential susceptibility of AKR, C57BL/6J and CF1 mice to 1-2 dimethylhydrazine induced colonic tumor formation predicted by proliferative characteristics of colonic epithelial cells. JNCI, pp 279-282.

Farber E (1982) Chemical carcinogenesis. Am J Pathol 106:271-291.

Gratzner HG (1982) Monoclonal antibody to 5-bromo and 5 iododeoxyuridine: a new reagent for detection of DNA replication. Science 218:474-476.

Herrera-Ornelas L, Porter C, Pera P, Greco W, Petrelli NJ, MiHelman A (1987) A comparison of ornithine decarboxylase and S-adenosyl methionine decarboxylase activity in human large bowel mucosa, polyps, and colorectal adenocarcinoma. J Surg Res 42:52-60.

Isbell GM, Hu PJ, Lynch P, Roubein L, Katz R, Cafferty S, Patel S, Wargovich MJ 1989 A comparison of tritiated thymidine and bromodeoxyuridine immunoperoxidase techniques for measuring epithelial proliferation in the human colon. Gastroenterology, 96(5), AB228.

Isbell, G, Hu, PJ, Bauer, A, Lanza, F, Shabot, M, Winn, R, Hochman, L, Michaletz, P, Levin, B, Wargovich, MJ (1989) Calcium modulation of mucosal proliferation in patients with sporadic adenoma or colon cancer. Gastroenterology, 96(5), A228.

Kolonel LN and LeMarchand L (1986) The epidemiology of colon cancer and dietary fat. In: Ip C, Birt DE, Roger AE, Mettlin C (eds) Dietary Fat and Cancer, Alan Liss, New York, pp 69-93.

LeVeen HH, Borek B, Axelrod DR, Johnson A (1967) Cause and treatment of diarrhea following resection of the small intestine. Surg Gyn Obst 127:766-770.

Lipkin M (1974) Phase I and phase 2 proliferative lesions of colonic epithelial cells in diseases leading to colonic cancer, Cancer (Phila) 34:878-888.

Lipkin M (1987) Proliferation and differentiation of normal and diseased gastrointestinal cells. In: Johnson LR (ed) Physiology of gastrointestinal tract, Raven Press, New York, pp 255-284.

Lipkin M, Newmark HL (1985) Effect of added dietary calcium on colonic epithelial cell proliferation in subjects at high risk for familial colon cancer N Engl J Med 313:1381-1384.

Lipkin M (1988) Biomarkers of increased susceptibility to gastrointestinal cancer: new application to studies of cancer prevention in human subjects. Cancer Res 48:235-245.

Luk GD, Hamilton SR, O'Ceallight D, Smith J, Natuzzi E, Baylin SB (1982) Azoxymethane (AOM) induces a bihphasic increase in intestinal ornithine decarboxylase (ODC) during colon carcinogenesis. Gastroenterol 82:AB 1121.

Newmark, HL, Wargovich MJ, Bruce, WR. (1984) Colon cancer and dietary fat, calcium, and phosphate: a hypothesis. JNCI 72:1323-1325.

Pegg AE (1986) Recent advances in the biochemistry of polyamines in eukaryotes. Biochem J 234:249-262.

Risio M, Coverlizza S, Ferrari A, Candelaseri GL, Rossini FP (1988). Immunohistochemical study of epithelial cell proliferation in hyperplastic polyps, adenomas, and adenocarcinomas of the large bowel. Gastroenterol 94:899-906.

Rogers AE and Nauss KM (1985) Contributions of laboratory animal studies of colon carcinogenesis. In: Mastromarino AJ and Brattain MG (eds) Large Bowel Cancer, Praeger, New York, pp 1-45.

Romagnoli P, Filiponi F, Bamdetteni L, Brugnola D (1986) Increase of mitotic activity in colonic mucosa of patients with colorectal cancer. Dis Colon Rectum 27:305-308.

Rozen P, Fireman Z, Wax Y, Ron E (1989) Oral calcium suppresses increased colonic mucosal proliferation of persons at risk for colorectal neoplasia. Gastroenterol 92:1603.

Simanoski UA, Wright NA, Seitz HK (1989) Mucosal cellular regeneration and colorectal carcinogenesis. In: Seitz HK, Simanoski UA, Wright NA (eds) Colorectal Cancer, Springer-Verlag, Berlin, pp 225-236.

Takasaki Y, Fishwild D, Tan EM (1984) Characterization of proliferating cell nuclear antigen recognized by autoantibodies in lupus sera. J Exp Med 159:981-992.

Vahouny GV, Satchithanandam S, Lightfoot F, Haas-Smith S, Kritchevsky D, Cassidy MM (1984) Morphological disruption of colonic mucosa by free or cholestyramine bound bile acids. Dig Dis Sci 29:432-442.

Wargovich MJ (1986). Dietary promoters and antipromoters. In: Shankel DM, Hartman PE, Kada T, Holaender A (eds) Antimutagenesis and anticarcinogenesis, Plenum, New York, pp 409-420.

Wargovich, MJ (1988) Calcium and colon cancer. J Amer Coll Nutr 7(4): 295-300.

Wargovich, MJ, Medline A, Bruce, WR. (1983) Early histopathological events to the evolution of colon cancer in C57BL/6J and CF-1 mice treated with 1,2-dimethylhydrazine. JNCI 71: 125-132.

Wright NA (1989) The control of cell proliferation in colonic epithelium. In: Seitz HK, Simanoski UA, Wright NA (eds) Colorectal Cancer, Springer-Verlag, Berlin, pp 237-243.

Yamada K, Yoshitake K, Ahnen DJ (1988) Proliferating cell nuclear antigen (PCNA) expression detects expansion of the proliferative compartment in carcinogen treated colonic mucosa in the rat. Gastroenterol 96:AB555.

Ornithine Decarboxylase (ODC) and S-Adenosylmethionine Decarboxylase (AdoMetDC) as Markers of Human Colonic Neoplasia

LEMUEL HERRERA, NICHOLAS J. PETRELLI, and GUSTAVO VIAL

ABSTRACT

Increased polyamine biosynthetic activity and raised levels of intracellular polyamines are commonly associated with normal, abnormal, and induced proliferative states. Ornithine Decarboxylase and S-adenosylmethionine Decarboxylase are known rate-limiting enzymes in polyamine biosynthesis. Herein, we report results from our group in relation to the activity of these enzymes in colonic neoplasias and their possible role as tumor markers.

Keywords: Ornithine Decarboxylase, S-Adenosylmethionine Decarboxylase, tumor markers, adenomatous polyps, colon cancer

Colorectal cancer is the second leading cause of cancer-related deaths in the United States. It is second only to cancer of the breast and lung in females and cancer of the lung in males. There were 140,000 new cases diagnosed in 1986.

Despite advances in the treatment of cancer in the colon and rectum, the 5-year survival rate for patients with cancer of the colon and rectum, has changed little in the last 30 years. A good predictor of survival has been the extent of the disease at a time of the diagnosis. The study of the involved lymph nodes remains the most significant parameter. The 5-year survival of tumors with serosal penetration but negative nodes is close to 80%; whereas, when the lymph nodes are positive, it is only about 50%. Therefore, it would seem reasonable that early detection would offer the main thrust in improving curability and longevity following cancer of the colon and rectum. Unfortunately, there is as yet no specific markers for the detection of early colorectal cancer. The current "gold standard" of colorectal cancer markers is the carcinomembryonic antigen (CEA). CEA is best used as a monitor of recurrence, but it is not useful for screening or as a test for early diagnosis.

Putrescine, Cadaverine, Spermidine, and Spermine are polyamines. They are ubiquitous substances in biologic materials. Polyamines are low molecular weight, highly charged organic cations. They are found in association with nucleic acids; thus, they are packaged with DNA. In Escherichia coli bacteriophage T4, they account for about 40% of the total cations in the phage. Prokaryotes generally have higher amounts of Putrescine, Cadaverine, Spermidine, and lack Spermine. Eukaryotes contain little Putrescine, but have both Spermidine and Spermine.

The enzymes Ornithine Decarboxylase (ODC) and S-Adenosylmethionine Decarboxylase (AdoMetDC) are the known rate-limiting steps in polyamine biosynthesis (Pegg 1982). The action of ODC produces Putrescine and requires pyridoxal phosphate as a co-factor. It is subject to feedback inhibition and repression by Putrescine and Spermidine. Methionine and Putrescine are the biosynthetic precursors of Spermidine and Spermine. S-Adenosylmethionine forms from Methionine and ATP after being acted upon by S-AdoMetDC to give decarboxylated S-Adenosylmethionine. S-AdoMetDC is devoid of pyridoxal phosphate, but the enzyme contains a covalently linked pyrovoyl residue (mw = 42,000 Daltons). This pyrovoyl group is required for enzymatic activity.

The excretion of polyamines is mainly urinary; however, the levels are low and total 5-10 mgs per 24-hours. Most of the urinary polyamines are monoacetyl derivatives and their site of synthesis is unknown. It is, however, of interest that although raised serum or urinary polyamine levels have been reported in up to 66% of patients with large bowel cancer (Moorehead 1987; Nishioka 1977), their clinical usefulness still remains unestablished.

Increased polyamine biosynthetic activity and raised levels of intracellular polyamines are comonly associated with normal, abnormal, and induced proliferative states. Our group has shown that the activity of both of the key enzymes for polyamine biosynthesis is elevated in neoplastic human colorectal tissues as compared to the normal controls (Herrera-Ornelas 1987). By biochemical localization studies, it has been previously determined that within the intestinal mucosa, ODC activity is located in the villous tips of differentiated cells, whereas S-AdoMetDC activity, by contrast, is highest in the crypt cells. Because proliferative states are associated with crypt cells activity and since the proportion of these particular cells is increased in polyps and adenocarcinomas, it was hoped that S-AdoMetDC activity would be a more sensitive an indicator of proliferative disorders than ODC activity. Contrary to these expectations, it was found that S-AdoMetDC activity exhibited the same general distribution as ODC, and that the differences between the normal, benign, and malignant neoplasias were less, rather than more, distinct (Porter 1987).

Levels of tissue polyamines are known to be affected by both transcription and translation mechanisms. Our group performed mRNA dot blot analysis using the probe PODC-934 (Berger 1984). This work revealed similar ODC mRNA content, while enzymatic activity varied by up to 3.3 fold among the samples of human colon cancer. These results suggest posttranscriptional regulation of ODC as a major determinant in ODC activity (Porter 1986).

We were very interested in the distribution of the polyamine biosynthesis and ODC activity among various premalignant diseases of the colon, looking for possible associations to their malignant potential. In fact, we were stimulated by the report of Luk and Baylin (1984) in that the progression from normal mucosa to adenoma and carcinoma was identifiable in patients with familial adenomatous polyposis (FAP). ODC levels were found useful for screening relatives at risk for FAP (Luk 1984). In the following study, we entered patients without a diagnosis of FAP. In our cases with no-known familial history of colonic neoplasms, we found no evidence for biochemical activation of the noninvolved colonic mucosa. Our results were: mean values (nmol/hour/mg/protein [± SEM = noninvolved mucosa,0.11 ± .02; polyps, 0.50 ± .11; and adenocarcinoma 0.88 ± .10). In addition, we measured levels of ODC activity in the distant nonaffected mucosa of patients harboring a carcinoma and compared these results to those obtained from colorectal biopsies from disease-free patients recruited at the Roswell Park Cancer Institute Screening Clinic (Table 1).

Table 1. ODC activity in subjects with and without colorectal cancer

	Non-involved Mucosa Patients Ca		Tumor	Colorectal Mucosa from Disease-free Subjects		
*Sigmoid	n=13	0.054	0.572	n=19	0.742	P<.001
*Rectum	n= 9	0.057	0.696	n=24	0.690	P<.001

*All Median Values
RESULTS in nmol/hr/mg/prot

It was clear that the nonaffected mucosa of patients harboring a colonic neoplasia exhibited a diminished level of Ornithine Decarboxylase activity as compared to the mucosa of disease-free patients. Results with similar trends have been reported by Moorehead and his group (Moorehead 1987). They have shown diminished levels of ODC activity in microscopically normal rectal mucosa of patients with colorectal tumors. Although performed in a group of patients without a defined contribution of inheritance, these results were also unexpected as the previous report by Luk (1984) in patients with FAP and their relatives at risk had demonstrated increased levels of this enzyme in the "normal" looking mucosa of those relatives-at-risk who eventually would develop the disease so that some biochemical changes were to be expected in the colonic mucosa. Although technical and artifactual reasons could be claimed as responsible for ours' and Moorehead's (1987) results, it is important to emphasize that these results were consistently obtained even though they were performed discontinuously in various specimens obtained at various times. The specimens were basically obtained either immediately upon surgical removal or at endoscopy, with comparable ischemia time, by the same surgeons, and processed by the same technician at Dr. Porter's laboratory. No sex differences were apparent in this group of individuals. We could speculate that the variability in the results may be related to possible changes in mRNA levels, not as yet identified, or due to ODC polymorphism; the latter is supported by experimental data generated by the androgen-regulated mouse kidney model where at least two nonhomologous ODC-DNA clones are recognized by different mRNAs in hybridization studies using plasmids. Interestingly, both ODC mRNAs are believed to be encoded, at least in part, by different nonhomologous genes (Berger 1984). In humans, we have already reported in the quantitative differences between the levels of ODC activity between primary colorectal cancers and liver metastases in the same host (Herrera 1988).

A recent report by Lawson et al (1989), focused on the proliferative and enzymatic activity in the transitional (within 2 cms) mucosa adjacent to colonic cancer; they concluded that transitional mucosa showed morphometric changes, but these changes were not reflected in the values for proliferative or enzyme markers to suggest a higher than expected risk for malignant change detectable prior to morphologic changes (Lawson 1989). Indeed, in two of our patients with FAP, we have been able to establish a significant gradient in ODC activity between the macroscopically observed and histologically documented adenomatous polyps and the noninvolved mucosa.

The ODC gene sequences in humans have been localized to chromosome regions 2pter→p23 and 7cen→qter. Our group has further defined the location of these sequences by sommatic cell and in situ techniques to 2p25 and 7q31-qter. It is believed that the ODC gene situated on chromosome 2, is the functional gene. Shows and Radford (1988) from our group have also mapped the S-AdoMetDC gene sequences to human chromosome

6 and X and have also established that there is no gene amplification in colon cancer and benign polyps; therefore, amplification is not the mechanism by which increased S-AdoMetDC activity occurs in colorectal neoplasia. As with ODC, it is likely that control of its regulation is at the transcriptional and posttranscriptional levels. Further work on the regulation of S-AdoMetDC in tumors will require cloning of the human gene (Radford 1988).

In summary, our previous work suggests the possibility of the existence of a paracrine effect of growth and other cellular factors possibly secreted by the colonic neoplasia. This possibility should be pursued as the potential for screening for colonic neoplasia utilizing a biopsy of the nonaffected colorectal mucosa and determinations of ODC isoforms which may be clinically significant.

REFERENCES

Berger FG, Szymanski P, Read E, Watson G (1984) Androgen-regulated Ornithine Decarboxylase in RNA of mouse kidney. J Biol Chem 259: 7941-7946

Herrera L, Petrelli N (1988) Ornithine Decarboxylase activity in hepatic and extrahepatic metastases from colorectal cancer. Dis Col Rectum 31:352-354

Herrera-Ornelas L, Porter C, Pera P, Greco W, Petrelli N, Mittelman A (1987) A comparison of Ornithine Decarboxylase activity in human large bowel mucosa, polyps and colorectal adenocarcinoma. J Surg Res 42:56-60

Lawson M, White L, Coyle P, Butler R, Roberts-Thomson I, Comyers R (1989) An assessment of proliferative and enzyme activity in transitional mucosa adjacent to colonic cancer. Cancer 64:1061-1066

Luk GD, Baylin SB (1984) Ornithine Decarboxylase as a biologic marker in familial colonic polyposis. New Engl J Med 311:80-83

Moorehead RJ, Hoper M, McKelvey STD (1987) Ornithine Decarboxylase activity in rectal mucosa as marker for colorectal adenomas and carcinomas. Br J Surg 87:364-365

Nishioka K, Romsdahl MN, McMurtrey MJ (1977) Serum polyamine alterations in surgical patients with colorectal carcinomas. J Surg Oncol 9:555-562

Pegg AE, McCann PP (1982) Polyamine metabolism and function. Am J Physiol 243:C212-221

Porter CW, Herrera-Ornelas L, Clark J (1986) Polyamine biosynthetic enzyme activities correlated with neoplastic progression in human colorectal tissue. Proc Amer Assn Cancer Res (abstract); Vol. 27, pp 159

Porter C, Herrera-Ornelas L, Pera P, Petrelli N, Mittelman A (1987) Polyamine biosynthetic activity in normal and neoplastic human colorectal tissues. Cancer 60:1275-1281

Radford DM, Eddy R, Haley L, Henry W, Pegg AE, Pajuney A, Shows TB (1988) Gene sequences coding for S-Adenosylmethionine Decarboxylase are present on chromosome 6 and the X and are not amplified in colon neoplasia. Cytogen & Cell Genetics 49:285-288

Dietary Fiber or Piroxicam as Potential Cancer Prevention Agents: Effects on Rectal Epithelial Cell Proliferation in Humans at Increased Risk of Colon Cancer

DAVID L. EARNEST, DAVID S. ALBERTS, LEE J. HIXSON, and FRANK L. MEYSKENS

INTRODUCTION

Over the past decade, there has been little improvement in outcome of treatment for advanced colon cancer. The best chance for cure remains early removal of a localized malignant tumor. Accordingly, much emphasis has been focused on screening, early detection and removal of recognized precursor lesions, namely adenomatous colon polyps. However, this approach is problematic in that current methods, such as testing of stool for occult blood and periodic examination of the rectum and colon by fiberoptic endoscopy, have either less than desired sensitivity or are expensive, entail some risk, detect only gross macroscopic lesions and do not address the persistence of abnormal colonic mucosal biology which imparts a continued cancer risk. However, the demonstration that colonic crypt epithelial cell proliferative activity (labeling index) which is increased in colon cancer was also abnormal in colon mucosa of patients with familial polyposis coli, who are known to be at high risk for developing cancer, provided a tool to assess for the presence of a subclinical or microscopic abnormality (Lipkin 1983, 1984). The subsequent reports that crypt cell proliferative activity was also increased in patients with sporadic colon adenomas, and that the labeling index in patients with familial polyposis could be changed toward normal by addition of calcium to the diet, provides evidence that this marker of crypt cell epithelial proliferative activity might be useful to evaluate cancer risk in certain patient groups and for assessing the effects of treatment interventions aimed at decreasing cancer risk (Lipkin 1985). We have used the tritiated thymidine labeling index to evaluate the effects of two proposed cancer prevention strategies, namely increased dietary fiber and treatment with the nonsteroidal anti-inflammatory drug (NSAID) piroxicam.

Epidemiological studies in humans and experimental cancer formation studies in animals strongly suggest that an increase in dietary fiber, especially wheat bran fiber, can exert a protective effect against colon cancer (Greenwald 1987, Reddy 1988). The proposed mechanism for a beneficial effect from fiber involves increased fecal bulk and decreased concentration in stool of soluble mutagenic substances. Another approach involves the use of drugs to decrease prostaglandin concentration in tissue. The rationale for this is based on the observation that concentration of prostaglandin E_2 is increased in benign and malignant colon neoplasms and that high levels of PGE_2 in a number of tumor models stimulate cell growth and depress immune system function (Bennett 1977, Han 1983, Goodwin 1984, Earnest 1989). We report the results of ongoing pilot studies at the University of Arizona Cancer Center which show improvement in colonic mucosal epithelial cell thymidine labeling index resulting from treatment with wheat bran fiber and with piroxicam.

METHODS

Wheat Bran Fiber Trial

Seventeen patients (11 female, 6 male) with a mean age of 70 years (range 54-78) who had undergone surgical resection of a colon cancer more than one year previous and subsequently remained free of apparent recurrence were entered into this one-arm, single-blind study. Patients were excluded if their normal diet contained 30gms/day or more fiber, if they were eating a special diet that might preclude compliance with study requirements, if they were in poor general health, or had significantly abnormal biochemical tests of renal and liver function.

The wheat bran cereal, All-Bran®, and a matching placebo cereal were provided by the Kellogg Company of Battle Creek, Michigan. All subjects were given the placebo cereal as a daily supplement to their regular diet for one month and then switched for an additional 2 months to treatment with the All-Bran cereal supplement. During the high fiber treatment period, the unit dose of All-Bran provided 13.5gms of wheat bran fiber daily. A previous study in a southern Arizona retirement community had documented that approximately 13gms/day of All-Bran for up to 3 months could be administered to a similar age group of subjects with acceptable compliance and side effects (Ho 1988). The purpose of the one-month run-in was to insure compliance with the cereal supplement and study procedures, to assure stable health, and to permit completion of all baseline procedures. Throughout the placebo run-in and fiber treatment periods, dietary intake was assessed monthly by standardized food intake questionnaires, and treatment compliance and evidence for toxicity evaluated by questionnaire and biochemical laboratory tests at scheduled clinic visits.

After completion of the one-month low fiber cereal supplement and again after 2 months of the high fiber cereal treatment, each subject had rectal mucosal tissue specimens obtained by forceps biopsy performed during fiberoptic sigmoidoscopy. The only preparation was two 150ml normal saline enemas without oral catharsis. Two mucosal biopsy specimens were incubated with 5μCi/ml [^{3}H]-thymidine (20Ci/mMol) for 90min and then processed for microautoradiography according to the method of Lipkin and others (1983, 1985). Proliferation of epithelial cells lining colonic crypts was measured by microscopic counting of cells labeled as a result of incorporation of [^{3}H]-thymidine into cellular DNA. Crypts longitudinally sectioned from base to lumen were analyzed according to the criteria of Lipkin and others (1983, 1984, 1985). An index of epithelial cell proliferation was also determined by a second method which assessed [^{3}H]-thymidine labeling of epithelial cell outgrowth from biopsy tissue maintained in culture. For this assay, two biopsy specimens were finely minced, and processed according to the method described by Buset and others (1986). The epithelial cell cultures were then fixed, developed by autoradiography, and the labeled cells counted.

Piroxicam Dose-Finding Study

Thirty patients (19 male, 11 female) with a mean age of 67 (range: 47 to 73) who had undergone colonoscopic removal of adenomatous colon polyps more than 1 month but less than 8 years previous were admitted into a single-blind protocol which evaluated the effects of 20mg, 10mg, and 5mg of piroxicam daily on changes in concentration of prostaglandin E_2 and epithelial proliferative activity in rectal mucosal biopsy specimens. Ten patients were assigned to each drug dose. The overall protocol was similar to that used in the fiber trial. All patients were given a matching placebo drug for the first month and then placed on one of the three doses of piroxicam for the next 3 months. Piroxicam and placebo drug were provided by Pfizer Laboratories, New York, NY. All patients had detailed diet evaluation and regular compliance assessment and toxicity monitoring.

The concentration of piroxicam in serum was measured by high pressure liquid chromatography (Finley 1989). Baseline or control biopsy specimens of rectal mucosa were obtained prior to and again at conclusion of the 1-month placebo drug run-in period as described above. Rectal biopsy was performed again after 4 and 12 weeks of active piroxicam treatment. Part of the tissue specimens were immediately frozen in liquid nitrogen and later processed for prostaglandin E_2 concentration. For this, frozen mucosal tissue (18-25mg) was thawed, homogenized in acid phosphate buffer, centrifuged, the supernate extracted with chloroform:methanol and PGE_2 quantitated by radioimmunoassay using a commercial kit (Seragen Laboratories, Boston, Massachusetts). Other mucosal specimens were incubated with [^{3}H]-thymidine as soon as obtained and processed for the epithelial cell labeling tritiated thymidine index as described above (Lipkin 1983, 1985).

RESULTS

Wheat Bran Fiber Trial

Table 1 presents dietary data for the 11 female subjects in the trial in whom dietary analysis is complete. There were absolute increases between study entry and study completion in the daily intakes of total calories, protein, carbohydrate, fat and calcium; however, intakes of these nutrients was not increased over baseline in terms of percent calories. The total dietary fiber intake in gms/day, exclusive of the supplemental cereal fiber, increased slightly between study entry and study completion.

Table 1. Nutrient Intakes (Mean) During Wheat Bran Fiber Trial (Estimated by Arizona Food Frequency Questionnaire Data)

Nutrients	Females (11) at Study Entry	Females (11) at Study Completion
Energy (kcal)	1533.0	1789.0
Protein (gms)	65.7	73.2
% kcal	17.4	16.5
Carbohydrate (gms)	188.0	215.0
% kcal	49.2	48.3
Fat (gms)	58.4	68.5
Calcium (mgs)	997.0	1034.0
Dietary Fiber (gms)		
From Grains	4.6	5.0
Other Diet	13.8	16.1
Fiber Supplement	0.0	13.5
Total	18.4	34.6

Compliance assessment showed that the cumulative average supplemental fiber intake was greater than 75% in 16 of the 17 subjects. In 55 evaluations in the 17 patients, toxicity monitoring showed no toxicity in more than 90% of the assessments; mild diarrhea was noted in 2%. The only moderate degree of toxicity was excessive intestinal gas, noted in less than 10% of assessments. There was no significant change in any of the blood tests, including serum chemistries and blood cell counts.

Table 2. [^{3}H]-Thymidine Labeling Indices (LI) by Crypt Organ Culture: Effects of Wheat Bran Fiber In Resected Colorectal Cancer Patients

LI Category	Decreased*	Increased	No Change	Total
Initial low+	1 Pt	2 Pts	6 Pts	9
Initial high+	4 Pts	1 Pt	3 Pts	8
Total	5	3	9	17

*p<.001, significant response, comparing labeling indices after two months of fiber to baseline control values for each patient
+median labeling index was used as cutoff between high and low labeling indices

The results of [^{3}H]-thymidine labeling index by crypt organ culture are available from 34 biopsies evaluated in the 17 patients. An average of 32 crypts were counted per biopsy. The average crypt column had 44.8 cells. An average of 2828 cells were counted per biopsy specimen. The cellular response to the 13.5gms/day wheat bran fiber supplement was evaluated statistically in each patient by comparing the baseline to the 3-month labeling indices. To be considered a significant response, the on-treatment labeling index had to be decreased or increased by a sufficient magnitude as compared to the baseline to compute a p value of less than 0.001. Patients were categorized as having initially low or initially high labeling indices by using the median baseline labeling index as a cutoff between high and low values. Of the 8 patients with initially high total labeling indices (Table 2), 4 had a significant decrease, 1 a significant increase, and 3 no change following 2 months of wheat bran fiber treatment. Of the 9 patients who had an initially low labeling index, 6 showed no change, 1 showed a significant decrease, and 2 showed a significant increase. Table 3 presents the individual thymidine labeling indices for compartments 1-5 in the eight patients who had an initially high value. There appears to be a trend toward lower on-treatment labeling indices in compartments 3, 4 and 5 with L_2/L_1 values of 0.60, 0.74 and 0.62 respectively.

Table 3. [^{3}H]-Thymidine Labeling Indices by Crypt Compartment in Resected Colorectal Cancer Patients

	Initial High Labeling Index (N=8)		
Compartment	L_1 (before)	L_2 (after)	L_2/L_1
1	.150	.140	.93
2	.171	.176	1.03
3	.128	.102	.60
4	.058	.043	.74
5	.013	.008	.62
Entire Crypt	.104	.094	.90

In the 16 patients for whom the 24hr epithelial cell outgrowth culture method of labeling index was performed at baseline and after 3 months of study, 11.6 (SD±7.8) outgrowths were counted per biopsy. This yielded an average of 2695 (SD±1272) cells per biopsy and an average of 431 (SD±351) cells per outgrowth. The labeling indices measured prior to and again after 2 months of wheat bran fiber treatment are shown in Table 4.

Table 4. [^{3}H]-Thymidine Labeling Index (LI) by 24-Hour Outgrowth in Resected Colorectal Cancer Patients: Effects of Wheat Bran Fiber

N	LI_1*±SD	LI_2*±SD	LI_2/LI_1	p Value
16	.100±0.03	.078±0.03	.78	<.001

*LI_1 = labeling index at baseline; LI_2 = labeling index after 2 months of wheat bran fiber supplementation

The 24hr [^{3}H]-thymidine labeling index data were again evaluated according to initially low versus initially high baseline values using the median baseline labeling index as a cutoff between high and low values, as described previously. Six of the 8 patients who had initially high baseline labeling indices showed a significant decrease in rectal mucosal biopsy labeling index in specimens obtained after 2 months of active fiber treatment (Table 5). Three of the 8 patients with initially low baseline labeling indices showed a decrease, whereas 1 increased and there was no significant change in the other four. Overall, there was a 22% decrease in the 24hr outgrowth labeling index following 2 months of dietary supplementation with 13.5gms/day wheat bran fiber. This change was highly significant with a p value less than .001.

Table 5. [^{3}H]-Thymidine Labeling Indices (LI) by 24-Hour Outgrowth in Resected Colorectal Cancer Patients: Effects of Wheat Bran Fiber

LI Category	Decreased*	Increased	No Change	Total
Initial low	3 Pts	1 Pt	4 Pts	8
Initial high	6 Pts	0 Pt	2 Pts	8
Total	9	1	6	16

*p<.001, comparing labeling indices after two months of fiber to baseline control values control values for each patient. Median labeling index was used as cutoff between high and low indices.

Piroxicam Trial

Throughout the piroxicam trial we observed excellent compliance with drug treatment and virtual absence of significant drug toxicity. The response in serum piroxicam concentration to treatment with each of the 3 drug dosages is shown in Table 6. Serum piroxicam levels reached a plateau within 2 weeks after starting active therapy and remained at a fairly constant level thereafter.

Table 6. Serum Piroxicam Concentration during Treatment with Placebo Followed by 5mg, 10mg or 20mg of Piroxicam Daily for 12 Weeks

Piroxicam	Mean Serum Concentration (μm/ml)					
Dosage	Placebo	2 Weeks	4 Weeks	6 Weeks	8 Weeks	12 Weeks
5mg/day (n= 9)	0	1.7	1.8	1.9	2.0	2.4
10mg/day (n=10)	0	3.2	3.4	3.3	3.4	3.8
20mg/day (n=10)	0	9.2	10.6	9.9	10.2	11.5

The effect of 20mg of piroxicam daily on PGE_2 concentration in rectal mucosa is shown in Fig. 1. Compared to control values, PGE_2 concentration was significantly decreased in rectal mucosal biopsies obtained after 4 and 12 weeks of drug treatment. A similar but less great reduction in mucosal PGE_2 concentration was also seen during treatment with 10mg piroxicam daily. Fig. 2 shows the percent reduction from baseline in concentration of prostaglandin E_2 in rectal mucosa induced by each of the three drug doses. The decrease in PGE_2 concentration during the 5mg/day dose of piroxicam was not statistically different from control values. However, the 10mg/day dose, which is only half that normally used to treat arthritis, gave significant ($p<.05$) reductions in mucosal PGE_2 concentrations.

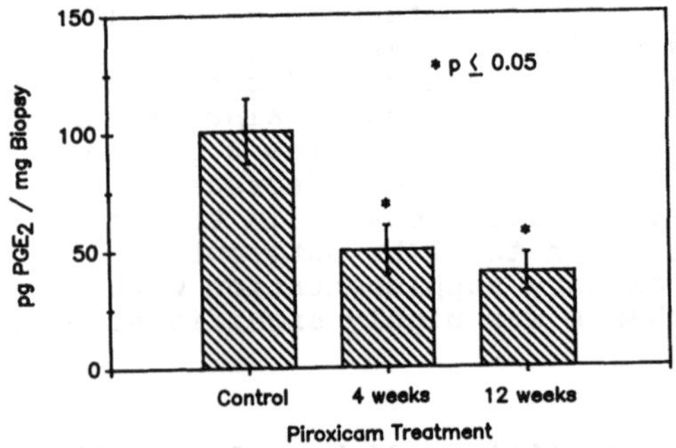

<u>Fig. 1</u> Concentrations of prostaglandin E_2 (PGE_2) in rectal mucosa of 10 subjects taking 20mg piroxicam per day.

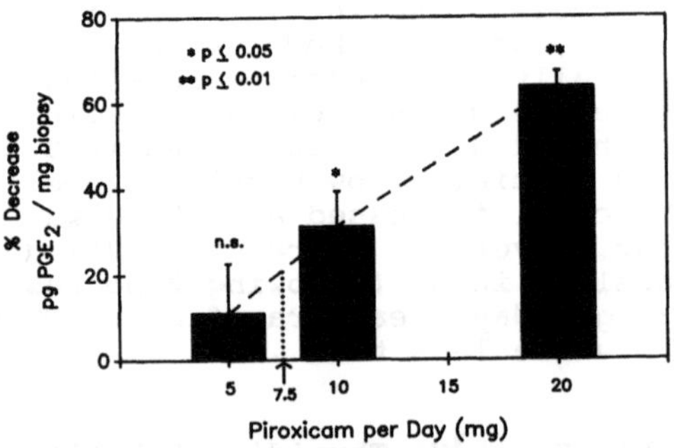

<u>Fig. 2</u> Percent decrease in concentration of PGE_2 in rectal mucosa induced by 3 different doses of piroxicam taken daily for 12 weeks. The vertical dotted line shows a predicted decrease for the 7.5mg/day piroxicam dose under current study.

Preliminary [^{3}H]-thymidine labeling index data (organ culture method) are available for 6 patients in the 20mg piroxicam/day arm of the study. For these results, a minimum of 36 crypt columns have been counted per treatment period. Fig. 3 shows that a small but consistent reduction in labeling index was present during piroxicam treatment in 5 of the 6 patients processed to date.

<u>Fig. 3</u>. [^{3}H]-Thymidine labeling index by crypt organ method before and during piroxicam (20mg/day) in 6 patients with resected adenomatous colon polyps.

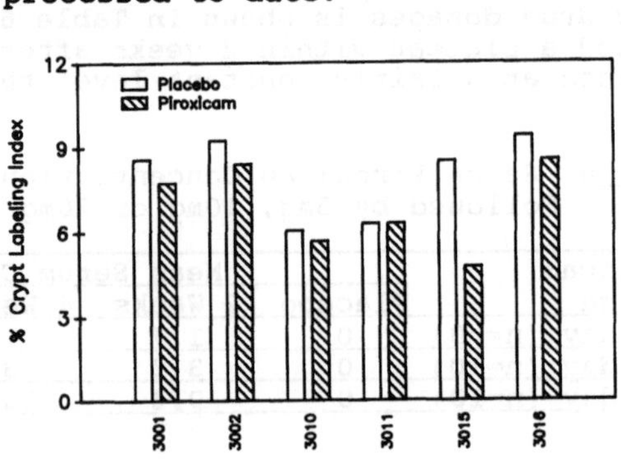

DISCUSSION

Several authors (Lipkin 1987, Terpstra 1987, Ponz de Leon 1988) have previously demonstrated a hierarchy of risk for colon cancer in relation to the proliferation rate of mucosal crypt epithelial cells. In these reports, patients with colorectal cancer and hereditary as well as sporadic adenomatous colon polyps had the highest [^{3}H]-thymidine labeling indices. Recent studies have shown that the increased thymidine labeling index in patients with familial polyposis coli can be reduced toward normal by addition of calcium to the diet (Lipkin 1985, Buset 1986). We utilized this index to carry out pilot studies of wheat bran fiber and the NSAID piroxicam as potential intervention treatments against development of colon cancer in high risk patients.

The 13.5gms/day dose of wheat bran fiber was taken with excellent compliance, was well tolerated and its use was associated with a significant decrease in rectal epithelial cell labeling index in those patients whose pretreatment index was increased above the median value for the group. These results as well as the recent observation by DeCosse (1989) that wheat bran fiber supplements significantly decreased the number of colorectal polyps in patients with familial polyposis, strongly support a beneficial role for wheat bran fiber in inhibiting abnormal colonic epithelial cell growth associated with increased risk of colon cancer.

Piroxicam and other NSAIDs which inhibit cyclooxygenase activity have been shown to exert a high degree of protection against experimental colon cancer in animal model studies (Pollard 1980, Reddy 1987). The exact mechanism for this beneficial effect is uncertain, but is presumed to be through a reduction in tissue prostaglandin synthesis. Although widely used to treat arthritis, high doses of an NSAID can produce significant injury to the gastric mucosa and impair renal function, side effects which appear to be dose-dependent in frequency and severity. In this pilot study, we attempted to determine that less than the 20-30mg/day dose of piroxicam used to treat arthritis could reduce prostaglandin E_2 in colon mucosa and also affect epithelial cell proliferative activity. The results show that as little as 10mg of piroxicam daily will significantly reduce PGE_2 concentration in rectal mucosal. Early results also show that piroxicam at 20mg/day can reduce DNA synthesis and proliferative activity in rectal mucosa. If the final results of this trial show a similar beneficial effect with the 10mg dose of piroxicam, they will provide strong rationale for a chemoprevention approach to intervention in patients at high risk for colon cancer.

The results of these pilot studies show that application of currently available dietary and drug treatments can improve abnormalities in a recognized risk factor associated with colon cancer. Ultimate confirmation of any cancer prevention effect as well as of the importance of the thymidine labeling index as a true predictive marker of cancer risk and response to interventional therapy will require randomized phase II-III clinical trials. Such are now underway or planned at the Arizona Cancer Center.

REFERENCES

Bennett A, Del Tacca M, Stamford IF, Zebro T (1977) Prostaglandins from tumors of human large bowel. Brit J Ca 35: 881-4

Buset M, Lipkin M, Winawer S, Swaroop S, Friedman E (1986) Inhibition of human colonic epithelial cell proliferation in vivo and in vitro by calcium. Ca Res 46: 5426-30

DeCosse JJ, Miller HH, Lesser ML (1989) Effect of wheat bran fiber and vitamins C and E on rectal polyps in patients with familial adenomatous polyposis. J Natl Cancer Inst 81: 1290-7

Earnest DL, Hixson LJ, Sim WW, Ahnen D, Alberts DS (1989) Piroxicam as an agent to inhibit colonic neoplasia. Gastroenterology 96: A134

Finley PR, Williams RJ, Earnest DL (1989) Rapid and sensitive HPLC assay for piroxicam in serum. (submitted)

Goodwin JS (1984) Immunologic effects of nonsteroidal anti-inflammatory drugs. Am J Med 77: 7-15

Greenwald P, Lanza E, Eddy GA (1987) Dietary fiber in the reduction of colon cancer risk. J Amer Dietic Assoc 87: 1178-88

Han T, Nemoto T, Ledesma EJ, Bruno S (1983) Enhancement of T lymphocyte proliferative response to mitogens by indomethacin in breast and colorectal cancer patients. Int J Immunopharmacology 5: 11-15

Ho EE, Atwood JR, Meyskens Jr FL (1988) Methodological development of dietary fiber intervention to lower colon cancer risk. In: Engstrom PF(ed) Advanced cancer control: the war on cancer -- 15 years of progress. Liss, New York, pp 263-81

Lipkin M, Blattner W, Fraumeni J, Lynch H, Deschner E, Winawer S (1983) Tritiated thymidine labeling distribution as a marker for hereditary predisposition to colon cancer. Ca Res 43: 1899-1904

Lipkin M, Blattner WA, Gardner EJ, Bert RW, Lynch H, Deschner E, Winawer S, Fraumeni JF Jr (1984) Classification and risk assessment of individuals with familial polyposis, Gardner syndrome and familial nonpolyposis colon cancer from [^{3}H]-dThd-labeling patterns in colonic epithelial cells. Ca Res 44: 4201-7

Lipkin M, Newmark H (1985) Effect of added calcium on colonic epithelial cell proliferation in subjects at high risk for familial colonic cancer. N Engl J Med 313: 1381-4

Lipkin M, Enker WE, Winawer S (1987) Tritiated-thymidine labeling of rectal epithelial cells in "non-prep" biopsies of individuals at increased risk for colonic neoplasia. Ca Letters 37: 153-61

Pollard M, Luckert P (1980) Indomethacin treatment of rats with dimethylhydrazine-induced intestinal tumors. Ca Treat Rep 64:1323-7

Ponz de Leon M, Roncucci L, Di Donato P, Tassi L, Smerieri O, De Maria D, Antonioli A, Chchin N, Perini M, Rigo G, Barberini G, Maneti A, Biasco G, Barbara L (1988) Pattern of epithelial cell proliferation in colorectal mucosa of normal subjects and of patients with adenomatous polyps or cancer of the large bowel. Ca Res 48: 4121-6

Reddy BS, Maruyama H, Kelloff G (1987) Dose-related inhibition of colon carcinogenesis by dietary piroxicam, a nonsteroidal antiinflammatory drug, during different stages of rat colon tumor development. Ca Res 47: 5340-6

Reddy BS, Engle A, Katsifis S, Simi B, Bartram H-P, Perrino P, Mahan C (1989) Biochemical epidemiology of colon cancer: effects of types of dietary fiber on fecal mutagens, acid and neutral sterols in healthy subjects. Ca Res 49: 4629-35

Terpstra OT, van Blankenstein M, Dees J, Eilers GAM (1987) Abnormal pattern of cell proliferation in the entire colonic mucosa of patients with colon adenoma or cancer. Gastroenterology 92: 704-48

Long-Term Effects of Dietary Calcium on Risk Markers for Çolon Cancer in Familial Polyposis Patients

HARTLEY S. STERN, ROGER C. GREGOIRE, HANOCH KASHTAN, TERI BERK, and W. ROBERT BRUCE

ABSTRACT

There is a conflicting evidence regarding the benefit of calcium in colon cancer prevention. In this study we evaluated the effect of long term calcium supplementation on colon cancer risk markers in homogeneous group of familial polyposis patients. Thirty-one patients, post subtotal colectomy, were randomized to two groups and received placebo or calcium 1200g daily. Intervention lasted 9 months, in which they underwent four 3 monthly evaluations that included food records, fecal pH, calcium and bile acids and rectal biopsy for thymidine labelling. Labelling index of placebo and calcium groups was similar before intervention and was significantly reduced after 3 months in the two groups. After 9 months it did not differ from the starting point in either group. In a long term intervention study with homogeneous group of familial polyposis patients, supplemental dietary calcium did not affect mucosal risk factors for colon cancer.
Key words: Familial polyposis, calcium supplementation, colorectal cancer.

INTRODUCTION

Some epidemiologists have suggested that high dietary levels of calcium are associated with low risk of colon cancer (Garland 1985) though others consider that this association is not yet established (Heilbrun 1986). Certainly, in experimental studies, calcium inhibits colonic mucosal damage induced by bile acids (Rafter 1986; Wargovich 1983,1984; Bird 1986a-b), by forming insoluble calcium soaps, that reduce the concentration of the potentially toxic bile acids reaching the mucosa (Wargovich 1983,1984; Newmark 1984; Graham 1983). Recently published data also suggest that calcium may reduce the rate and alter the pattern of colonic mucosal hyperproliferation that can be found in individuals of familial colon cancer kindreds (Lipkin 1989). However, a randomized controlled study in patients previously operated on for colon cancer has failed to confirm an effect of calcium on proliferation and showed no difference between the calcium and placebo supplemented groups (Gregoire 1989).
Familial polyposis coli is a disease inherited as an autosomal dominant trait in which hundreds of adenomatous polyps develop throughout the colon. Polyps usually begin appearing during the

second decade (Bussey 1975). If left untreated, most patients will develop an adenocarcinoma by age forty (Aitken 1986). Thus, patients are advised to have their colon removed. In those individuals with only a few rectal polyps, a sub-total colectomy and ileorectal anastomosis is usually performed (Jarvinen 1985). This latter cohort has proved a useful model in which to study chemopreventive interventions on adenomatous polyps because of the abnormalities in mucosal proliferation in these individuals (Stern 1986) and because these abnormalities may precede polyp development. Previous attempts at inducing regression of such rectal polyps have been reported. In a study with vitamin C, some investigators found a trend toward a reduction in the number of polyps but this was not significant (DeCosse 1975). They also showed some stabilization on tritiated thymidine labelling in the rectal mucosa.

In this randomized double-blind controlled trial, we investigated the effect of supplemental dietary calcium on mucosal proliferation in polyposis coli patients having previously undergone a subtotal colectomy and ileorectal anastomosis over a nine month period. Dietary intakes of the subjects as well as various demographic parameters were evaluated to assess group comparability. Mucosal proliferation was assessed by tritiated thymidine labelling of biopsy specimens. Fecal calcium and bile acid concentrations and fecal pH were also measured to assess compliance and to determine if any relationship existed between these measures and labelling index.

STUDY DESIGN

Thirty-one subjects with familial polyposis coli were recruited from the Familial Polyposis Registry based at Toronto General Hospital. All these individuals had previously undergone a subtotal colectomy and ileorectal anastomosis with a 12-15 cm rectal stump retained. The volunteers were randomly allocated to one of two groups. The first group, received placebo capsules containing lactose and cellulose (Novopharm Ltd, Scarborough, Ontario, Canada) while second, took calcium carbonate capsules containing 200 mg elemental calcium (Calcium carbonate 500 mg, Novopharm Ltd, Scarborough, Ontario, Canada). Each volunteer was instructed to take two capsules three times a day at mealtime so the total amount of calcium added in the calcium group was 1200 mg/day. The intervention period lasted 9 months. While on the study, the volunteers were asked to stay on their regular diet.

During the intervention period, the volunteers were seen at 4 visits to our research institute i.e. 0, 3, 6, 9 months. On each visit, they underwent a rectal examination without preparation during which biopsies were taken in the rectal stump distal to the ileorectal anastomosis. They also provided a stool sample which was immediately frozen. Also, sets of 3-day food records were taken before intervention and on the last three days of each three-month period. Compliance to the assigned regimen was assessed by pill count and measurement of calcium concentration in the aqueous phase of stools. The study protocol was approved by the Human Subject Committee of the University of Toronto. Two individuals dropped out voluntarily for personal reasons; another one was excluded because he developed a bleeding duodenal ulcer.

LABORATORY ANALYSIS

Labelling index technique and measurement:

The method for processing and incubating the biopsies was similar to that previously published by us (Stadler 1988).

A cell was considered labelled when five or more grains were seen overlying the nucleus. Labelling index (LI) in percentage was computed for each specimen and each subject as the number of labelled cells devided by the total number of cells.

Cell position in the longitudinal axis was assessed in each crypt column by dividing the ordinal number of the cell counted, starting at the base of the crypt, by the total number of cells in the column and assigning that cell a decimal coordinate ranging from 0 to 1. Each cell was then included into one of five equally determined segments. Because of differences in size of the biopsies, the number of crypts and cells scored varied greatly among the different biopsies.

Biochemical analysis of feces:

Stool sample analysis for pH, bile acid concentration in total feces, bile acid concentration in the aqueous phase of feces and fecal calcium concentration was carried out according to the following procedure. The specimen was thoroughly homogenized and pH was measured using a special electrode (Orion #8163). An aliquot of each sample was assayed for bile acid concentration in total feces by a method previously published (Rafter 1987) with a few modifications. A second aliquot of homogenized feces was centrifuged at 20000 xg for 2 hours at 2-5C. The supernatant was carefully removed and 200 μl were used to assay bile acid concentration in the aqueous phase of feces according to the method described above. Calcium concentration was measured in the supernatant by standard calorimetric methods.

Nutrient analysis:

Three-day food records were evaluated by the Nutrition Coding Centre (NCC) at the University of Minnesota, Minneapolis. Daily intakes of major macro and micronutrients were determined by computerized nutrient data base.

RESULTS

Several constitutional and dietary variables were measured initially to asess group comparability (Table 1). Age, height, weight and elapsed time since operation were similar. Despite randomization, there were more males in the calcium group. This aspect was reflected in the dietary pattern. The calcium group consumed more calories. However, on the percentage of calories derived from fat, carbohydrate and protein, as well as on other nutrients, the two groups were similar. They remained essentially comparable throughout the trial although some minor differences could be seen in some micronutrients at one return visit or another (Table 2).

Compliance was assessed by two methods: pill count on the return visits and calcium measurements on the aqueous phase of stool. On

TABLE 1

Comparison of sex, age, height, weight and time from surgery between treatment groups.

	PLACEBO (n=14)	CALCIUM (n=17)
MALE/FEMALE	4/10	11/6
MEAN AGE	39 (14.6)	37 (11.6)
HEIGHT (cm)		
male	167 (13.8)	177 (9.5)
female	158 (7.8)	160 (2.9)
WEIGHT (kg)		
male	73 (7.0)	72 (12.7)
female	66 (12.7)	61 (8.4)
TIME FROM OPERATION (months)		
median	92.0	98.5
range	4-216	11-360

TABLE 2

Comparison of dietary pattern between the two groups before and throughout the study.

DAY	0	90 (S.D.)	180 (S.D.)	270 (S.D.)	(S.D.)
TOTAL CALORIES	P	2378 (762)	2283 (833)	2562 (747)	2268 (74)
	C	2714 (702)	2057 (998)	2362 (933)	2521 (779)
FAT AS % OF T CALORIES	P	39 (9.1)	35 (7.4)	39 (9.6)	39 (9.9)
	C	39 (5.9)	35 (9.0)	38 (6.8)	38 (6.1)
PROTEIN AS % OF T CALORIES	P	14 (2.5)	15 (2.7)	14 (2.6)	14 (1.7)
	C	14 (2.7)	16 (4.2)	15 (2.6)	15 (3.3)
CARBOHYD AS % OF T CALORIES	P	45 (10.6)	49 (9.9)	46 (12.8)	47 (11.5)
	C	47 (6.3)	49 (10.7)	47 (8.5)	48 (8.9)
STARCH (g/day)	P	132 (60.9)	128 (52.0)	136 (68.0)	130 (69.0)
	C	131 (43.2)	108 (50.0)	119 (39.6)	123 (39.0)
DIETARY FIBER (g/day)	P	16.7 (7.1)	17.3 (7.5)	18.7 (8.3)	16.9 (7.6)
	C	18.5 (7.2)	12.3 (5.2)	17.5 (5.4)	15.4 (5.8)
CALCIUM (mg/day)	P	908 (444)	834 (309)	842 (266)	783 (342)
	C	1102 (398)	904 (486)	1097 (526)	1107 (596)

the average, more than 92% of the pills were taken by the volunteers in the placebo group throughout the study similar to the pill intake of the calcium group (N.S.). Calcium concentration in the aqueous phase of stool was comparable at the start of the trial (P:16.1+8.4 vs C:22.3+13.1, NS). On each of the return visit, this measurement was significantly higher in the calcium group ($p<0.05$ in all cases, Table 4).
Results for total labelling index i.e. including all segments as well as values measured for each of the five segments are summarized in Table 3. All values for the groups were comparable on starting the study. On the second visit (90 days), we observed a significant decrease in values for total as well as for segments 1 and 2 indices for both groups. On the third visit (180 days), this observation remained true for the calcium group only when compared to visit one. On the fourth visit (270 days), all values were lower than on initial examination but statistical significance was not seen in either group. Comparing the reductions seen within each group for the three return visit, we were unable to find a difference between the groups.

TABLE 3

Labelling index (LI) measurements in both groups in all segments and 20% subsequents.

DAY		0 L.I. (S.D.)	90 L.I. (S.D.)	180 L.I. (S.D.)	270 L.I. (S.D.)
ALL SEGMENTS	P	4.8 (1.9)	*3.1 (2.0)	3.7 (2.7)	3.4 (2.5)
	C	6.1 (2.9)	*4.4 (2.5)	*3.4 (2.2)	4.0 (3.0)
SEGMENT I	P	8.7 (4.9)	*6.3 (4.1)	5.1 (4.0)	6.0 (4.7)
	C	11.9 (5.7)	*6.9 (3.8)	*6.6 (4.5)	7.1 (5.8)
SEGMENT II	P	10.1 (3.8)	*5.9 (4.0)	7.0 (4.8)	6.5 (4.8)
	C	11,7 (5.8)	*8.5 (5.2)	*6.5 (4.7)	8.6 (5.8)
SEGMENT III	P	4.2 (2.7)	2.3 (2.3)	4.3 (4.5)	3.4 (2.8)
	C	4.7.(4.1)	4.6 (4.4)	3.3 (3.1)	3.3 (2.7)
SEGMENT IV	P	0.8 (0.7)	0.9 (0.8)	1.5 (3.0)	0.8 (0.8)
	C	1.6 (2.8)	1.7 (2.2)	0.6 (0.8)	0.8 (1.0)
SEGMENT V	P	0.2 (0.3)	0.2 (0.3)	0.3 (1.0)	0.2 (0.2)
	C	0.2 (0.3)	0.3 (0.3)	0.1 (0.1)	0.3 (0.3)

(I = basal 20% of crypt)
(V = surface 20% of crypt)
* $p < 0.05$

Table 4 shows the results for fecal pH, total bile acid concentration and soluble bile acid concentration. All these variable were comparable at the beginning of the trial. The values remained essentially similar within each group throughout the study and comparison between the groups were not statistically significant.

TABLE 4

Effect of intervention in both groups on fecal: bile acids, total and soluble; pH and calcium concentration

DAY	0	90 (S.D.)	180 (S.D.)	(S.D.)	270 (S.D.)
BILE	P	7.3 (2.8)	6.7 (1.5)	6.2 (0.9)	7.0 (1.4)
ACIDS	C	6.2 (0.9)	6.2 (0.8)	6.7 (1.0)	6.3 (1.0)
mmol/L					
SOLUBLE	P	1.63 (0.7)	1.97 (0.92)	1.61 (0.77)	1.52 (0.42)
B. ACIDS	C	1.53 (0.8)	1.62 (0.92)	1.66 (0.74)	1.48 (0.75)
mmol/L					
pH	P	5.88 (0.67)	5.94 (0.81)	6.03 (0.88)	5.87 (0.56)
u	C	5.60 (0.56)	6.00 (0.87)	5.62 (0.62)	5.72 (0.68)
CALCIUM	P	16.2 (8.4)	13.4 (10.6)	15.7 (18.2)	20.6 (15.2)
mmol/L	C	22.2 (13.1)	*34.5 (15.8)	*51.6 (21.6)	*45.9 (13.5)

* $P<0.05$

DISCUSSION

In this randomized double-blind controlled trial, we evaluated the effect of oral calcium supplementation on colonic mucosal proliferation and fecal biochemical variables. Prior to randomization, the calcium and placebo groups were essentially comparable with respect to the demographic and dietary variables except for an uneven distribution of males and females, a difference that can be attributed to the randomization process. The groups were also similar for the study variables, labelling index, total bile acid and soluble bile acid concentration. Following the intervention, pill count and calcium concentration showed that the groups complied to the supplementation. Both groups also showed a significant reduction in labelling index as well as labelling in segment 1 and 2 at the second visit a difference persisted for the group receiving the calcium to the third visit. There was, however, no significant difference in labelling index reductions between the calcium and the placebo groups. There was also no influence of the intervention on fecal pH, total bile acid or soluble bile acid concentrations. Thus this study did not demonstrate any measureable benefit of calcium supplementation on the colon cancer risk markers in familial polyposis patients.

The results of the study both complement and contrast with earlier studies with calcium supplementation (Lipkin 1989; Gregoire 1989). We observed a drop in the labelling index of our patients following the introduction of the supplement. A similar drop was observed by Lipkin and Newmark (1989). In our case the drop was similar in the intervention and control subjects, raising the possibility that the earlier study may have observed a change that was not strictly a consequence of the calcium supplementation itself. In this respect the results presented here are consistent with those obtained in our earlier study with patients with previous colonic resections for colon cancer (Gregoire 1989). That randomized control trial also failed to demonstrate an effect of calcium supplementation on colonic proliferation patterns.

A second difference between the results repeated here and ealier studies is evident in the biochemical measures. Here we observed a change of calcium concentration but no change in the pH or in the concentration of the bile acids following the intervention. This is in contrast to the result obtained earlier with individuals with largely intact colons where the calcium led to an increased pH and bile acid concentration (Gregoire 1989). This could be a consequence of the fact that the pH was much lower in this group of patients than it was in the cancer patients (5.7 vs 6.8) and that the colon which normally affects pH through reabsorption, secretion and fermentation was removed or because of frequent bowel movements associated with the ileorectal anastomosis.

The study design can also be contrasted with earlier studies that observed polyp regressions in patients treated with subtotal colectomy and ileorectal anastomosis after long term follow-up of the rectal remnant (Watne 1983). At the Cleveland Clinic, 38% of patients showed complete disappearance and 26% partial regression on the first sigmoidoscopic examination after surgery (median time, 6 months). However, 55% of those with complete regression subsequently redeveloped polyps (Jagelman 1983). Some investigators have used various drugs in an attempt to induce polyp regression in the rectal remnant. In a prospective randomized controlled trial, Bussey compared ascorbic acid to a placebo in 36 patients. The polyp area was reduced in the ascorbic acid group, particularly in the middle of the trial, but this was not statistically significant (Bussey 1982). We did not carry out any polyp count in our study because of the subjectivity and lack of precision of this measure and because we wished to take our biopsies without bowel preparation in order to avoid a possible influence on proliferation.

Familial polyposis patients remain a good model for carcinogenesis studies because of the consistent pattern of phenotypic expression (Bussey 1975; Decosse 1975; Jagelman 1983; Stern 1986). In this study, we could not prove a beneficial influence of calcium on mucosal proliferation in the rectum of these individuals and cannot support the contention that calcium has a chemoprotective effect in this disease. Recent studies have identified the defective gene in familial polyposis to be located on chromosome 5 (Bodmer 1987). Until one can find what this gene normally codes for or what triggers its expression, chemoprevention will remain highly speculative. Even if this information becomes available, agents should be tested in a randomized prospective controlled fashion to confirm their effectiveness.

REFERENCES

Aitken RJ, Elliot MS, Torrington M, Louw JH. Twenty year experience with familial polyposis coli in Cape Town. Br J Surg 1986; 73:210-213.

Bird RP. Effect of dietary components on the pathobiology of colonic epithelium: Possible relationship with colon tumorigenesis. Lipids 1986; 21:289-291.

Bird RP, Schneider R, Stamp D, Bruce WR. Effect of dietary calcium and cholic acid on the proliferative indices of murine colonic epithelium. Carcinogenesis 1986; 7:1657-1661.

Bodmer WF, Bailey CJ, Bodmer J et al. Localization of the gene for familial adenomatous polyposis on chromosome 5. Nature 1987; 328:614-616.

Bussey HJR. Familial polyposis coli: Family studies, histopathology, differential diagnosis and results of treatment Baltimore: John Hopkins University Press, 1975:73-74.

Bussey HJ, DeCosse JJ, Deschner EE et al. A randomised trial of ascorbic acid in polyposis coli. Cancer 1982; 50:1434-1439.

DeCosse JJ, Adams MB, Kuzma JF et al. Effect of ascorbic acid on rectal polyps of patients with familial polyposis. Surgery 1975; 78:608-612.

Heilbrun LK, Hankin JH, Nomura AMY, Stemmerman GN. Colon cancer and dietary fat, phosphorus and calcium in Hawaiian-Japanese men. Am J Clin Nutr 1986; 43:306-309.

Garland C, Barrett-Connor E, Rossof AH, Shekelle RB, Criqui MH, Paul O. Dietary vitamin D and calcium and risk of colorectal cancer: a 19-year prospective study in men. Lancet 1985; i:307-309.

Graham DY, Sackman JW. Solubility of calcium soaps of long-chain fatty acids in simulated intestinal environment. Dig Dis Sci 1983; 28:733-736.

Gregoire RC, Stern HS, Yeung KS, Stadler J, Langley S, Furrer R, Bruce WR. Effect of calcium supplementation on mucosal cell proliferation in high risk patients for colon cancer. Gut 1989; 30:376-382.

Jagelman DG. Familial polyposis coli. Surg Clin North Am 1983; 63:117-128.

Jarvinen HJ. Time and type of prophylactic surgery for Familial adenomatous coli. Ann Surg 1985; 202:93-97.

Lipkin M, Friedman E, Winawer SJ, Newmark. Colonic epithelial cell proliferation in responders and nonresponders to supplemental dietary calcium. Cancer Res 1989; 49:248-254.

Newmark HL, Wargovich MJ, Bruce WR. Colon cancer and dietary fat, phosphate and calcium: a hypothesis. J Natl Cancer Inst 1984; 72:1323-1325.
Rafter JJ, Eng VWS, Furrer R, Medline A, Bruce WR. Effects of calcium and pH on the mucosal damage produced by deoxycholic acid in the rat colon. Gut 1986; 27: 1320-1329.
Rafter JJ, Child P, Anderson AM, Alder R, Eng VWS, Bruce WR. Cellular toxicity of fecal water depends on diet. Am J Clin Nutr 1987; 415:13-26.
Stadler J, Stern HS, Yeung KS, McGuire V, Furrer R, Marcon N, Bruce WR. Effect of high fat consumption on cell proliferation activity of colorectal mucosa and on soluble fecal bile acids. Gut 1988; 29:1326-1331.
Stern HS. New research on the effect of calcium in familial polyposis. Newsletter GI. Polyposis & related conditions. Fall 1986.
Waddell WR, Loughry RW. Sulindac for polyposis of the colon. J Surg Oncol 1983; 24:83-87.
Wargovich MJ, Eng VWS, Newmark HL, Bruce WR. Calcium ameliorates the toxic effect of deoxycholic acid on colonic epithelium. Carcinogenesis 1983; 4:1205-1207.
Wargovich MJ, Eng VWS, Newmark HL. Calcium inhibits the damaging and compensatory proliferative effects of fatty acids on mouse colon epithelium. Cancer Lett 1984; 23:253-258.
Watne AL, Carrier JM, Durham JP, Hrabovsky EE, Chang W. The occurrence of carcinoma of the rectum following ileoproctostomy for familial polyposis. Ann Surg 1983;197:550-554.

Chemoprevention Using Wheat Fiber and Vitamins C and E in Patients with Familial Adenomatous Polyposis

JEROME J. DECOSSE and JUDITH S. JACOBSON

ABSTRACT

Fifty-eight patients with familial adenomatous polyposis participated in a four-year, randomized, double-blind, placebo-controlled chemoprevention trial. Twenty patients were treated with ascorbic acid (vitamin C) 4 g/day, plus alpha tocopherol (vitamin E) 400 mg/day, plus a high-fiber supplement (22.5 g/day). Sixteen patients were treated with the vitamins and a low-fiber supplement (2.2 g/day). Twenty-two were treated with placebo capsules and the low-fiber supplement. The endpoint of the study was change in number and area of rectal polyps. Analysis by patient compliance showed a significant benefit for patients who ingested more than 11 g/day of the wheat fiber supplement.

KEY WORDS: chemoprevention, dietary fiber, neoplasia, polyposis, vitamins

1. INTRODUCTION

In the past decade, a number of studies have placed the concept of pharmacologic or nutritional intervention to prevent cancer on a firm scientific basis (Bertram et al 1987; Jones et al 1981). This concept originated with epidemiologic surveys that found vast differences between countries in incidence of and mortality from most common cancers (Doll et al 1966), and related these differences, especially in gastrointestinal malignancy rates, to diet (Boyd et al 1964).

The incidence of colon cancer in most industrialized countries is more than three times that in most developing countries, where people consume diets much higher in fiber and lower in fat (Bjelke 1974). The importance of diet or environment, rather than genetic factors or ethnicity, to colorectal cancer risk emerges clearly in migrant studies, which show, for example, that the age-standardized incidence rate of colorectal cancer is 17.9 per 100,000 population for male residents of rural Miyagi, Japan, but 52.0 per 100,000 -- one of the highest rates in the world -- for men of Japanese origin living in Hawaii (Muir et al 1987).

In case control studies, the role of specific dietary components in colorectal carcinogenesis has been difficult to pinpoint. Moreover, in laboratory studies, the effect of fiber supplements on carcinogenesis has varied with the design of the study and the type of fiber (Reddy, 1987). In the laboratory, wheat fiber, citrus fiber, and cellulose have been found most frequently to be protective against chemical carcinogenesis (Goldin et al, 1988). Despite conflicting results in observational studies, it is widely believed today that dietary fiber or some component(s) of it inhibit, and that dietary fat or some component(s) of it stimulate, colorectal carcinogenesis. (Committee on Diet, Nutrition, and Cancer, 1982).

Observational studies have generally used incident cancer as their endpoint. Familial adenomatous polyposis (FAP), an autosomal dominant disorder, is characterized by large numbers of adenomatous polyps of the large bowel and progression to cancer in virtually all patients left untreated. Treatment consists generally of total colectomy and ileorectal anastomosis. In patients who have undergone this procedure, rectal polyps can be readily observed and counted. Intervention trials in which the subjects are patients with FAP can use as their endpoint changes in area and number of rectal polyps. The polyps in these patients are morphologically indistinguishable from sporadic polyps arising in patients with no known genetic susceptibility to colorectal cancer.

In the 1970s, we conducted a randomized trial of ascorbic acid (4 g/day) in patients with familial adenomatous polyposis. Our findings suggested that this agent could reduce polyp formation (DeCosse et al, 1975; Bussey et al, 1982). Because alpha tocopherol had been shown to inhibit experimental colon tumors when used in conjunction with ascorbic acid, and because of the widespread interest in dietary fiber as a preventive agent in colorectal cancer, we decided, in the early 1980s, to study the effects of ascorbic acid plus alpha tocopherol, with and without wheat fiber supplements, on rectal adenomas in patients with familial adenomatous polyposis. The results of this study have been published (DeCosse et al 1989); what follows summarizes the methodology, findings, and inferences from that study.

2. METHODS

2.1 Patients and Clinical Methods

From our familial adenomatous polyposis registry population of more than 200 patients we recruited 72 adults to participate in the trial. All patients had had a total colectomy and ileorectal anastomosis at least one year before they entered the trial. The study protocol was approved by the institutional review boards at the Memorial Sloan-Kettering Cancer Center and The New York Hospital-Cornell Medical Center, and each patient was asked for and gave informed consent for participation. The protocol called for a run-in period, in which each patient took placebo for 3 months and was asked not to take vitamin supplements.

During the run-in period, 6 patients dropped out of the trial, and 4 patients failed to meet the study criteria for compliance with the placebo, leaving 62 to be randomized to treatment.

Eligibility for trial participation was verified by an initial proctosigmoidoscopy and confirmed by a second one at the end of the run-in period. At both of these examinations, rectal polyps were counted and measured. The polyp counts and measurements were averaged and the averages constituted the baseline for each patient. During the four-year trial, patients underwent proctosigmoidoscopy every three months -- a total of 18 examinations per patient, all conducted by the principal investigator, using identical instruments.

In almost every case, the rectal segment that remained following colectomy measured 15 cm. The patient's preparation for each examination consisted of one Fleets enema. At each examination, the investigator examined the patient's rectum, counted and recorded the number and location of the polyps, and estimated the diameter of each polyp by reference to the 16-mm inner width of the proctosigmoidoscope. The area of each polyp was calculated as πr^2, and for each examination for each patient, polyp areas were summed to arrive at total polyp area.

The treatments were distributed to the patients by the hospital pharmacist, and only the pharmacist, who was in a separate part of the building from the clinical investigators, and the statistician, who was located in another town, knew the treatment allocations. One participant, who was a nurse, obtained a chemical analysis of her placebo capsule; the other patients and all the clinical investigators remained blind to treatment allocation throughout the trial.

The treatment consisted of a daily allotment of 8 capsules and 2 boxes of cereal. Each capsule contained either lactose (placebo) or 500 mg of ascorbic acid and 50 mg of alpha tocopherol. Hoffmann-La Roche Inc. (Nutley, NJ) provided the vitamin and identical-appearing lactose capsules. Each box contained either 1.1 g of fiber in a cereal base or a commercial bran cereal with 11.25 g of fiber. Each box (whether treatment or control) also contained 30 mg of ascorbic acid, 2,000 IU of Vitamin A, and small amounts of other vitamins and minerals, providing close to 30% of the Recommended Daily Allowance of these nutrients. The Kellogg Company (Battle Creek, MI) provided both the high- and the low-fiber cereals in specially designed, identical, unlabeled boxes.

The patients were randomized to three treatment groups. The high-fiber group's treatment allocation was two boxes of high-fiber cereal and eight vitamin capsules daily. The vitamin group's treatment allocation was two boxes of low-fiber cereal and eight vitamin capsules daily. The control group's allocation was eight placebo capsules and two boxes of low-fiber cereal daily. The patients were instructed to take two capsules four times a day and to ingest the contents of the two boxes in the course of each day either as cereal with milk or in the form of muffins, cookies, or other variants, for which recipes were provided.

We urged the study participants not to take nutritional supplements other than their treatment allocations, but we did not supply them with specific complete dietary protocols. In order to include in our analyses information on all dietary components that might influence polyp formation, we asked the patients to keep a 3-day diet record encompassing 2 weekdays and 1 weekend day during the week before each quarterly examination. In addition, at each patient visit, a nutritionist reviewed the record with the patient, completed a food frequency questionnaire, and advised the patient on nutrition, supplying new recipes for the fiber supplements whenever possible. Average intake of nutrients of interest was calculated from the 3-day records by using the Michigan State University Nutrient Data Bank.

At each visit, we monitored compliance with treatment allocation by interview, review of a daily calendar on which the patients had been asked to record each day's intake, count of the unused capsules and boxes which the patients were instructed to bring with them, and urine test for ascorbic acid. We also used random telephone calls and a trial newsletter to reinforce adherence to treatment. We monitored adverse side effects of the treatment by interview and serologic tests.

2.2 Statistical Methods

On the basis of our previously described randomized trial of ascorbic acid vs. placebo, we determined that with 20 patients per treatment arm, the study would have 90% power to distinguish a 30% decrease in number of polyps in the control group from a 75% decrease in the treatment group. We established as the principal endpoint variable the ratio of the number of polyps at each visit after the patient began treatment to the number of polyps at the baseline, which in all but one case was the mean of the counts at two pretreatment visits.

Given the complexity and duration of this preventive intervention trial in an outpatient population, we expected that patients would not be consistent either as a group or individually over time in their adherence to the treatment. For this reason, we analyzed the data both by randomization and according to the patients' actual consumption of both treatment fiber and vitamins and dietary fiber and fat from unprescribed food intake.

3. RESULTS

3.1 Patients

Of the 62 patients randomized to treatment, 2 from the vitamin group and 2 from the control group withdrew or were withdrawn from the treatment. One patient in the vitamin group and one in the control group withdrew from the trial at three months. A second patient in the vitamin group developed cancer of the duodenum after 9 months of trial participation. A second patient in the control group, who had no rectal polyps, was reviewed at 9 months and found not to have polyposis.

The 58 patients who remained in the trial throughout its four-year duration were randomized as follows: 22 to the control group, 16 to the vitamin group, and 20 to the high-fiber group. The groups were comparable in demographic characteristics (except gender), previous treatment for FAP, and previous dietary habits. These assessable patients represented 235 years of patient follow-up and had a total of 966 endoscopies.

During the four years of the trial, several events caused postponement of examination or endoscopy. These events included 12 pregnancies among 8 of the 37 women participants. Four patients, all with normal levels of serum calcium, had seizures. One elderly patient had a cerebral vascular accident with hemiplegia, and another had a cholecystectomy.

Other events appeared to result from FAP. One patient in the high-fiber group had a proctectomy for a Dukes stage A carcinoma of the rectum. Four patients (3 in the high fiber group) had a laparotomy for adhesive small bowel obstruction. Three patients underwent laparotomy for ovarian cysts.
Two had a thyroidectomy for papillary thyroid carcinoma, and one had surgery for duodenal adenomas.

Twenty-three patients underwent 37 diathermies or excisional biopsies of rectal polyps. None of the polyps was larger than 10 mm, and all proved on histopathological examination to be adenomas. Of the 5 patients who had one polyp removed, one was in the control group and two were in each of the vitamin groups. Of the 18 patients who had more than one polypectomy, 9 were in the control group, 4 in the vitamin group, and 5 in the high fiber group. Because these procedures were distributed among all three study groups and had little effect on polyp count at the next visit, they were disregarded in the data analysis.

3.2 Treatment Adherence

As expected, adherence to the treatment allocations generally varied and diminished over the course of the trial (P<.005). Capsule ingestion declined from 90.2% to 63.4% in the control group, from 92.7% to 49.9% in the vitamin group, and from 92.2% to 79.0% in the high fiber group. Presecribed cereal ingestion declined from 84.8% to 43.5% in the control group, from 79.1% to 38.9% in the vitamin group, and from 66.8% to 62.0 percent in the high fiber group.

3.3 Dietary Patterns

The 2,806 daily dietary records completed during the trial showed substantial interpatient and intervisit variability in all three treatment groups. Dietary fiber (as distinguished from treatment fiber) ingestion fluctuated, but not seasonally, and declined over the four years (P<.0001). From visit 3 to visit 18, average dietary fiber consumption declined from 10.6 g/day to 8.1 g/day in the control group, from 10.9 g/day to 9.1 g/day in the vitamin group, and from 9.5 g/day to 7.7 g/day in the high-fiber group. Because both treatment fiber and dietary fiber intake declined, total fiber intake declined in all three groups during the trial, but overall fiber intake was highest in the high-fiber group. Average total fiber intake throughout the trial was 12.2 g/day for the control group, 11.3 g/day for the vitamin group, and 22.4 g/day for the high-fiber group.

Fat consumption also varied considerably among patients and between visits in all three groups but did not change significantly over time, nor did the groups vary significantly in their fat consumption. From visit 3 to visit 18, total fat consumption increased slightly, from 85.2 g/day to 93.8 g/day in the control group, from 102.7 g/day to 99.0 g/day in the vitamin group, and from 96.4 g/day to 103.0 g/day in the high-fiber group.

3.4 Effect of Treatment on Polyps

We began our statistical analysis by comparing the randomization groups median polyp numbers at each visit. The medians for the high fiber group were lower than for the other two groups at all but one visit. The medians for the control group were higher than for the other groups. However, the differences were statistically significant only at visit 4 ($P<.07$) and visit 13 ($P<.07$). Adjustment for age, gender, dietary fiber consumption, total fat consumption, percentage of calories from fat, and total calories did not affect this analysis.

Adjustment for compliance with prescribed fiber did affect the analysis. Polyp number decreased significantly and consistently as ingestion of prescribed fiber increased. Table 1 shows the correlations generated by multiple regression analysis between four nutritional factors and ratio of polyp number at each examination to the baseline measurement. The negative correlations with ingestion of prescribed fiber were statistically significant as follows: visit 5, $P<.028$; visit 7, $P<.061$; visit 8, $P<.072$; visit 9 $P<.016$; visit 10, $P<.070$; visit 11, $P<.32$; visit 13, $P<.052$; and visit 17, $P<.076$. The positive correlations with total fat were statistically significant as follows: visit 3, $P<.09$; visit 5, $P<.023$; visit 8, $P<.039$; visit 11, $P<.057$.

Another analytical approach involved dividing mean daily prescribed fiber intake into two categories: less than 11 g and 11 g or more. We chose this cutpoint because it represented approximately 50% compliance. Patients were then divided into those whose polyp counts were lower than the baseline number and those whose polyp counts were not lower than the baseline number at each visit. At all 16 visits, patients who had consumed an average of at least 11 g of prescribed fiber were more likely to have fewer polyps than the baseline than those who had consumed less fiber. These associations were statistically significant as follows: visit 4, $P<.015$; visit 5, $P<.075$; visit 6, $P<.028$; visit 7, $P<.078$; visit 8, $P<.049$; visit 9, $P<.045$; visit 10, $P<.006$; visit 11, $P<.010$; visit 12, $P<.089$; visit 15, $P<.083$; and visit 16, $P<.019$. Stratification of this analysis by gender did not affect the results. A separate data analysis was aimed at determining whether or not treatment was associated with a shift in polyps toward the distal one-third of the rectum; no such association emerged.

4. DISCUSSION

The findings of this study constitute evidence for a significant effect of nutritional intervention on benign large bowel neoplasia. In a study population consisting of relatively young patients with FAP, who had undergone colectomy, negative correlations between polyp number and ingested prescribed fiber were consistently observed. Vitamin intake also was negatively correlated, but not significantly so, with reduction in polyp number, at 14 of 16 visits. The possibility of a weak independent treatment effect of alpha tocopherol and ascorbic acid is suggested by these findings. The study design precluded identifying an interactive effect of fiber with vitamins; no study participants took prescribed fiber and no vitamins. However, prescribed fiber intake remained significant in the regression analysis even after adjustment for vitamin intake, as well as total caloric intake and consumption of polyunsaturated fat.

The selection of patients with familial adenomatous polyposis as subjects permitted us to study a smaller sample for a shorter time than studies involving patients with sporadic polyps or patients with a family history of colorectal cancer but no clinical evidence of disease at baseline.

However, FAP patients who fulfilled the criteria for eligibility were scarce; colleagues in distant states helped us to recruit study participants, many of whom had to travel great distances to keep their appointments with us. In addition, there is some evidence that the low-fiber supplement was less palatable than the high-fiber supplement. Under these circumstances, missed appointments and difficulty in maintaining adherence to the trial over its 4-year duration were not surprising. Known and unknown patient factors and dietary variables also may have confounded our analysis by compliance. Even in patients in the control group, with few, easily counted rectal polyps, counts waxed and waned as if regulated by some secular phenomenon.

Patients in the high-fiber group consumed an average of 22.4 g/day of total prescribed and dietary fiber. This quantity is not unusual for populations of other countries, but in the United States, according to a recent study, only about 10% of the population consumes more than 20 g/day of dietary fiber (Lanza et al, 1987). The mean dietary fiber consumption in our control group was 12.2 g/day, which is consistent with reported means of 11/1 g/day (Lanza et al) and 13.3 g/day (Paul et al, 1978) in industrialized countries.

The chemistry of fiber and its components is not fully understood. We may hypothesize that the treatment effect is associated with the relative insolubility of bran and its high content of noncellulose polysaccharides and pentose polymers. Bran consumption might therefore decrease the exposure of the colonic mucosa to deoxycholate (Pomare et al, 1973) or increase generation of butyric acid (Parish et al, 1986). Our results confirm laboratory findings that of all dietary fibers studied, wheat bran exerts the most consistent protection against experimentally induced colon cancer (Kritchevsky, 1988) and epidemiological findings of an inverse correlation between colorectal cancer incidence and intake of fiber pentosans (Bingham et al, 1979).

Our findings are evidence that the environment can affect neoplasia and alter the course of a genetically initiated disease. It is well known that after FAP patients undergo colectomy, their rectal polyps often regress spontaneously (Dunphy et al, 1959; Feinberg et al, 1988). This phenomenon is attributed to exposure of the rectal mucosa to ileal contents (Cole et al, 1959). The predominance of distal sites of both adenomas and cancer of the large bowel in FAP patients (as well as other colorectal cancer patients), even though genetic influences on the mucosa are presumably uniform, may prove to be due to environmental influences.

Given the design of this study, we cannot assert that grain fiber other than wheat fiber would have the effect we observed in our high-fiber treatment group. A recent report (Reddy et al, 1989) on the effect of different types of dietary fiber on fecal mutagens and bile acids suggests that other forms of fiber may be less effective in reducing the production and/or excretion of mutagens in the stools and the concentration of fecal secondary bile acids in humans.

Nor can we assert that wheat fiber would have the same beneficial effect on patients with sporadic colorectal polyps that we have observed in patients with FAP. The effect would certainly require a longer intervention to become apparent in a patient population with sporadic polyps. Although some benefit of prescribed fiber in our study could be observed within 6 months of the start of treatment, the significant findings took close to two years to emerge. However, the data suggest that a dietary modification in adults can have benefits; lifelong or childhood exposure to the high-fiber diet was not required.

Table 1. Change in number of polyps*

Visit No.***	Trial Mo.	Ingested Prescr. Fiber	Ascorbic acid & alpha tocopherol	Ingested dietary fiber	Total fat
		Variable**			
3	3	-.10	-.10	-.10	+.23§
4	6	-.19	-.20	-.21	-.02
5	9	-.31¶	-.12	-.13	+.26§
6	12	-.23	-.13	-.12	+.06
7	15	-.27§	+.05	+.03	-.00
8	18	-.25§	-.14	-.22	+.26§
9	21	-.35‡	-.08	-.14	+.30¶
10	24	-.26§	-.13	-.00	+.11
11	27	-.31¶	-.12	+.06	+.28
12	30	-.16	-.13	-.04	+.15
13	33	-.29¶	-.16	-.04	+.24
14	36	-.20	-.13	-.07	+.20
15	39	-.13	-.13	-.24	+.07
16	42	-.21	-.12	+.04	+.03
17	45	-.26§	+.04	+.05	+.05
18	48	-.18	-.04	+.06	+.04

*Correlation coefficient for named variable after adjustment for remaining three variables.
**Values = correlation coefficients.
***Sample sizes at each visit ranged from n=44 to n=57.
§ $.05 \leq P < .10$
¶ $.02 \leq P < .05$
‡ $P < .02$

REFERENCES

Bertram JS, Kolonel LN, Meyskens FL Jr (1987) Rationale and strategies for chemoprevention of cancer in humans. Cancer Res 47: 3012-3031

Bingham S, Williams DRR, Cole TJ et al (1979) Dietary fibre and regional large bowel cancer mortality in Britain. Br J Cancer 40:456-463

Bjelke E (1974) Epidemiologic studies of cancer of the stomach, colon, and rectum; with special emphasis on the role of diet. Scand J Gastroenterol 9: 1-235.

Boyd J, Landman M, Doll R (1964) The epidemiology of gastrointestinal cancer with special reference to causation. Gut 5: 196-200.

Bussey HJR, DeCosse JJ, Deschner EE et al (1982) A randomized trial of ascorbic acid in polyposis coli. Cancer 50: 1434-1439

Committee on Diet, Nutrition, and Cancer, National Research Council (1982) Diet, Nutrition, and Cancer. National Academy Press, Washington, DC, chap 5, pp 1-33; chap 8, pp 1-8

DeCosse JJ, Adams MB, Kuzma JF, et al (1975) Effect of ascorbic acid on rectal polyps of patients with familial polyposis. Surgery 78:608-612

DeCosse JJ, Miller HH, Lesser ML (1989) Effect of wheat fiber and vitamins C and E on rectal polyps in patients with familial adenomatous polyposis. J Natl Cancer Inst 81: 1290-1297

Doll R, Payne P, Waterhouse J (eds) (1966) Cancer incidence in five continents. Vol 1. Tech Rep Int Union Against Cancer. UICC, Geneva

Dunphy JE, Patterson wB, Legg MA (1959) Etiologic factors in polyposis and carcinom a of the colon. Ann Surg 150: 488-496

Feinberg SM, Jagelman DG, Sarre RG et al (1988) Spontaneous resolution of rectal polyps in patients with familial polyposis following abdominal colectomy and ileorectal anastomosis. Dis Colon Rectum 31: 169-175

Goldin BR (1988) Chemical induction of colon tumors in animals: An overview. In: Steele G Gr, Burt RW, Winawer SS et al (eds) Basic and clinical perspectives of colorectal polyps and cancer, Alan R Liss, New York, pp 319-333

Jones FE, Komorowski RA, Condon RE (1981) Chemoprevention of 1,2-dimethylhydrazine-induced large bowel neoplasms. Surg Forum 32: 435-437

Kritchevsky D (1988) Diet and nutrition research. Cancer 62:1839-1843

Lanza E, Jones DY, Block G et al (1987) Dietary fiber intake in the U.S. Population. Am J Clin Nutr 46: 790-797

Muir C, Waterhouse J (1987) Cancer incidence in five continents. Vol 4. UICC, Geneva

Parish PD, Lupton JR (1986) The effect of wheat bran and pectin supplementation on luminal pH and short chain fatty acid production in the rat large intestine. Fed Proc 45:349

Paul AA, Southgate DAT (1978) McCance and Widdowson's The Composition of Foods, HM Stat Office, London.

Pomare EW, Heaton KW (1973) Alteration of bile salt metabolism by dietary fibre (bran) Br Med J 4: 262-264

Reddy BS (1987) Dietary fiber and colon cancer: Animal model studies. Prev Med 16: 559-565

Reddy B, Engle A, Katsiis, et al (1989) Biochemical epidemiology of colon cancer: Effect of types of dietary fiber on fecal mutagens, acid, and neutral sterols in healthy subjects. Cancer Res 49:4629-4635.

Ornithine Decarboxylase (ODC) and S-Adenosylmethionine Decarboxylase (AdoMetDC) as Markers in Human Colonic Neoplasia

LEMUEL HERRERA, NICHOLAS J. PETRELLI, and GUSTAVO VIAL

ABSTRACT

Increased polyamine biosynthetic activity and raised levels of intracellular polyamines are commonly associated with abnormal and induced proliferative states. Ornithine Decarboxylase and S-Adenosylmethionine Decarboxylase are the known rate-limiting enzymes in polyamine biosynthesis. Herein, we report results from our group in relation to the activity of these enzymes in "normal looking" mucosa and neoplasias of the colon. Both enzymes tend to reflect neoplastic progression (mucosa < polyp < carcinoma). During these studies, we observed low levels of activity in the "normal looking" mucosa of colons containing a neoplasia, but high levels of ODC in "normal looking" mucosa of the same colons after the removal of their neoplasias. These observations suggest a role of ODC as a possible biochemical marker of a colon harboring a neoplasia.

Keywords: Ornithine Decarboxylase, S-Adenosylmethionine Decarboxylase, tumor markers, adenomatous polyps, colon cancer

Colorectal cancer is the second leading cause of cancer-related deaths in the United States. It is second only to cancer of the breast and lung in females and cancer of the lung in males. There were 140,000 new cases diagnosed in 1986.

Despite advances in the treatment of cancer in the colon and rectum, the 5-year survival rate for patients with cancer of the colon and rectum, has changed little in the last 30 years. The best predictor of survival has been the extent of the disease at a time of the diagnosis. The status of the draining lymph nodes remains as the most significant prognostic parameter. The 5-year survival of tumors with serosal penetration but negative nodes is close to 80%; whereas, when the lymph nodes are positive, it is only about 50% (Herrera 1987). Therefore, it is reasonable to postulate that early detection of colorectal cancer would offer the main thrust in improving curability and longevity. Unfortunately, there is as yet no specific markers useful in the detection of early colorectal cancer. The current "gold standard" of colorectal cancer markers is the carcinomembryonic antigen (CEA); while CEA is best used as a monitor of postoperative recurrence, it is not useful for screening or as a test for early diagnosis.

Putrescine, Cadaverine, Spermidine, and Spermine are polyamines, and ubiquitous substances in biologic materials. Polyamines are low molecular weight, highly charged organic cations. They are found in association with nucleic acids; thus, they are packaged with DNA; for instance, in the Escherichia coli bacteriophage T4, they account for about 40% of the total cations in the phage. Prokaryotes generally have higher amounts of Putrescine, Cadaverine, Spermidine, and lack Spermine. Eukaryotes contain little Putrescine, but have both Spermidine and Spermine.

The enzymes Ornithine Decarboxylase (ODC) and S-Adenosylmethionine Decarboxylase (ADOMetDC) are the known rate-limiting steps in polyamine biosynthesis (Pegg 1982). The action of ODC produces Putrescine and requires pyridoxal phosphate as a co-factor.

It is subject to feedback inhibition and repression by Putrescine and Spermidine. Methionine and Putrescine are the biosynthetic precursors of Spermidine and Spermine. S-Adenosylmethionine forms from Methionine and ATP after being acted upon by S-AdoMetDC to give decarboxylated S-Adenosylmethionine. S-AdoMetDC is devoid of pyridoxal phosphate, but the enzyme contains a covalently linked pyrovoyl residue (mw = 42,000 Daltons). This pyrovoyl group is required for enzymatic activity.

The excretion of polyamines is mainly urinary; however, the levels are low and total 5-10 mgs per 24-hours. Most of the urinary polyamines are monoacetyl derivatives and their site of synthesis is unknown. It is, however, of interest that although raised serum or urinary polyamine levels have been reported in up to 66% of patients with large bowel cancer (Moorehead 1987; Nishioka 1977), their possible clinical usefulness, still remains unestablished.

Increased polyamine biosynthetic activity and raised levels of intracellular polyamines are commonly associated with abnormal and induced proliferative states. Our group has shown that the activity of both of the key enzymes for polyamine biosynthesis is elevated in neoplastic human colorectal tissues as compared to controls provided by "normal looking" mucosa from the same colons (Herrera-Ornelas 1987). By biochemical localization studies, it has been previously determined that within the intestinal mucosa of some species, ODC activity is located in the villous tips of differentiated cells, whereas S-AdoMetDC activity, by contrast, is highest in the crypt cells. Because proliferative states are associated with crypt cells activity and since the proportion of these particular cells is increased in polyps and adenocarcinomas, it was hoped that S-AdoMetDC activity would be a more sensitive an indicator of proliferative disorders than ODC activity. Contrary to these expectations, it was found that S-AdoMetDC activity exhibited the same general distribution as ODC, and that the differences between the normal, benign, and malignant neoplasias were less, rather than more, distinct (Porter 1987).

Levels of tissue polyamines are known to be affected by both transcription and translation mechanisms. Our group performed mRNA dot blot analysis using the probe pODC-934 (Berger 1984). This work revealed similar ODC mRNA content, while enzymatic activity varied by up to 3.3 fold among the samples of human colon cancer. These results suggest posttranscriptional regulation of ODC as a major determinant in ODC activity as detected in surgical specimens (Porter 1986).

We were very interested in the distribution of the polyamine biosynthesis and ODC activity among various premalignant states of the colon, looking for possible predictions for their malignant progression. In fact, we were stimulated by the report of Luk and Baylin (1984) in that the progression from normal mucosa to adenoma and carcinoma was identifiable in patients with familial adenomatous polyposis (FAP) biochemically prior to a distinct morphologic picture. ODC levels were reported as useful for screening relatives at risk for FAP and effective in segregating patients (Luk 1984). In the study herein reported, we entered patients without a diagnosis of FAP. There was also no-known familial history of colonic neoplasms in first-degree relatives (sporadic type). We found no evidence to suggest biochemical activation of the adjacent noninvolved ("normal looking") colonic mucosa. Our results were: mean values (nmol/hour/mg/protein [± SEM = noninvolved mucosa, 0.11 ± 0.02; adenomatous polyps, 0.50 ± .11; and adenocarcinoma 0.88 ± .10). In addition, we measured levels of ODC activity in the distant nonaffected mucosa of patients harboring a carcinoma and compared these results to those obtained from ("normal looking") colorectal biopsies from disease-free patients recruited at the Roswell Park Cancer Institute Screening Clinic (Table 1). These patients would undergo a physical examination 66cm flexible sigmoidoscopy and air contrast barium enema.

Table 1. ODC activity in subjects with and without colorectal cancer

	Non-involved Mucosa Patients Ca		Tumor	Mucosa from Disease-free Subjects		
*Sigmoid	n=13	0.054	0.572	n=19	0.742	P<.001
*Rectum	n= 9	0.057	0.696	n=24	0.690	P<.001

*All Median Values
RESULTS in nmol/hr/mg/prot

It was clear that the nonaffected mucosa of patients harboring a colonic neoplasia exhibited a diminished level of Ornithine Decarboxylase activity as compared to the "normal looking" mucosa of disease-free patients. Results with similar trends have been reported by Moorehead and his group (Moorehead 1987). They have shown diminished levels of ODC activity in microscopically normal adjacent mucosa in patients harboring colorectal tumors. Although performed in a group of patients without a defined contribution of inheritance, these results were surprising. A previous report by Luk (1984) in patients with FAP and their relatives at risk had demonstrated increased levels of this enzyme in the "normal looking" mucosa of those relatives-at-risk who eventually developed the phenotypical features of the disease so that some increased values were also expected in the colonic "normal looking" but adjacent mucosa. Although technical and artifactual reasons could be claimed as responsible for ours' and Moorehead's (1987) results, it is important to emphasize that these results were consistently obtained even though they were performed discontinuously in various specimens obtained at various times. Specimens obtained either immediately upon surgical removal or at endoscopy, with comparable ischemia time, by the same surgeons, and processed by the same technician at Dr. Porter's laboratory at Roswell Park produced consistent results (Table 2).

Table 2.

SURGICAL SPECIMEN		POST-SURGICAL SAMPLE*
Normal Mucosa	Tumor	Normal mucosa
0.179	0.746	1.407

Average values expressed in nmol/hr/mg/prot
39 samples obtained from 18 patients, post-surgical sample obtained after 12 weeks of original large bowel surgery.

We could speculate that the differences in the biochemical results may be related to possible changes in mRNA levels, not as yet identified, or due to ODC polymorphism; the latter view could be supported by experimental data generated by the androgen-regulated mouse kidney model where at least two nonhomologous ODC-DNA clones are recognized by different mRNAs in hybridization studies using plasmids. Interestingly, both ODC mRNAs are believed to be encoded, at least in part, by different nonhomologous genes (Berger 1984). In humans, we have already reported in the quantitative differences between the levels of ODC activity between primary colorectal cancers and liver metastases in the same host (Herrera 1988).

A recent report by Lawson et al (1989), focused on the proliferative and enzymatic activity in the transitional (within 2 cms) mucosa adjacent to colonic cancer; they concluded that transitional mucosa showed morphometric changes, but these changes were not reflected in the values for proliferative or enzyme markers to suggest a higher than expected risk for malignant change detectable prior to morphologic changes (Lawson 1989). In two of our patients with FAP who were intensely studied, we were able to establish a significant gradient in ODC activity between histologically documented adenomatous polyps and the "normal looking" adjacent noninvolved mucosa, demonstrating low levels of activity in the latter (Figure 1) regardless of its distance to the polyp.

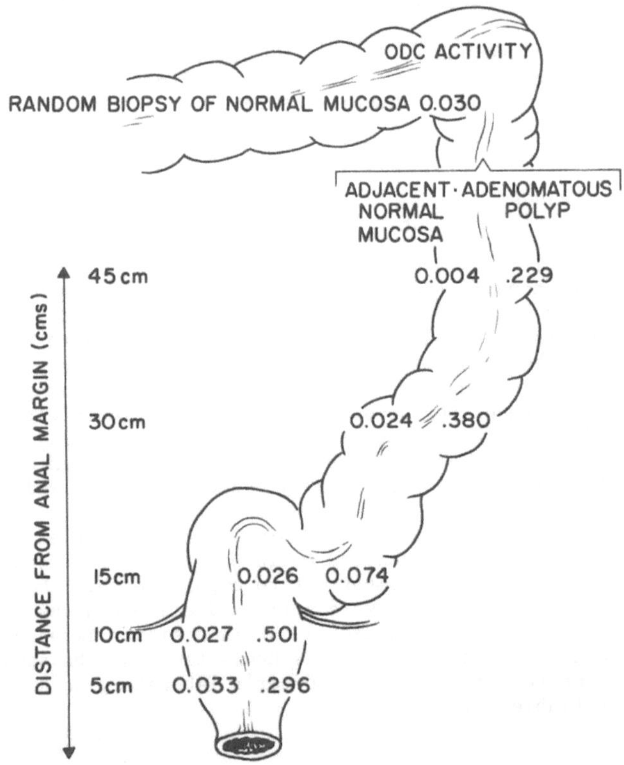

Figure 1.

The ODC gene sequences in humans have been localized to chromosome regions 2pter→p23 and 7cen→qter. The group at Roswell Park has further defined the location of these sequences by sommatic cell and in situ techniques to 2p25 and 7q31-qter. It is believed that the ODC gene situated on chromosome 2, is the functional gene. Furthermore, Shows and Radford (1988) have also mapped the S-AdoMetDC gene sequences to the human chromosome 6 and X and have also established that there is no gene amplification in colon cancer and benign polyps; therefore, amplification is not the mechanism by which increased S-AdoMetDC activity occurs in colorectal neoplasia. As with ODC, it is likely that control of its regulation is at the transcriptional and post-transcriptional levels. Further work on the regulation of S-AdoMetDC in tumors will require cloning of the human gene (Radford 1988).

In summary, our previous work suggests the possibility of the existence of a paracrine effect of growth and other cellular factors possibly secreted by the colonic neoplasia detectable by determinations of ODC in adjacent and/or distant "normal looking" colorectal mucosa. This possibility should continue to be explored as the potential for screening for early colonic neoplasia utilizing a rectal biopsy of nonaffected mucosa may suggest the coexistence of a more proximal neoplasia. Determinations of ODC isoforms and of the ODC gene and gene regulation, may be of clinical significance.

REFERENCES

Berger FG, Szymanski P, Read E, Watson G (1984) Androgen-regulated Ornithine Decarboxylase in RNA of mouse kidney. J Biol Chem 259:7941-7946

Herrera L, Petrelli N (1988) Ornithine Decarboxylase activity in hepatic and extrahepatic metastases from colorectal cancer. Dis Col Rectum 31:352-354

Herrera OL, Justiniano J, Castillo N, Petrelli N, Stulc J, Mittelman A (1987) Metastases in small lymph nodes from colon cancer. Arch Surg 122:1253-1256

Herrera-Ornelas L, Porter C, Pera P, Greco W, Petrelli N, Mittelman A (1987) A comparison of Ornithine Decarboxylase activity in human large bowel mucosa, polyps and colorectal adenocarcinoma. J Surg Res 42:56-60

Lawson M, White L, Coyle P, Butler R, Roberts-Thomson I, Comyers R (1989) An assessment of proliferative and enzyme activity in transitional mucosa adjacent to colonic cancer. Cancer 64:1061-1066

Luk GD, Baylin SB (1984) Ornithine Decarboxylase as a biologic marker in familial colonic polyposis. New Engl J Med 311:80-83

Moorehead RJ, Hoper M, McKelvey STD (1987) Ornithine Decarboxylase activity in rectal mucosa as marker for colorectal adenomas and carcinomas. Br J Surg 87:364-365

Nichioka K, Romsdahl MN, McMurtrey MJ (1977) Serum polyamine alterations in surgical patients with colorectal carcinomas. J Surg Oncol 9:555-562

Pegg AE, McCann PP (1982) Polyamine metabolism and function. Am J Physiol 243:C212-221

Porter CW, Herrera-Ornelas L, Clark J (1986) Polyamine biosynthetic enzyme activities correlated with neoplastic progression in human colorectal tissue. Proc Amer Assn Cancer Res (abstract); Vol. 27, pp 159

Porter C, Herrera-Ornelas L, Pera P, Petrelli N, Mittelman A (1987) Polyamine biosynthetic activity in normal and neoplastic human colorectal tissues. Cancer 60: 1275-1281

Radford DM, Eddy R, Haley L, Henry W, Pegg AE, Pajuney A, Shows TB (1988) Gene sequences coding for S-Adenosylmethionine Decarboxylase are present on chromosome 6 and the X and are not amplified in colon neoplasia. Cytogen & Cell Genetics 49: 285-288

Chemoprevention Trials in Patients with Familial Adenomatous Polyposis (FAP) at Roswell Park Cancer Institute

LEMUEL HERRERA and THERESA M. SPEERS

ABSTRACT

Two chemoprevention trials have recently been started in patients with FAP registered and ascertained at the Roswell Park Familial Polyposis Registry. The first one is a Phase I study based in the oral administration of α-difluoromethylornithine (DFMO), an irreversible inhibitor of ornithine decarboxylase, a key enzyme for polyamine biosynthesis. Patients with adenomatous polyps diffusely distributed throughout their gastrointestinal tract and patients who have undergone surgery for cancer, but who possess characteristics related to a high risk of relapse, are candidates for the DFMO study. The second trial, randomizes patients to either oral administration of calcium carbonate versus a placebo. Patients with adenomatous polyps in the rectal remnant are the candidates for the calcium study. Herein, we present the rationale and the experimental design, but as both studies have recently began, it would be inappropriate to draw any conclusion.

Keywords: adenomatous polyps, colorectal cancer, α-difluoromethylornithine, calcium carbonate, chemoprevention

Colorectal cancer remains as the leading cause for cancer mortality affecting to both sexes in the United States. It is also a major cause of morbi-mortality in the Western World. Inherited and environmental factors are known both to play a role in colorectal carcinogenesis, but their interactions in humans are far from being completely elucidated.

Clinical observations indicate that many colorectal cancers arise from a previous adenomatous polyp. Polyps are frequently incidental findings in the elderly, but when present in individuals younger than 40 years of age, they are probably a representation of a phenotypical expression of an inherited trait. Regardless of the age of presentation, adenomatous polyps denote a population at a higher risk for colorectal cancer. Adenomatous polyps vary significantly in their malignant potential; whereas, a small (<1 cm) tubular polyp, the commonest type found in the human colon, has a rather miniscule risk of developing into cancer ($<1\%$), larger polyps (>1 cm), and especially those with villous formations are prone to develop into cancers ($>10\%$). In fact, we have previously reported that most villous adenomas equal or larger than 4 cm, will contain foci of carcinoma ($>80\%$), most of them invasive; fortunately, the overall incidence of these type of polyps is small (Stulc 1987). Interestingly, a small but well defined number of these polyps will not become cancerous despite being large, sessile, and villous. As a general statement, it can be said that the majority of adenomatous polyps occurring in the general population, will never become malignant. Markers reflecting unequivocal growth and a biological commitment towards malignant transformation of a given polyp, are greatly needed, keenly searched for, but still at large.

Familial adenomatous polyposis (FAP), also known by geneticists as Adenomatous Polyposis Coli, is considered a classic prototype for colonic neoplastic studies because it has a relatively predictable clinical behavior once its phenotypic manifestations have been diagnosed. FAP is characterized by the appearance of multiple neoplastic gastrointestinal polyps with preferential localization to the colon in the second or third decade of life. This characteristic is inherited in a dominant Mendelian autosomal fashion and it is often associated to extracolonic manifestations (Herrera 1987). The transformation of one or several of these adenomatous polyps into invasive carcinomas, is an accepted phenomenon. However, the frequency, time lapse, and possible underlying operating etiologic factors, are still far from being understood. Malignant changes, often multiple, are usually diagnosed at an average age of 40 years in untreated patients, but often earlier. It must be again emphasized that although FAP is a premalignant condition associated with multiple carcinomas, cancer will occur only in a few of the hundred(s) of polyps present. Colorectal cancer develops in FAP patients at a much younger age than at the usual 6th-7th decade in the general population. At Japan, where there is a low incidence of colon cancer in the general population as compared to the U.S., once patients are diagnosed with FAP, they have the same risk for increased colorectal cancer at the same age than their Western counterparts. This finding clearly supports the premalignant evolution of FAP in a selected polyp-population (Utsonomiya 1989).

The ability to induce colonic tumors in experimental animals has provided us with the opportunity to study various aspects of large bowel carcinogenesis. Colorectal carcinogenesis seems to proceed through distinct and identifiable stages of initiation, promotion, and progression. These stages can be studied by a number of enzymatic and biochemical differences between normal mucosa, premalignant adenomatous polyps, and colon carcinomas; furthermore, one could also expect to identify differences in the multiple cellular genes involved in the mechanisms of colorectal carcinogenesis (Guillem 1988). This knowledge has a great potential for diagnostic or therapeutic purposes. The chemopreventive trials presented here, are constructed in part, taking into consideration knowledge acquired through some of these studies.

POLYAMINES

Polyamines are ubiquitous substances widely distributed in nature. Biosynthesis of polyamines can be significantly increased in response to external stimuli including hormones and various growth factors in experimental tumors. Our group has previously reported that ornithine decarboxylase (ODC) - the key rate-limiting enzyme in the biosynthesis of polyamines that converts ornithine into putrescine, displays a gradient of enzymatic activity (i.e.: adenocarcinoma > polyp > mucosa) that correlates positively with the neoplastic status of the colon (Porter 1987).

Experimental data indicates that there is a critical role for polyamines in mediating the proliferation and tumor promotion in experimental human colon cancer. Although the precise mechanisms for the regulation of colonic proliferation by polyamines is not known, it has been well established that the inhibition of ODC exerts beneficial effects in experimental models of induced proliferative diseases of the colon and that cellular multiplication in eukaryotes can be significantly reduced by depleting putrescine and spermidine (Celano 1988; Zhang 1988).

Studies have been performed producing depletion of intracellular polyamines utilizing α-difluoromethylornithine (DFMO), an irreversible inhibitor of ODC, and MAP [(2R,5R)-6-heptyne-2,5-diamine]. Recently, the anti-tumor properties of the methyl and ethyl esters of MFMO [(E)-2-(fluoromethyl) dehydroornithine] have been reported. These compounds, prodrugs of MFMO, are also irreversible inhibitors of mammalian 1-ODC. In "in vitro" studies, they have been found 14 times more potent than DFMO and equipotent to MAP. These products seem to possess longer duration of action, higher potency, and in some cases, better anti-tumor efficiency than other inhibitors of ODC (Claverie 1989); however, their use in humans has not yet been studied.

High levels of ODC activity and increased polyamine biosynthesis, are seen mainly in the early phase of tumor growth (Luk 1989). As the growth fraction is inversely related to the tumor size, requirements for polyamine biosynthesis diminish as the tumoral mass increases its size; thus, inhibition of ODC activity in states of low proliferation is unlikely to produce significant anti-tumor effect since ODC inhibitors are cytostatic rather than cytotoxic (Pegg 1988).

Experimentally, ODC inhibitors have been found to be more effective as anti-tumor agents when treatments are begun prior to, concommitant, or shortly after tumor inoculation; therefore, they are believed to play a role in the promotion phase. While the results do not support the use of ODC inhibitors as single agents, nevertheless, they raise the possibility of therapeutic value when used in combination with other antiproliferative and/or cytotoxic drugs (Claverie 1989).

Phase I and Phase II studies in humans have demonstrated that DFMO can be given by mouth q 6 hours for a total treatment of 28 days with a maximum tolerated dose of 12 grams/M^2/day. Thrombocytopenia and gastrointestinal disturbances were the observed dose-limiting toxicities (Abeloff 1984). In another study, DFMO was given q 8 hours for 5 days q 2 weeks orally, for a maximum tolerated dose of 27 grams/M^2/day; again, gastrointestinal toxicity manifested by diarrhea and mucositis, were dose-limiting toxicities (Natale 1985). In a Phase II study, 2-4 grams/M^2/q 8 h of DFMO p.o., were given for up to 5 months with side effects of hearing loss and thrombocytopenia (Meyskens 1986); whereas, the administration of oral DFMO, 2.25 grams/M^2/q 6 hours, 3 weeks/month, for an average of 49 days, produced thrombocytopenia, auditory changes, nausea, vomiting, and diarrhea (Abeloff 1986).

Detailed pharmocokinetics have previously been reported by Haegele (1981) and Abeloff (1984).

The data clearly demonstrates that DFMO is well tolerated even in high doses for prolonged periods of time with tolerable and reversible toxicity.

As it is the case of ODC, polyamine pools in normal and neoplastic colorectal tissues reflect a significantly increased level in malignancy versus normal mucosa in the resected surgical specimen. The following are results obtained by Dr. Porter (1987) at Roswell Park (Table 1).

Table 1. Polyamine pools of normal and neoplastic colorectal tissues

Tissue	Patient samples	Putrescine	Spermidine	Spermine	Total
Adenocarcinoma	21	72 ± 12	358 ± 27	678 ± 47	1608
Adenomatous polyps	2	16 ± 9	232 ± 64	517 ± 89	765
Adjacent mucosa	19	14 ± 2	115 ± 7	291 ± 14	420

*Mean ± SEM in nmol/g wet weight.

It has previously been observed that DFMO has a significant effect on decreasing the levels of ODC activity and diminishing the pools of putrescine and spermidine, but not of spermine. Thus, we began to collaborate with Dr. Patrick Creaven of the Department of Clinical Pharmacology and Therapeutics in a Phase I trial utilizing oral DFMO as a chemopreventive agent. This trial is mainly directed towards patients with FAP with diffuse gastrointestinal polyposis, although patients at a high risk of cancer recurrence are also considered for this study. DFMO is given orally, daily, in 4 divided doses. We aim to study DFMO pharmacokinetics in the FAP population and to relate the steady state pharmacokinetics to the observed toxicities. A primary endpoint of the study will be the recurrence of adenomatous polyps. Upon their recurrence, polyps will be again removed endoscopically and assessed for ODC activity and polyamine pools. In the case of adenomatous polyps in the duodenum that cannot be removed, changes in the histology or in the size may be used for assessment of drug effectiveness. Additionally, this Phase I study will allow us to establish the safety and the side effects of prolonged administration of DFMO, as well as the assessing of the biological effects of prolonged dosing in the selected candidates. Starting dose is 200 mgs/M^2/d in 4 divided doses/4 weeks. If no side effects or measurable toxicity are seen, then the dose is increased to 400 mgs/M^2/4 weeks. The procedure is continued with doubling of the dose every 4 weeks to a finite period (6 weeks), when the dose is 6,400 mgs/M^2/d. If side effects are seen or abnormalities in hematology or serum chemistries attributed to the drug, then the dose will be reduced to the next lowest dose and the patient continued on the study.

The patients will continue with their regular FAP follow-up as per the following algorithm (Table 2).

Table 2. Algorithm

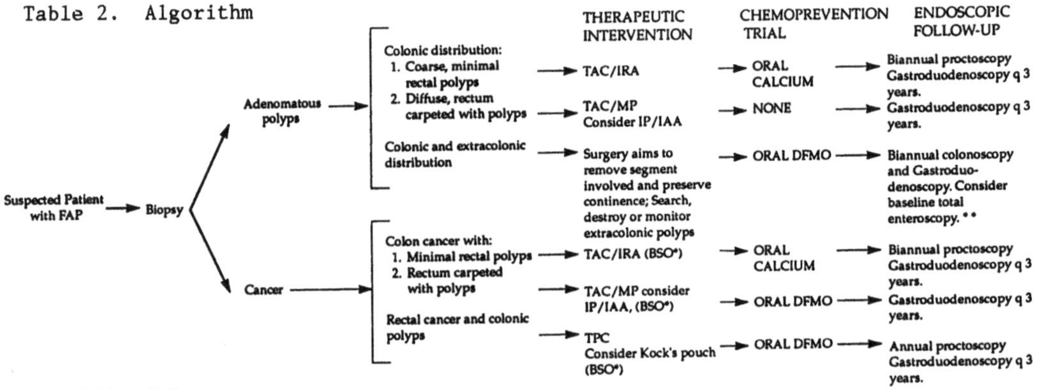

TAC = Total abdominal colectomy.
IRA = Ileorectal anastomsis.
MP = Mucosal proctetomy.
IP = Ileal pouch.
IAA = Ileoanal anastonsis.
TPC = Total protocolectomy.
BSO* = Bilateral salpingoophorectomy complementary to a cancer operation.

** = Total enteroscopy is considered in the search of bleeding sources in the GI tract.

Recent observations by Porter and Libby (unpublished), suggest that enzymes involved in the degradation of polyamines, as opposed to their synthesis, might be of relevance. Tumor samples of various sources have been found devoid of MTA phosphorylase, an enzyme which degrades the toxic by-product of polyamine biosynthesis, S-Methylthioadenosine, whereas increased "in vitro" activity of spermidine/spermine acetyltransferase (SSAT) of up to 5,000 fold over a 24-hour period have been observed in response to certain polyamine analogs. Initial results in 13 surgical specimens from a single surgical unit at Roswell Park from patients with colorectal cancer,are expressed in mean values (nmol/hr/mg/prot); MTA; non-involved "normal" mucosa, 978.4; adenomatous polyp, 1001.3; tumor, 1411.8. SSAT; non-involved mucosa, "normal", 29.9; adenomatous polyps, 31.3; tumor, 47.4. Thus far, trends indicate a decline in polyamine amino oxidase (PAO), an increase in SSAT, and no deficiency in MTA phosphorylase; however, as the sample-size is small, these results need validation.

Continued analysis of a larger number of samples by the Roswell Park Group should provide a better understanding about the role of MTA phosphorylase, SSAT, and PAO in colorectal cancer for their possible role in future chemopreventive or therapeutic trials.

DIETARY CALCIUM CARBONATE

Studies about proliferation and differentiation of cells within the gastrointestinal tract have identified stages of abnormal development that are associated with increased susceptibility to gastrointestinal cancer, such is the case of FAP. In FAP patients, the epithelial cells of the colon continue to synthesize DNA with delayed onset of normal terminal differentiation as they migrate to the mucosal surface (Lipkin 1989).

Even if asymptomatic in patients with FAP, the colonic crypts exhibit an abnormally high fraction of the proliferating cellular compartment (Friedman 1989). Recent studies have indicated that oral calcium supplementation decreases significantly such cell proliferation to levels approaching those found in subjects at a lower risk for colonic cancer. Therefore, in collaboration with Dr. Martin Lipkin from Memorial Sloan-Kettering Cancer Center, a chemopreventive trial that searches for the effect of calcium carbonate on growth and development of gastrointestinal epithelial cells, has been started. Patients are randomized to receive either calcium or placebo in a double-blind fashion following a detailed 3-day dietary questionnaire including amounts of ingested fat, carbohydrate, protein, calories, calcium, Vitamin D, and other dietary supplements. All of them have scheduled rectoscopies every three months. At each visit, information regarding number, location, size, and appearance of polyps is recorded. Seven patients have been started since July 1989; however, although it is too early to draw conclusions, none of them has developed recurrent polyps so far.

REFERENCES

Abeloff MD, Slavik M, Luk GD, Griffin CA, Hermann J, Blanc O, Sjoerdsma A, Baylin SB (1984) Phase I trial and pharmacokinetic studies of α-Difluoromethylornithine - An inhibitor of polyamine biosynthesis. J Clin Oncol 2:124-130

Abeloff MD, Rosen ST, Luk GD, Baylin SB, Zeltzman M, Sjoerdsma A (1986) Phase II trials of α-Difluoromethylornithine, an inhibitor of polyamine synthesis, in advanced small cell lung cancer and colon cancer. Ca Treat Rep 70:843-845

Celano P, Baylin SB, Giardiello FM, Nelkin BD, Casero P (1988) Effect of polyamine depletion on c-myc expression in human colon carcinoma cells. J Biol Chem 263(12): 5491-5498

Claverie N, Mamont PS (1989) Comparative antitumor properties in rodents of irreversible inhibitors of l-ornithine decarboxylase, used as such or as prodrugs. Ca Res 49:4466-4471

Freidman E, Lipkin M, Winawer S, Buset M, Newmark H (1989) Heterogeneity in the response of familial polyposis epithelial cells and adenomas to increasing levels of calcium in vitro. Cancer 63:2486-2491

Guillem JG, Hsiel LL, O'Toole K, Ford K, LoGerfo P, Weinstein BI (1988) Changes in expression of oncogenes and endogenous retroviral-like sequences during colon carcinogenesis. Ca Res 48:3964-3971

Haegele KD, Alken RG, Grove J, Schechter PJ, Koch-Weser J (1981) Kinetics of α-difluoromethylornithine: An irreversible inhibitor of ornithine decarboxylase. Clin Pharmacol Ther 30:210-217

Herrera OL, Elsiah S, Petrelli N, Mittelman A (1987) Causes of death in patients with familial polyposis coli. Sem Surg Onc 3:109-117

Lipkin M, Friedman E, Winawer SJ, Newmark H (1989) Colonic epithelial cell proliferation in responders and nonresponders to supplemental dietary calcium. Ca Res 49: 248-254

Luk GD, Zhang S-Z, Hamilton SR (1989) Effects of timing of administration and dose of Difluoromethylornithine on rat colonic carcinogenesis. JNCI 81(6):421-427

Meyskens FL, Kingsley EM, Glattke T, Loescher L, Booth A (1986) A phase II study of α-difluoromethylornithine (DFMO) for the treatment of metastatic melanoma. Investigational New Drugs 4:257-262

Natale RB, Meyer K, Forastiere A (1985) Phase I trials of α-Difluoromethylornithine (DFMO) alone and in combination with Methylglyoxal Bis-Guanylhydrazone (MGBG). Proceedings ASCO (C-532) 4:137

Pegg AE (1988) Polyamine metabolism and its importance in neoplastic growth and as a target for chemotherapy. Ca Res 48:759-774

Porter CW, Herrera OL, Pera P, Petrelli NJ, Mittelman A (1987) Polyamine biosynthetic activity in normal and neoplastic human colorectal tissues. Cancer 60:1275-1281

Stulc JP, Petrelli NJ, Herrera LO, Mittelman A (1987) Colorectal villous and tubulovillous adenoma equal to or greater than four centimeters. Ann of Surg 207:65-71

Utsonomiya J, Miki Y, Kuroki T, Iwama T (1990) Phenotypic expressions of Japanese patients with Familial Adenomatous Polyposis. In: Herrera L (ed) Familial Adenomatous Polyposis. Alan R. Liss, New York, pp 101-107
Zhang S-Z, Luk GD, Hamilton SR (1988) α-Difluoromethylornithine-induced inhibition of growth of autochthonous experimental colonic tumors produced by Azoxymethane in male F344 rats. Ca Res 48:6498-6503

Chapter 5

Clinicopathological Aspects of Hereditary Colorectal Cancer Syndrome

Summary of Chapter 5: Clinicopathological Aspects of Inherited Colorectal Cancer Syndromes

STANLEY R. HAMILTON

This workshop dealt with clinical and pathological aspects of various inherited syndromes which predispose to colorectal carcinoma. The speakers addressed intestinal and extraintestinal tumors in adenomatous polyposis syndrome, and malignancy in Peutz-Jeghers syndrome. The characteristics of flat adenomas of the large bowel were presented. Three papers relating to hereditary nonpolyposis colorectal cancer discussed the histopathological features of the tumors, and crypt atrophy and cellular immune responses in the large bowel mucosa of patients with the syndrome. The final presentations dealt with carbohydrate-associated antigens and interphasic nucleolar organizer regions in neoplastic and non-neoplastic colorectal mucosa.

Dr. Stanley R. Hamilton from The Johns Hopkins University, U.S.A., discussed the definition and inheritance of Turcot syndrome (adenomatous polyposis associated with tumor of the central nervous system), based upon 12 cases from the Johns Hopkins and Toronto General Hospital polyposis registries along with an analysis of 58 additional cases from the literature. In the Hopkins and Toronto cases, 10/11 patients had a parent and/or sibling with polyposis, but only one had a family history of brain tumor. Medulloblastoma accounted for 8/11 cases. The temporal relationship between the development of brain tumor and of adenomatous polyposis of the large bowel was variable, with brain tumor preceeding polyposis in some patients but subsequent to polyposis in others. Extraintestinal lesions of Gardner syndrome were frequently present in the patients with brain tumor or their family members (10/12 cases). In the analysis of the Hopkins and Toronto cases along with those from the literature, patients were categorized on the basis of their colorectal findings and family history as adenomatous polyposis (>100 adenomas and/or adenomatous polyposis in a parent or sibling) or as nonpolyposis adenomas. Medulloblastoma and glial cell tumors were the most common central nervous system tumors associated with polyposis, accounting for 63% (20/32) and 38% (12/32), respectively, of tumors of known histology. By contrast, glial cell tumors accounted for a higher proportion of tumors in patients with colorectal adenomas but not polyposis than in polyposis patients (22/25, 88% vs. 12/38, 32%, $p < .0001$). The majority of non-polyposis patients with brain tumor (14/22, 64%) had another family member with a central nervous system tumor. The investigators concluded that Turcot syndrome is medulloblastoma or glial cell tumor occurring as a pleiotropic extra-intestinal manifestation in a patient who has the gene for adenomatous polyposis. Discussion of the paper emphasized that the association of glial cell tumors and nonpolyposis adenomas remains unexplained. The report at the Symposium by Dr. Ray White of two polyposis families with members having small numbers of colorectal adenomas but linkage to probes near the polyposis gene on the long arm of chromosome 5 are of particular interest in this regard. The limitations of phenotypic analysis emphasized the need for molecular genetic studies of pedigrees with members having Turcot syndrome and of the brain tumors themselves to define more precisely the spectrum of the syndrome. The occurrence of various abnormalities of pigmentation in patients with inherited conditions predisposing to colorectal neoplasia was pointed out, including congenital hypertrophy of the retinal pigment epithelium in adenomatous polyposis patients, mucocutaneous pigmentation in Peutz-Jeghers syndrome, and cafe au lait spots in patients reported as Turcot syndrome. Studies of tryptophane metabolism may therefore be of interest. It is hoped that this International Symposium will stimulate collection of specimens from patients with Turcot syndrome and their families for collaborative analyses.

Dr. Hidenobu Watanabe from Niigata University, Japan, discussed the pathology of upper gastrointestinal lesions in familial adenomatosis coli. Among 34 affected patients, 24 (70.6%) had gastric lesions, including adenoma in 13, fundic gland polyps in 11, carcinoma in 4, and microcarcinoid in 3. The characteristics of the lesions in polyposis patients differed from those in the general population: fundic gland polyps occurred at younger age and with a predominance of females in polyposis patients, and gastric adenomas in polyposis patients were characterized by younger age of the patients, smaller size and multiplicity of the adenomas, and less frequent association with intestinal metaplasia in the gastric mucosa as compared with "ordinary" gastric adenomas. All 25 patients in whom the duodenum was examined had lesions, consisting of adenoma in 24, carcinoma in an adenoma in 1, and microcarcinoids in 2. The entire jejunum and ileum were investigated by endoscopy or autopsy in 16 patients; 8 (50%) showed small polyps which were limited to the proximal jejunum. Five of these patients had jejunal adenoma, but the histopathology of the polyps in the remaining 3 was unknown. The distal ileum rarely showed lesions, which were present in only 4 patients (25%); three patients had adenoma and 1 a malignant lymphoma. This presentation emphasized that gastroenteric lesions occur frequently in patients with adenomatous polyposis. The investigators suggested that special attention should be given to the stomach and small intestine in patients with adenomatous polyposis, particularly in those with previous colectomy. The opportunity to develop cancer of extracolonic sites due to removal of the high-risk large bowel suggests the importance of surveillance in enhancing patient survival. Studies of the potential benefits of surveillance are needed.

Dr. Takeo Iwama, Research Center for Polyposis, Tokyo Medical and Dental University, presented their experience with and a literature review of malignancy in Peutz-Jeghers syndrome. Among their 19 cases, 4 (21%) had a malignant tumor: adenocarcinoma of the jejunum in a 30 year old male and a 38 year old male; endometrial carcinoma in a 31 year old female; and adenocarcinoma of the uterine cervix and a tumor of the head of the pancreas in a 49 year old female. Among 420 cases of Peutz-Jeghers syndrome (PJS) in the Japanese literature through December, 1988, 70 (17%) had gastrointestinal carcinoma. Their mean age was only 34.4 years. Forty-five of the 70 carcinomas (64%) were locally extended or metastatic. Colorectal carcinoma was the most common gastrointestinal carcinoma, occurring in 23 patients (5%). Five gastric carcinomas, 3 duodenal carcinomas, and 3 jejunal or ileal carcinomas were also reported. Seven of the 18 cases in which the histopathologic classification was reported had mucus-producing adenocarcinoma. Twenty-one cases of extra-gastrointestinal neoplasms were identified with a mean age of 41.2 years. The most common site was uterus (9 cases), while there were 2 cases each of carcinoma of the lung, pancreas, gallbladder, and ovary. The authors emphasized that the mean age of development of malignant tumors in patients with PJS was young, that colorectal carcinoma was the most frequent cancer,and that mucus-producing carcinoma was common among gastrointestinal carcinomas. Uterine cancer also had unusual characteristics in PJS in that cervical adenocarcinoma accounted for two-thirds of the 9 cases whereas 95% of cervical carcinoma in Japan is epidermoid carcinoma. The authors concluded that PJS cannot be considered merely as a benign condition which only causes intussusception. During the discussion, the association of gynecologic tumors with PJS was again emphasized. The problem of distinguishing pseudocarcinomatous epithelial invasion in PJ polyps from invasive carcinoma was discussed. The lack of molecular genetic studies of patients with PJS and of their tumors was noted, emphasizing the need for collection of specimens for molecular analysis when cases become available.

Dr. Hidenobu Watanabe of Niigata University, Japan, discussed the histogenesis of gastrointestinal carcinomas in Peutz-Jeghers syndrome (PJS). The investigators found that 6 of 27 patients (22%) with PJS had intestinal carcinoma. This prevalence was similar to that in Dr. Iwama's study. Three patients had an advanced jejunal carcinoma accompanied by intramucosal and submucosal carcinoma in Peutz-Jeghers (PJ) polyps with adenoma (dysplasia). The other 3 patients had a colorectal carcinoma including 1 with an advanced carcinoma, 1 with intramucosal carcinoma in a PJ polyp, and 1 with intramucosal carcinoma in an adenoma. In addition to the carcinomas, 4 patients had adenomas in the duodenum or the colon. The differences between patients with PJS (mucocutaneous pigmentation and hamartomatous polyps) as compared to those with harmatomatous polyps alone were also discussed: the patients without PJS were older and had a higher proportion of males and of colonic hamartomatous polyps than PJS patients. The authors proposed that malignancy in PJS polyps can occur by 4 possible mechanisms: (1) Malignant transformation of an adenoma (dysplasia) arising in a PJ polyp. (2) Malignant transformation in the PJ polyp itself. (3) Malignant change in a pure adenoma. (4) De novo carcinoma. From their data the authors favored the first and third mechanisms.

Dr. Tetsuichiro Muto, University of Tokyo, Japan, presented the clinical and pathological features of flat adenoma of the large bowel. During a 17 year period, 1437 polyps were removed via colonoscopy at his institution. 972 were neoplastic polyps, including 858 adenomas with mild or moderate dysplasia, 78 adenomas with severe dysplasia, and 36 invasive carcinomas. Among the adenomas, there were 92 (6.4% of all polyps and 9.5% of neoplastic polyps) which were classified as "flat adenomas", characterized by macroscopically slightly elevated lesions with occasional central depression. Thirty-one additional flat adenomas from 21 patients were collected from surgical resection specimens, providing a study group of 123 lesions in 98 patients. The male to female ratio was 3.4:1, and the average age of the patients was 58 years. 35 patients (35.7%) had a solitary flat adenoma whereas the flat adenoma in 32 was associated with polypoid adenoma, in 14 with carcinoma, and in 17 with both adenoma and carcinoma. Most of the flat adenomas were located in the left colon, including the rectum, but the frequency in the right colon was much higher than that of polypoid adenomas. About 94% of the flat adenomas were under 1 cm in diameter and only a few lesions exceeded 2 cm. On routine colonoscopy, flat adenomas appeared as slightly elevated flat lesions with reddish mucosa but became sessile with central depression when the colon was deflated. At this stage the lesions could be easily and safely removed by snare polypectomy. On histopathologic examination, all of the flat adenomas were tubular adenomas. The lesions showed lateral spread of adenomatous tubules, rather than luminal growth. The adenomatous component was less than twice as thick as the surrounding mucosa. The muscularis mucosae usually showed no thickening. The most striking histopathologic feature of the flat adenomas was a high frequency of severe dysplasia despite their small size: 14% of small flat adenomas under 1 cm in diameter showed severe dysplasia. In addition, abnormal DNA content was strongly associated with the severity of dysplasia in flat adenomas: those with mild atypia were diploid whereas those with severe dysplasia were aneuploid; about half of the flat adenomas with moderate dysplasia were diploid while the others were aneuploid. The authors suggested that flat adenomas, particularly with severe dysplasia, play an important role in the development of colorectal carcinoma and should be considered a new type of precursor deserving of careful investigation. During the discussion, the importance of recognition and removal of flat adenomas was emphasized. Polypectomy was recommended, although hot biopsy obliteration of 3 mm or smaller flat lesions was regarded as satisfactory. The problem of recurrence of or failure of detection of flat adenomas in patients with hereditary nonpolyposis colorectal cancer syndrome was discussed.

Dr. Thomas Smyrk from Creighton University, U.S.A., discussed the histopathologic features of hereditary nonpolyposis colorectal cancer (HNPCC). The clinical features of HNPCC are well established: autosomal dominant transmission pattern, early age of cancer onset, predominance of proximal colonic involvement, and predilection for multiple carcinomas, including both synchronous and metachronous cancers. A previous study from the Finnish registry suggested that a higher proportion of mucinous and poorly differentiated carcinomas occurred in HNPCC than in sporadic colorectal cancers. Dr. Smyrk's study included 86 tumors from 66 patients in 15 families. The mean age of first colonic cancer diagnosis was 47.5 years with a range of 22 to 80 years. 71% of the cancers occurred proximal to the splenic flexure. Six patients (9%) had multiple synchronous cancers, and another 6 developed metachronous tumors. 35% of the HNPCC carcinomas were graded as poorly differentiated based on the absence of gland lumens, as compared to only 13% of sporadic cases ($p<.01$). In addition, the HNPCC group more frequently showed marked lymphocytic response (35% vs. 15%, $p<.04$), and marked formation of lymphoid nodules at the periphery of the tumor, termed Crohn's-type reaction to the tumor (42% vs. 20%, $p<.04$). In addition, the HNPCC cases showed a lower proportion of tumors with extension through the muscularis propria (69% vs. 87%, $p<.03$), lower prevalence of cases with lymph node metastasis (25% vs. 48%, $p<.02$), and a smaller number of examined lymph nodes in the specimens. HNPCC cases had a lower Jass score, which is associated with better prognosis, than "ordinary" colorectal carcinomas. During the discussion, the Finnish group reported that their HNPCC tumors rarely showed aneuploid DNA content, another feature associated with better prognosis. The authors' study confirmed the previous report of an excess of poorly differentiated tumors with HNPCC. On the other hand, lymphocytic response and Crohn's-like reaction, which were more common in HNPCC, have been reported to be associated with improved prognosis of colorectal cancer. These histopathologic findings may be reflected in the clinical paradox that HNPCC cancers appear to have better survival by stage than "sporadic" cancers, despite having a greater proportion of poorly differentiated tumors. On the other hand, the less advanced nature of the HNPCC tumors may also provide the explanation. Further studies of the pathologic features of HNPCC cancers are needed. Molecular genetic analyses of this type of colorectal carcinoma for comparison with "sporadic" colorectal cancers are also of great interest, and may be spurred by this Symposium.

Dr. Pantaleo Bufo, Bari University, Italy, presented a study of the mucosa in 12 patients from 2 Italian kindreds with hereditary nonpolyposis colorectal cancer. Pathologic examination revealed crypt atrophy associated with an excess of macrophages, and the investigators therefore carried out a morphometric stereological evaluation. They found that the mean volume fraction of crypts was considerably below that of colonic mucosa in healthy subjects, and their data on crypt density of control colorectal mucosa were similar to those of other researchers (Eide, 1986). They pointed out that crypt atrophy also occurred in the late stages of idiopathic inflammatory bowel disease such as ulcerative colitis, which is associated with the development of colorectal carcinoma, often of the mucinous type as has been reported to be increased in frequency with HNPCC. The authors suggested that the crypt atrophy in HNPCC reflected genetically determined increased susceptibility of the colonic epithelium to damage produced by some still unknown environmental factors. During the discussion, the importance of site-matched specimens in such studies was emphasized because the right colon in human beings normally shows more crypt distortion, more inflammatory cells in the epithelium and lamina propria, higher mitotic rate in the epithelium, lower epithelial mucin content, and more frequent presence of Paneth cells in the bases of crypts than does the remainder of the large bowel.

Dr. Silvano Senatore, di Summa Brindisi Hospital, Italy, presented a study of the cellular immune response in cancer family syndrome (Lynch syndrome II). Previous immunological studies using mixed leukocyte cultures of hereditary nonpolyposis colorectal cancer patients showed deficient cellular immune reaction, and immunoenzymatic studies of gastrointestinal specimens showed polyclonal B cell activation. Because immunoregulatory cell interactions and macrophages appear to play a role in the modulation of colon cancer growth, the author studied GI biopsies from 18 members of the first family with Lynch syndrome II (cancer family syndrome) identified in Italy. The male-to-female gender ratio was 1.25, and ages ranged from 21 to 55 years with a mean of 39.6 years. Immunohistochemical morphometric evaluations for macrophages and T cell populations were carried out using immunoperoxidase with polyclonal and monoclonal antibodies. The investigators found that both the T-helper and T-cytotoxic suppressor cell distributions were similar in the whole material and per subject, as shown by their experimental ratio, i.e. 1.1. Macrophages were 5 times less frequent than each tested lymphocyte subset, with T-helper cells to macrophages ratio of 5.1 and T-cytotoxic suppressor cells to macrophages ratio of 5.1. Furthermore, the investigators found that there was a significant correlation between the increase of macrophages, T-cytotoxic suppressor cells, as well as of macrophages to T-helper cells ratio and of macrophages to T-cytotoxic suppressor cells ratio and age. The authors hypothesized that the activated macrophage pool stimulated T-helper cells, whereas no such reaction occurred in T-cytotoxic suppressor cells. They also proposed that both macrophages and T-helper cells activated B cells. They suggested that further investigations will be required to determine whether immune functions and/or immunological abnormalities are primarily involved in the pathogenesis of cancer family syndrome.

Dr. Young S. Kim, University of California, San Francisco, U.S.A., discussed carbohydrate-associated antigens in neoplastic and preneoplastic colon. Three main types of changes in glycoconjugates may occur in colon cancer: (1) Expression of an antigen not usually found in normal tissues, such as incompatible expression of A,B,H and Lewis^b blood group antigens. (2) Deletion of an antigen usually expressed by normal tissues with or without accumulation of precursors, such as deletion of A, B, and H and the expression of precursor antigens such as T and Tn antigen. (3) Modification of existing structures such as Lewis^x and Lewis^y antigens (positional isomers of Lewis^a and Lewis^b). Studies using monoclonal antibodies showed that short chain Lewis^x and Lewis^y antigens are expressed in all types of colonic tissues, whereas all types of extended Lewis^x and Lewis^y antigens are absent from normal colonic mucosa and hyperplastic polyps, but are present in colorectal adenomas and carcinomas. In studies of adenomas, expression of extended Lewis^x and Lewis^y antigens correlated with histopathologic parameters of malignant potential, including size, villous architecture, and grade of dysplasia. Studies of cancers showed that extended Lewis^x and Lewis^y with or without addition of terminal sialic acids or internal fucoses were expressed. T, Tn and sialyl Tn antigens represent incomplete glycosylation of mucin type carbohydrate side chains. These antigens are expressed in colorectal cancer and fetal colonic epithelial cells, but not in normal colonic mucosa. Studies of adenomas showed that expression of T antigen was associated with histopathologic features favoring malignant potential. Several carbohydrate structures behaved as tumor markers, although none was specific for colon cancer. Studies of these antigenic alterations in preneoplastic colonic mucosa are in progress in the flat mucosa of patients with adenomatous polyposis, cancer family syndrome, and ulcerative colitis. Preliminary data suggest that extended Lewis^x and Lewis^y related antigens may be expressed in these conditions.

Dr. Pietro L. Mingazzini, La Sapiienza, Italy, presented a paper on interphasic nucleolar organizer regions in dysplastic and neoplastic colorectal lesions. Nucleolar organizing regions (NORs) are ribosomal DNA loops mainly located in the fibrillar centers of the nucleolus. These can be identified by silver staining (Ag) due to their argyrophilic non-histone proteins. Changes in NORs distribution and number reflect variations in ribosomal transcription activity. In a previous study, the authors demonstrated a striking difference in number and distribution of Ag-NORs among hyperplastic polyps, adenomatous polyps, and adenocarcinoma of the colon. In the present study, the authors investigated Ag-NORs in different grades of colonic epithelial dysplasia using computerized image analysis. They found that the mean number of argyrophilic dots increased progressively from mild to severe dysplasia to adenocarcinoma although with a wide overlap in the ranges. In dysplastic lesions, the dots were mainly arranged in one or more large clumps, whereas in carcinomas a large number of small-sized clumps containing few dots was observed. The percentage of mean nuclear area occupied by Ag-NORs increased from dysplastic to carcinomatous lesions. The overlap among number, distribution, and ratio of nuclear area/dots area made it impossible to identify a single cell as malignant except for those cells showing a striking increase in number of dots. The authors concluded that the Ag-NORs technique was useful in distinguishing different grades of dysplasia and in distinguishing severe dysplasia from infiltrating adenocarcinoma, although the predictive value was reliable only when a suitable number of cells was observed.

An important theme of this Workshop was the importance of clinical and pathological aspects of various inherited syndromes which predispose to colorectal carcinoma, particularly as molecular genetics emerges as a tool. Evaluation and validation of probes associated with these conditions, and ultimately of probes for the genes causing these conditions, can only be carried out in carefully defined clinical and pathological situations. The classification of cases is often difficult in syndromes other than adenomatous polyposis, but misclassification of patients or lesions can be detrimental (e.g. in linkage analysis of families). The importance of collecting and classifying appropriate specimens for molecular genetic studies is obvious and represents an important short-term goal for investigators. In the long term, the challenge is to use the verified molecular technology to improve the management of patients with the inherited syndromes. The move of molecular genetics from the research arena to the clinical arena has barely begun. Therapeutic applications of molecular genetics are in the conceptual phase at present. We hope this International Symposium will provide the impetus for advances toward these short-term and long-term goals.

Pathology of Gastroenteric Lesions in Familial Adenomatosis Coli

HIDENOBU WATANABE, MITSUO IIDA, MITSUYA IWAFUCHI, YOICHI AJIOKA, YUTAKA NODA, and TEIICHI MOTOYAMA

ABSTRACT

This paper reports on the findings of high incidences, predominantly neoplastic nature and follow-up data of gastroenteric lesions in Japanese patients with familial adenomatosis coli. Prior to, during or after the colectomy, careful attention should be paid especially to the stomach, duodenum including the papillary region, upper jejunum and lower ileum as well as the thyroid because of high incidences of carcinoma, adenoma and carcinoid.

Keywords: familial adenomatosis coli, gastroenteric lesions, carcinoma, adenoma, fundic gland polyposis, carcinoid

Since 1974, the high incidences of the gastroenteric lesions in familial adenomatosis coli (FAC) has been clarified systematically first by Japanese investigators (Utsunomiya 1974; Ohsato 1974; Ushio 1976; Yao 1977; Watanabe 1977, 1978) and later by the Americans and Europeans (Hamilton 1979; Ranzi 1981; Jarvinen 1983; Burt 1984; Sivak 1984; Bulow 1985; Tonelli 1985; Shemesh 1985; Sarre 1987; Kurtz 1987). In this paper I would like to show our data on the incidences, histological natures and follow-up data of gastroenteric lesions in Japanese FAC.

1. GASTRIC LESIONS

Gastric lesions excluding erosion and peptic ulcer were found in 24(71%) of 34 Japanese FAC patients examined either by endoscopic, radiograghic and biopsy examinations, or with surgically resected or autopsy materials. They consisted of adenoma in 13 cases, fundic gland polyposis in 11, carcinoma in four and microcarcinoid in three. The age distribution of the patients with each kind of gastric lesions was shown in Table 1. The features of gastric lesions in FAC were; (1)younger age of the patients with each gastric disease than that of general population, (2)multiplicity of each gastric lesion, and (3)occurrence of multiple kinds of diseases in a stomach.

1.1 Gastric Adenoma

This was found in 38% (13 cases) of all 34 FAC patients and in 54% of 24 patients with gastric lesions. The older the patient-age, the higher the incidence of gastric adenoma (Table 1). The adenoma predominantly occurred in the pyloric mucosa or intestinal metaplastic mucosa and rarely in the cardiac mucosa, but not in the fundic mucosa. The number of gastric adenoma was one tumor in 3 patients and 3-43 in 10 patients. Macroscopically, 103 gastric adenomas, which were detected in seven resected stomachs of FAC patients, was IIa-like (slightly elevated sessile polypoid) type in 32%, IIb-like flat type in 27%, IIc-like (slightly depressed) type in 6% and erosion-like type in 35%. Size of the adenomas was 10mm or less in 93%. Gastric intestinal metaplasia was severe only in a 57-year-old man with 43 adenomas, three carcinomas and a microcarcinoid in his partially resected stomach, and the size of his gastric adenomas generally was larger than that in other FAC patients with mild gastric intestinal metaplasia.

Table 1 Age distribution of patients with gastric diseases in familial adenomatosis coli

Disease \ Age	0-9	10-19	20-29	30-39	40-49	50-59	Total No. of patient
Carcinoma	0	1	0	1	1	1	4
Carcinoid	0	1	0	1	0	1	3
Adenoma	0	1	3	4	3	2	13
Fundic gland plyposis	0	3	5	2	1	0	11
No. of patient with lesion/ total No. of patient examined	0/1	5/9	8/10	6/7	3/5	2/2	24/34

The comparison of gastric adenoma between these FAC patients and Japanese general population was shown in Table 2 (Enjoji 1975; Watanabe 1986). In addition to these features shown in Table 2, erosive gross type of adenomas and their predominant occurrence in pyloric mucosal area without intestinal metaplasia were characteristic of gastric adenoma of FAC patients. However, histology of gastric adenoma itself was the same between FAC and non-FAC patients.

Twenty six patients including many of the patients from the group of 34 mentioned above were followed for an average of 6.8 years (1 year 5 months to 15 years 4 months) and examined repeatedly by gastric radiography, endoscopy and biopsy (Iida 1988). Gastric adenomas were present in 13 (50%) at the last follow-up period. During the follow-up period, there was a new appearance of gastric adenomas in six patients, but no distinct change in number, size and histologic features in the remaining seven patients. A 51-year-old man in the former group had a 13mm sessile polypoid gastric adenoma with an irregular central depression at the initial examination. It did not change in size and morphology during 4 years 1 month, but at the same time malignant change was confirmed by endoscopic biopsy, which was reconfirmed 8 month later at autopsy.

Table 2 Comparison of gastric adenoma between FAC patients and general population in Japanese

	Gastric adenoma in	
	FAC patients	general population
Average age(range)	36 (15-57)	62 (37-81)
Sex ratio(M:F)	8:5	129:39
Incidence	13/34(38%)	188/126,358(0.15%)
Multiplicity	10/13(77%)	36/168(21%)
Size(mm) ≦5	60/103(58%)	35/218(16%)
5<X≦10	36/103(35%)	61/218(28%)
10<X≦20	5/103(5%)	75/218(34%)
20<	1/103(1%)	47/218(22%)
Intestinal metaplasia (mod.+ severe)	1/7 (14%)	149/168(89%)

1.2 Fundic Gland Polyposis

This was found in 32 % (11 cases) of all 34 FAC patients and in 46% of 24 patients with gastric lesions. The incidence by age was 50% in twenties, 33% in tens, 29% in thirties, 20% in forties, but 0% in fifties (Table 1). Fundic gland polyposis occurred only in the fundic mucosa and were numerous in the anterior and posterior wall as well as on the greater curvature, but a few on the lesser curvature. The number of the polyp were from hundreds to 1880 in each case, the size generally was 5mm or less, and the polyps usually were sessile, white-yellow ones with a pattern of area gastricae and no erosion. Histologically the polyps consisted of hyperplasia of tortuous fundic glands and many microcysts.

The comparison of fundic gland polyp between FAC patients (Watanabe 1977,1978) and general population (Iida 1984) was shown in Table 3. It is keypoints to make a diagnosis of FAC by fundic gland polyp that its number exceeds hundreds, and that the patient is younger.

Twenty three patients including many of the patients from the group of 34 mentioned above were examined over a follow-up period ranging from 17 months to 13 years (average 6 years). Examinations included gastric radiography and endoscopy with biopsy. Fundic gland polyps were found in 10 individuals. During the follow-up period, there was an increase in the number or size of polyps, or both, in 5 patients (aged 8-27 years), a decrease or disappearance in 2 patients (aged 36 and 41 years), an initial decrease or disappearance followed by a late-occurring increase in 2 patients (aged 28 and 35 years), and a new appearance in 1 patient (aged 23 years). Malignant or adenomatous changes of fundic gland polyps were not observed in any patients. Therefore, when the FAC patients with the polyps reach up to their thirties, there is a gradual increase in number and size of polyps and then their proliferation ceases and polyps may even decrease in number and size.

Table 3 Comparison of fundic gland polyp between FAC patients and general population in Japanese

	Fundic gland polyp	
	FAC patients	general population
Average age(range)	26 (18-41)	50 (32-70)
Sex ratio(M:F)	6:5	5:16
Incidence	11/34(32%)	23/27,000(0.085%)※
Number of polyp	hundreds-1,880	1-less than 100
Prevalent site	Fundic mucosa of greater curvature, anterior and posterior wall	Same as the left
Size	Usually less than 5mm	Same as the left
Gross type	Sessile,sometimes pedunculated polyp	Same as the left
Histology	Hyperplasia of tortuous fundic glands, and many microcysts Shortening of foveolae	Same as the left

※ Iida (1984)

1.3 Carcinoma and Carcinoid

This was found in 12% (4 cases) of all of the 34 FAC patients and in 17% of 24 patients with gastric lesions. Table 4 summarized our four cases with gastric carcinoma and carcinoid. Eleven microcarcinomas in case 1 (Table 4), two IIc type carcinomas in case 2 and a IIc type 6mm carcinoma in case 4 were not pointed out clinically, but were detected with precise macroscopic and microscopic examinations of the surgically resected specimens. Three of the carcinomas occurred in adenoma.

It is characteristic of gastric carcinoma of FAC patients that the carcinoma was very high in incidence, multiple, and differentiated type adenocarcinoma in many patients, and that it occurred in younger generation as well as in Japanese prevalently. It is suggested that gastric carcinoma of FAC patients may arise in adenoma in many cases and that its high incidence in Japanese is related not only to a genetic factor but also to environmental factors.

Microcarcinoids were incidentally found in the deep layer of the pyloric and junctional mucosa in three out of eight stomachs resected surgically. Gastric carcinoid is usually rare (0.4%) in general

Table 4 Gastric carcinoma and carcinoid tumor in FAC patients

Case No.	Age & Sex	Carcinoma: Gross type	size(mm)	Depth of invasion	Histologic type	Carcinoid	Others
1	17.f.	IIc-like	25	Serosa	sig※	Microcarcinoid, two,0.2mm and 0.4mm	Intestinal metaplasia, mild
		IIc	20	Submucosa	sig		
		IIc	9	Submucosa	sig		
		Microcarcinoma	0.1-3.0	Mucosa	sig		
2	36.m.	Expansive ulcerating	35	Proper muslce	tubl+	Microcarcinoid, one,1.5mm	Adenoma,one, Intestinal metaplasia, mild
		IIc	5	Mucosa	tubl		
		IIc	2.5	Mucosa	tubl		
3	56.m.	IIc+IIa	10	Mucosa	Car(tubl) in adenoma		Adenoma,13 Intestinal metaplasia, mild
4	57.m.	IIc	27	Submucosa	tubl	Microcarcinoid, one,6mm	Adenoma,43 Intestinal metaplasia, severe
		IIc	18	Mucosa	Car(tubl) in adenoma		
		IIc	6	Mucosa	Car(tubl) in adenoma		

※ Signet-ring cell carcinoma, + Well differentiated tubuar adenocarcinoma population (Watanabe 1989) as well as duodenal and rectal carcinoid. However, in FAC patients a high incidence or multiplicity of duodenal or rectal carcinoids is reported (Watanabe 1986; Iwafuchi 1984). From this data, it is more than coincidental that gastric carcinoid occurred in FAC patients.

2. DUODENAL LESIONS

Twenty five of 26 patients examined had sessile polyps of the duodenum on endoscopy, which were verified as adenomas in 24 cases, carcinoma in adenoma in a case (autopsy) and an advanced carcinoma (surgical material) by histologic examination following the endoscopic biopsy, surgical resection and/or autopsy. In the remaining one, endoscopic biopsy taken for caution's sake from the ampulla of the duodenal major papilla disclosed an adenoma.

Lesions of the duodenal major papilla were found in 14 of 26 cases examined, and certified as adenoma in all cases by histologic examination. The adenomas were detected by endoscopy as white protrusions in 12 cases. In the remaining two cases, however, neither radiography nor endoscopy showed any abnormality, although endoscopic biopsy taken by way of precaution from the ampulla of the duodenal major papilla revealed an adenoma.

Twenty patients were followed for an average of 7.1 years (range 1 year 7 months to 12 years 2 months) and repeatedly examined by hypotonic duodenography, duodenofiberscopy and biopsy. Tubular adenomas of the duodenum less than 8 mm in diameter were present in 18 (90%). During the follow-up period, there was a slight increase or decrease in number of the duodenal adenomas in four patients but no distinct change in 13. No histologic changes were found on biopsy of all of the 17 patients. In the remaining patient, 49-year-old woman, a 17mm polypoid lesion of the duodenal bulb, which had been over looked at the initial examination, developed into an advanced carcinoma (50x30 mm in size) during 22 months. Tubular adenoma of the duodenal major papilla was detected in 11 patients (55%) on biopsy. Follow-up study of the lesions disclosed no change in endoscopic and histologic findings in all but one patient, in whom there was a slight enlargement of the duodenal papilla without any histologic change.

Duodenal microcarcinoid were incidentally found in two of 26 patients with FAC. A 41-year-old man had a 1.3 mm carcinoid in the duodenal bulb of autopsy material, and a 57-year-old man two 0.2 mm carcinoids in the duodenal bulb attached to the stomach surgically resected for gastric carcinomas.

3. JEJUNAL AND ILEAL LESIONS

In order to precisely analize the jejunal and ileal lesions, FAC cases were examined by endoscopic biopsy and endoscopy passed through the ileal stump or enteric stoma at the time of colectomy or in case of autopsy by inspection of specimen fixed immediately after death. Out of 16 patients investigated eight patients (50%) had one to 242 adenomas located within the limits of less than 120 cm jejunum from the ligament of Treitz, and four (25%) revealed ileal lesions (a malignant lymphoma in one case, and adenomas in three) restricted to the terminal ileum. Benign lymphoid polyposis was found in 9 of 16 patients.

4. SUMMARY AND CONCLUSION

Table 5 is our data on the incidences and histologic kinds of gastroenteric lesions of patients with familial adenomatosis coli. It is evident that the gastroenteric neoplastic lesions are very high in incidence in FAC patients. However, frequency of carcinoma is higher in the colon and rectum than in the stomach and small intestine. Therefore, the site of main phenotype is the colon and rectum (Table 6).

Recent advances in clinical diagnosis and surgery can save the FAC patients from death of carcinoma of the colon and rectum. The patients have been living longer than before. In such a circumstance, they have a lot of chances to suffer from the second or the third malignant tumors of extracolonic sites.

Table 5 Incidence and diseases of extracolonic lesions in familial adenomatosis coli

Site	Indicence	Diseases	
Stomach	71%(24/34)	Adenoma	38%(13/34)
		Fundic gland polyposis	32%(11/34)
		Carcinoma	12%(4/34)
		Carcinoid	9%(3/34)
Duodenum	96%(25/26)	Adenoma	96%(25/26)
		Carcinoma	8%(2/26)
		Carcinoid	8%(2/26)
Major papilla	54%(14/26)	Adenoma	54%(14/26)
		(Carcinoma)※	
Jejunum	50%(8/16)	Adenoma	50%(8/16)
		(Carcinoma)	
		(Carcinoid)	
		Malignant lymphoma	(1/16)
Ileum	25%(4/16)	Adenoma	25%(4/16)
		(Carcinoma)	
Thyroid	44%(4/9)+	Carcinoma	22%(2/9)
		Adenoma	22%(2/9)
Soft tissue tumor	33%		
Bone tumor	67%(-95%)		

※:Lesions in parentheses are reported in the literature.
+:Our date at autopsy

Table 6 Different phenotypes responsible for familial adenomatosis coli

1. Main phenotype : Multiple colonic adenomatosis with or without carcinomas

2. Extracolonic phenotypes :

Entodermal :	Adenomas	; Stomach, Duodenum, Duodenal major papilla, Jejunum, Ileum, Thyroid, Gallbladder, Adrenal gland, ets.
	Fundic gland polyposis	; Stomach
	Carcinomas	; Stomach, Duodenal major papilla, Duodenum, Thyroid, Jejunum, Ileum, etc.
	Carcinoid	; Rectum and sigmoid colon, Stomach, Duodenum, Ileum, Thymus
Ectodermal :	Epidermal cysts, sebaceous cysts, Brain tumors, etc.	
Mesodermal :	Soft tissue tumors	; Desmoid tumor, Fibroma, Lipoma, etc.
	Hard tissue tumors	; Osteoma, Odontoma, etc.

As you can see from Table 5 and 6, the subsequent or coexistent malignant tumors are prone to occur in the stomach, duodenum, duodenal major papilla, thyroid gland, upper jejunum, and lower ileum. In addition, these organs have multiple adenomas in a high frequency. Usually the adenomas are small, but have a probability to transform into malignant tumor. Therefore, we should thoroughly follow-up gastroenteric adenomas by endoscopy and endoscopic biopsy, and inspect susceptible extracolonic organs listed in the Table 5 and 6.

REFERENCES

Bulow S, Lauritsen KB, Johansen A, Svendsen LB. Sondergaard JO (1985) Gastroduodenal polyps in familial polyposis coli. Dis Colon Rectum 28: 90-93

Burt RW, Berenson MM, Lee RG, Tolman KG, Freston JW, Gardner EJ (1984) Upper gastrointestinal polyps in Gardner's syndrome. Gastroenterology 86: 295-301

Enjoji M, Watanabe H (1975) Adenoma of the stomach. Stomach and Intestine 10: 1443-1447 (in Japanese)

Hamilton SR, Bussey HJR, Mendelsohn G, Diamond MP, Pavlides G, Hutcheon D, Harbison M, Shermeta D, Morson BC, Yardley JH (1979) Ileal adenomas after colectomy in nine patients with adenomatous polyposis coli/Gardner's syndrome. Gastroenterology 77: 1252-1257

Iida M, Yao T, Itoh H, Watanabe H, Kohrogi N, Shigematu A, Iwashita A, Fujishima M (1988) Natural history of fundic gland polyposis in patients with familial adenomatosis coli/Gardner's syndrome. Gastroenterology 89: 1021-1025

Iida M, Yao T, Itoh H, Watanabe H, Matsui T, Iwashita A, Fujishima M (1988) Natural history of gastric adenomas in patients with familial adenomatosis coli/Gardner's syndrome. Cancer 61: 605-611

Iida M, Yao T, Itoh H, Watanabe H, Matsui T, Iwashita A, Fujishima M (1989) Natural history of duodenal lesions in Japanese patients with familial adenomatosis coli (Gardner's syndrome). Gastroenterology 96: 1301-1306

Iwafuchi M, Watanabe H, Itsuno M, Suda T, Enjoji M (1984) Familial adenomatosis coli associated with multiple microcarcinoids in the colon and rectum. Stomach and Intestine 19: 679-683 (in Japanese)

Jarvinen H, Nyberg M, Peltokallio P (1983) Upper gastrointestinal tract polyps in familial adenomatosis coli. 24: 333-339
Jones TR, Nance FC (1977) Periampullary malignancy in Gardner's syndrome. Ann Surg 185: 565-573

Kurtz RC, Sternberg SS, Miller HH, Decosse JJ (1987) Upper gastrointestinal neoplasia in familial polyposis. Dig Dis Sci 32: 459-465

Ohsato K, Watanabe H, Itoh H, Yao T, Nishimura M (1974) Simultaneous occurrence of multiple gastric carcinomas and familial polyposis of the colon. Jpn J Surg 4: 165-174

Pauli RM, Pauli ME, Hall JG (1980) Gardner syndrome and periampullary malignancy. AM J Med Genet 6: 205-219

Ranzi T, Gastagnone D, Velio P, Bianchi P, Polli EE (1981) Gastric abd duodenal polyps in familial polyposis coli. Gut 22:363-367

Sarre RG, Frost AG, Jagelman DG, Petras RE, Sivak MV, McGannon E (1987) Gastric and duodenal polyps in familial adenomatous polyposis: a prospective study of the nature and prevalence of upper gastrointestinal polyps. Gut 28: 306-314

Shemesh E, Bat L (1985) A prospective evaluation of the upper gastrointestinal tract and periampullary region in patients with Gardner's syn
drome. Am J Gastroenterology 80: 825-827

Sivak MV, Jagelman DG (1984) Upper gastrointestinal endoscopy in polyposis syndromes: familial polyposis coli and Gardner's syndrome. Gastrointest Endosc 30: 102-104

Tonelli F, Nardi F, Bechi P Taddei G, Gozzo P, Romagnoli P (1985) Extracolonic polyps in familial polyposis coli and Gardner's syndrome. Dis Colon Rectum 28: 664-668

Ushio K, Sasagawa M, Doi H, Yamada T, Ichikawa H, Hojo K, Koyama Y, Sano R (1976) Lesions associated with familial polyposis coli: studies of lesions of the stomach, duodenum, bones, and teeth. Gastrointest Radiol 1: 67-80

Utsunomiya J, Maki T, Iwama T, Matsunaga Y, Ishikawa T, Shimomura T, Hamaguchi E, Aoki N (1974) Gastric lesion of familial polyposis coli. Cancer 34: 745-754

Watanabe H, Enjoji M, Yao T, Iida M, Ohsato K (1977) Accompanying gastro-enteric lesions in familial adenomatosis coli. Acta Pathol Jpn 27: 823-839

Watanabe H, Enjoji M, Yao T, Ohsato K (1978) Gastric lesions in familial adenomatosis coli. Human Pathol 9: 269-283

Watanabe H (1986) Extracolonic lesions in familial adenomatosis coli. In: Takayama S, Ushio K (ed) Colon cancer in progress in cancer clinics. Medical View, Tokyo, pp188-195 (in Japanese)

Watanabe H (1989) Carcinoid tumor of the intestine. Stomach and Intestine 24: 853-857

Yao T, Iida M, Ohsato K, Watanabe H, Omae T (1977) Duodenal lesions in familial polyposis of the colon. Gastroenterol 73: 1086-1092

The Peutz-Jeghers Syndrome and Malignant Tumor

TAKEO IWAMA, HIDEYUKI ISHIDA, MAHITO IMAJO, KATSUJI TAKEMURA, NOZOMU AOKI, and YOSHIO MISHIMA

ABSTRACT

In our 19 cases of the Peutz-Jeghers (P-J) syndrome, we experienced two cases of carcinoma of the small intestine and two cases of uterine carcinoma. In 420 reported cases the of the P-J syndrome in Japanese literature there were 70 cases of gastrointestinal carcinoma (mean age of 34.4 years) and 21 cases of extra gastrointestinal cancer (mean age of 41.2 years). Mucus producing adenocarcinoma was common patho-histological subdivision of gastrointestinal carcinoma (39%). Twelve of 20 cases of extra gastrointestinal cancer were uterine (9 cases) or ovarial (2 cases) carcinoma. Cervical adenocarcinoma (6 cases) was thought to be a specific cancer associated with the P-J syndrome.

KEY WORDS

Peutz-Jeghers syndrome, Cervical adenocarcinoma, Mucus producing adenocarcinoma, Ovarial sex cord tumor.

Peutz (1921) reported in his original paper that in some polyps, which was usually composed of normal columnar cells, he found dysplastic parts with nuclear hyperchromatism which was considered to be adenoma or even carcinoma. There have been some controversies about potentiality of the development of cancer in the Peutz-Jeghers (P-J) syndrome since Berkowitz (1955), Bailey (1957) and Bartholomew (1957). We experienced four cases of malignant tumors in the P-J syndrome. Recently, in Japan, increasing number of case reports of malignant tumors associate with the P-J syndrome have appeared and we have realized that there are certain characteristic features in these gastrointestinal or extra gastrointestinal malignant tumors.

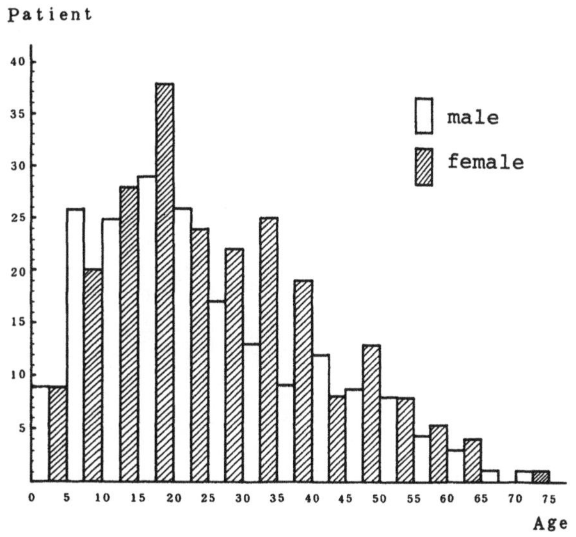

Fig.1. Age distribution of the Peutz-Jeghers syndrome ;
420 cases in Japanese literature.

MATERIALS

In our institute we experienced 19 cases of the P-J syndrome. We also used 420 cases of the P-J syndrome which have been reported in Japanese literature up to Decem. 1988 in which multiple booking was carefully avoided. Their mean age was 25.3 years (Fig. 1). We picked up the cases with malignant neoplastic lesions out of them.

RESULTS

Of our 19 cases of the P-J syndrome, which showed characteristic mucocutaneous pigmentation and gastrointestinal polyposis, we experienced four cases of malignant tumors (21%). Case 1. A 30 year old male. At his second operation in Sept. 1972 jejunal polyps were resected and in one of them, marked cellular and constructive atypism and mucus producing parts were observed (Fig. 2a). They were considered to be reversed growth of hamartoma. Three years after the operation, he died of peritoneal dissemination of carcinoma (Fig.2b). Case 2. A 38 year old male. In 1972 at his sixth operation the jejunum was resected and in one of the polyps, mucus producing carcinoma with invasion into the muscle wall was detected (Fig. 3). Case 3. A 31 year old female underwent intestinal polypectomy in Oct. 1976. Three years after the operation she underwent hysterectomy because of uterine endometrial carcinoma. Case 4. A 49 year old female. Since Feb. 1986 she complained of general

a

b

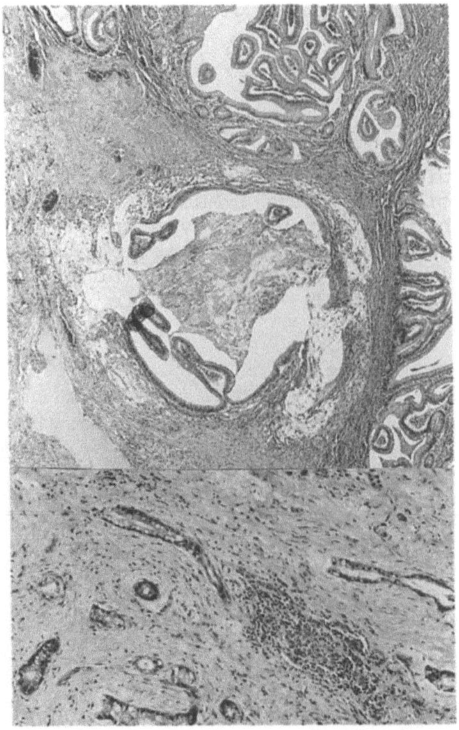

Fig. 2 .

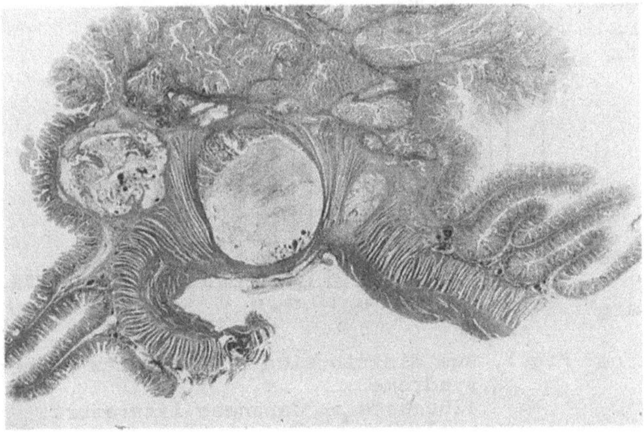

Fig.3.

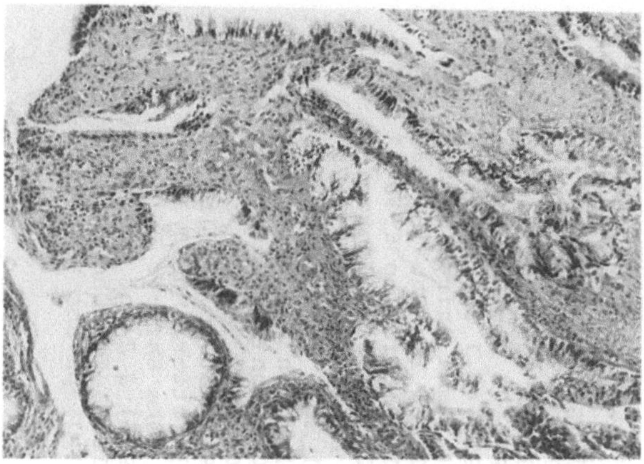

Fig. 4.

fatigue, jaundice and bloody mucus discharge from the vagina. Many polyps were found in the stomach, the small intestine and the colon. A colonic polyp was P-J type polyp. Examination revealed mucus producing adenocarcinoma of the cervix (Fig. 4) and peritoneal dissemination.

In 420 reported cases in Japanese literature, we found 75 gastrointestinal carcinoma (Table 1). Their mean age was 34.4 years and it is 10 years older than that of the background cases. Of these tumors, ten were located in the stomach, seven in the duodenum, 18 in the small intestine and 40 in the colo-rectum. Forty of 75 carcinomas were locally extended or carcinoma with metastasis. They were eight stomach carcinoma, four duodenal carcinoma, five carcinoma of small intestine and 23 colo-rectal carcinoma.

Table 1. Gastrointestinal carcinoma in the Peutz-Jeghers syndrome.

Stage of carcinoma	Stomach	Duodenum	Small intestine	Colon and Rectum
Focal or limited to submucosa	2	3	13	17
Locally extended or with metastasis	8	4	5	23

from Japanese literature, 1988.

Histological subdivision was described in 20 of the 40 cases and they consisted of six well differentiated adenocarcinoma, nine moderately or poorly differentiated adenocarcinoma, seven mucus producing adenocarcinoma and an alpha-fetoprotein producing carcinoma (five tumors contained mixed histological findings , Table 2).

Including our two cases of uterine carcinoma, we found 20 cases of extra gastrointestinal malignant neoplasms (Table 3). The mean age of them was 41.2 years. They included nine cases of uterine carcinoma, two cases of pulmonary carcinoma, two cases of pancreatic carcinoma, two cases of gall bladder carcinoma, two cases of ovarian carcinoma and other malignant tumors which included cerebellum, nasal mucosa, leukemia and choriocarcinoma. Twelve of 21 extra gastrointestinal malignant tumors occurred in the uterine and the ovary. In nine cases of uterine carcinoma six were adenocarcinoma of the cervix. One of two pancreatic cancer and the nasal mucosal tumor were mucus producing adenocarcinoma.

Table 2.
Histological subdivision of gastrointestinal carcinoma in the Peutz-Jeghers syndrome.

Case	Age	Sex	Location	Metastasis	Subdivision well	mod	poor	muc	Reporter
1	26	F	stomach	+	o				Taira(1975) Gann no Rinnsyo 21:208
2	13	M	stomach	-	o	o			Mishima(1978)J J Soc Clin Surg 39:9872
3	24	F	stomach	+			o		Yasui(1982) J J Soc Clin Surg 43:168
4	28	M	duodenum	+			o		Watanabe(1966) J Jpn Soc Pathol 55:234
5	26	F	duodenum	+			o		Kurimoto(1973) J J G S 6:191
6	48	F	duodenum	-	o				Shitu(1977) Geka Chiryo 19:349
7	26	F	small intestne	-	o				Sakaguchi(1978) Ito Cho 13:1089
8	45	F	asc. colon	+		o	o		Yamaguchi(1970) Ito Cho 5:1541
9	36	F	sigma	+			o		Ito(1972) J Jpn Soc Coloproct 25:47
10	53	F	asc. colon	+				o	Aoki(1976) Kanagawa Med J 4:75
11	26	F	colon	+				o	Kouzu(1978) Bull Fukuoka Univ 5:232
12	32	F	rectum	-		o			Tutui(1978) J Jpn Soc Coloproct 31:295
13	46	M	rectum	+				o	Kimura(1980)J Jpn Soc Coloproct 33:344
14	43	M	sigma	+				o	Kimura(1980)
15	39	M	asc. colon	+				o	Kurihara(1981) J Jpn Soc Int Med 70:605
16	22	M	desc. colon	+	o				Inoue(1982) Tottori Med J 10:300
17	39	M	desc. colon	+		o	o		Sato(1984) Geka Shinryo 26:527
18	40	M	desc. colon	+		o		o	Kuramoto(1986) J J Soc Coloproct 39:527
19	42	M	desc. colon	+	o			o	Takahashi(1986) Ito Cho 21:321
20	34	M	desc.colon	-	AFP,HCG pdoducing				Ehara(1987) J Jpn Soc Pathol 76:237

well: well differentiated. mod: moderately differentiated.
poor: poorly differentiated. muc: mucus producing.
AFP: alpha fetoprotein. HCG: human cholionic gonadotropin.

Table 3.
Extra gastrointestinal malignant tumor associated with the Peutz-Jeghers syndrome (mean age of 41.2 years).

Cerebellar schwannoma	1	Choriocarcinoma	1
Adenocarcinoma of the nasal mucosa	1	Ovarial carcinoma	2
Pulmonary squamous cell carcinoma	2	Uterine carcinoma	9
Leukemia	1	;endometrial carcinoma	(2)
Pancreatic carcinoma	2	;cervical-; squamous cell carcinoma	(1)
Carcinoma of the gall bladder	1	; adenocarcinoma	(6)

DISCUSSION AND CONCLUSION

Dozois (1969) reported that if polyps in the P-J syndrome were a premalignant factor, more cases of cancers should have been reported in view of the multitude of polyps, especially in the small intestine. Morson (1972) described that an oversecretion of mucin which becomes trapped between mucosal fold in the polyp and causes misplacement of epithelium, with histological appearances which may be misinterpreted as invasive carcinoma.
Although their description seems to be reasonable, our Case 1. warns us to pay attention to so called pseud invasion of polyp and we can also find several features in malignant tumor which associates with the P-J syndrome.
1) The mean age of development of malignant tumor is young. The mean age of gastrointestinal carcinoma was 34.4 years and that of extra gastrointestinal carcinoma was 41.2 years.
2) Colo-rectal carcinoma was the most prominent cancer and locally progressed small intestinal cancer was only three. Considering the occurrence of small intestinal cancer in general population being very rare it is understandable that even in the P-J syndrome this tendency is kept.
3) Mucus producing carcinoma was very common in gastrointestinal carcinoma (7/20). It may reflect the feature of polyps of the P-J syndrome in which goblet cell is the most prominent component.
4) Uterine cancer seems to have special meaning in the P-J syndrome. It is very specific that cervical adenocarcinoma consisted 67 percent of cervical carcinoma considering that, in general population, 95 percent of cervical cancer is epidermoid carcinoma. Dozois (1970) pointed out a high incidence (15%) of ovarian tumors in 115 reported women cases with the P-J syndrome and among them, granulosa cell tumor was the most common. Scully (1970) reported a high incidence of ovarian sex cord tumors among ovarian tumors of patients with the P-J syndrome and said that it indicates a unique relationship of them. In Japanese literature, Yamaguchi (1986) reported a case of the P-J syndrome associated with cervical adenocarcinoma and ovarial sex cord tumor. The P-J syndrome seems to have specific relationship with tumors from ovary and uterus.
Despite of all these evidences, prevalence of malignant tumor in the P-J syndrome is not so high as expected from its large and numerous polyps as Dozois (1969) stated. Age distribution of the P-J syndrome which is deviated to younger generation may explain the reason. After 20 years of age the reported cases decreased linearly. This may also prove that after 20 years of age polyps of the P-J syndrome do not progress so rapidly to produce intussusception as do before 20. Utsunomiya (1975) reported that the P-J syndrome indicated a much shorter survival than in the control population and that death occurring after age 30 was attributed to neoplastic disease in approximately 60% of cases. Long

term follow up is necessary to confirm these facts and recently Giardiello (1987) reported that cancer developed in 15 of 31 patients with P-J syndrome (48%)- gastrointestinal carcinoma in 4, extra gastrointestinal carcinoma in 10 and multiple myeloma in 1. Their relative risk of development of cancer was 18 times grater than expected in the general population.

Our conclusions were as following; 1) The mean age of developing malignant tumor is young. 2) Gastrointestinal polyps may develop carcinoma and we should pay attention to the phenomenon so called glandular pseudo-invasion particularly when the polyp shows any atypism. When a polyp is large or hard or fixed to the intestinal wall, it is necessary at least to resect the base of the polyp including the serosa. 3) Mucus producing carcinoma is a common type of malignant tumor either intra or extra gastrointestinal carcinoma. 4) The P-J syndrome has strong relationship with cervical adenocarcinoma.

REFERENCES

1) Bailey D. (1957) Polyposis of gastrointestinal tract: The Peutz syndrome. Br Med J 2:433-439.
2) Bartholomew LG, Dahlin DC, Waugh JM. (1957) Intestinal polyposis associated with mucocutaneous melanin pigmentation (Peutz-Jeghers syndrome). Gastroenterology 32(3):434-451.
3) Berkowitz SB, Peard MJ, Shapiro NH. (1955) Syndrome of intestinal polyposis with melanosis of the lips and buccal mucosa: A study of the incidence and location of malignancy. Ann Surg 141(1):129-133.
4) Dozois RR, Judd ES, Dahlin DC, Bartholomew LG. (1969) The Peutz-Jeghers syndrome. Arch Surg 98:509-517.
5) Dozois RR, Kempers RD, Dahlin DC, Bartholomew LG. (1970) Ovarian tumors associated with the Peutz-Jeghers Syndrome. Ann Surg 172(2):133-238.
6) Giardiello FM, Welsh SB, Hamilton SR, Offerhause GJA, Gittersohn AM, Booker SV, Krush AJ, Yardley JH, Luk GD. (1987) Increased risk of cancer in the Peutz-Jeghers syndrome. New Engl J Med 316(24):1511-1514.
7) Morson BC, Dawson IMP. (1972) Gastrointestinal pathology. Blackwell Scientific Publications, Oxford.
8) Peutz JLA. (1921) Over een zeer merkwaardige, gecombineerde familiare polyposis van de slijimvliezen van den tractus intestinalis met die van de neuskeelholte en gepaard met eigenaardige pigmentaties van huid- en slijmvliezen (from a translation to English). Nedel Maandschr voor Geneeskunde 10:134-146.
9) Scully RE. (1970) Sex cord tumor with annular tubules : A distinctive ovarian tumor of the Peutz-Jeghers syndrome.
10) Utunomiya J, Gocho H, Miyanaga T, Hamaguchi E, Kashimura A, Aoki N, Komatu I. (1975) Peutz-Jeghers syndrome: Its natural course and management. Johns Hopkins Med J 136(2):71-82.
11) Yamaguti T, Kutuzawa T. (1986) A case of the Peutz-Jeghers syndrome complicated by cervical adenocarcinoma and ovarial sex cord tumor. J Jpn Clin Cytology 25(2):353.

(Grant-in-Aid for Cancer Research from The Ministry of Education, Science and Culture, Fund from the Sagawa aid for Cancer Research)

Histogenesis of Gastrointestinal Carcinoma in Peutz-Jeghers Polyp

HIDENOBU WATANABE, YOICHI AJIOKA, MITSUYA IWAFUCHI, TEIICHI MOTOYAMA, NORIKO ISHIHARA, and JIRO HITOMI

ABSTRACT

Peutz-Jeghers (P-J) polyps (n=367) from 27 patients were histologically examined. There are seen five P-J polyps with adenoma, two P-J polyps with carcinoma in adenoma, a P-J polyp with independent foci of adenoma and carcinoma, a P-J polyp with carcinoma, two advanced primary carcinomas without any remnant of P-J polyp, a carcinoma in adenoma and a pure adenoma in eight patients. Four processes of malignant change of P-J polyp are proposed; (1) malignant transformation of adenoma arisen in P-J polyp, (2) malignant transformation of P-J polyp itself, (3) malignant change in pure adenoma, and (4) de novo carcinoma in normal mucosa. From our data, the first process seems to be the most frequent, and the third to be common in the colon and rectum.

Keywords: Peutz-Jeghers polyp(syndrome), histogenesis of neoplastic lesions, carcinoma, adenoma

The histogenesis of gastrointestinal carcinoma in P-J polyps is not clear. Because many of the gastrointestinal carcinoma in P-J syndrome reported hitherto have been advanced carcinomas which are inadequate for their precise histogenetic study. In addition misplacement or pseudoinvasion of the epithelium of P-J polyp was misdiagnosed as carcinoma (Bartholomew 1957; Reid 1974; Watanabe 1983, 1984). Here we studied the histogenesis using an early stage of gastrointestinal carcinoma of P-J polyp.

1. MATERIAL AND METHOD

Our material consisted of three groups; a group with both P-J polyps and pigmentation (P-J syndrome), a group with P-J polyps and without pigmentation, and a group with P-J polyps but with unknown history about pigmentation (Table 1). The P-J polyps showed the same histologic findings among three groups. Therefore we dealt three groups here as P-J polyps.

2. NEOPLASTIC LESIONS IN PATIENTS WITH P-J POLYPS

Gastrointestinal carcinoma was detected in 6 (22%) of 27 patients with P-J polyps, and in P-J polyps in 3 (11%) of the 27 patients. Out of six patients, two patients had a carcinoma of the jejunum, one patient two carcinomas of the duodenum (not papillary region), one patient carcinoma of the sigmoid colon and the remaining two patients had a carcinoma of the rectum, respectively (Table 2). It is surprising that 50% of the gastrointestinal carcinoma occurred in the small intestine.

There were seven gastrointestinal carcinomas in all of the six patients. Two carcinomas (jejunum and rectum) were advanced and did not have any remnant of P-J polyp and/or adenoma in themselves. Two carcinomas were each intramucosal or submucosal carcinoma, and occurred in adenomatous area of P-J polyp (Fig 1a-1b). A carcinoma (duodenum) arose de novo (ab initio) in a P-J polyp measuring 10mm in the largest diameter (Fig 2). Furthermore, a 30mm P-J polyp of the sigmoid colon had two foci of intramucosal adenocarcinomas and three foci of tubular adenomas independently in itself (Fig 3a-3d). The last carcinoma (rectum, case 26) was a carcinoma in adenoma without any trace of P-J polyp, and this case had two P-J polyps in the rectum.

Table 1 Cases with Peutz-Jeghers polyp

No. of cases	Age & sex	Polyp(s) in			Pigment.
		Stomach	Small intes.	Large intes.	
1	2 F	+	?	+	+
2	7 F	+	-	-	+
3	8 F	+	+	+	+
4	12 F	+	+	?	+
5	13 F	+	+	+	+
6	13 F	+	+	+	+
7	15 M	+	+	+	+
8	15 F	-	+	-	+
9	17 M	+	+	+	+
10	19 F	+	+	+	+
11	20 F	+	+	+	+
12	20 F	+	+	+	+
13	25 F	+	-	-	+
14	31 M	-	+	-	+
15	38 M	+	+	+	+
16	43 M	-	+	+	+
17	29 M	-	-	+	-
18	33 M	-	?	+	-
19	53 F	+	+	+	-
20	57 M	-	-	+	-
21	79 F	-	+	-	-
22	11 F	?	?	+	?
23	27 F	?	+	?	?
24	41 F	?	?	+	?
25	43 M	?	?	+	?
26	56 M	?	?	+	?
27	69 M	?	?	+	?

* Age at the initial diagnosis of P-J polyps.
* Case 1-27 are all an independent family.

Table 2 Gastrointestinal neoplastic lesions of the patients with Peutz-Jeghers polyp

No. of case in Table 1		Material	Site	Size and histology
9	20y. M	Surgical,	Jejunum	:30mm. Carcinoma (s), ulcerating
	21y.	〃	〃	:43mm. Carcinoma (s), ulcerating, metastatic (?)
	23y.	Necropsy,	Ileum	:20mm. Carcinoma (s), polypoid, metastatic (?)
	〃	〃	〃	: 6mm. Carcinomas (pm), polypoid, metastatic (?)
12	20y. F	Surgical,	Jejunum	:45mm. P-J polyp with carcinoma (m) in adenoma
16	43y. M	Polypectomy,	Duodenum	:35mm. P-J polyp with carcinoma (sm) in adenoma
	〃	〃	〃	:10mm, P-J polyp with carcinoma (sm)
	〃	〃	〃	:30mm. P-J polyp with adenoma
	〃	〃	〃	:10mm. P-J polyp with adenoma
	〃	〃	〃	:10mm. P-J polyp with adenoma
17	29y. M	Surgical,	Sigmoid	:30mm. P-J type polyp with independent foci of carcinomas (m) and adenomas
	〃	〃	〃	: 4mm. Adenoma
19	53y. F	Polypectomy,	Transverse	:50mm. P-J type polyp with adenoma
24	41y. F	Polypectomy,	Sigmoid	:15mm. P-J type polyp with adenoma
25	43y. M	Surgical,	Rectum	:42mm. Carcinoma (s), ulcerating
26	56y. M	Polypectomy,	Rectum	: 8mm. Carcinoma (m) in adenoma

The small letter in parenthesis indicates depth of invasion of carcinoma; serosal(s), submucosal(sm) and mucosal(m).

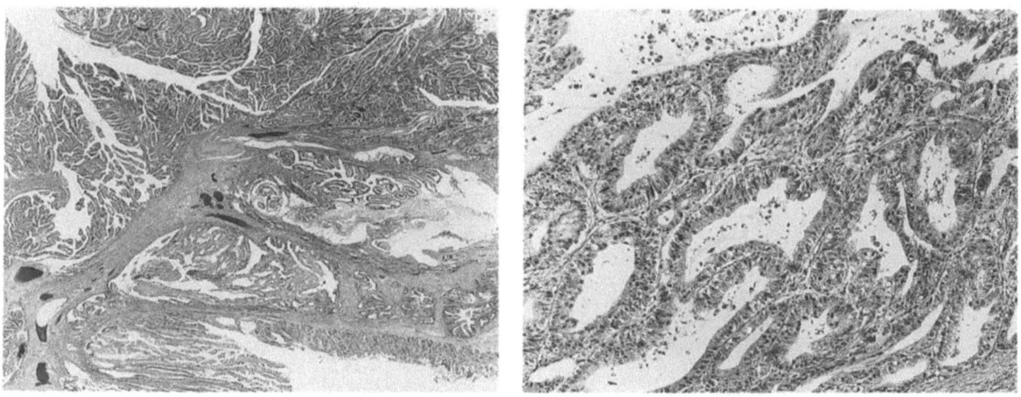

a b

Fig. 1a-1b. A Peutz-Jeghers polyp with carcinoma (sm) in adenoma, duodenal polyp 35mm in size (case 16). (1a, x8), Carcinoma in submucosa (1b, x88).

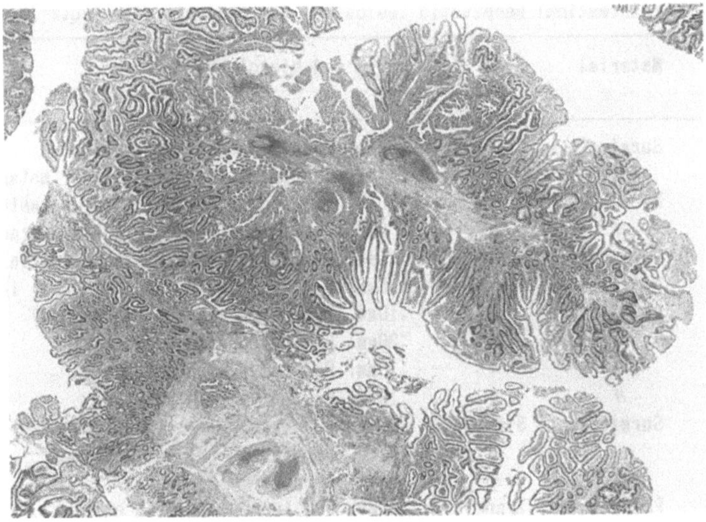

Fig. 2. A peutz-Jeghers polyp with a small focus of papillary adenocarcinoma invading down to the submucosa, duodenal polyp, 10mm in size (case 16)(2a-2d, x 20).

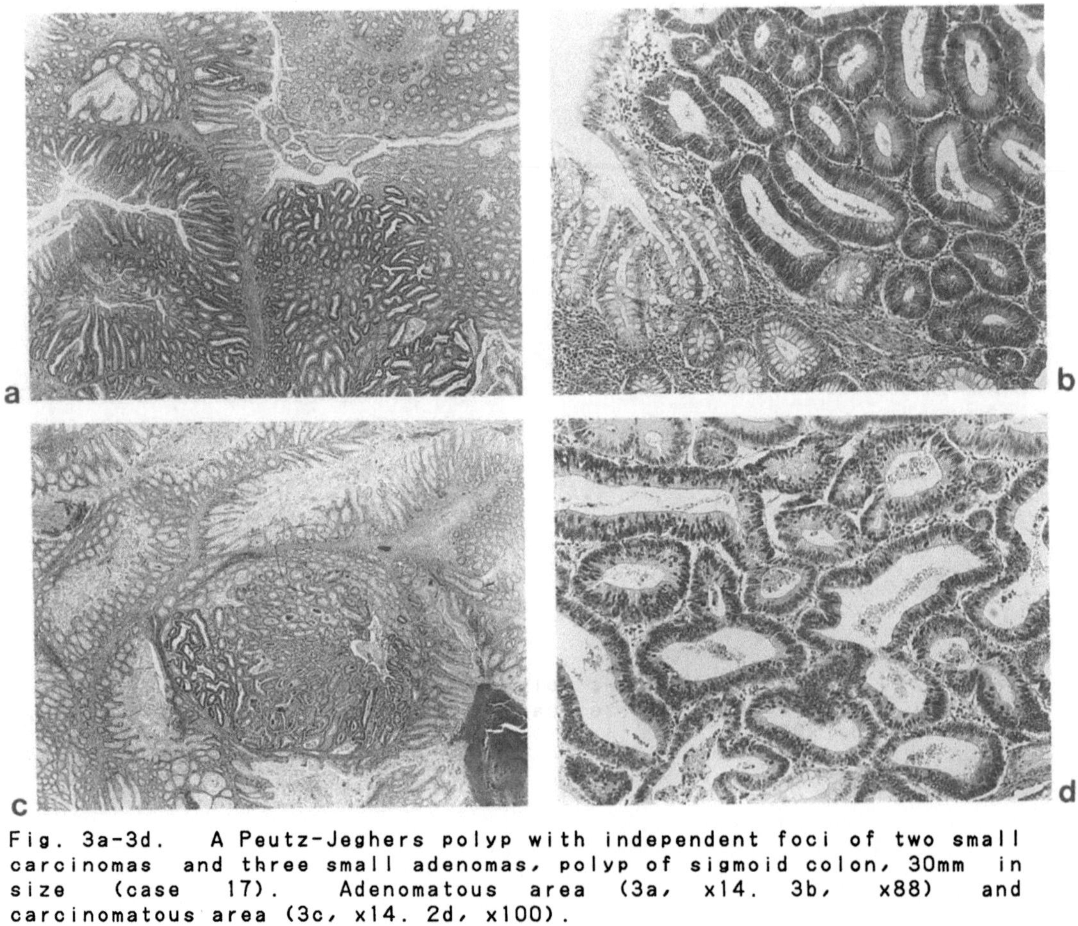

Fig. 3a-3d. A Peutz-Jeghers polyp with independent foci of two small carcinomas and three small adenomas, polyp of sigmoid colon, 30mm in size (case 17). Adenomatous area (3a, x14. 3b, x88) and carcinomatous area (3c, x14. 2d, x100).

In addition to carcinoma or carcinoma in adenoma arising in P-J polyps, other neoplastic lesion, adenoma, was found in P-J polyps or in patients with P-J polyps. Five P-J polyps, three in the duodenum (case 17) and two in the colon (case 19, 24), contained adenomatous area which was various in amount among polyps. Case 17 had a pure adenoma, four P-J polyps (size; 20, 20, 10, 10mm) and a P-J polyp with carcinomas and adenomas. Therefore, at least 8 of 27 patients with P-J polyps had neoplastic lesions in the gastrointestinal tract. Three (11%) of the 27 patients distinctly showed a malignant change of P-J polyps (case 12, 16, 17).

3. INCIDENCE OF NEOPLASTIC CHANGE OF P-J POLYPS BY SIZE

Table 3 indicated an incidence of neoplastic change of P-J polyps by their size in the stomach, small intestine and large intestine. The neoplastic change showed a positive correlation with the size of P-J polyps in the small and large intestine. There was no neoplastic transformation of P-J polyps less than 1 cm, but 5.2% in the small intestinal polyps and 7.1% in the large intestinal polyps in 1 centimeters in size, respectively and 8.6% in the small intestinal polyps and 20% in the large intestinal polyps in 2cm or more in size, respectively.

Table 3 Incidence of neoplastic change of P-J polyps by size

Site	Size					Total
	<1cm	1cm～		2cm～		
		Car.	Adenoma	Car.	Adenoma	
Stomach	0/17	0/4				11
Small intestine	0/219	1/58 (1.7%)	2/58 (3.4%)	2/35 (5.7%)	1/35 (2.9%)	312
Large intestine	0/20	0/14	1/14 (7.1%)	1/10 (10%)	1/10 (10%)	44

4. HISTOGENESIS OF GASTROINTESTINAL CARCINOMA IN P-J POLYPS

From our data, four processes of malignant transformation of P-J polyps are proposed (Watanabe 1983, 1984); (1) malignant transformation of adenoma arisen in P-J polyp, (2) Malignant transformation of P-J polyp itself, (3) malignant change in pure adenoma, and (4) de novo carcinoma in normal mucosa of P-J patients.

The first process is suggested to be the most common as a histogenesis of gastrointestinal carcinoma in P-J polyps. Because five P-J polyps of the small intestine contained adenoma, and two of them had carcinoma in adenoma, and also three colonic P-J polyps contained adenoma (Table 2). On the contrary to the colon and rectum, the small intestine has a very low incidence of adenoma in the general population as well as in the patients with P-J polyps. It is also one of the reasons why the first process is the main as a histogenesis of carcinoma of the small intestine.

The second process is certified by two P-J polyps (case 16, 17) in which cancers were very small in size. The third process is surely present in the patient with P-J polyps as seen in case 26, and is probably seen more frequently in the large intestine than in the small intestine, because of prevalent occurrence of pure adenoma in the colon and rectum.

REFERENCES

Bartholomew LG, Dahlin DC, Waugh JM (1957) Intestinal polyposis associated with mucocutaneous melanin pigmentation (Peutz-Jeghers syndrome). Proc Staff Meet Mayo Clin 32: 675-680

Reid JD, Petrelli M (1974) Intestinal cancer in the Peutz-Jeghers syndrome. A re-evaluation. Ohio State Med J 70: 231-235

Watanabe H, Nashimoto A, Ishihara N, Itoh M (1983) Histopathological study of gastrointestinal lesions with skin manifestation. Stomach and Intestine 18: 465- 473 (in Japanese)

Watanabe H, Suda T (1984) Precancerous lesions of the colon and rectum. Jpn J Cancer Chemother. 11: 1-9 (in Japanese)

Pathology of Polyposis Syndromes with Special Reference to Juvenile Polyposis

JEREMY R. JASS

ABSTRACT

At this time, the final diagnosis of gastrointestinal polyposis rests on the histopathological examination of biopsy or surgical material. The main diagnostic clinical and pathological features of the various polyposis syndromes will be compared and contrasted. Particular emphasis will be placed on juvenile polyposis. The fact that juvenile polyposis is a precancerous syndrome which is inherited on an autosomal dominant basis has been appreciated only recently.

Keywords: gastrointestinal polyposis, juvenile polyposis, pathology, diagnosis, classification.

1. INTRODUCTION

The classification of gastrointestinal polyposis syndromes will surely become clearer within the next few years as we begin to understand the nature of the molecular and genetic events underlying the development of mucosal polyps. However at this time polyps and polyposis syndromes are classified according to the epithelial abnormalities observed through histopathological examination of biopsy or surgical material. Thus polyps are described as neoplastic (adenomas), metaplastic (hyperplastic), hamartomatous (juvenile and Peutz-Jeghers polyps) and inflammatory. A more fundamental division would be the separation of epithelial (as above) from non-epithelial polyps. It is worth stressing that the commonest form of polyposis is benign lymphoid polyposis. Simple hyperplasia of lymphoid tissue is common in young children and adults and may be confused with familial adenomatous polyposis on the basis of endoscopic or radiologic examination. This emphasises the importance of establishing a tissue diagnosis in all cases and it is prudent to obtain a representative sample, say five polyps. Epithelial polyposis syndromes may be further classified into those that are hereditary and those that are non-hereditary. However, whilst it is clear that some forms of polyposis are inherited on an autosomal dominant basis, we are uncertain about the role of inherited factors in Turcot syndrome and in the multiple adenoma syndrome. The picture is further confused by the description of families showing particular extra-gastrointestinal manifestations. Gardner syndrome is now regarded as a variant of familial adenomatous polyposis. Cowden syndrome and the Ruvalcaba-Myhre-Smith syndrome may be variants of juvenile polyposis. Molecular genetic studies will doubtless shed some light on these problems in the future.

In this presentation particular emphasis will be placed on the pathology of juvenile polyposis. The fact that this syndrome is inherited on an autosomal dominant basis and is associated with an increased risk of large bowel cancer has been appreciated only relatively recently.

2. NATURE OF JUVENILE POLYPS

The juvenile polyp is regarded as a hamartoma or malformation in which tissues indigenous to the organ of origin are essentially normal but are arranged in a haphazard manner. One of the striking features of the polyp on histological examination is the excessive amount of lamina propria. It may be conjectured that the lamina propria in affected individuals is especially prone to overgrowth at a particular developmental stage (ie in childhood). Furthermore it would seem that this overgrowth is caused by a relatively trivial inflammatory stimulus. When these polyps are examined at an early stage they comprise oedematous and hyperaemic lamina propria with minor ulceration of the overlying epithelium. Gradually the lamina propria expands and the glands embedded within it become coiled, branched and cystic.

3. CLINICAL FEATURES OF SOLITARY JUVENILE POLYPS

Juvenile polyps usually present in childhood with rectal bleeding. Children are aged from 1-10 with a peak at 4-5 years. They may occur in as many as 1% of children. Although traditionally regarded as solitary lesions and mainly confined to the rectum, over half the children in a colonoscopic survey had more than one polyp and these were distributed evenly throughout the colon (Mestra 1986). The polyps may undergo spontaneous amputation with passage of the head per rectum.

4. PATHOLOGY OF JUVENILE POLYPS

Macroscopically the typical lesion has a smooth spherical red head and a narrow stalk. The cut surface showed cysts filled with mucin. The thin stalk and head lacks muscularis mucosae. This distinguishes the lesion from another type of hamartoma, the Peutz-Jeghers polyp. The latter is characterised by a tree-like branching of bands of muscle extending up from the muscularis mucosae. In addition Peutz-Jeghers polyps have a papillary configuration.

Microscopically, juvenile polyps consist of epithelial tubules which may be dilated or cystic and embedded in an excess of lamina propria. The tubules are lined by an essentially normal epithelium. The surface is frequently ulcerated and there may be inflammation of the lamina propria. This results in reactive or regenerative change within the epithelium which may be mistaken for dysplasia.

5. MALIGNANT CHANGE WITHIN JUVENILE POLYPS

There are only two descriptions of malignant change within an isolated juvenile polyp (Schilla 1954; Liu et al. 1978). On reviewing the material it would seem that only the latter is a genuine example of malignant change within a juvenile polyp. Adenomatous change within a solitary juvenile polyp is equally rare having been reported only once (Friedman & Fechner 1982).

6. CLINICAL FEATURES OF JUVENILE POLYPOSIS

In this condition numerous polyps of juvenile type are found in the large intestine. They may also occur in the small bowel and stomach. One form occurs in infancy and is associated with diarrhoea, haemorrhage, malnutrition, intussusception and death at an early age. No family history is found (Sachatello et al. 1974). The remaining cases vary in their age of onset, but a typical presentation would be brisk rectal bleeding occurring in the second decade. The distribution of polyps and clinical features distinguish juvenile polyposis and the Peutz-Jeghers syndrome. In the last, polyps are most numerous in the stomach and small bowel and patients usually present in the first decade with colicky abdominal pain and intussusception. In familial adenomatous polyposis symptoms do not occur until the third or fourth decade and are then associated with the development of malignancy.

In juvenile polyposis there may be a family history indicating an autosomal dominant pattern of inheritance (Smilow et al. 1966). Associated congenital defects are described including abnormalities of the heart, cranium, cleft palate, polydactyly and malrotations of the gut. These abnormalities may be more frequent in cases with no family history of juvenile polyposis. Ganglioneuromatous polyposis has been described in association with juvenile polyposis (Mendelsohn & Diamond 1984).

7. PATHOLOGY OF JUVENILE POLYPOSIS

Patients with juvenile polyposis usually have between 50 and 200 colorectal polyps. Some patients seem to have relatively few polyps, but these tend to be the parent of the propositus. It is conceivable that juvenile polyps are produced only within the first few decades and are subsequently lost through auto-amputation. The polyps may be relatively large and multilobated, though the lobes themselves may be rounded and similar to typical solitary juvenile polyps. The intervening mucosa is entirely normal. Careful inspection of the mucosa in familial adenomatous polyposis often discloses numerous minute polyps between the larger adenomas.

Histological examination allows juvenile polyps to be separated into two broad types. The majority resemble typical solitary type polyps. However about 20% show a multilobated or papillary configuration. The lamina propria may not be particularly obvious and careful examination may show areas of epithelial dysplasia. Mixed polyps may be encountered in which part resembles typical or atypical juvenile polyp whereas the remainder shows the appearance of an adenoma. Some polyps may include features reminiscent of the metaplastic polyp.

8. DIFFERENTIAL DIAGNOSIS OF JUVENILE POLYPOSIS

8.1 Familial Adenomatous Polyposis (FAP)

Juvenile polyposis can usually be distinguished from FAP because the polyps are relatively few in number (50-200) and are separated by entirely normal mucosa. Confusion may arise in patients with numerous atypical juvenile polyps showing adenomatous change. Careful examination of a representative sample should avoid this pitfall.

8.2 Multiple Adenoma Syndrome

Occasionally adult patients may be encountered with multiple adenomas, say between 10 and 100. Little is known of the genetics of this condition or the magnitude of risk of development of cancer. Careful histological examination should distinguish this from juvenile polyposis.

8.3 Turcot Syndrome

Some reports of Turcot syndrome may be describing examples of familial adenomatous polyposis in association with brain tumours, particularly medulloblastoma. However there does appear to be a separate distinct syndrome characterised by an autosomal recessive mode of inheritance (Haggitt & Reid 1986). Adenomas are multiple but do not occur in the same numbers as found in familial adenomatous polyposis. Tumours of the central nervous system including astrocytomas as well as other malignancies tend to occur at a young age. The malignancies may be of relatively low biological aggressiveness.

8.4 Metaplastic (Hyperplastic) Polyposis

In this condition perhaps 50 or a few hundred metaplastic polyps are scattered throughout the large intestine. The polyps may be relatively large and there may be associated adenomas or mixed polyps. The genetics of this condition is not understood and the risk of malignancy may be increased but is not thought to be high. Careful examination of a representative sample should distinguish metaplastic polyposis from juvenile or other forms of polyposis.

8.5 Cronkhite-Canada Syndrome

Biopsy material from this condition may show some resemblance to the juvenile polyp. However the changes are essentially a diffuse nodularity of the mucosa though large discrete polyps may be formed also. This is a disorder of the entire gastrointestinal tract with no familial tendency. There are a number of associated features including alopecia, pigmentation of the skin, dystrophy of the nails, diarrhoea, protein-losing enteropathy and severe electrolyte disturbance.

8.6 Cowden Syndrome

This was named after the family in which it occurred. It is characterised by the presence of gastrointestinal and cutaneous hamartomas together with proliferative lesions of the breast and thyroid (Haggitt & Reid 1986). The gastrointestinal hamartomas may resemble juvenile polyps. Sometimes the polyps may be recognisable as hamartomatous but lack typical juvenile appearance. Many patients with this disease do not have gastrointestinal polyps at all. The syndrome is inherited as an autosomal dominant condition and it is possible that it represents a variant of juvenile polyposis. More research is required.

8.7 Ruvalcaba-Myhre-Smith Syndrome

This is characterised by the combination of macrocephaly, mental deficiency and unusual craniofacial appearance, pigmented macules on the shaft and glans of the penis and hamartomatous intestinal polyposis. The polyps in this condition appear to be typical juvenile polyps. An autosomal dominant mode of inheritance has been suggested. It is likely that this is a variant of juvenile polyposis (Haggitt & Reid 1986).

8.8 Inflammatory Polyposis

Inflammatory injury of the colorectal epithelium may result in diffuse or solitary mucosal proliferation. The polyps range in their gross appearance from finger-like projections to rounded masses. There may be cystic dilatation of glands producing an appearance resembling the juvenile polyp. This is especially true for inflammatory polyps arising at the site of the ureterosigmoidostomy. Careful histological examination, the appearance of the surrounding mucosa and the clinical history should together distinguish inflammatory polyposis from juvenile polyposis.

8.9 Peutz-Jeghers Syndrome

There should be little difficulty distinguishing this from juvenile polyposis. The main distinguishing features have been noted above.

9. CANCER IN JUVENILE POLYPOSIS

At the time of its first description, patients with juvenile polyposis were not considered to be at increased risk of large bowel cancer because the polyps were understood to be hamartomas rather than neoplasms. Even today there are only seven case reports of unequivocal colorectal cancer occurring in association with histologically confirmed juvenile polyposis (Smilow et al. 1966; Stemper, Kent & Summers 1975; Restrepo et al. 1978; Goodman, Yardley & Milligan 1979; Grigioni et al. 1981; Rozen & Baratz 1982; Jarvinen & Fransilla 1984). One of these reports describes a large kindred in which there were 10 patients with single or multiple juvenile polyps and 11 with carcinomas of the gastrointestinal tract including pancreas (Stemper et al. 1975). However, only one patient had both juvenile polyposis and colorectal cancer. The authors concluded that regular follow-up surveillance of patients with juvenile polyposis was not warranted. This assessment was based on the fact that the risk of malignancy was apparently higher in family members without polyposis and that malignant change occurred anywhere within the gastrointestinal tract and not necessarily within juvenile polyps.

There are, however, grounds for questioning the view put forward by Stemper et al. (1975). The alleged absence of juvenile polyposis in family members cannot be taken at face value unless the condition has been excluded by careful examination. Furthermore, the presence of precancerous dysplasia has been documented in colorectal polyps from patients with juvenile polyposis. This change has been observed within juvenile polyps (Haggitt & Pitcock 1970; Kaschula 1971; Velcek et al. 1976; Restrepo et al. 1978; Goodman et al. 1979; Lipper et al. 1981; Grigioni et al. 1981; Mills & Fechner 1982; Grotsky et al. 1982; Jarvinen & Fransilla 1984) and in co-existing adenomas lacking residual features of juvenile polyp (Kaschula 1971; Velcek et al. 1976; Chevrel, Amouroux & Guerad 1976; Barge et al. 1977; Restrepo et al. 1978; Rabin et al. 1984). Thus, there is a well documented histogenetic mechanism for the evolution of colorectal cancer in juvenile polyposis. Finally, although there are only seven fully documented cases of colorectal cancer complicating juvenile polyposis, five of the patients developed cancer below the age of 50 and two were in their twenties.

The St Mark's Polyposis Registry includes 87 patients with juvenile polyposis (Jass et al. 1988). Histopathological material from 80 of these patients was reviewed. Eighteen of the 87 patients have developed large bowel cancer. There were 15 males and 3 females with an average age of 34 years (range 15-59 years). In the patients who developed cancer there was no obvious weighting of particular clinical or pathological features. Thus there was no increased familial instance of juvenile polyposis or of colorectal cancer and the associated juvenile polyps did not show increased dysplasia. Interestingly the cancers from these patients tended to be mucinous or poorly differentiated or both. The cumulative risk of cancer is likely to exceed 50%.

10. HISTOGENESIS OF CANCER IN JUVENILE POLYPOSIS

There is little direct information on the histogenesis of cancer in juvenile polyposis. Dysplasia has been shown to occur in two forms: (1) a focus of adenomatous change within a juvenile polyp and (2) an adenoma showing no residual juvenile features. It is not known whether such adenomas arise de novo or through the total conversion of a pre-existing juvenile polyp. The absence of small adenomas would speak against a de novo origin (Goodman et al. 1979) and our own observations support this view. Furthermore, out of a total of 1032 polyps, only 21 were adenomas with no residual juvenile features. It is clear that dysplasia occurs relatively frequently, especially within juvenile polyps that adopt an atypical configuration. The demonstration of various grades of dysplasia within a series of juvenile polyps provides indirect but important evidence that carcinoma originates within a juvenile polyp. Furthermore, the series includes two malignant polyps one of which was an atypical juvenile polyp and the other a large villous adenoma showing only equivocal evidence of juvenile origins (though the patient himself was only 15 years old).

11. MANAGEMENT OF JUVENILE POLYPOSIS

The first stage of management is correct diagnosis and a working definition of the condition is given below.

1 At least five juvenile polyps and/or
2 Juvenile polyps throughout the gastrointestinal tract and/or
3 Any number of juvenile polyps and a positive family history.

It is clear that the increased malignant potential of juvenile polyposis warrants some form of clinical intervention. The familial nature of the disease means that management should be directed not simply towards the patient but towards the whole family as has been described for familial adenomatous polyposis. Prophylactic colectomy in affected individuals has been advocated (Jarvinen & Fransilla 1984). However regular colonoscopic surveillance would be an acceptable alternative measure. The choice wil be influenced by the severity of the associated symptoms and the feasibility of achieving endoscopic clearance.

12. SPECULATIONS ON THE NATURE OF THE UNDERLYING GENETIC DEFECT

As noted above examination of early polyps suggests that they arise on the basis of faulty overgrowth of the lamina propria. It is possible that the underlying fault centres on the genetic control of interactions between epithelium and stroma. Hence following a relatively trivial stimulus such as mild inflammation or ulceration, there is an excessive and uncoordinated overgrowth of the lamina propria and associated epithelium. It is possible that adenomatous change is secondary and not a genetically determined event. The architectural disorder displayed by juvenile polyps may be accompanied by alterations in the spatial relationship of generative cells which may in turn accelerate the development of adenomatous change. The preceding suggestions are in keeping with the associated developmental defects that may be found in patients with juvenile polyposis.

13. REFERENCES

Barge J, Desvignes G, Maillard J-N, Potet F (1977) Polypose colique associant des aspects juveniles et adenomataux. Presentation d'un cas. Gastroenterol Clin Biol 1: 159-164

Chevrel JP, Amouroux J, Guerad JP (1976) La polypose juvenile. Med Chir Dig 5: 47-54

Friedman CJ, Fechner RE (1982) A solitary juvenile polyp with hyperplastic and adenomatous glands. Dig Dis Sci 27: 946-948

Goodman ZD, Yardley JH, Milligan FD (1979) Pathogenesis of colonic polyps in multiple juvenile polyposis. Report of a case associated with gastric polyps and carcinoma of the rectum. Cancer 43: 1906-1913

Grigioni WF, Alampi G, Martinelli G, Piccaluga A (1981) Atypical juvenile polyposis. Histopathology 5: 361-376

Grotsky HW, Rickert RR, Smith WD, Newsome JF (1982) Familial juvenile polyposis coli. Gastroenterology 82: 494-501

Haggitt RC, Pitcock JA (1970) Familial juvenile polyposis of the colon. Cancer 26: 1232-1238

Haggitt RC, Reid BJ (1986) Hereditary gastrointestinal polyposis syndromes. Am J Surg Pathol 10: 871-887

Jarvinen H, Fransilla KO (1984) Familial juvenile polyposis coli; increased risk of colorectal cancer. Gut 25: 792-800

Jass JR, Williams CB, Bussey HJR, Morson BC (1988) Juvenile polyposis - a precancerous condition. Histopathology 13: 619-630

Kaschula ROC (1971) Mixed juvenile adenomatous and intermediate polyposis coli. Dis Colon Rectum 14: 368-374

Lipper S, Kahn LB, Sandler RS, Varma V (1981) Multiple juvenile polyposis. A study of the pathogenesis of juvenile polyps and their relationship to colonic adenomas. Hum Pathol 12: 804-813

Liu T-H, Chen M-C, Tseng H-C (1978) Malignant change of juvenile polyp of colon. A case report. Chin Med J 4: 434-439

McColl I, Bussey HJR, Veale AMC, Morson BC (1964) Juvenile polyposis coli. Proc Roy Soc Med 57: 896-897

Mecklin J-P, Sipponen P, Jarvinen HJ (1986) Histopathology of colorectal carcinoma and adenomas in cancer family syndrome. Dis Colon Rectum 29: 849-853

Mendelsohn G, Diamond MP (1984) Familial ganglioneuromatous polyposis of the large bowel. Report of a family with associated juvenile polyposis. Am J Surg Pathol 8: 515-520

Mestre J (1986) The changing pattern of juvenile polyps. Am J Gastroenterol 81: 312-314

Mills SE, Fechner RE (1982) Unusual adenomatous polyps in juvenile polyposis coli. Am J Surg Pathol 6: 177-183

Rabin ER, Patel T, Chen F-H, Gunalp S, Brown HW (1984) Juvenile colonic polyposis coli with villous adenoma and retroperitoneal fibrosis: report of a case. Dis Colon Rectum 27: 393-398

Restrepo C, Moreno J, Duque E, Cuello C, Amsel J, Correa P (1978) Juvenile colonic polyposis in Columbia. Dis Colon Rectum 21: 600-612

Rolles CJ (1987) Juvenile intestinal polyps - are they always benign? Br Med J 294: 529

Rozen P, Baratz M (1982) Familial juvenile polyposis with associated colon cancer. Cancer 49: 1500-1503

Sachatello CR, Hahn IS, Carrington CB (1974) Juvenile gastrointestinal polyposis in a female infant. Report of a case and a review of the literature of a recently recognised syndrome. Surgery 75: 107-113

Schilla FW (1954) Carcinoma in a rectal polyp. Am J Surg 4: 434-439

Smilow PC, Pryor CA, Swinton NW (1966) Juvenile polyposis coli. A report of three patients in three generations. Dis Colon Rectum 9: 248-254

Stemper TJ, Kent TH, Summers RW (1975) Juvenile polyposis and gastrointestinal carcinoma. Ann Int Med 83: 639-646

Velcek FT, Coopersmith IS, Chen CK, Kassner EG, Klotz DH, Kottmeir PK (1976) Familial juvenile adenomatous polyposis. J Ped Surg 11: 781-787

Clinicopathologic Features of Flat Adenoma of the Large Bowel

TETSUICHIRO MUTO, MIKI ADACHI, KENICHI SUGIHARA, TOSHIO SAWADA, TADAHIKO MASAKI, and YASUHIKO MORIOKA

ABSTRACT

One hundred and twenty-three "flat adenomas" in 98 patients were collected from the polypectomy and surgically resected specimens, and colonoscopic & histologic characteristics were described. They consisted 9.5% of ordinary polypoid adenomas removed colonoscopically and tended to situate more evenly in the colon than ordinary polypoid adenomas although the commonest site was in the left colon and the rectum. More than 90% of them were under 1cm in diameter and 15% of them showed severe atypia. The importance of recognizing the presence of these small "flat adenomas" as a new precursor of colonic carcinoma was stressed.

Keywords: flat adenoma, adenoma-carcinoma sequence, de novo carcinoma, colonic carcinogenesis, polypectomy

INTRODUCTION

It has been widely accepted that most carcinomas of the large bowel arise from pre-existing adenomas, and adenoma size is the most important factor in determining malignancy; the larger the adenoma, the higher the malignancy rate, the concept being known as adenoma-carcinoma sequence (Muto 1975). The adenomas mentioned here are mostly polypoid in shape and are amenable to endoscopic polypectomy. However, recently non-polypoid adenoma coined as "flat adenoma" has been detected during routine colonoscopy which has not been recognized before (Muto 1985). Our purpose is to present the clinicopathologic features of "flat adenomas" with special reference to its role in the carcinogenesis of colonic carcinoma.

MATERIALS AND METHODS

A total of 123 "flat adenomas"in 98 patients, 92 in 77 polypectomy patients and 31 in 21 surgical patients were collected for the study. They were removed at the Department of Surgery, University of Tokyo between 1972 and 1988. Clinical and colonoscopic features were analyzed in detail and histologic characteristics were investigated with special reference to their relation to small colonic carcinoma.

RESULTS

Colonoscopic Features

The characteristic features of "flat adenoma" are slight elevation with reddish and rather flat surface(Fig.1).

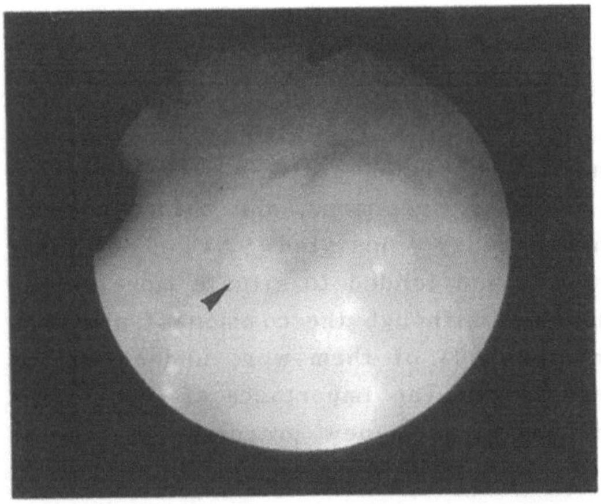

Fig.1. Colonoscopic view of a small "flat adenoma", 5mm in diameter. Note slight central depression with reddish color.

A central depression can be seen when air is properly deflated whereas it becomes entirely flat with too much air inflation. The shape of "flat adenoma" tends to change from "flat" to "sessile" with differing content of air insufflation. Dye spread (methylene blue or indigo carmine) facilitates observation of the central depression (Fig.2).

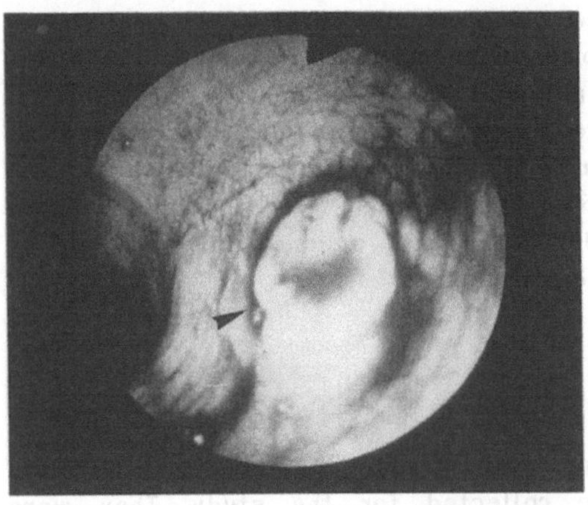

Fig.2 A small "flat adenoma" strikingly demonstrated using less air inflation and dye (methylene blue) spread (same example as shown in Fig.1).

Histologic Features

They were all tubular adenomas with different degree of atypia, 102 adenomas with either mild or moderate atypia and 18 adenomas with severe atypia. Adenomatous tubules tend to occupy the full thickness of the lamina propria with the thin and loose muscularis mucosae. The adenomatous component is less than twice as thick as surrounding normal mucosa. Adenomatous tubules particularly with moderate atypia tends to spread laterally by proliferating between normal glands (Fig.3).

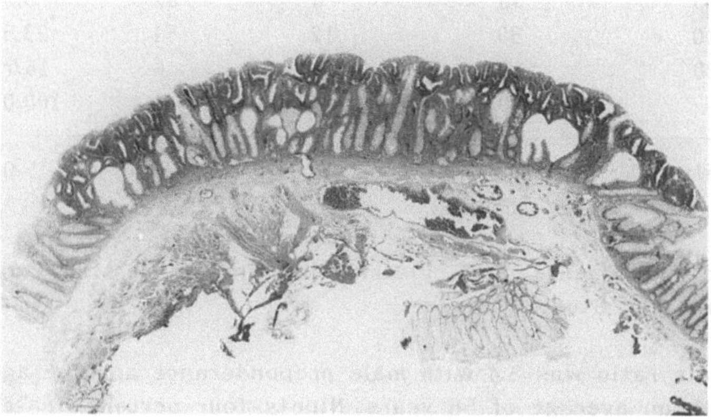

Fig.3. Histology of a "flat adenoma" with moderate atypia (6mm). Note the slight elevation which is occupied by adenomatous tubules showing lateral spread between normal glands and the thin muscularis mucosae.

Sixteen adenomas with severe atypia contained microcarcinomas surrounded by benign tubular adenoma and remaining 2 showed no coexisting benign adenoma which are equivalent to intramucosal carcinomas (Fig.4).

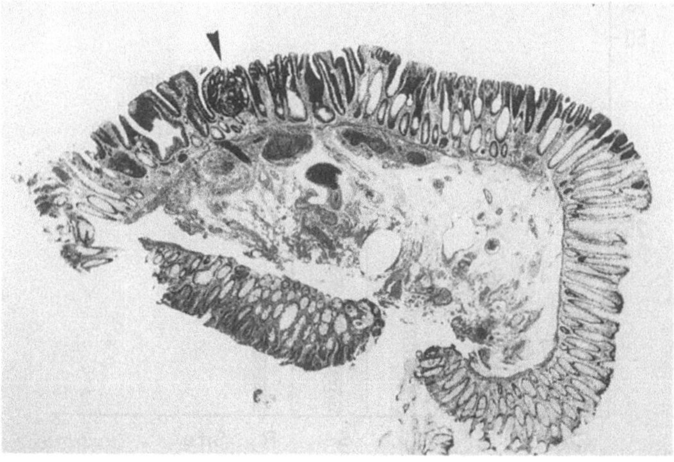

Fig.4. Histology of a "flat adenoma" with severe atypia (7mm). Note the presence of intramucosal carcinoma (arrow).

The frequency of severe atypia in the whole "flat adenomas" examined was as high as 15%. The muscularis mucosae in "flat adenomas" is always thin and loose regardless of the grade of atypia (Table 1).

Table 1. Size and Grade of Atypia

Size (mm)	Grade of atypia: Mild/Moderate	Grade of atypia: Severe	Total	Percentage of Severe Atypia
~ 5	58	4	62	6.5
6~10	39	12	51	23.5
11~20	5	1	6	16.7
21~	0	1	1	100.0
Total	102	18	120	15.0

Sex and Age of Patients, Size, Distribution and Associated Lesions of "Flat Adenomas" in the Study

Male to female ratio was 3.4 with male preponderance and the age ranges from 36 to 82 with an average of 58 years. Ninety-four percent of "flat adenoams" were under 1cm in diameter, more than half being less than 5mm and the frequency of severe atypia increased with increasing size except the lesions more than 1cm in diameter which consist only 6% of "flat adenomas". (Table 1). Thirty-two "flat adenomas" were assciated with polypoid adenoma, 14 with carcinoma, 17 with adenoma & carcinoma and 35 lesions (35.7%) were solitary. They were mostly situated in the left colon and the rectum, however, the frequency in the right colon was much higher than that of polypoid adenomas (Fig.5).

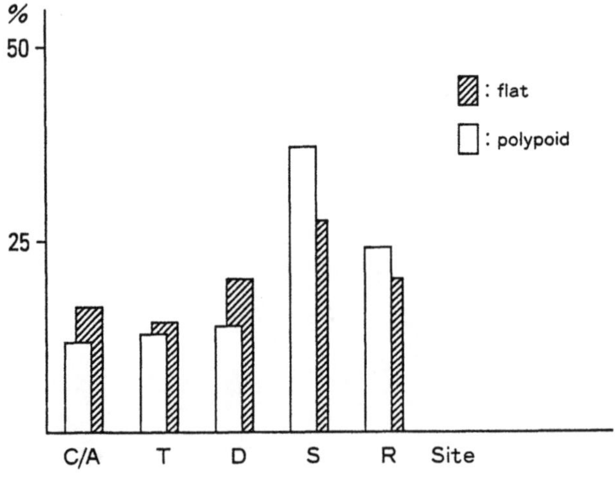

Fig.5. Distribution of flat and polypoid adenoma.

DISCUSSION

Over the past 20 years much attention has been paid to only polypoid adenomas and the concept of adenoma-carcinoma sequence has been established (Muto 1975). Adenoma size is the most important factor in determining potential malignancy. It can be concluded that the larger the adenoma, the higher the malignancy rate. However, these data were based mainly upon surgically resected specimens, which included rather large specimens with advanced disease. However, recent advances in colonoscopy and colonoscopic polypectomy enabled us to collect small polypoid adenomas with severe atypia and moreover, revealed the presence of "flat adenomas " which have not been recognized in the past (Muto 1980,1985).

Clinically they can be easily missed during routine colonoscopy because of their small size and flat shape. The characteristic colonoscopic feature is a plaque like reddish spot of the mucosa which may not be detected by inexperienced eyes. However, once one gets used to the colonoscopic appearances recognition of "flat adenoma" during routine coloscopy is not so difficult (Muto 1987). For colonoscopic detection of "flat adenomas" it is essential to recognize the presence of such tiny lesions and not to miss every tiny reddish spots of the mucosa during routine colonoscopy. It is assumed that the frequency of "flat adenoma" in general population seems to be much higher than might be expected when the increasing frequency from 3% to 9% in our polypectomy series over the past 10 years is taken into consideration (Muto 1987). Two-third of them were associated with either adenoma or carcinoma but remaining one-third was detected by chance as a solitary lesion without any clinical symptoms. Although the most frequent site is the left colon and the rectum they tend to distribute more evenly than polypoid adenomas. In recent years special attention is being paid to "flat adenomas" as they tend to be found in the colon with cancer family syndrome, however, family history was not carefully taken in our series and any detailed information concerning family history was not obtained in this study (Lynch 1988).

Histologically they have quite characteristic features in terms of growth pattern of adenomatous tubules. Interestingly they were all tubular adenomas and tend to grow laterally instead of growing towards the lumen which is the case in ordinary polypoid adenomas. The growth pattern is more similar to that of sessile adenomas, particularly sessile villous adenomas, however, the adenomatous component of "flat adenomas" is always less than twice as thick as surrounding normal mucosa and the surface appeared flat with occasional central depression. The most striking feature of "flat adenoma" is the frequency of severe atypia being as high as 15% and most of them contains coexisting adenomatous component. Considering the small size ,more than 90% being under 1cm in diameter, the rate of severe atypia is extremely high as compared to that of polypoid adenoma with the same size (2.8%). As adenoma with severe atypia is equivalent to the stage of intramucosal carcinoma and considered to be a precursor of invasive carcinoma, it is assumed that "flat adenoma" with severe atypia plays an important role in

carcinogenesis of colorectal carcinoma through adenoma-carcinoma sequence. It is not unreasonable to assume that carcinoma arising from "flat adenoma" may destroy and replace preexisting adenomatous tissue in a short time, then invade the submucosa through the thin, loose muscularis mucosae. In another words, carcinoma arising in a small "flat adenoma" seems to become invasive carcinoma more easily and rapidly than carcinomas in a small polypoid adenoma. Although there is no clinical data as to the natural history of "flat adenomas", it is most likely for "flat adenoma" to become small invasive carcinoma. Recent reports suggest that small carcinomas under 1cm in diameter without residual adenomatous tissue are considered to be carcinomas arising "de novo", however, they might have arisen from pre-existing small "flat adenoma" described here (Kuramoto 1989).
Furthermore, DNA study of adenomas with moderate atypia showed that some of them already had non-diploid character suggesting nuclear changes towards malignancy (unpublished data). Therefore, it can be assumed that "flat adenomas" may have much higher malignant potential as currently estimated. As to the management of "flat adenoma" colonoscopic polypectomy is safe and adequate treatment. When forceps biopsy is taken from "flat adenoma" the chance of sampling adenomatous tissue with severe atypia is considerably high which would make erroneous diagnosis of carcinoma and mislead patients management. They can be easily and safely treated by colonoscopic polypectomy as their size is rather small. After deflating the air they tend to become sessile in shape and are amenable to safe colonoscopic removal.

REFERENCES

Kuramoto S, Oohara T (1989) Flat early cancers of the large intestine. Cancer 64:950-955

Lynch HT, Lanspa SJ, Boman BM, Smyrk T, Watson P, Lynch JF, Lynch PM, Cristofaro G, Bufo P, Tauro AV, Mingazzini P, DiGiulio E (1988) Hereditary nonpolyposis colorectal cancer - Lynch syndromes I and II. In: Luk GD(ed) Gastroenterology Clinics of North America. W B Saunders, Philadelphia London Toronto Montreal Sydney Tokyo, 17:679-712

Muto T, Bussey HJ, Morson BC (1975) The evolution of cancer of the colon and rectum. Cancer 36:2251-2270

Muto T, Kamiya J, Sawada T, Kusama S, Itai Y, Ikenaga T, Yamashiro M, Hino Y, Yamaguchi S (1980) Colonoscopic polypectomy in diagnosis and treatment of early carcinoma of the large intestine. Dis Colon Rectum 23:68-75

Muto T, Kamiya J, Sawada T, Konishi F, Sugihara K, Kubota Y, Adachi M, Agawa S, Saito Y, Morioka Y, Tanprayoon T (1985) Small "flat adenoma" of the large bowel with special reference to its clinicopathologic features. Dis Colon Rectum 28:847-851

Muto T, Adachi M, Sawada T, Kubota Y, Saito Y, Ooya T, Sunouchi K, Masaki T, Morioka Y (1987) Endoscopic and histological features of small early carcinomas of the colon with special reference to flat elevation and II. type carcinoma. Stomach Intestine 22:397-406 (in Japanese with English abstract)

Histologic Features of Hereditary Nonpolyposis Colorectal Carcinoma

THOMAS C. SMYRK, HENRY T. LYNCH, PATRICE A. WATSON, and HENRY D. APPELMAN

ABSTRACT

The clinical features of Hereditary Nonpolyposis Colorectal Cancer (HNPCC) are well established, but less is known about the histology of the carcinomas that occur in the syndrome. We reviewed 86 colorectal cancers from 66 patients belonging to 15 HNPCC families and compared them to a series of 40 sporadic tumors.

The hereditary group was remarkable for the number of carcinomas with absent gland lumens, a marked peritumoral inflammatory infiltrate and a marked Crohn's-like reaction in the region of the tumor. The hereditary group also had fewer patients with local spread through the muscularis propria and fewer with lymph node metastases. The latter four features contribute to the apparently improved survival of patients affected with HNPCC.

Key words: hereditary colon cancer, histology, prognosis

INTRODUCTION

The characteristic clinical features of HNPCC - autosomal dominant transmission, early age of cancer onset, proximal colonic involvement and a propensity for multiple tumors - have been described by authors from several countries (Lynch 1988, Mecklin 1986, Vasen 1989). Of these, only Mecklin has provided a detailed description of tumor histology. He found an excess of poorly differentiated carcinomas and mucinous carcinomas in cancer family patients compared to controls. Mecklin remarked on the discrepancy between these aggressive histologic features and reports of favorable prognosis in patients with HNPCC (Albano, 1982).

We reviewed 86 colorectal carcinomas from 66 HNPCC patients. In addition to recording the site and stage of all tumors, we utilized parameters summarized by Jass (1987) to develop a more complete description of the lesions. The parameters analyzed included tubule configuration, growth pattern, host inflammatory response, vascular and perineural invasion, and the Crohn's-like reaction recently described by Graham (1989). The histologic features of HNPCC were compared to those of 40 consecutive carcinomas resected from patients with no known family history of colon cancer.

MATERIAL AND METHODS

The Hereditary Cancer Center at Creighton University has on file the pedigrees of more than 25 families that have been designated as HNPCC based on the presence of multiple colorectal cancers in multiple generations. As part of the pedigree analysis, efforts are made to obtain pathologic material on all affected patients from the hospital at which surgery was performed. The fifteen families that make up this report were chosen using two criteria: colorectal cancer in at least three first-degree relatives (the criterion used by Mecklin for inclusion in his 1986 study of Finnish cancer families), and at least two tumors available for histologic review. Six of these families have been described in a previous publication (Lynch 1988) as Families 2, 3, 4, 8, 9 and 10.

Information about patient age and site of colorectal cancer were taken from the pathology report. Survival data was ascertained by interview with family members and review of medical records.

Histopathologic review of HNPCC cases was accomplished using slides provided by contributing hospitals, or slides cut from contributed paraffin blocks. The control group consisted of 40 consecutive cases of colorectal cancer resected at Creighton's affiliated hospital during 1987-88; none was known to come from a cancer family. Reviewers were not blinded to the source of the slides being reviewed. Histologic parameters were scored according to the definitions below.

Local spread: The deepest point of invasion was recorded as being either mucosa, submucosa, into muscularis propria, through muscularis propria or to the serosal surface. Direct invasion into adjacent organs was not recorded.

Lymph node spread: The total number of lymph nodes dissected from the specimen and the number involved by metastatic tumor were noted.

Tubule pattern: Simple tubules are round or oval tubules lined by a single layer of epithelium. Complex tubules have a similar outline, but contain multiple secondary spaces. Irregular tubules have distorted outlines and small, irregular lumens. Tumors with absent tubules form sheets of tumor cells. Tubule pattern was graded according to the worst area present.

Growth pattern: Tumors with a sharply circumscribed, "pushing" margin were designated as having expanding growth. Infiltrative growth was defined as diffuse permeation of normal structures such that tumor margins were difficult to define.

Inflammatory response: The inflammatory mantle of lymphocytes, plasma cells, eosinophils or neutrophils at the advancing edge of the tumor was graded as marked if a distinct cap of inflammatory cells was present. The infiltrate was usually composed of lymphocytes, but there were cases with dense eosinophilic inflammation. A slight or absent inflammatory infiltrate was considered a negative response.

Vascular invasion: Only invasion of extramural veins with muscular walls was recorded. No special stains were used to help identify vessels.

Perineural invasion: Both perineural and endoneural invasion were noted; if either was present, positive perineural invasion was recorded.

Crohn's reaction: A marked Crohn's reaction was defined as numerous lymphoid aggregates in advance of the tumor margin. Germinal centers were sometimes present, but were not required. Small numbers of lymphoid aggregates (one or two per tissue section) or absent lymphoid aggregates indicated a negative Crohn's reaction.

Some parameters were combined to create the prognostic score described by Jass and Morson (1987). One point was assigned for a tumor that extended through the muscular wall of the bowel, one point for metastases to lymph nodes, another point if more than four nodes were involved, one point for an infiltrative growth pattern, and one point if a marked lymphocytic mantle was not seen at the advancing tumor edge. The minimum score for a particular carcinoma was 0, the maximum was 5. The scores were used to assign tumors to one of four groups: Score 0 or 1 = group I, 2 = II, 3 = III, and 4 or 5 = IV.

Cumulative survival curves were constructed based on information gathered from interviews with family members, review of medical records and retrieval of death certificates. Information about disease status in those patients still living, and cause of death in those who have died, was only partially available and was not included in the analysis. For patients with multiple colon cancers, survival was calculated from the date of diagnosis of the first malignancy.

Statistical analysis: Most variables were analyzed by cross tabulation into 2 x 2 tables, and significance of the association was evaluated using Fisher's Exact Test (two-tailed). The groups derived from the Jass and Morson scores were crosstabulated with source (HNPCC or control) and significance of association was tested using the Chi-square test.

RESULTS

The clinical features of the HNPCC group paralleled those previously reported. The mean age at first diagnosis was 47.5 years. Sixty of the 85 tumors for which location was known were proximal to the splenic flexure (71%). In contrast, the average age of the control group was 67.5 years and 50% of tumors arose in the right colon.

As shown in Table 1, the HNPCC group had significantly more tumors with absent tubules, marked inflammatory response and marked Crohn's reaction. There were also more tumors with expanding growth, although the difference was not significant. In contrast to Mecklin's experience (1986), we did not see an excess of mucinous carcinomas. Seven carcinomas in the hereditary group contained signet cells, compared to one of the control cases. The extent of spread was different in the two groups: fewer tumors in the HNPCC families had breached the muscularis propria and fewer had metastasized to regional lymph nodes.

Neither absent tubules, expanding growth, or Crohn's reaction were more common in right-sided tumors. A marked lymphocytic response was seen in 34% of proximal tumors versus 15% of distal ones ($p<0.05$), but the difference in lymphocyte response between HNPCC and controls was seen regardless of site (39% vs 20% in the right colon and 21% vs 10% in the left colon).

Table 2 shows the effect of consolidating parameters in the Jass scoring system. The hereditary tumors were much more likely to have a low score and the control cases were more likely to have a high score.

Table 1: Histologic Features of colorectal carcinoma

Parameter	HNPCC	Controls	
Absent tubules	35	13	$p<0.01$
Expanding growth	65	48	$p<0.08$
Marked inflammation	35	15	$p<0.04$
Crohn's reaction	42	20	$p<0.04$
Mucinous (1)	11	8	$p<0.75$
Through wall	69	87	$p<0.03$
Nodal metastases	25	48	$p<0.02$

(1) Mucinous carcinoma defined as tumors with more than 60% extracellular mucin.

Table 2 Distribution of Jass scores

Group	HNPCC	Controls
I	40%	15%
II	25%	18%
III	21%	40%
IV	14%	27%

$p<0.01$ for the difference in distribution

Table 3: Five Year Survival (%) in HNPCC

Dukes Stage	Jass Score	Inflammatory Response	Crohn's Reaction	Grade
A 100	I 97	Marked 100	Marked 95	Well 80
B 82	II,III 79			Mod 77
C 71	IV 64	Negative 74	Negative 82	Poor 92

The first colorectal cancer diagnosed was available for review in 63 of the 66 HNPCC patients. Followup was achieved for 62 of these; the mean length of followup was 10.5 years. The overall five-year survival was 83%. Among the individual histologic parameters reviewed, only lymphocyte response gave statisically different survival curves. (Table 3) Poor histologic grade, as evidenced by absent tubules, did not adversely affect survival. Both Dukes' stage and Jass score gave some some prognostic information, but the Jass score identified a larger subset of patients with good prognosis: only 14% of HNPCC patients presented with a Dukes A tumor, but 47% of them fell into Jass Group I.

DISCUSSION

Previous work with HNPCC has yielded two disparate observations: There is an excess of poorly differentiated carcinomas (Mecklin 1986) and there is improved survival compared to patients with apparently sporadic colorectal cancer (Albano 1982). Our findings provide support for both observations, and offer an explanation for the apparent incongruity.

Histologic grade is accepted as an independent predictor of survival (Chapuis 1985, Phillips 1984). Grade is usually based on the degree of glandular differentiation. Thus, our observation that 35% of carcinomas in HNPCC families have areas lacking gland lumens is in keeping with Mecklin's 1986 report that 24% of such carcinomas are poorly differentiated.

Other histologic features, ignored in most grading schemes, may affect prognosis. Inflammation at the advancing edge of tumor is regarded as indicative of host resistance; several studies have shown that such a response confers improved survival (Jass 1986, Murray 1975). A particular type of inflammatory response, termed the Crohn's reaction by Graham and Appelman (1989), also appears to confer favorable prognosis. Both types of inflammation were significantly more common in the HNPCC group than in controls.

An expanding growth pattern has also been associated with favorable prognosis (Carlon 1985). The increased number of tumors with expanding growth in the HNPCC falls short of statistical significance.

Tumor stage is an independent predictor of survival in colorectal cancer. In our review, carcinomas from HNPCC patients were significantly less likely than controls to have breached the muscularis propria or to have metastasized to regional lymph nodes.
There are several potential sources of bias in this study. First, histologic assessment of the parameters described above is unavoidably subjective. This inherent subjectivity, combined with the fact that the pathologists were aware of the source of the slides under review makes bias possible. Future studies should be designed so that coded slides are reviewed blindly. Second, the retrospective nature of the study makes the lymph node status of HNPCC cases dependent on the care with which other pathologists have searched for nodes. One marker of the pathologists' diligence is the number of nodes recovered from each specimen: In the HNPCC group, dissected at more than 30 institutions over a 40 year period, an average of 9.5 nodes were reported for each case. In the control group, dissected at one institution over a six month period, the average was 14.5 nodes per specimen ($p<0.05$). Finally, the apparent differences revealed by using the scoring system of Jass and Morson (1987) are dependent on both lymph node dissection and histologic grading, so that both sampling differences and reviewer subjectivity may affect the results.

The prognosis of HNPCC is remarkably good; the 5-year survival of 83% is particularly impressive when one considers that 10% of the patients developed additional colon tumors during the 5 year period. While improved survival may be partly accounted for by early stage at diagnosis, the presence of a marked peritumoral inflammatory infiltrate identified a group with favorable prognosis and the Jass score, based on a combination of staging and histologic parameters, identified a large subset (47%) of HNPCC patients with a particularly good prognosis.

Are the histologic differences described here inherent in the tumors of HNPCC or are they related to the tendency for right-sided distribution? Among the histologic parameters we analyzed, only lymphocytic response was significantly associated with proximal tumors. Of great interest for the future will be the correlation of site, histology and genetic alterations.

CONCLUSION

The colorectal carcinomas that arise in the setting of HNPCC appear to behave less aggressively than sporadic cancers. This difference is reflected both in patient survival and in the histologic appearance of the tumors. A study utilizing blinded review of cases is necessary to confirm that these histologic differences exist.

Albano WA, Recabaren JA, Lynch HT, Campbell AS, Mailliard JA, Organ CH, Lynch JF, Kimberling WJ (1982) Natural history of hereditary cancer of the breast and colon. Cancer 50:360-363

Carlon CA, Fabris G, Arslan-Pagnini C (1985) Prognostic correlations of operable carcinoma of the rectum. Dis Colon Rectum 28;47-50

Chapuis PH, Dent OF, Fisher R (1985) A multivariate analysis of clinical and pathological variables in prognosis after resection of large bowel cancer. Br J Surg 72:698-702

Graham D, Appelman HD (1989) Crohn's type lymphoid reaction in colon carcinoma. Modern Pathol 2:34A

Jass JR (1986) Lymphocytic infiltration and survival in rectal cancer. J Clin Pathol 39:585-589

Jass JR and Morson BC (1987) Reporting colorectal cancer. J Clin Pathol 40:1016-1023

Lynch HT, Watson P, Lanspa SJ, Marcus J, Smyrk T, Fitzgibbons RJ, Kriegler M, Lynch JF (1988) Natural history of colorectal cancer in hereditary nonpolyposis colorectal cancer (Lynch syndromes I and II). Dis Colon Rectum 31:439-444

Mecklin J-P, Sipponen P, Jarvinen HJ (1986) Histopathology of colorectal carcinomas and adenomas in Cancer Family Syndrome. Dis Colon Rectum 29:849-853

Murray D, Hreno A, Dutton J, Hampson LG (1975) Prognosis in colon cancer. A pathologic reassessment. Arch Surg 110:908-913

Phillips RKS, Hittinger R, Blesovsky L (1984) Large bowel cancer: Surgical pathology and its relationship to survival. Br J Surg 71:604-610

Vasen HFA, Hartog Jager FCA, Menko FH, Nagengast FM (1989) Screening for hereditary nonpolyposis colorectal cancer: A study of 22 kindreds in the Netherlands. Am J Med 86:278-281

Crypt Atrophy of Colorectal Mucosa in Lynch Syndromes I and II: Its Characteristics and Meaning, Preliminary Observations

PANTALEO BUFO, FLORIANO FRASSANITO, HEIKE MÜLLER, GIUSEPPE CRISTOFARO, SILVANO SENATORE, HENRY D. APPELMAN, and HENRY T. LYNCH

SUMMARY

In twelve young patients (7 males and 5 females, mean age 30.5 years) with findings of Lynch syndromes, crypt atrophy with macrophage excess in colorectal mucosa have been noted. The authors tried to support the simple subjective observation with morphometrical data. Evaluation of the specimens of colonic mucosa was performed, using a semiautomatic Video-Assistence-Unit attached to a microscope. In our set, the mean of the Volume Fraction of crypts is 37.43 (S.D. 9.6), considerably below the values found in 15 healthy subjects used as control group (Mean=58.75, S.D.=12.7).
Our results suggest that crypt atrophy in young relatives at risk could be considered a premonitory phenotipic manifestation, advising to put under special control patients who show this pattern and to investigate, whether they are more likely to develop carcinomas than the general population.

Keywords: hereditary colorectal cancer, Lynch syndromes, crypt atrophy, stereology.

INTRODUCTION

Hereditary nonpolyposis colorectal cancer (HNPCC) includes two henceforth well known entities, the Lynch syndromes I and II (Lynch 1966, Lynch et al 1971; Lynch, Lanspa, Smyrk, Bowman et al 1988). Both are characterized by susceptibility to nonpolyposis colorectal cancer, with a striking predilection to the proximal colon and early age of onset. In addition, the Lynch syndrome II also shows a susceptibility to carcinoma of the endometrium, ovary, pancreas, stomach and possibly cancer of other anatomic sites (Lynch, Lanspa, Smyrk et al 1988).
As already stated, both syndromes apparently lack distinctive feature of non neoplastic colonic mucosa or a characteristic premalignant lesion which allows to identify, on the ground of phenotipic manifestation, subjects at risk (Lynch, Smyrk, Lanspa et al 1988).
Some interest has been rousen by the presence of so-called "flat adenomas" (Muto 1985) in some members of these families (Lynch, Smyrk, Lanspa, Marcus et al 1988), because of the possible relationship between these morphological precursors and the conclamated cancer.

Of the two lines of investigation, suggested by Lynch et al (1988), we have privileged that of prospective screening of patients at risk for the syndrome. Cristofaro et al (1985) discovered a large Italian family (329 members, 7 generations) with well documented Lynch syndrome II, and then another family (22 members), which showed a Lynch syndrome I. In ten asymptomatic subjects, who underwent colonscopy, an atrophy of colonic mucosa was detected, characterized by rarefication of crypts and an excess of macrophages in the lamina propria. Two other cases were added recently (See Fig. 1 and 2) Therefore it seemed interesting to support the subjective findings of atrophy with stereological study, since our remarks await confermation and extention to other families (Lynch, Smyrk, Lanspa, Marcus et al 1988).

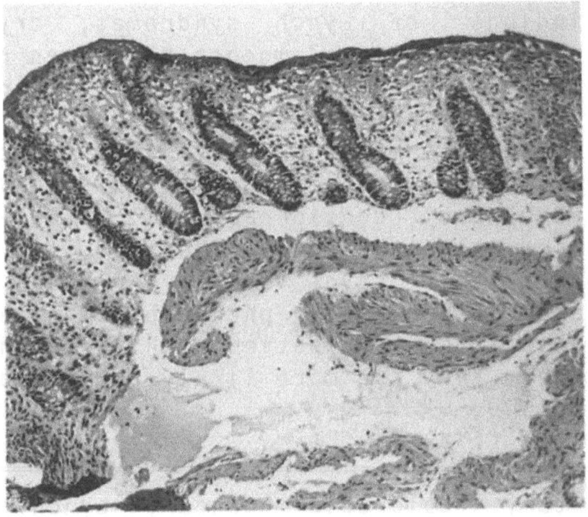

Fig. 1. Lynch syndrome II. Colonic mucosa: atrophy and rarefication of crypts (H&E, 25X).

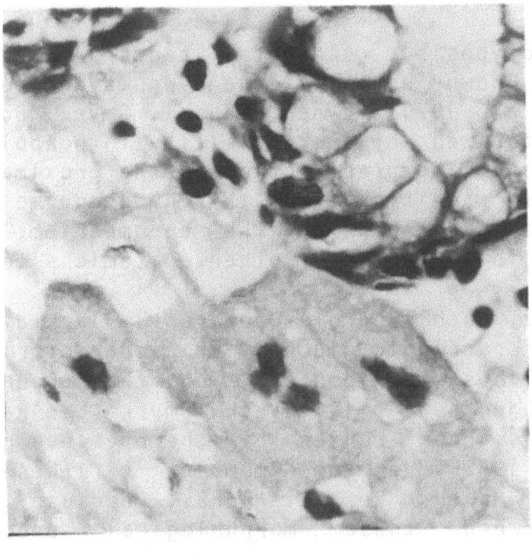

Fig. 2. Small group of muciphages in the lamina propria of the colonic mucosa. (H&E, 400X).

MATERIAL AND METHODS

The endoscopical specimens, used for the study, were obtained from twelve asymptomatic subjects, members of two large Italian kindreds with Lynch syndromes I e II (22 and 328 members respectively), in whom were found some interesting pathological findings, such as crypt atrophy and macrophage excess of colorectal mucosa. All the subjects, 7 males and 5 females, were young (mean age 30.5 years), therefore the presence of a marked crypt atrophy was unexpected.
The fragments of mucosa were first fixed in 10% neutral buffered formalin and then adeguately oriented and embedded in paraffin. One 5 micron section of each specimen, stained with H & E, was processed, in order to evaluate the Volume Density of crypts in each case.
The stereological analysis was performed by point counting method with a semiautomatic Video Assistence Unit (V.A.U.- Metamorphosis s.r.l. Bari-Italy) attached to a Olympus BH-2 microscope.
On the monitor screen of the Video Assistence Unit was displayed the image of the colorectal mucosa, taken from the slide by a CCD camera at the standardized linear magnification of 100X. An electronically synthesized test grid was superimposed on the analogic image and, to evaluate the accuracy of our work, the relative standard error of Point Density was calculated with the following formula:

$$RSE(Pp)=\sqrt{(1-Pp)/(Pc*Pp)}$$

where:
RSE(Pp) is the relative standard error of Pp, Pp is the rate Pa/Pc, Pa is the number of test points in the object space, Pc is the number of test points of the containing space (Selkainaho 1982).
The RSE value, in our set, remains under 0.1, which confirms, that the number of test points was sufficiently large.
The same stereological analysis was performed in 15 specimens of normal colorectal mucosa of unaffected adult subjects. The results were used for comparison.
No correction of the Volume Density of crypts has been necessary, because the shrinkage of the colonic mucosa on the basal side (due to contraction of the muscolaris mucosae) was constant, as the specimens were all fixed in phosphate buffered formalin.

RESULTS

In our set of 12 subjects (Table I) the mean of the Volume Fraction of the crypts was 37.43 (S.D. 9.62). The Volume Fraction of crypts in the control group (15 specimens) was 58.75 (S.D. 12.7). The differences between the two groups were statistically significant ($P<0.001$).

Table I. Mean and standard deviation of crypt (epithelial) fraction and stromal fraction in specimens of subjects with Lynch syndromes and normal

	LYNCH SYNDROME (n= 12)		NORMAL (n= 15)	
	Mean	s.d	Mean	s.d
Crypt (epithelial) Fraction	37.43	9.6	58.75	12.7
Stroma Fraction	62.57	9.6	41.25	12.7

Difference highly significant ($P<0.001$) in the comparison between the two groups.

DISCUSSION

The role of primary genetic factors in the etiology of colon cancer has been emphasized by the profitable research in this direction done in the last twenty years (Lynch 1966; Lynch, Lanspa, Boman, Smyrk 1988).
Hereditary Nonpolyposis Colorectal Cancer (HNPCC) represents a challenge to the researchers involved in the field of hereditary colorectal cancer. In fact, phisicians often neglect investigating the cancer family history of affected patients and, furthermore, it is difficult to individualize the families affected. Nevertheless there has been a sharp increase of interest on this issue which is leading to a more extensive identification of subjects at risk, using the family history as the most gainful method.
The enormous progress in the field of genetics and biomolecular studies will allow to easily recognize the affected or at risk subjects in the general population, hopingly in a few years (Cristofaro, Lynch, Caruso, Attolini et al 1987, Lynch, Smyrk, Lanspa, Markus et al 1988).
Pathologists, on the other hand, have highlightened the increased frequency of mucinous adenocarcinoma in the Lynch syndromes (Mecklin et al 1986, Budd and Fink 1982).
Moreover, a certain interest has been rousen by the observation of Muto et al. (1985) of a new entity, which he called "flat adenoma". This histological lesion has been observed in excess in colon-cancer-prone families by some investigators (Lynch, Smyrk, Lanspa, Markus, Kriegler et al 1988; Adachi et al 1988), even though without the high grade dysplasia, frequently seen in the Muto series (1985). Therefore it is impossible to infer conclusive remarks, but, if flat adenomas will be observed in most or even all of the studied kindreds, they could be an important phenotipic marker of hereditary colon-cancer-prone families.

Another recent morphological finding is that of Cristofaro and associates (1987), who observed in young adult members of an Italian family with HNPCC, crypt atrophy and excess of mucosal macrophages.
These remarks were based only on subjective evaluation of the specimens, that is why we carried out our work, using a stereological approach in order to obtain an unbiased judgement.
Our results make evident that there is a statistically significant difference between the subjects whith HNPCC and the control group. The data concerning the control group are very similar to those of the control group of Eide (1986), which confirms the correctness of our method.
As known, the lower portion of the crypts is the proliferative compartment, and the upper portion is the site of cellular differentiation where the exaustion of cells seems to be prevailingly localized (DeSchryver-Kecskemety 1986). Loss of glands is associated to an attempt to regenerate the missing epithelial cells, therefore flat adenomas might represent the abnormal morphological expression of this proliferative process in the upper part of the crypt.
Crypt atrophy is also present in the late stages of inflammatory bowel disease as ulcerative colitis. When carcinoma occurs, it is generally mucinous and arises from atrophic mucosa like that we observed in HNPCC. Furthermore, glandular disruption and epithelial misplacement both seem to play an important role in promoting the development of carcinoma, and could explain the growth of submucosal, flat, infiltrating cancer (Allen and Biggart, 1986).
Although destruction of the mucosa has never been observed in HNPCC the objective demonstration of crypt atrophy and the concomitant presence of muciphages in our cases could be interpreted as expression of an increased, genetically determinated susceptibility of the colonic epithelium to the damage produced by some, still unknown, environmental factors. Consequently, a pathway similar to that postulated for ulcerative colitis might be put forward to explain the infiltrating, mucinous carcinomas often reported in Lynch syndromes.
Our results suggest to put under special control patients who show crypt atrophy and to investigate whether they are more likely than expected to develop carcinomas.

REFERENCES

Adachi M, Muto T, Morioka Y, Ikenage T, Hare M (1988) Flat adenoma and flat mucosa carcinoma (II type) - a new precursor of colorectal carcinoma? Report of two cases. Dis Colon Rect 31: 236-243

Allen DC, Biggart JD (1986) Misplaced epitelium in ulcerative colitis and Crohn's disease of the colon and relantionship to the colon to malignant mucosal changes. Histopathology 10: 37-52

Baak JPA, Oort J.(1983) Practical Morphometry. In: A manual of morphometry in diagnostic pathology. Spinger-Verlag. Berlin Heidelberg New York Tokyo, pp.159-187

Budd DC, Fink DL (1982) Autosomal dominant mucoid colon carcinoma: a study of a case and a kindred. Am Surg 48: 180-188

Cristofaro G, Lynch HT, Caruso ML, Attolini A, Dimatteo G,

Giorgio P, Senatore S, Argentieri A, Sbano E, Guanti G, Fusaro R and Giorgio I(1985) Cancer Family Syndrome (Lynch Syndrome II): preliminary report of new phenotipic findings. Familiar Cancer; Müller & Weber Eds. Karger, Basel. 85-87

Cristofaro G, Lynch HT, Caruso ML, Attolini A, Dimatteo G, Giorgio P, Senatore S, Argentieri A, Sbano E, Guanti G, Fusaro R and Giorgio I(1987) Excess of gastric cancer and precancerous condition in a family with Lynch syndrome II. Epidemiology prevention and early detection of gastric cancer. In: Scientific Committee (ed) CIC Eds. Intern. Roma. 287-289

Cristofaro G, Lynch HT, Caruso ML, Attolini A, Dimatteo G, Giorgio P, Senatore S, Argentieri A, Sbano E, Guanti G, Fusaro R and Giorgio I (1987) New phenotipic aspects in a family with Lynch syndrome II. Cancer. 60: 51-58

DeSchryver-Kekscкemety K (1986) Large intestine. In Henson DE, Albores Saavedra J (ed) The pathology of incipient neoplasia. WB Saunders Company Philadelphia London Toronto Mexico City Rio De Janeiro Sydney Tokyo Hong Kong, pp 147-166

Eide TJ (1986) A morphometrical analysis of dysplasia in small adenomas of the large intestine. Virchows Arch. A 410:119-124

Lynch HT, Shaww MW, Magnuson CW (1966) Hereditary factors in two large midwestern kindreds. Arch Intern Med 117: 206-215

Lynch HT, Krush AJ (1971) Cancer Family "G" Revisited: 1895-1970. Cancer. 27: 1505-1511

Lynch HT, Lanspa SJ, Smyrk T, Boman BM, Watson P, Lynch JF, Cristofaro G (1988) Colorectal Cancer And The Lynch Syndromes. In Lise M, Infantino A, Pucciarelli S (ed) II Congresso Nazionale di Colonproctologia. 9 Sett. - 1 Ott. Cleup, Padova, pp 9-15

Lynch HT, Smyrk T, Lanspa SJ, Marcus JN, Kriegler M, Lynch JF, Appelman HD(1988) Flat Adenomas in a Colon Cancer-Prone Kindred. Journal of the National Cancer Institute. 80 (4): 278-282

Lynch HT, Lanspa SJ, Boman BM, Smyrk T, Watson P, Lynch JF, Lynch PM, Cristofaro G, Bufo P, Tauro AV, Mingazzini P, Di Giulio E (1988) Hereditary Nonpolyposis Colorectal Cancer - Lynch Syndromes I and II. Gastroent Clin North Am 17 (4) 679-712

Lynch HT, Smyrk T, Lanspa SJ, Marcus JN, Boman BM, Watson P, Lynch JF, Boland CR, Appelman H, Cristofaro G, Bufo P, Mingazzini P, Di Giulio E, Tauro AV, Pathology and Genetic Markers of Colorectal Cancer in Lynch Syndromes I and II. Journal of Tumor Marker Oncology 3 (4): 341-350

Mecklin JP, Sipponen P, Jarvinen HJ (1986) Histopathology of colorectal carcinomas and adenomas in Cancer Family Syndrome. Dis Colon Rectum 29: 849-853

Muto J, Kamyia J, Sawada T, (1985) Small "flat adenoma" of the large bowel with special referece to its clinicopathologic features. Dis Colon Rect 28: 847-851

Selkainaho K.(1982) Statistics in stereology and morphometry. Morphometry in morphological diagnosis. Y.Collan,T.Romppanen. Kuopio University Press, Kuopio pp. 1-11

Cellular Immune Response in Lynch Syndrome II on Gastrointestinal Biopsy

SILVANO SENATORE, MASSIMO LONGO, GIUSEPPE CRISTOFARO, GIANNI CAPANO, MICHELE TANCREDI, FRANCA DETA, CATERINA BLASI, SIMONA RINALDI, PANTALEO BUFO, EMILIO DI GIULIO, and HENRY T. LYNCH

ABSTRACT

Immunoregulatory cell interactions between macrophages and T-cell subpopulations suggest the need for evaluation of the cellular immune response in gastrointestinal mucosa of asymptomatic subjects with Lynch Syndrome II. It was observed that macrophages pool coexists with T-cell subsets which had almost the same cellularity. However, an interesting movement of the immune cells distribution correlated to age were observed.

Keywords: Lynch Syndrome II; Immunocytochemistry; Tissue immune cells distributions.

INTRODUCTION

Lynch Syndrome II is a hereditary precancer disorder characterized by hereditary colorectal cancer without florid adenomatosis, a proximal colonic cancer predominance, an excess of metachronous cancer and a significant association with carcinoma of the endometrium, ovary, stomach, and in certain families, pancreas and other forms of cancer (Lynch 1985). This cancerous condition, which affects joung family members (Boland 1984, Lynch 1985), presents early age at cancer onset (Lynch 1985).

At present particular attention has been given to both the problems of phenotypic variation and genetic heterogeneity of hereditary colonic cancer (Lynch 1985) as well as to the assessment of immunological characteristics and their significance in these patients. In particular, previous immunological studies in hereditary non-polyposis colorectal cancer (HNPCC) patients using mixed leucocyte cultures (Lynch 1981, Twomey 1972) showed a deficient cellular immune reaction (Lynch 1981), as did a polyclonal B-cell activation (PBA) in gastrointestinal (g.i.) specimens, detected by immunoenzymatic methods (Senatore 1986).

Both immunoregulatory cell interactions (Cristofaro 1985, Lynch 1981) and macrophages rôle in the modulation of colon cancer growth (Martin 1983) suggest the need for evaluation of the cellular immune response in the g.i. mucosa of asymptomatic subjects with Lynch Syndrome II.

In this study, immunopathologic findings in these subjects were described in order to elucidate their rôle in the most frequent tumor site-related expression.

SUBJECT AND METHODS

Eighteen members of the first family with Lynch Syndrome II observed in Italy (Cristofaro 1985) with a sex ratio, male to female of 1.25 and an age ranging from 21 to 55, with an average of 39.6, underwent g.i. biopsies during follow-up examinations. 58 bioptic specimens were obtained from different g.i. sites, i.e. both proximal colonic and gastric mucosa. In particular, 2 biopsies per each site, which were treated using different technical procedures, were considered. Both formalin fixed and unfixed material were employed. The former was subjected to routine procedures, the latter was cryosected. Both morphological and immunocytochemical evaluations were made on 5 micron serial sections H.E. staining as well as immuno-cytochemical evaluation for both macrophages (M) and T-cell sub-populations, i.e. T helper (Th), T cytotoxic-suppressor (Tc-s) and Pan-T ones, using a PAP method were formed. In particular M were detected by the use of a primary polyclonal anti-human lysozime antibody and a rabbit universal immunocytochemical kit from Byk Gulden Italy. T-cell subpopulations were investigated employing monoclonal antibodies, i.e. Tec-T4 CD4, Tec-T8 CD8, Tec-T11 CD2 from Technogenetics Italy and a mouse universal immunocytochemical kit from Byk Gulden. The immune cell populations were evaluated on the entire cut biopsy surface.

CYTOMETRY

Both M and T-cell subpopulations were considered. The cell count was performed on the entire g.i. serial sections with an average thickness (e) of 5 micron, using an optic apparatus, i.e. a Leitz Orthoplan microscope connected to a Hitachi camera, projecting images onto a monitor at a final magnification of 800 x. Although a 121 point square grid was located in the camera-microscope connecting tube, an 8·11 points grid was observed on the screen at the set magnification, covering an area measuring 0.0212^2 mm^2 (a^2) which responded to a tissue volume of 0.0006374 mm^3 The number of cells (N) falling on the test grid and the number of grid points (P) falling on cells, as well as total grid points covering each biopsy were counted. The total number of counts performed in each subjects varied from 4 to 16 for M and from 5 to 10 for T lymphocyte subpopulations. Cell density (Nv) per mm^3 of g.i. mucosa was calculated using the formula:

$$[\, Nv = (N/P \cdot e \cdot a^2) \cdot 10^9 \,]$$

(Duclert 1974). Further volumetric analysis of various cytotype volume fraction (Vvi) was separately performed by differential point-counting volumetry (Weibel 1966). The collective number of test points lying in "i" (Pi) together with the number of test point (Pt) were also considered to obtain Ppi, i.e. the fraction of test points enclosed in "i", as stated by the formula:

$$Vvi = Pi/Pt = Ppi$$

The results indicated the number of cells per cubic millimeter of g.i. mucosa and the M and T-cells volumetric densities (M- and TVD).

STATISTICS

In the statistical analysis mean values ± SE per subject as well as per cell populations were considered. Both Student's T test, Fisher's variance analysis as well as the relationship between MVD and TVD values were performed. The age-related distributions of immune cell densities and their ratios were assessed by a simple linear correlation coefficient (r).

RESULTS

Though in our cases, one asymptomatic patient with colonic cancer was found, both the disease-free subjects and the patient with cancer showed overlapping characteristics in immune populations. Immune cells had a uniform distribution in the investigated gastrointestinal sites.
Both Th and Tc-s cell distributions were statistically identical, as shown by Th/Tc-s experimental ratio, i.e. 1.1. Moreover lymphocyte subsets distribution appeared analogous both in the whole material and per subject (Fig. 1). On the other hand, M

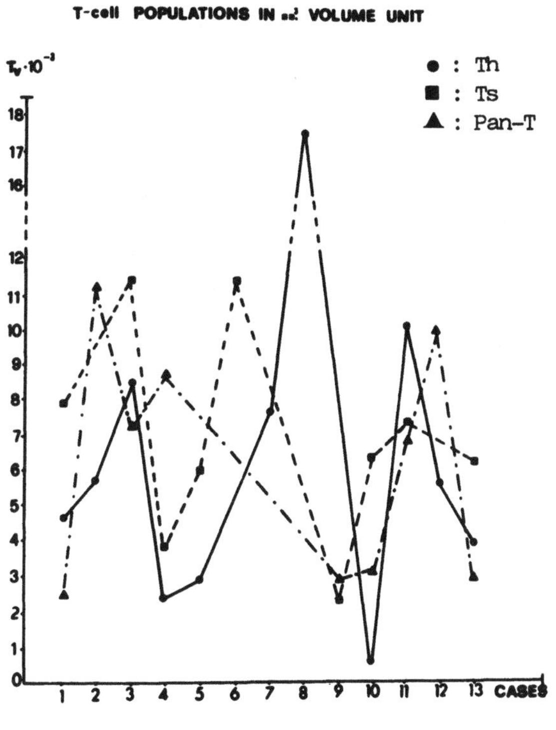

Fig. 1.

detected, which were well represented in the immune population of these subjects (Fig. 2), were 5 times less frequent than each tested lymphocyte subset, as confirmed by Th/M and Tc-s/M experimental ratios, i.e. 5.1 and 5.1, respectively. Such a distribution of immune populations was also revealed by their volumetric analysis (Fig. 3). The linear correlation coefficient (r) between the increase of immune cells, obtained by differential point-counting volumetry, and age was significant for M (r = 0.876), Tc-s (r = -0.0919) cells, as well as for M/Th (r = 0.955), M/Tc-s (r = 0.976) experimental ratios (Fig. 4).

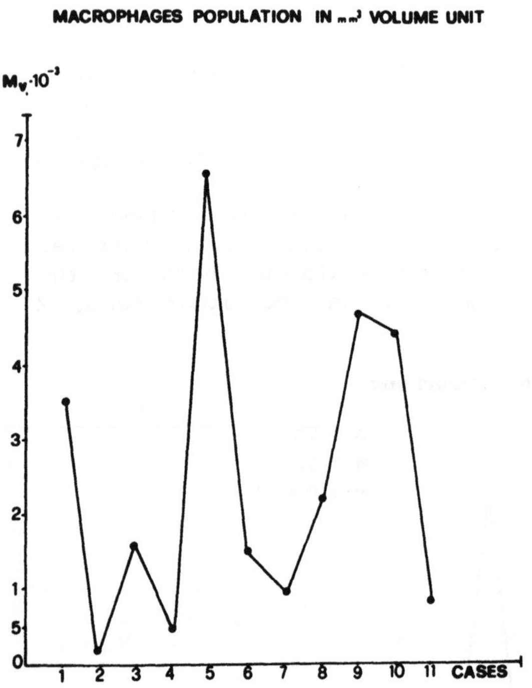

Fig. 2.

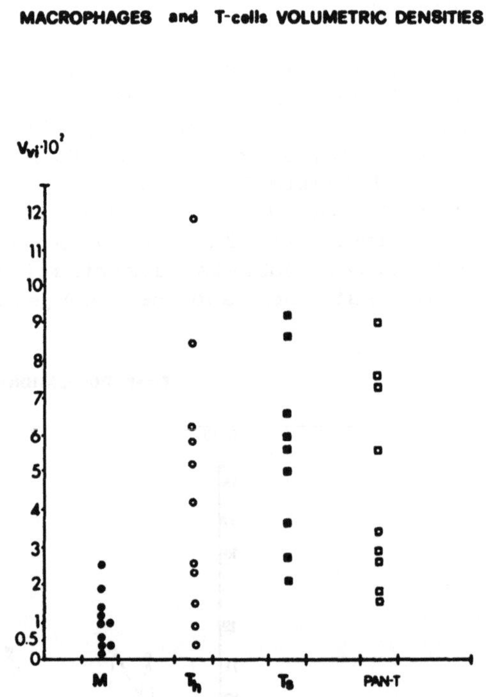

Fig. 3.

● : M; o : Th; ■: Ts; □: Pan-T

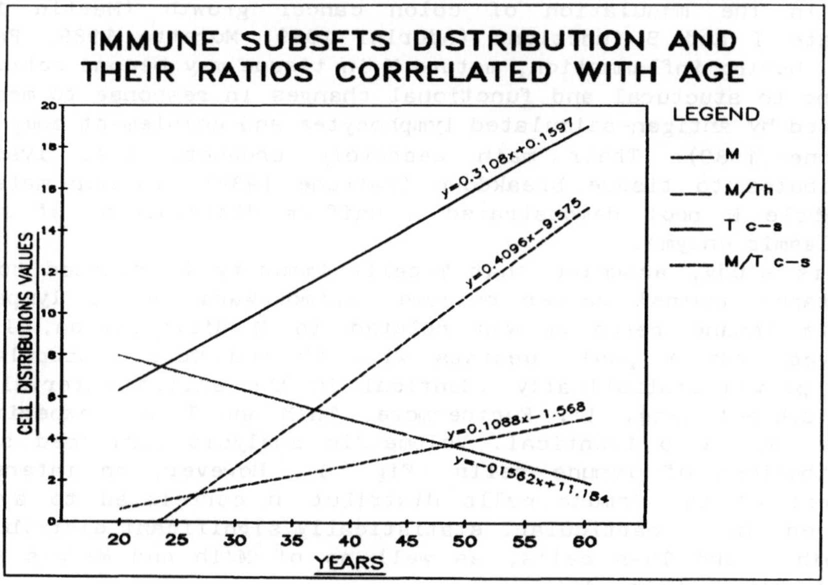

Fig. 4.

DISCUSSION

At present, biomarker systems have been studied in the cancer family syndrome with different results (Lynch 1981). In particular immunocytochemical analysis of T and B lymphocytes distribution in g.i. tissue gave no correlation with the mean sera values observed in vitro (Lynch 1981).

Our previous results suggested a polyclonal B-cell activation (PBA) which appeared to be preheminent, probably related to both the immune functions and distribution (Senatore 1986). Such a finding which could be occasional or the expression of a promoting action in B-cell proliferation and differentiation, provided no specific information concerning the management of the subjects with Lynch Syndrome II (Senatore 1986).

An impaired cellular immunity was also reported in patients with HNPCC (Lynch 1981) which may be related to T-cells distribution as a consequence of the tumor. Colon cancer was, however, hypothesized among disorders with a possible immunological pathogenesis (Dionigi 1978). On the basis of these apparently contradictory findings, it appears necessary to evaluate the interactions between T and M cells, which have a particular significance during the response to foreign histocompatibility antigens (Lynch 1981).

In accordance with the literature (Cristofaro 1985), this study showed that M appeared to be in excess in the g.i. mucosa of asymptomatic subjects (Fig. 2). These cells, which may also play a rôle in the modulation of colon cancer growth (Martin 1983), regulate T and B functions (Adorini 1989, Moretta 1989, Patrone 1989). During inflammation, mature M in tissue may become activated-loading to stuctural and functional changes in response to mediator released by antigen-stimulated lymphocytes and complement components (Patrone 1989). Their main secretory product, i.e. lysozime, contributes to tissue breakdown (Patrone 1989). In our material, the whole M pool demonstrated a uniform distribution of such a cytoplasmic enzyme.

In this study, assuming that T-cells immunity is related to host resistance against cancer outcome (Shimokawara 1982), lymphocyte subsets immune response was related to M distribution. It was observed that M pool coexists with Th and Tc-s subpopulations which proved statistically identical in the entire material, and per subject (Fig. 1). Furthermore, Th/M and Tc-s/M experimental ratios were also identical. Volumetric analysis confirmed such a distributions of immune cells (Fig. 3). However, an interesting movement of the immune cells distribution correlated to age was observed. In particular, statistically significant distributions of both M and Tc-s cells, as well as of M/Th and M/Tc-s ratios were assessed (Fig. 4).

M pool appeared to increase with age as well as M/Th ratio. Such a finding was probably due to a parallel increase of M and Th populations. Conversely Tc-s distribution as well as M/Tc-s ratio decreased with age. This suggests an inverse age-related relationship between M and Tc-s cell densities, that could be considered either an abnormality of the g.i. tract, or a pathogenetic factor responsible for the increased susceptibility to cancer outcome with age increase. It shoud be remembered that Tc-s seem to play a significant rôle concerning the host defense against tumors (Dionigi 1978).

Furthermore it could be emphasized that the activated M pool stimulates Th subpopulation, whereas no such reation occurs in Tc-s as has been revealed by our cross-checking.

The described PBA (Senatore 1986), however, could presumably be initiated by both M and Th subsets, which increases B-cell growth and secretion. In this condition the activation of both B and T cell functions and proliferation appears to be an M-dependent process, probably supported by IL-1 secretion.

At present, on the basis of our results, we maintain that the immune background, which appears to be uniform in g.i. areas, suggest a particular T-cell immune response supported by an active M pool. In this cancerous condition, it seems possible that the construction of orientative "fingerprints" could reveal a particular individual internal environment, at tissue level. It could be further hypothesized that the surveillance of M, Th and Tc-s interactions could help to identify different biological situations in the natural history of the disease.

More investigations will be required to prove whether immune functions and/or immunological abnormalities are primarily involved in the pathogenesis of the disease.

REFERENCES

Adorini L. (1989), Interleuchine. In: Dammacco F. (ed) Immunologia in medicina, Edi-Ermes, Milano, vol. I: 127-142.

Boland C.R., Troncale F.J. (1984), Familial colonic cancer in the absence of antecedent polyposis. Ann. Int. Med. 100: 700-701.

Cristofaro G., Caruso M.L., Attolini A., Di Matteo G., Giorgio P., Trabucco M., Senatore S., Giocoli Nacci G., Argentieri A., Sbano E., Giorgio I. (1985), Cancer Family Syndrome (Lynch Syndrome II): Preliminary Report of New Phenotipic Findings. In: Müller H.J., Weber W. (eds.) Familial Cancer, Karger, Basel-München-Paris-London-New York-New Delhi-Singapore-Tokyo-Sydney, 85-87.

Dionigi R., Zonta A. (1978), Immunobiologia delle neoplasie, Piccin Padova.

Duclert N.C., Degott C.L., Brousse N., Hippeau R., Potet F. (1974), Analyse morphologique quantitative: technique simplifiée appliable à des examens de routine. Nouv. Press. Med. 3: 245-246.

Lynch H.T., Lynch J.F. (1985), Genetics and colorectal cancer. In: Müller H.J., Weber W. (eds.), Familial Cancer, Karger, Basel-München-Paris-London-New York-New Delhi-Singapore-Tokyo-Sydney, 72-77.

Lynch H.T., Lynch P.M., Albano W., Lynch J.F. (1981), The Cancer Syndrome: a status report. Dis. Col. and Rect. 24: 311-322.

Lynch H.T., Kimberling W.J., Albano W. (1985), Hereditary non-polyposis colorectal cancer. I Clinical description of resource. Cancer 56: 934-938.

Martin F., Caignard A., Jeannin J.F., Olsson O., Martin M.S. (1983), Rôle of host-tumor interaction in the growth control of chemically induced colon cancer. In: Sherlock P., Morson B.C., Barbara L., Veronesi U. (eds.), Precancerous lesions of the gastrointestinal tract. Raven Press, New York, 237-240.

Moretta L., Mingari M.C. (1989), I linfociti. In: Dammacco F. (ed.), Immunologia in medicina. Edi-Ermes, Milano, vol. I: 1-22.

Patrone F. (1989), Granulociti neutrofili, eosinofili e cellule del sistema monocito-macrofagico. In: Dammacco F. (ed.), Immunologia in medicina, Edi-Ermes, Milano, vol. I: 63-79.

Senatore S., Saccani Jotti G., Liguori D., Chetrì M., Attolini A., Cristofaro G., Gabrielli M. (1986), Lymphocyte subpopulations in Lynch Sindrome II: an immunocytochemical study on gastro-intestinal biopsies. Preliminary report. Int. J. Bio. Mark. 1 (3): 137-140.

Shimokawara I., Imamura M., Yamanaka N., Ishii Y., Kikuchi K. (1982), Identification of lymphocyte subpopulations in human breast cancer tissue and its significance: an immunoperoxidase study with anti-human T- and B-cell sera. Cancer 49 (7): 1456-1464.

Twomey J.J., Sharkey D. (1972), An adaptation of the mixed leucocyte culture test for use in evaluating lymphocyte and macrophage function. J. Immunol. 108: 984-990.

Weibel E.R., Kistler G.S., Scherle W.F. (1966), Practical stereological methods for morphometric cytology. J. Cell Biol., 30: 23-38.

Glycoconjugate Expression in Familial Colorectal Cancer: Polyposis Syndromes and Hereditary Nonpolyposis Syndromes

C. RICHARD BOLAND

ABSTRACT

Different forms of glycoconjugates are expressed in epithelial tissues during the process of normal cell differentiation, and during neoplastic transformation. Traditional histochemical dyes, monoclonal antibodies, and lectins have been used to identify different forms of glycoconjugates that are expressed in histological sections of tissues. These probes have been used to study colorectal tissues from patients with the familial colorectal cancer syndromes. Lectins and histochemical stains identify modifications in glycoconjugate structure that occur during normal cellular differentiation in the colon. Monoclonal antibodies and lectins have been used to demonstrate that cancer-association antigens appear in benign adenomatous polyps in the colon. One of these antigenic structures, the T-antigen is discussed in detail. This antigen tends to first appear in larger adenomatous polyps, and is abundantly expressed in cancers. Other more subtle abnormalities in glycoconjugate expression are found in colons of patients with familial polyposis coli, including decreased expression of certain glycoconjugate structures and enhanced expression of others. Attempts to identify glycoconjugate abnormalities in the tissues of patients with hereditary nonpolyposis colorectal cancer syndromes is a major challenge, and is discussed.

Key words: Glycoconjugates, lectins, mucin, colonic polyps, and colonic cancer

INTRODUCTION

The development of neoplasia is accompanied by the abnormal synthesis, assembly, and trafficking of a wide variety of cellular macromolecules. It has been know for several decades that glycoconjugates, that is, glycoproteins, glycolipids, proteoglycans, and other complex molecules containing carbohydrate residues, play a central role in mediating cellular behavior, including response to external stimuli, cell-cell interactions, and growth regulation, just to name a few. Furthermore, it has long been appreciated that certain patterns of abnormal glycoconjugate synthesis are common to a wide variety of neoplastic cells. These abnormalities include the reexpression of glycoconjugates previously expressed in fetal tissues (the so called onco-developmental antigens), expression of incomplete or otherwise inappropriate blood group antigens (such as the deletion of normally expected blood group activity or the expression of immunologically incompatible blood group antigens), enhanced expression and abnormal cellular distribution of a normal cellular glycoconjugate (such as occurs with carcinoembryonic antigen), or other perturbations in the post-translational modification of glycoproteins or other glycoconjugates (such as, changes in the patterns of oligosaccharides synthesis).

The number of possible modifications in glycoconjugate structure that may accompany changes in cell behavior is bewildering. In order to detect these changes, one must anticipate the molecule that might undergo a structural change, develop probes to the normal and abnormal variants, and measure the changes in glycoconjugate structure as they occur hand in hand with emerging cellular behavior. Because of the inherent difficulties in a direct approach to this question, strategies have been devised to identify generalized modifications in glycosylation, even when the full molecular identities of the target macromolecules are unknown.

The focus of this paper is the development of cancer in the colon and rectum. Colorectal neoplasia is thought to be a process whereby normal tissue is first gradually replaced by benign neoplastic tissue; malignant tissue later emerges from this setting. This process is thought to take place over a period of many years, and perhaps even decades. If the above hypothetical model is accurate, it might be possible to identify neoplastic tissue at an early stage by the use of biochemical markers for the modified glycoconjugates that mediate neoplastic behavior. This paper will focus upon attempts to identify specific forms of cellular glycoconjugates that accompany normal cellular differentiation and the abnormal forms of maturation that make up the process of early neoplasia in the setting of the familial colonic cancer syndromes.

Familial Colorectal Cancer Syndromes

Colorectal neoplasia generally occurs on a sporadic basis depending upon environmental factors encountered by the individual. Within this context, certain individuals in the general population are somewhat more susceptible, presumably on a genetic basis, to environmental carcinogens. These people are prone to develop adenomatous polyps, but their susceptibility is relative and probably influenced by the diet. Furthermore, not all patients who develop these polyps will eventually have a colon cancer.

A smaller percentage of the population appears to develop colorectal cancer on a somewhat different basis. These individuals are virtually assured of developing colorectal cancer, often at a very early age. These hereditary variants include familial polyposis coli (FPC) and hereditary nonpolyposis colonic cancer (Lynch syndrome).

FPC: Patients who inherent the gene for FPC (or its sister entity, Gardner's syndrome) all experience the development of small, benign adenomatous polyps as the first neoplastic manifestation of disease in the colon. These gradually increase in number, and the degree of neoplasia in individual polyps increases. At least three different approaches have indicated that even the flat, apparently normal-appearing colonic epithelium, these patients may already manifest a disturbance in the regulation of its proliferation (Danes, 1978; Deschner and Raicht, 1981; Luk and Baylin, 1984). The florid development of multiple adenomatous polyps in the colon permits the facile identification of this syndrome. Because of the orderly appearance of benign neoplasia followed by the later emergence of malignancy, it is possible to limit the morbidity and mortality of cancer from this disease. Furthermore, it is an informative model by which to study the predictable, stepwise emergence of neoplasia.

The Lynch Syndromes: Hereditary nonpolyposis colonic cancer is a disease that appears to be inherited as an autosomal dominant genetic characteristic, but it is impossible at present to identify this disorder with certainty in an individual patient. Lynch syndrome families do not develop antecedent polyposis, but are at extremely high risk to develop cancer of the colon or rectum at uncharacteristically early ages, typically from ages 25-50, with a median age of onset in the early forties. Members of these kindreds have an unusual distribution of cancers in the colon, in which over two thirds occur proximal to the splenic flexure. In addition, a large proportion of these tumors are mucinous cancers. These patients are at increased risk to have multiple synchronous primary tumors, and will develop additional metachronous in any residual colon or rectum. This disease is very different from FPC, but our understanding of it is limited by the fact that there have been no reliable phenotypic markers for this disease. Thus, the diagnosis is usually made by inference based upon family history. The identification of a reliable phenotypic marker would represent the first step in understanding the biological defect that underlies this syndrome. As is discussed elsewhere in this symposium, the Lynch syndrome has at least two variants; patients in Lynch syndrome I families develop colorectal neoplasms, and those with Lynch syndrome II are also at risk to develop neoplasms in the endometrium, ovaries, stomach, and elsewhere (Boland and Troncale, 1984).

Glycoconjugate Expression In The Colon And Its Recognition Using Lectins

Lectins: Countless glycoconjugates are synthesized in any epithelium such as the colon. Nonetheless it is possible to identify certain glycoconjugates on histochemical sections of tissue using lectins, if specific carbohydrate configurations are present in adequate abundance. Lectins are naturally occurring proteins or glycoproteins that will "recognize" and bind to specific terminal glycosylation structures. Although there are only six different monosaccharides residues present in mammalian glycoproteins, and a few more that may occur in glycolipids and proteoglycans, the number of different possible structures is amplified by the sequential combinations and anomeric linkages between the sugars. In many instances, the carbohydrate-binding specificity of a lectin has been assumed to involve a single sugar residue or specific anomeric linkage (Goldstein and Poretz, 1986). However, when studied in detail, the lectin binding specificity has often been found to be very complex, may require di-or tri-saccharide structures, and the lectin-sugar interaction may involve only specific portions of each carbohydrate molecule (Rinderle and Goldstein, 1989). This degree of specificity may be used to advantage, since the lectin may select unique glycoconjugates within a tissue section. Lectins have been used as histochemical probes to identify modifications in glycoconjugates that accompany changes in the behavior of the tissue, such as normal cellular differentiation or malignant transformation (Boland, et al., 1982a; Cooper, 1982).

Glycoconjugate Expression in the Normal Colon: Specimens of histologically normal colon were studied by rehydrating parrafin embedded tissues, incubating with tagged lectins, washing unbound lectin off the slide, and examining using fluorescence or light microscopy. The lectins used and the carbohydrate specificity of each are listed in **Table 1.**

TABLE 1: LECTINS USED TO IDENTIFY TISSUE GLYCOCONJUGATES

Lectin	Carbohydrate Structure(s) Identified
Ricinus communis agglutinin$_1$ (RCA$_1$)	β-Galactose (β-Gal)
Bauhinia purpurea agglutinin (BPA)	β–Gal
Dolichos biflorus agglutinin (DBA)	α-N-acetylgalactosamine (α-GalNAc)
Soybean agglutinin (SBA)	GalNAc
Wheat germ agglutinin (WGA)	N-acetylglucosamine (GlcNAc), or, sialic acid
Succinylated - WGA (s-WGA)	Only GlcNAc
Ulex europeus agglutinin$_1$ (UEA$_1$)	α–L-fucose
Concanavalin A (ConA)	Mannose
Peanut agglutinin (PNA)	Gal β1, 3 GalNAc (T-antigen)
Amaranthus caudatus agglutinin (ACA)	T-antigen, or sialylated variants of T-antigen

In the normal colon, a difference in lectin labeling of the goblet cell mucin was found between the lower and upper portions of the colonic crypt. The lower portion of the crypt is the proliferative zone for colonic epithelium, and the upper portion of the crypt is the location of mature cells which are ultimately sloughed into the lumen. Goblet cell mucin in lower portion of the crypt was bound by the lectins that labeled terminal β–linked galactose residues (RCA$_1$ and BPA-see **Table 1**). A transition occurred in the mid portion of the colonic crypt; in the mature cells, goblet cell mucin was labeled by lectins that recognize α-linked GalNAc residues (DBA and SBA). Since goblet cell mucin is secreted into the lumen, a mixture of mucins from mature and immature cells could be found in this location, creating a more complex picture. Mucin from all portions of the crypt were bound by the lectins WGA and sWGA. However, no mucin was bound by PNA, a lectin which recognizes the T-antigen (Boland, et al., 1982).

The lectin UEA$_1$ is expressed selectively throughout the colon, appearing some of the time in the proximal colon, but not in the distal colon (Yonezawa, et al., 1982). Lectins were also useful in identifying selective expression of glycoconjugates based upon location in the colonic crypt and location throughout the colon (Bresalier, et al., 1985).

Glycoconjugate Expression in Human Colonic Neoplasia: Glycoconjugate expression in the colon is modified in neoplastic tissues. The earliest neoplastic tissue in the colon may consist of portions of an individual colon crypt in which nuclear aberrations are identifiable as adenomatous. This cluster of cells, which represents the clonal expansion of a single neoplastic progenitor, slowly grows, and soon develops a polypoid configuration. Adenomatous polyps usually lose the goblet cell mucin vacuole, and appear to secrete smaller amounts of glycoprotein. When an adenomatous polyp is small, it tends to synthesize glycoconjugates that have the same lectin-binding characteristics as those found in the normal colon (Boland, et al., 1982b). At some point in the life history of an adenomatous polyp, individual glands begin to synthesize, and in some instances secrete, glycoconjugates bearing the Thomsen-Freidenreich antigen (T-antigen), which may be identified by the binding of peanut agglutinin (PNA). In a histochemical study of 31 benign tubular adenomas, a mean of 2% of the glands were labeled with a fluorescein-tagged PNA in the 16 smallest polyps, and most of the polyps had no labeling. However, 24% of the glands were labeled in the 15 largest polyps. Greater amounts of labeling were found in polyps containing villous adenoma or carcinoma-in-situ. Of interest, the focus of carcinoma-in-situ (or invasive cancer) in adenomatous polyps was *always* labeled by PNA.

Virtually every cancer secretes PNA-binding glycoconjugates. However, this characteristic is stage-dependent, may be lost in larger tumors, and is typically lost in metastases (Bresalier, et al., 1984). The appearance of this class of glycoconjugates occurs in the same time frame as the more recently described genetic alterations in colon cancer (Vogelstein, et al., 1988). It is not unusual, and in fact it is generally the rule, that tumor-associated glycoconjugates are expressed in benign colonic adenomas. Examples of this include the antigen recognized by monoclonal antibody B72.3 (Stramignoni, et al., 1983), and modifications of the ABO and Lewis blood group antigen families (Itzkowitz, et al., 1986; Kim, et al., 1986; Yuan, et al., 1987; Ruggiero, et al., 1988).

GLYCOCONJUGATE EXPRESSION IN FPC

Traditional Histochemistry

The traditional approach to glycoconjugate histochemistry has been to use variations on the periodic acid-Schiff technique. These variations can detect increases in glycoconjugate sulfation, and changes in acylation of the "tail" of sialic acid groups. In 1980, Filipe, et al. , reported a predominance of sialomucins in neoplastic tissues compared to the normal colon, in which sulfomucins typically predominate, and similar changes were found in the colons of patients with FPC. These changes were more extensive in the distal colon, were consistently present immediately adjacent to cancers and large polyps, but were also seen in flat mucosa not involved by obvious neoplasia. This approach was extended by Muto, et al. (1985), who demonstrated that the sialomucins in cancers, adenomas, and flat mucosa in patients with FPC tended to have decreased acylation of the sialic acid residues compared to normal colons. FPC tissues were studied by Sugihara and Jass (1987), who used additional techniques to uncover modifications in sialic acid residues. They found heterogeneous forms of sialomucins in control colons, but were unable to demonstrate specific associations between sialic acid modifications and neoplastic tissues.

Lectin Histochemistry

As described above, lectins can be used to detect families of terminal carbohydrate structures expressed in tissue glycoconjugates, and can provide structural details not detectable using traditional histochemistry. Yonezawa, et al. (1983) used the lectin UEA_1 to study FPC tissues obtained from the distal colon, where the lectin had proved to be most informative in normal tissues. In a small number of specimens, UEA_1 staining was observed in the adenomatous epithelium and also the intervening non-neoplastic tissue between the polyps. Sugihara and Jass (1987) found more binding by UEA_1 in the distal colon of control patients than others had previously reported, but found no differences between FPC tissues and controls using this lectin.

Our group has studied a group of 22 colectomy specimens obtained from patients with FPC. The specimens included polypoid tissue as well as "normal tissue", i.e., flat epithelium between obvious adenomatous tissue. Control tissues were obtained from patients who had undergone colonoscopy for a variety of symptoms and were found to have a normal colonoscopy, and a negative family history for colorectal cancer. The colonic specimens were stained with five lectins: PNA, DBA, UEA_1, sWGA, and WGA. In order to detect subtle differences in glycoconjugate expression, each individual colonic crypt was given a score from 0 to 4+, based upon a subjective visual estimate. Zero indicated no labeling, and 4+ represented maximal intensity of labeling. Scores of 1+ - 3+ represented intermediate grades of fluorescent labeling. After a representative number of colonic crypts were counted (usually 100-200), the sum of the scores was expressed per 100 colonic crypts. Thus, the scores could range from 0 (zero labeling for all crypts) to 400 (all crypts 4+).

The labeling scores were very high for the lectins DBA and WGA, which was expected from prior work. The scores were of an intermediate level for sWGA (in all instances being less than that seen for WGA, as expected), and the scores were substantially lower for the lectins PNA and UEA_1.

As indicated in **Table 2**, the polypoid lesions in FPC colons bound significantly less DBA, WGA, and sWGA than seen in control colons. The reduction in labeling by DBA might not have been detected using a less rigorously quantitative system of scoring. It suggests the possibility that the epithelium is less mature than that seen in the normal colon, since fewer terminal GalNAc residues are expressed. The reduction in labeling by WGA and sWGA suggests either a total reduction in glycoconjugate synthesis in these tissues, or a modification in oligosaccharide synthesis that results in a reduction of terminal sialic acid and GlcNAc residues.

Labeling with PNA and UEA_1 were not significantly different than that seen in the normal colon. The findings with PNA were not unexpected, since the polypoid lesions in this tissue are all rather tiny, and small adenomatous polyps that occur on a sporadic basis do not produce abundant amounts of PNA-binding glycoconjugates. The findings with UEA_1 were not expected, since at least one prior group had demonstrated increased UEA_1 binding in adenomas (Yonezawa, et al., 1982). A review of the individual data indicated that the control tissues had uniformly low scores (1.0 ± 0.2). Although most of the scores in polypoid tissues were also low, 3/22 of the tissues had very high scores. Thus, marked discrepancies in reported data could reflect selection bias of the polyps. Our study did not include any large polyps from FPC patients.

TABLE 2: LECTIN BINDING SCORES: FPC POLYPS VS. CONTROL

Lectin	Control	FPC Polyps
DBA	362 ± 6	220 ± 22 ($p = .0001$)
WGA	375 ± 4	279 ± 15 ($p = .0001$)
sWGA	133 ± 15	61 ± 16 ($p = .0254$)

PNA, UEA-not significantly different

Table 3 demonstrates the lectin binding scores in flat FPC tissues compared with controls. Significantly increased levels of binding were found with UEA_1, together with significant reductions in binding by WGA and sWGA. The results with WGA and sWGA are similar to those found in the FPC polyps. The data obtained with UEA_1 are similar to those previously reported by

Yonezawa, et al.(1983), but were somewhat unexpected because of the failure to find enhanced binding in polypoid lesions. Labeling by DBA indicated that reduced expression of terminal α-GalNAc residues does not occur until the tissue becomes morphologically neoplastic. The absence of PNA binding in normal-appearing FPC tissues was consistent with our observation that T-antigen expression is an event that occurs later in the natural history of neoplastic tissue.

TABLE 3: LECTIN BINDING SCORES: FPC FLAT VS. CONTROL

Lectin	Control	FPC-Flat Colon
UEA_1	1 ± 0.2	30 ± 14 (p =.0315)
WGA	375 ± 4	259 ± 15 (p =.0006)
sWGA	188 ± 8	133 ± 15 (p =.0335)

PNA, DBA-not significantly different

HEREDITARY NONPOLYPOSIS COLONIC CANCER (LYNCH SYNDROMES I AND II)

Several pedigrees have been identified by Henry Lynch, M.D., at Creighton University, for the suspected presence of hereditary nonpolyposis colon cancer. At present, it is not known whether this represents a uniform genetic disorder or a heterogeneous collection of high risk families. A group of 47 individuals were subjected to colonoscopic surveillance because they were first degree relatives of a person identified with HNPCC. This is a difficult group of patients to study; if ascertainment of HNPCC were perfect, only half of these study patients would actually carry the abnormal gene, making it even more difficult to identify. Rectal biopsies were labeled with PNA, DBA, UEA_1, and sWGA, and compared with control tissues.

As demonstrated in **Table 4**, significant differences in labeling were found with the lectins PNA and DBA. It was quite unexpected that HNPCC patients would have significantly less labeling with the lectin PNA, so the presence of confounding variables was sought. HNPCC patients were significantly younger than control patients, and PNA binding was found to be affected by increasing age. Thus, this finding does not serve as a biological marker of this condition. A significant reduction was found in labeling by DBA, and labeling by this lectin appeared to have a bimodal distribution in the "at risk" population. Although the labeling scores are significantly different between the HNPCC and control groups, the scores actually represent a rather subtle reduction in labeling that may have been overlooked if the quantitative labeling score had not been used. As such, if reduced binding by DBA actually predicts the carriage of the gene for Lynch syndrome, it still may not be a powerful biomarker for the gene using this approach. Nonetheless, it suggests the possibility that a preneoplastic modification in glycoconjugate synthesis may be occurring in these tissues.

TABLE 4: LECTIN BINDING SCORES: HNPCC VS. CONTROL

Lectin	Control	HNPCC
PNA	19 ± 7	4 ± 2 (p =.0059*)
DBA	362 ± 6	287 ± 15 (p =.0001)

UEA and sWGA-not significantly different
*PNA scores affected by age; HNPCC patients significantly younger than controls

OLIGOSACCHARIDE MODEL

A model may be proposed to explain the observations made in neoplastic colonic tissues and in the familial colorectal cancer syndromes. Podolsky (1985a, 1985b) isolated and sequenced 26 different O-linked oligosaccharides prepared from nonneoplastic human colonic mucin. The chains ranged from two to twelve sugars in length, and included linear and branched structures. The non-reducing terminal sugar residues were β-Gal, β-GlcNAc, α-GalNAc, α-fucose and α(2,6) sialic acid, which correlated with the lectin histochemistry.

Our data suggest the following generalizations. Ten of the sequenced oligosaccharides terminate with an unsubstituted β-galactose residue, in each instance either as part of a lactosamine disaccharide (i.e., Galβ1,4 GlcNAc) or a Galβ1,3 linkage distal to it. These chains range from three to ten sugar units in length. The lectin histochemistry suggests that these β-Gal structures predominate in the proliferating and less mature epithelial cells at the bottom of the colonic crypt where RCA_1 and BPA bind most avidly. Nine of the oligosaccharides terminate in α(1,3) GalNAc residues at the end of an extended chain, slightly longer than the β-Gal chains and ranging from seven to twelve sugars in length. These chains are expressed in the more fully differentiated chains at the top of the crypt. All but one of the chains contains at least one GlcNAc residue (which may be bound by WGA and sWGA even when not in a terminal position), which explains why the wheat germ lectins bind throughout the colon.

Podolsky did not describe any oligosaccharides in the normal colon that would bind PNA, so it is reasonable to conclude that novel biosynthetic processes are responsible for the production of the T-antigen in cancers and larger adenomatous polyps.

The reduction in labeling by WGA and sWGA in FPC tissues (flat and polypoid) suggests a reduction in total mucin synthesis by these tissues. The appearance of UEA_1 binding in neoplastic and normal-appearing FPC tissues is not as easily explained by the structural data; UEA_1 binding should be abundant throughout normal colonic tissues, but this does not occur in the distal colon. ABO blood group antigens are not normally expressed in the distal human colon, although the structural work suggests that blood group A activity should be found.

The most interesting finding is the significant reduction in DBA binding in the presence of normal WGA and sWGA binding in the HNPCC patients. This suggests that the colonic tissues may be immature, and share phenotypic characteristics with tissues normally found at the bottom of the colonic crypt.

Figure 1 demonstrates a model, from Podolsky, of normal and abnormal oligosaccharide synthesis in colonic mucins.

FUTURE PROSPECTS

New lectins are under development that might be useful in the identification of biomarkers of abnormal biological behavior in colorectal epithelial. One such lectin is amaranthin, or ACA (see **Table 1**) that has recently been isolated and characterized by Rinderle and Goldstein (1989). This lectin binds to T-antigen and to both sialylated variants, i.e., T-antigen with sialic acid on the Gal, GalNAc, or both residues. This variation in binding specificity makes it useful in a different way in the human colon. This lectin binds to mucins secreted by cancers, and it binds diffusely throughout adenomatous polyps (Rinderle et al., 1988). In the normal colon it selectively binds in the lower portion of the colonic crypt, which is the proliferative region of this epithelium. It appears to bind to a cytoplasmic glycoprotein other than goblet cell mucin in the normal colon, however the molecular identity of the target is not yet know. Preliminary data in our laboratory indicates that increased binding of this lectin is seen in flat FPC tissues, both in the lower and upper portions of the colonic crypts, making it potentially more valuable than the lectins used previously to study this disease. We are currently exploring the potential use of this lectin as a biomarker in tissues from patients at risk for HNPCC. Additional new lectins are under development that have the ability to distinguish the different sialic acid linkages that may be present in these tissues.

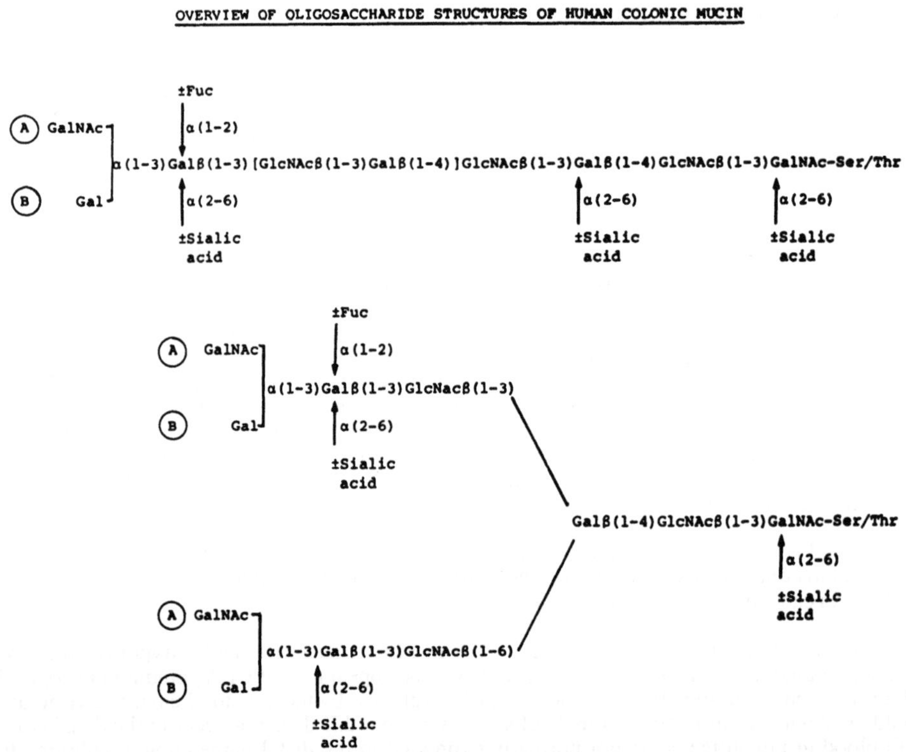

Figure 1 Legend: Model of linear and branched oligosaccharide structures, used by permission from D.K. Podolsky, M.D. The sugar chain consists of an O-linked GalNAc residue at the reducing terminus (at the right), extended by one or more lactosamine disaccharides (i.e., Galβ1,4 GlcNAc). Much of the variation in oligosaccharide structure involves: (a) extension of the basic backbone; (b) addition of terminal GalNAc or Gal residues; and (c) addition of sialic acid residues, as outlined in the figure. Addition of GalNAc or Gal residues to the non-reducing terminal Gal residue (on the left) together with the fucose (Fuc) residue would produce an ABO blood group structure. The failure to add either GalNAc or Gal (i.e., A or B), or fucose/sialic acid (arrows), would leave an exposed β-Gal residue, which we have hypothesized to be the case in immature colonocytes. The addition of terminal GalNAc is characteristic of more mature cells.

In summary, normal and abnormal varieties of cell maturation are characteristically accompanied by different classes of glycoconjugates. We have attempted to identify classes of glycoconjugates that may be associated with specific types of cellular behavior. Examples of cancer-associated carbohydrates sequences or linkages have been identified using traditional histochemical stains and their modifications, monoclonal antibodies, and lectins. Many of these tumor-associate antigens are expressed to varying degrees in premalignant tissues such as adenomatous polyps. In general, most of these tumor antigens are absent from small adenomatous polyps, begin to appear in larger adenomas, and are abundantly expressed in carcinoma. We are attempting to find abnormalities in glycoconjugate synthesis that precede these better defined tumor-associated oligosaccharide structures. Candidate probes are available that appear to identify abnormal glycoconjugates in normal-appearing but possibly preneoplastic tissue in FPC. HNPCC, or the Lynch syndromes, are a more enigmatic problem because it is difficult to definitively identify affected individuals, and it is at present impossible to identify putative gene carriers before they develop a tumor. The first step in understanding these syndromes is to thoroughly identify the phenotypic abnormality associated with the carriage of the HNPCC gene. Only then will it be possible to attempt to locate the gene responsible for this disease and to understand the mechanism by which these individuals develop precocious tumors in the colon and other sites.

REFERENCES

Boland CR, Montgomery CK, Kim YS (1982a) Alterations in human colonic mucin occurring with cellular differentiation and malignant transformation. Proc Natl Acad Sci, USA 79:2051-2055

Boland CR, Montgomery CK, Kim YS (1982b) Cancer-associated mucin alterations in benign colonic polyps. Gastroenterology 82:664-672

Boland CR, Troncale FJ (1984) Familial colonic cancer without antecedent polyposis. Ann Int Med 100:700

Bresalier RS, Boland CR, Kim YS (1984) Characteristics of colorectal cancer cells with high metastatic potential. Gastroenterology 87:115-122

Bresalier RS, Boland CR, Kim YS (1985) Regional differences in normal and cancer-associated glycoconjugates of the human colon. J Natl Cancer Inst 75:249-260

Cooper HS (1982) Peanut lectin-binding sites in large bowel carcinoma. Lab Invest 47:383-390

Danes BS (1978) Increased *in vitro* tetraploidy: tissue specific within the heritable colorectal cancer syndromes with polyposis coli. Cancer 41:2330-2334

Deschner EE, Raicht RF (1981) Kinetic and morphologic alterations in the colon of a patient with multiple polyposis. Cancer 47:2440-2445

Filipe MI, Mughal S, Bussey HJ (1980) Patterns of mucus secretion in the colonic epithelium in familial polyposis. Invest Cell Pathol 3:329-343

Goldstein IJ, Poretz RD (1986) Isolation, physicochemical characterization, and carbohydrate-binding specificity of lectins. In: Liener IE, Sharon N, Goldstein IJ (eds) The lectins properties, functions and applications in biology and medicine. Academic Press, Inc., Orlando, Florida, pp 35-247

Itzkowitz SH, Yuan M, Ferrell LD, Palekar A, Kim YS (1986) Cancer-associated alterations of blood group antigen expression in human colorectal polyps. Cancer Res 46:5976-5984

Kim YS, Yuan M, Itzkowitz SH, Sun Q, Kaizu T, Palekar A, Trump BF, Hakomori S (1986) Expression of Le^y and extended Le^y blood group-related antigens in human malignant, premalignant, and nonmalignant colonic tissues. Cancer Res 46:5985-5992

Luk GD, Baylin SB (1984) Ornithine decarboxylase as a biologic marker in familial colonic polyposis. N Engl J Med 311:80-83

Muto T, Kamiya J, Sawada T, Agawa S, Morioka Y, Utsunomiya J (1985) Mucin abnormality of colonic mucosa in patients with familial polyposis coli. Dis Colon Rectum 28:147-148

Podolsky DK (1985a) Oligosaccharide structures of human colonic mucin. J Biol Chem 210:8262

Podolsky DK (1985b) Oligosaccharide structures of isolated human colonic mucin species. J Biol Chem 260:15510.

Rinderle SJ, Goldstein IJ, Luk GD, Resau J, Rigot WL, Boland CR (1989) Development of a new lectin, amaranthin (ACA), as a marker for epithelial cell differentiation in the human colon. Gastroenterology 96:A417

Rinderle SJ, Goldstein IJ, Matta KL, Ratcliffe RM (1989) Isolation and characterization of amaranthin, a lectin present in the seeds of amaranthus caudatus, that recognizes the T-(or cryptic T)-antigen. J Biol Chem 264:16123-16131

Ruggiero F, Cooper HS, Steplewski Z (1988) Immunohistochemical study of colorectal adenomas with monoclonal antibodies against blood group antigens (sialosyl-Le^a, Le^a, Le^b, Le^x, Le^y, A, B, and H). Lab Invest 59:96-103

Stramignoni D, Bowen R, Atkinson BF, Schlom J (1983) Differential reactivity of monoclonal antibodies with human colon adenocarcinomas and adenomas. Int J Cancer 31:543-552

Sugihara K, Jass JR (1987) Colorectal goblet cell mucins in familial adenomatous polyposis. J Clin Pathol 40:608-611

Vogelstein B, Fearon ER, Hamilton SR, Kern SE, Preisinger AC, Leppert M, Nakamura Y, White R, Smits AMM, Bos JL (1988) Genetic alterations during colorectal-tumor development. N Engl J Med 319:525-530

Yonezawa S, Nakamura T, Tanaka S, Maruta K, Nishi M, Sato E (1983) Binding of Ulex europaeus agglutinin-1 in polyposis coli: comparative study with solitary adenoma in the sigmoid colon and rectum. JNCI 71:19-24

Yonezawa S, Nakamura T, Tanaka S, Sato E (1982) Glycoconjugate with Ulex europaeus agglutinin-1-binding sites in normal mucosa, adenoma, and carcinoma of the human large bowel. JNCI 69:777-785

Yuan M, Itzkowitz SH, Ferrell LD, Fukushi Y, Palekar A, Hakomori S, Kim YS (1987) Expression of $Lewis^x$ and sialylated $Lewis^x$ antigens in human colorectal polyps. JNCI 78:479-488

Carbohydrate Associated Antigens in Neoplastic and Preneoplastic Colon

YOUNG S. KIM

ABSTRACT

In colorectal cancer, several major alterations in glycosylation of glycoproteins and glycolipids occur resulting in the expression of cancer associated antigenic epitopes. These changes can occur either in the outer peripheral or inner core regions of the carbohydrate side chains. The major changes are inappropriate expression, deletion or modification of antigenic structures present in normal colorectal tissues. These changes are illustrated by recent studies on the expression of several blood group antigens such as A,B,H, and Le^b antigens, modified blood group related antigens such as sialosyl Le^a, Le^x (X) and Le^y (Y) antigens and inner core carbohydrate antigen such as T, Tn and Sialyl Tn antigens. These changes also occur in adenomatous polyps and appear to correlate with parameters of malignant potential. Thus, these carbohydrate antigens may serve as preneoplastic markers which may be useful in identification and screening of subjects at high risk for developing colorectal cancer.

Keywords: carbohydrate antigen, glycoprotein,glycolipid, colorectal cancer, adenomatous polyp

INTRODUCTION

It is now apparent that the best hope for improving the outcome of colorectal cancer is early diagnosis. There are two approaches to early detection; primary and secondary prevention. Primary prevention involves identification and management of groups at high risk due to environmental factors and to genetic susceptibility. Secondary prevention involves screening and management of patients to prevent premalignant lesions and early cancers from developing into metastatic cancer.

Screening of the general population for colorectal cancer is currently impractical. However, recent observations that inherited susceptibility may be a factor in the majority of colonic neoplasms seen clinically offers the possibility of identification and screening of subjects at high risk for developing colorectal cancer.

There appears to be two pathways involved in the development of colorectal cancer. One predominant pathway is the progression of hyperproliferative epithelium to adenoma and carcinoma. Another pathway is the progression of hyperproliferative epithelium to dysplasia and carcinoma without going through the adenomatous stage as in the case of inflammatory bowel diseases and familial colon cancer syndromes.

Since the earliest changes in carcinogenesis is impaired growth regulation and differentiation, phenotypic or genotypic markers that reflect these altered states in various stages of carcinogenesis are not only important in identifying subjects at high risk, but these markers have also been demonstrated to be useful in assessing the efficacy of chemopreventive measures. To what extent these stages are reversible is unclear at present. However, identification of stage-specific markers may help clarify these processes in the future.

Altered glycosylation in colonic neoplasia

Among many potential tumor or preneoplastic markers that have been investigated, glycoconjugate markers, proliferative markers and molecular markers appear to be potentially useful (Table 1). Many of the known phenotypic markers for colorectal cancer are carbohydrate-containing molecules such as glycoconjugates (Kim 1989; Hakomori 1985, 1986). The antigenic specificity of these markers may reside either in the carbohydrate moiety or in the protein portion of the molecule.

Table 1. Biochemical markers of preneoplastic and neoplastic colon cells

I. Glycoconjugate Markers

- A. Carbohydrate Epitopes
  1. Peripheral region carbohydrate changes
     A, B, H, Le^a, Le^b
     Sialosyl Le^a (19-9)
     Sialosyl Le^x, Extended Le^x
     Extended Le^y
  2. Core region carbohydrate changes
     Sialosyl Tn (TAG 72), Tn and T
- B. Peptide Epitopes
  1. CEA
  2. MAM-6

II. Proliferative Markers

- A. Polyamine metabolic enzymes
  1. Ornithine decarboxylase
  2. S-adenoxyl methionine decarboxylase
- B. Crypt-labeling index

III. Molecular markers

- A. Oncogene
- B. Suppressor genes
- C. Chromosomal abnormalities

The carbohydrate side chains of glycoprotein and glycolipids consist of several types of sugars in various types of linkages and chain lengths (1 to over 20) thereby generating considerable variety of antigenic specificities. Carbohydrate changes that occur in colorectal cancer can be divided into three categories; 1) inappropriate expression of antigenic structures not normally present in a particular location in the colon and rectum which may occur due to reactivation of a fetal gene. 2) deletion of normally expressed antigens, with or without precursor accumulation which arises as a result of incompletion of the carbohydrate side chains. 3) neosynthesis which occurs as a result of either extension or modification of existing carbohydrate structures or synthesis of new structures (Table 2) (Abe 1986; Atkinson 1982; Itzkowitz 1986; Kim

1986; Magnani 1982; Yuan 1985, 1986, 1987). These changes are illustrated by recent studies on the expression of several normal blood group antigens and modified blood group-related antigens that are expressed in colorectal cancer. These changes in carbohydrates occur either in the peripheral (outer), or inner core regions of oligosaccharide side chains of glycoproteins and glycolipids.

Table 2. Altered carbohydrate antigen expression in colorectal cancer

1. Inappropriate expression of antigenic structures not normally present in a particular location in the colon and rectum (e.g. incompatible expression of A,B,H and Le^b).

   Mechanism: reactivation of a fetal gene function

2. Deletion of normally expressed antigens, with or without precursor accumulation (e.g. deletion of A,B,H antigens, expression of T and Tn).

   Mechanism: decreased or altered glycosyltransferase activity.

3. Neosynthesis

   A. Modification of existing structure (e.g. Le^x, Le^y).
   B. New antigenic structure (?)

Peripheral and Backbone Region Carbohydrate Changes

After birth, the major blood group antigens ABH and Le^b disappear from the distal normal colon. However, re-expression of these antigens occur in distal colorectal cancer in 90% of the cases (Yuan 1985). Another finding is that 60-80% of colorectal cancer of both proximal and distal colon expressed blood group antigen activity incompatible with host's blood type. Deletion of the host's blood type also occurred in nearly half of colorectal cancers in the proximal colon. Adenomatous polyps frequently re-expressed ABH antigens or expressed incompatible blood group A or B in 27% of polyps (Table 3) (Itzkowitz 1986). Reappearance of ABH antigens in distal polyps was significantly correlated with increasing grade of dysplasia but was not significantly correlated with polyps size or histologic type. Thus, incompatible expression of blood group A or B antigens occurs only in adenomatous polyps and cancer tissues but not in fetal colonic mucosa, adult normal colonic mucosa or hyperplastic polyp suggesting that this may be a premalignant and malignant phenomenon.

An example of the modification of existing structure is the gastrointestinal cancer-associated antigen (GICA), which is recognized by monoclonal antibody 19-9 (Magnani 1982; Atkinson 1982). This antigen, a sialylated Le^a blood group antigen, occurs as an acidic glycolipid in tissues, but in serum and pancreatic juice it is found on mucin type glycoproteins. Most specimens of colon cancer and second trimester fetal colon expressed this antigen, whereas normal mucosa rarely expressed it. However, the majority of adenomatous polyps and hyperplastic polyps expressed this antigen (Table 3). Thus, a modification of the Le^a epitope by the addition of sialic acid appears to produce an oncodevelopmental antigen in colorectal cancer tissues, but it did not discriminate between the polyps of malignant and non-malignant potential.

Table 3. Carbohydrate antigen markers in normal colon, hyperplastic and adenomatous polyps and colorectal cancer*

Antigen Alteration+	Normal	Hyperplastic Polyps	Adenomatous Polyps	Cancer
Reappearance (Distal)				
A,B,H	1	15	73	70-100
Le^b	5	0	90	95
Incompatibility				
A,B,H,Le^b	0	0	38	61
Deletion (Proximal)				
A,Le^b	0	60	18	43
Incompletion				
T	0	60	54	76
Tn	14	-	-	81
Sialyl Tn (TAG-72)	0	0	50	96
Neosynthesis				
Sialyl Le^a (19-9)	0-45	82	51-81	59-82
Sialyl - extended Le^x	8-15	0	45-56	60-67
Difucosyl - extended Le^x	0-8	0-5	45-48	96
Extended - Le^y	0-6	0	33-66	79-83

*Data obtained from References 1,2,5,6,7,9,11,15,16,17
+Expressed as the percentage of specimens positive by immunohistochemical methods
-Not determined

Le^x and Le^y antigens are positional isomers of Le^a and Le^b respectively, and the respective epitopes reside on peripheral trisaccharides or tetrasaccharides of the carbohydrate side chains (Abe 1986; Itzkowitz 1986; Kim 1986; Yuan 1987). Recently, several monoclonal antibodies have been established which recognize these antigenic epitopes on extended carbohydrate side chains with or without further modification of the antigens. Recent studies show that the short chain Le^x antigen is expressed in the normal (lower colonic crypt cell membrane), cancerous and fetal colon and in hyperplastic and adenomatous polyps. In contrast, all types of extended Le^x antigens were absent from normal colonic mucosa and hyperplastic polyps, but were present in cancerous and fetal colons, and in adenomatous polyps (Table 3). Among adenomatous polyps, extended and polyfucosylated antigen expression tended to correlate with three measures of malignant potential; larger polyp size, villous histology, and severe dysplasia (Itzkowitz 1986; Yuan 1987). Le^y antigen showed a similar pattern of expression in various types of colorectal tissues (Abe 1986; Kim 1986).

<u>Core Region Carbohydrate Changes</u>
Recently, many carbohydrate alterations have been shown to occur in colon cancer mucins. For example, T, Tn, and Sialosyl Tn antigens which represent the inner core carbohydrate structures of mucin glycoproteins are oncodevelopmental antigens in the colon and rectum. Our studies indicate that Tn, Sialosyl Tn or T antigens were not expressed in normal colonic mucosa but were expressed in colon cancers (Tn 81%, Sialosyl Tn 96%, and T 71%) (Table 3). While T antigen was preferentially expressed by moderately well and well differentiated adenocarcinomas, both Tn and Sialosyl Tn antigens appear to be useful

markers of poorly differentiated adenocarcinomas and mucinous carcinomas, two histological subsets that often fail to express other cancer-associated antigens and that are often associated with a poor clinical outcome (Itzkowitz 1989; Yuan 1986).

In addition, the frequency of expression of T antigens in adenomatous polyps was 54% and its expression appeared to correlate with all three parameters (size, histological type and dysplasia) of malignant potential (Yuan 1986). Therefore, T antigen appears to ba a potentially useful premalignant and malignant marker. The expression of these antigens provides additional evidence for incomplete glycosylation in malignant and premalignant colon cells, and suggests the altered regulation of mucin carbohydrate side chain synthesis in these cells.

Peptide antigens (peptide moiety of glycoproteins)
The most widely studied serum glycoprotein tumor marker, carcinoembryonic antigen (CEA), has its antigenic determinant in the peptide moiety. It has limited clinical utility which may be due largely to the existence of a number of closely related glycoproteins that often cross-react with CEA in the commonly available clinical assays (Kam 1985; Shively 1985). The extensive glycosylation of CEA has prevented full investigation of its antigenic protein structure. Recently, however, several primary sequences of the protein moiety have been predicted as a result of the molecular cloning of several cDNA and genomic DNA probes (Neumaier 1988; Oikawa 1987). It is hoped that better characterization of the structure, properties, and tissue distribution of CEA-related antigens will allow development of more specific assays for the neoplasia-related CEA family members.

A series of monoclonal antibodies raised against human milk fat globule membranes recognized a peptide backbone of high molecular weight mucin type glycoprotein. One of these monoclonal antibodies, MAM-6, identifies an epitope that is present on 99% of 123 colon carcinomas but is totally absent from all 50 normal specimens tested. In addition, this epitope is expressed in 0 of 64 adenomas with mild dysplasia and 2 of 32 samples of colonic inflammation (Zotter 1987). MAM-6 expression is found in 61% of adenomas with foci of severe dysplasia or carcinoma *in situ*. If further studies confirm the high sensitivity and specificity of MAM-6, it may have considerable potential utility in diagnostic and therapeutic applications.

SUMMARY

Several carbohydrate structures behave as tumor and premalignant markers in human colorectal tissues, although none is specific only for colon cancer. These antigens are expressed heterogenously in colorectal cancer tissues due to tumor cell heterogeneity, and therefore the use of multiple monoclonal antibodies will enhance the potential clinical usefulness of these reagents. The expression of some carbohydrate antigens by colon cancers is considered rather "cancer-specific", since normal colorectal mucosa does not express these antigens. Most of these cancer-specific alterations may also be markers of premalignancy since adenomatous polyps, but not hyperplastic polyps are capable of exhibiting these changes, and antigenic expression often correlates with malignant potential in adenomatous polyps. However, it has not been determined whether or not similar antigenic alterations are observed in preneoplastic colonic conditions such as normal appearing "flat mucosa" of affected individuals of familial polyposis coli, or family cancer syndrome, or in the dysplastic cells of ulcerative colitis.

Although these carbohydrate tumor and preneoplastic markers appear to be useful in immunohistochemical studies of malignant and premalignant colorectal tissues, thus making them potential candidates in immunodetection, staging, and therapy, their clinical utility as serological markers for colorectal cancer have not yet been demonstrated.

REFERENCES

Abe K, Hakomori S, Ohshiba S (1986) Differential expression of difucosyl type 2 chain (Le^y) defined by monoclonal antivody AH6 in different locations of colonic epithelia, various histological types of colonic polyps, and adenocarcinomas. Cancer Res 46:2639-2644.

Atkinson BF, Ernst CS, Herlyn M, Steplewski Z, Sears HF, Koprowski H (1982) Gastrointestinal cancer-associated antigen in immunoperoxidase assay. Cancer Res 42:4820-4823.

Hakomori S (1985) Aberrant glycosylation in cancer cell membranes as focussed on glycolipids: Overview and perspectives. Cancer Res 45:2405-2414.

Hakomori S (1986) Glycosphingolipids. Sci Am 254:44-53.

Itzkowitz SH, Yuan M, Ferrell LD, Palekar A, Kim YS (1986) Cancer-associated alterations of blood group antigen expression in human colorectal polyps. Cancer Res 46:5976-5984.

Itzkowitz SH, Yuan M, Fukushi Y, Palekar A, Phelps PC, Shumsuddin AM, Trump BF, Hakomori S, Kim YS (1986) $Lewis^x$- and sialylated $Lewis^x$-related antigen expression in human malignant and nonmalignant colonic tissues. Cancer Res 46:2627-2632.

Itzkowitz SH, Yuan M, Montgomery CK, Kjeldsen T, Takahashi HK, Bigbee WL, Kim YS (1989) Expression of Tn, sialosyl Tn and T antigens in human colon cancer. Cancer Res 49:197-204.

Kam W, Itzkowitz SH, Kim YS (1985) Production and characterization and clinical utility of CEA. Advancer in Biotechnological Processes. Alan R. Liss, Inc., New York pp 151-181.

Kim YS, Yuan M, Itzkowitz SH, Sun Q, Kaizu T, Palekar A, Trump BF, Hakomori S (1986) Expression of Le^y and extended Le^y blood group-related antigens in human malignant, premalignant and nonmalignant colonic tissues. Cancer Res 46:5985-5992.

Kim YS (1989) Altered carbohydrate antigen expression in colorectal cancer and polyps. Modern Concepts in Gastroenterology. Vol 2 Raven Press, New York, pp. 197-208.

Magnani JL, Nilsson B, Brockhaus M, Sopf D, Steplewski Z, Koprowski H, Ginsburg V (1982) A monoclonal antibody-defined antigen associated with gastrointestinal cancer is a ganglioside containing sialylated lacto-N-fucopentaose II. J. Biol. Chem. 257:14365-14369.

Neumaier M, Zimmermann W, Shively L, Hinoda Y, Riggs AD, Shively JE (1988) Characterization of a cDNA clone for the nonspecific cross-reacting antigen (NCA) and a comparison of NCA and carcinoembryonic antigen. J. Biol. Chem. 263:3202-3207.

Oikawa S, Nakasato H, Kosaki G (1987) Primary structure of human carcinoembryonic antigen (CEA). Biochem. Biophys. Res. Comm. 142:511-518.

Shively JE, Beatty JD (1985) CEA-related antigens: Molecular biology and clinical significance. CRC Crit Rev Oncol Hematol 2:355-367.

Yuan M, Itzkowitz SH, Palekar A, Shumsuddin AM, Phelps PC, Trump BF, Kim YS (1985) Distribution of blood group antigens A,B,H, $Lewis^a$ and $Lewis^b$ in human normal, fetal and malignant colonic tissue. Cancer Res 45:4499-4511.

Yuan M, Itzkowitz SH, Boland CR, Kim YD, Tomita JT, Palekar A, Bennington JL, Trump BF, Kim YS (1986) Comparison of T-antigen expression in normal, premalignant, and malignant human colonic tissue using lectin and antibody immunohistochemistry. Cancer Res 46:4841-4847.

Yuan, M, Itzkowitz SH, Ferrell LD, Fukushi Y, Palekar A, Hakomori S, Kim YS (1987) Expression of $Lewis^x$ and sialylated $Lewis^x$ antigens in human colorectal polyps. J. Natl. Cancer Inst. 78:479-488.

Zotter S, Lossnitzer A, Hageman PC, et al. (1987) Immunohistochemical localization of the peithelial marker MAM-6 in invasive malignancies and highly dysplastic adenomas of the large intestine. Lab Invest 57:193-

Interphasic Nucleolar Organizer Regions in Colorectal Dysplastic and Neoplastic Lesions

P.L. MINGAZZINI, L. SCUCCHI, D. DI STEFANO, ALBEDI F. MALCHIODI, F. CIARALLI, M. FALCHI, and G. CRISTOFARO

ABSTRACT

The behaviour of silver-binding Nucleolar Organizer Regions (Ag-NORs) in interphasic nuclei was investigated in six cases of normal colonic mucosa, six cases each of mild, moderate and severely dysplastic colonic adenomatous polyps and six cases of colonic adenocarcinomas. The silver-stained dots were counted directly from slides using a 100X oil-immersion lens and from micrographs of the same fields using an image analyzer at a final magnification of 1,700X. The mean number of argyrophilic dots and the mean nuclear area occupied by argyrophilic proteins increased progressively from mild to severe dysplasia to adenocarcinoma with both methods. The Ag-NORs technique has a predictive value only when a suitable number of cells are examined because a wide overlap between the ranges of different parameters does not allow to consider the Ag-NOR method as a marker of malignant transformation in a single cell.

Keywords: interphasic nucleolar organizer regions, colorectal dysplastic lesions, colorectal adenocarcinomas

INTRODUCTION

Nucleolar Organizer Regions (NORs) are ribosomal DNA loops, mainly located in the fibrillar centers of the nucleolus, stained by virtue of their argyrophilic associated non-histone proteins (Angelier 1982; Hernandez-Verdun 1983; Hernandez-Verdun 1986; Hubell 1979; Ploton 1986), whose exact biochemical nature is still under discussion (Busch 1982; Hubell 1979; Lischwe 1981; Ochs 1983; Williams 1982). Changes in NORs distribution and number reflect variations in ribosomal transcriptional activity (Derenzini 1987; Morton 1983).

In a previous study we demonstrated the striking differences in number and distribution of NORs between hyperplastic polyps, adenomatous polyps and adenocarcinomas of the colon (Derenzini 1988).

The present study compares the behaviour of silver-binding nucleolar organizer regions in paraffin sections in different grades of colonic epithelial dysplasia. We investigated the mean number of interphasic NORs, the mean nuclear area occupied and their structural arrangement.

MATERIALS AND METHODS

The material examined was obtained from six samples of normal colonic mucosa, six colonic adenomatous polyps with mild epithelial dysplasia, six with moderate dysplasia and six with severe dysplasia and from six colonic adenocarcinomas.
Tissue samples were routinely fixed in formalin and processed to paraffin. Four micron thick paraffin sections were dewaxed, postfixed for 20 min in a 3:1 ethanol/acetic acid solution, rehydrated and stained using a solution of one volume of 2% gelatin in 1% acqueous formic acid and two volumes of 50% silver nitrate for 20 min at room temperature in the dark.
The number of interphasic Ag-NORs was counted both from slides using a 100X oil-immersion lens and from micrographs of the same fields using an image analyzer IBAS 2 at a final magnification of 1,700X. Moreover, the nuclear area and the area of argyrophilic dots were measured by means of the same image analyzer to obtain the percentage of nuclear area occupied by Ag-NOR proteins.
Statistical analysis was performed using Kolmogoroff-Smirnoff's non parametric test.

RESULTS

The mean number of argyrophilic dots increased progressively from mild to severe dysplasia to adenocarcinoma with both methods ($p<0.0001$). The increase was not significant in moderate versus severe dysplasia.
For each class of lesions the mean number of dots observed through micrographs was smaller when compared to the numbers counted with light microscope which allows a finer resolution through continuous focusing (Figs. 1 and 2).

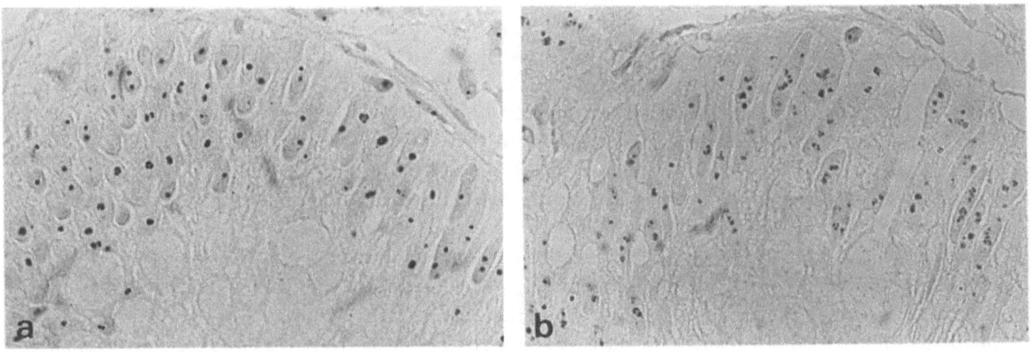

Fig. 1 Patterns of black dots distribution in colonic adenomatous polyps with mild (a) and moderate (b) dysplasia. Ag-NORs stain 750X.

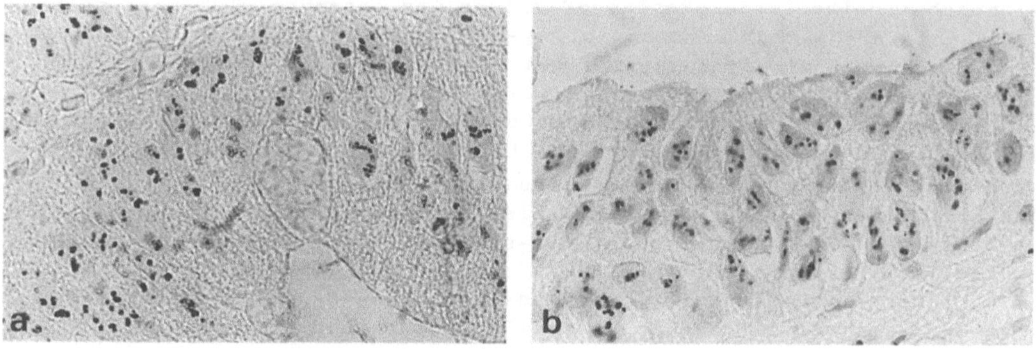

Fig. 2 Patterns of black dots distribution in colonic adenomatous polyps with severe dysplasia (a) and adenocarcinomas (b). Ag-NORs stain 750X.

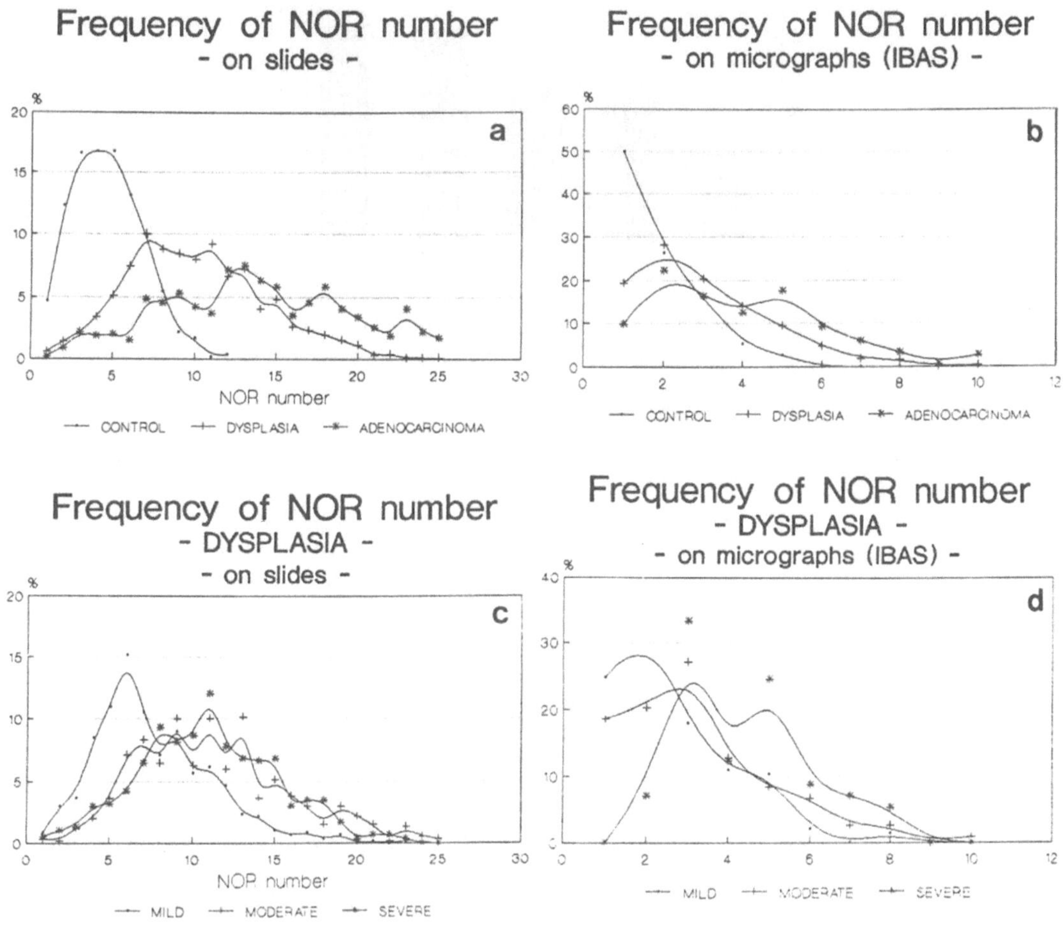

Fig. 3 Diagrams showing the frequency of Ag-NORs number counted from slides and from micrographs.

Although a rather wide overlap of values was observed with both methods, it is noteworthy that a number of Ag-NORs greater than 8 or 32 was counted by means of micrographs or light microscope respectively only in infiltrating malignant epithelial cells (Fig. 3).
The percentage of mean nuclear area occupied by Ag-NORs increased from dysplastic to carcinomatous lesions (Fig. 4). No significant changes were observed between severe dysplasia and adenocarcinoma.
The comparison of the results revealed an overlap of ranges in the percentage of mean number of silver-staining black dots and in the mean nuclear area occupied by Ag-NORs.
In carcinomas we observed an increase in the number of clumps which were small sized and made up of smaller numbers of silver-stained dots.

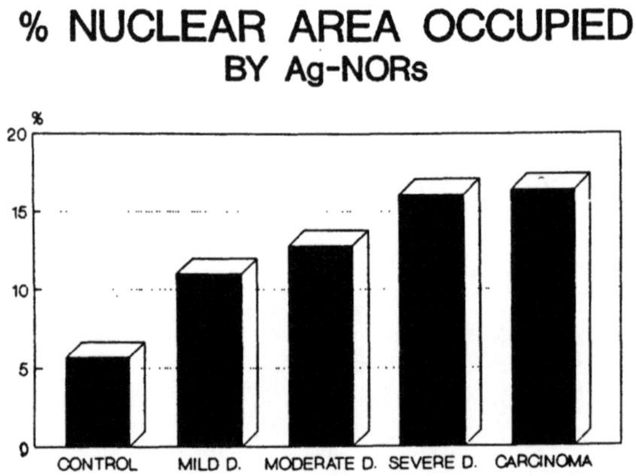

Fig. 4 Modifications of the percentage of mean nuclear area occupied by Ag-NORs in normal colonic mucosa, dysplastic and neoplastic lesions.

DISCUSSION

A recent study (Ploton 1986) showed that the Ag-NOR method can be applied to routinely processed paraffin sections and therefore used in diagnostic histopathology (Crocker & Nar 1987; Crocker & Skilbeck 1987; Derenzini 1986; Derenzini 1988).
The present study compared the behaviour of silver-binding nucleolar organizer regions in different grades of colonic epithelial dysplasia revealing significant relations between the mean number of Ag-NORs, the nuclear area occupied and their distribution compared to the different levels of cellular atypia.
Although the mean number of dots counted through micrographs was smaller when compared to that counted with the light microscope, both methods showed a progressive increase in the mean number of argyrophilic dots from mild to severe dysplasia to adenocarcinoma ($p<0.0001$). Such a correlation was not confirmed for moderate versus severe dysplasia.
An increase in the percentage of the mean nuclear area occupied by silver-stained dots was observed from dysplastic lesions to adenocarci-

nomas, it resulted significant for moderate versus severe dysplasia too. The arrangement of dots differed in different lesions, resulting in one or more large clumps in dysplastic epithelium and in numerous, small size clumps containing only few dots in carcinomas.
We observed a wide overlap of ranges between number of dots, nuclear area/dots area ratio and between different patterns of distribution. Such an overlap made it impossible to identify a single cell as malignant except for those cells showing a marked increase in dot number.
Our data suggest that the Ag-NOR technique is a useful tool in evaluating different grades of epithelial dysplasia and infiltrating colonic adenocarcinomas although its predictive value is reliable only when a suitable number of cells are observed in a tissue context.

REFERENCES

Angelier N, Hernandez-Verdun D, Bouteille M (1982) Visualization of Ag-NOR proteins on nucleolar transcriptional units in molecular spreads. Chromosoma 86: 661-672

Busch H, Lischwe MA, Michalik J, Chan PK, Busch RK (1982) Nucleolar Proteins of special interest: silver-staining proteins B23 and C23 antigens of human tumour nucleoli. In the Nucleolus. Jordan EG and Cullis CA, Cambridge University Press, pp 43-71

Crocker J, Nar P (1987) Nucleolar organizer regions in lymphomas. J Pathol 151: 111-118

Crocker J, Skilbeck N (1987) Nucleolar organizer regions in melanotic lesions of the skin. A quantitative study. J Clin Pathol 40: 885-889

Derenzini M, Betts CM, Ceccarelli C, Eusebi V (1986) Ultrastructural organization of nucleoli in benign naevi and malignant melanomas. Virchows Arch (Cell Pathol) 52: 343-352

Derenzini M, Farabegoli F, Pession A, Novello F (1987) Spatial redistribution of ribosomal chromatin in the fibrillar centres of human lymphocytes after stimulation of transcription. Exp Cell Res 170:31-41

Derenzini M, Romagnoli T, Mingazzini P, Marinozzi V (1988) Interphasic nucleolar organizer region distribution as a diagnostic parameter to differentiate benign from malignant epithelial tumors of human intestine. Virchows Arch (Cell Pathol) 54: 334-340

Hernandez-Verdun D, Derenzini M (1983) Non-nucleosomal configuration of chromatin in nucleolar organizer regions of metaphase chromosomes in situ. Eur J Cell Biol 31: 360-365

Hernandez-Verdun D (1986) Structural organization of the nucleolus in mammalian cells. Meth Arch Exp Pathol 12: 26-62

Hubbell HR, Rothblum LI, Hsu TC (1979) Identification of a silver binding protein associated with the cytological silver staining of actively transcribing nucleolar regions. Cell Biol Int Rep 3: 315-322

Lischwe MA, Richards RL, Busch RK, Busch H (1981) Localization of phosphoprotein C23 to nucleolar structures and to the nucleolus organizer regions. Expl Cell Res 136: 101-109

Morton CC, Brown JA, Holmes WM, Nance WE, Wolf B (1983) Stain intensity of human nucleolus organizer region reflects incorporation of uridine into mature ribosomal RNA. Exp Cell Res 145: 405-413

Ochs R, Lischwe M, O'Leary P, Busch H (1983) Localization of nucleolar phosphoproteins B23 and C23 during mitosis. Expl Cell Res 146:139-149

Ploton D, Menager M, Jeannesson P, Himber G, Pigeon F, Adnet JJ (1986) Improvement in the staining and in the visualization of the argyrophilic proteins of the nucleolar organizer region at the optical level. Histochem J 18: 5-14

Williams MA, Kleischmidt IA, Krohne G, Franke WW (1982) Argyrophilic nuclear and nucleolar proteins of Xenopus laevis oocytes identified by gel electrophoresis. Expl Cell Res 137: 341-351

Cultured Skin Fibroblasts from Hereditary Colorectal Cancer Patients: Susceptibility Mechanisms, Genetics, and Biomarkers

LEVY KOPELOVICH

ABSTRACT

The present studies illustrate the utility of biomarkers that occur systemically in skin fibroblasts of patients with hereditary adenomatosis of the colon and rectum, an autosomal dominant trait. These biomarkers provide insight into the initiated cell phenotype, susceptibility mechanisms, genetic alterations during colorectal cancer, and potential therapeutic approaches.

Keywords: biomarkers, susceptibility mechanisms, genetic predisposition, cultured fibroblasts, colorectal cancer.

INTRODUCTION

Here is a dilemma: specific chromosomes have been assigned to each of several distinct autosomal dominant forms of inherited cancer (Friend et al., 1988; Sandberg 1980; White and Caskey 1988); experiments, however, show a systemic expression of abnormal biomarkers that are commonly shared by these syndromes, viz, hereditary adenomatosis of the colon and rectum (ACR), Von Recklinghausen's neurofibromatosis (VRNF), bilateral retinoblastoma (bRB), and lung and breast cancer. The occurrence of abnormal biomarkers in clinically unaffected skin cells from patients who are predisposed to different forms of cancer suggested to us the concept of a global expression for the cancer trait (Kopelovich 1988, 1989). While each distinct form of cancer may represent a single and specific gene defect (tissue-specific differentiation genes), an additional gene or class of genes may pleiotropically control the expression of distinct forms of inherited cancer. In line with epidemiological findings (Knudson 1985; Lynch 1985), an underlying assumption is that, while more than one hierarchy of control is proposed, the combined outcome vis a vis cancer predisposition must be manifested clinically as an autosomal dominant trait (Kopelovich 1988, 1989).

To suggest another example, in the case of bRB, the RB1 locus, presumed to be bRB specific, is widely expressed and may contribute to the physiology of many cell types. Yet clinical cancer due to the RB gene is limited to only a few tissues among bRB patients, and among patients having no obvious predisposition to bRB and no previous evidence of bRB. Significantly as well, bRB has never been observed in any other mammalian species where it may be associated with a range of tumors quite distinct from that seen in humans (Bernards et al., 1989; Buckhkovich et al., 1989; DeCaprio et al., 1989; Knudson 1985). Whether these observations can also be used to support the existence of a senior hierarchy of control in cancer development has yet to be established.

---

[1] In this article familial polyposis coli is referred to as hereditary adenomatosis of the colon and rectum (ACR).

These considerations suggest, as one possibility, that the cancer trait can be regulated by homeotic genes (Akam 1989). An added dimension would include the concept of modularity in promoters/enhancers (Dynan 1989) vis a vis the homeotic gene system. Involvement by a homeotic class of genes may account for the fact that similar phenotypic alterations are shared by several distinct cancer syndromes. A homeotic protein associated with DNA binding activity would have the potential for recognition and differential control of a specific cancer "differentiation" gene that was altered, e.g., the ACR mutation. The tumor type would presumably be determined by the proliferative potential and the cell lineage of the "target organ(s)", including epigenetic mechanisms.

THE EXPERIMENTAL SYSTEM

As part of our study of genetic mechanisms that predispose to cancer, we investigated cultured skin fibroblasts from ACR patients. Knowledge that an autosomal dominant pattern of inheritance in ACR is manifested by a tendency toward colorectal cancer as well as other tumors, including those arising from skin (Gardner and Richards 1953; Morson and Bussey 1970), led us to consider the use of skin fibroblasts to study genetic determinants of cancer predisposition in ACR patients. Using only cultured skin fibroblasts from patients and from healthy individuals, we were able to examine a single cell type under comparable conditions in vitro. Clearly, it is an easier task to scan cultured fibroblasts than it is to obtain cells from most of the tissues at high risk for a variety of cancers.

From our observations, a terminology of basic concepts has developed (Kopelovich 1986, 1987, 1988, 1989). **Transformed cell** describes cells with an abnormal phenotype in vitro. The term **cancer initiation,** or **cancer predisposition,** describes the transformed cell phenotype in conjunction with genetic susceptibility in vivo. The term **biomarker** describes the abnormal expression of a specific biological parameter associated with the neoplastic process. As used here, the term **oncogene** describes a genetic sequence whose expression within a cell may induce that cell to convert from one cell phenotype to another. The term **protooncogene** describes a genetic sequence which, if altered in the appropriate manner, has the potential to become an oncogene. Cancer-specific expressions, or **global expression** of the cancer trait, as distinct from cancer-specific genes, suggests the existence of a senior hierarchy of control in cancer development that results in the occurrence of similar biomarkers in cells from patients who are predisposed to different dominantly inherited forms of cancer.

BIOMARKERS AND THE INITIATED CELL PHENOTYPE

To date, many abnormal phenotypic expressions have been identified in fibroblastic cells from ACR patients (Table 1). The abnormalities include growth parameters, increased life-span in vitro, changes in DNA content, deformed cytoarchitecture, alterations of membrane-associated parameters, augmented expression of host-cell coded transformation-associated proteins, increased susceptibility to further transformation by a variety of physical, chemical, and viral agents, and decreased cytotoxic response to a variety of physical and chemical agents. Extension of these experiments in a number of laboratories has confirmed the occurrence of these alterations not only in cells from ACR patients but also in VRNF, bRB, the Li-Fraumeni Syndrome, and lung and breast cancer patients (For review see Kopelovich, 1986, 1988; Tainsky et al., 1989). In general, the abnormal phenotypic expressions seen in fibroblasts from persons predisposed to cancer were further amplified during cancer progression (spontaneous or experimentally-induced (Kopelovich 1988).

One example of an abnormal biomarker as it pertains to our understanding of cancer initiation is cytoskeletal-actin. In the cytoplasm of well-spread cultured normal cells, cytoskeletal-actin is organized into a network of cables adherent to the inside of the cell membrane. Fibronectin and collagen represent principal components which, in association with other extracellular factors, are responsible for the formation of organized cell adhesions.

Using indirect immunofluorescence, we found a disruption of actin organization in unperturbed cultured skin fibroblasts from ACR patients (Kopelovich et al., 1977, 1980). These cells were normal with regard to other cytoskeletal structures such as microtubules and intermediate filaments (Kopelovich L., and Fusenig N., unpublished observations, (1978)). The possibility that ACR cells express high amounts of actin-depolymerizing proteins (Norberg et al., 1979), or an abnormal form of the actin gene(s) (Chou et al., 1987; Kakunaga et al., 1984), has yet to be observed. However, an increased level of ^{35}S- methionine incorporation into G-and F-actin and a faster turnover of F-actin were subsequently demonstrated in ACR cells (Antecol et al., 1986; Higgins P., and Kopelovich L., in preparation, 1989).

ACR cells were indistinguishable from normal fibroblasts with respect to both synthesis and surface retention of fibronectin, indicating that alterations involving fibronectin appear later in the transformation process (Kopelovich et al., 1985). However, since ACR cells did not respond to the addition of exogenous fibronectin and/or collagen by a normalization of their morphology and reorganization of their cytoskeletal-actin filaments, it is conceivable that a constitutive alteration of the actin-containing cables in ACR skin fibroblasts renders the attachment plaques insensitive to the addition of exogenous fibronectin and collagen (Kopelovich et al., 1985).

Along similar lines, experiments using cis-hydroxyproline showed an appreciable toxicity to proliferating normal skin fibroblasts (50% at 100 ng/ml, and 100% at about 400 ng/ml), but not to proliferating ACR cells (up to 1 ug/ml) (Kopelovich 1985). These results suggest that, although collagen synthesis may be normal, final assembly of extracellular collagen matrices (tertiary structure) is defective in ACR cells. Similar results were observed by electron microscopy (Gardner and Rogers 1980).

Recent data showed significant decrease in ACR cells of a 52Kd cell-attachment glycoprotein, a serine protease inhibitor (Higgins and Ryan 1989). This finding appears to represent an early event leading to the abnormal expression of cytoskeletal-actin within ACR cells (Higgins P., and Kopelovich L., in preparation, 1989).

In this instance, therefore, our data show that an initiated ACR cell can be characterized through its defective cytoskeletal-actin, defective extracellular collagen matrix, and lack of response to exogenous fibronectin or collagen. The regulation of fibronectin and procollagen expression in virus-transformed cells in vitro and in spontaneous cancer in vivo is thought to be effected through a similar sequence, including loss of fibronectin from the cell periphery as a consequence of decreased levels of actin cables and an alteration in the anchoring collagen molecules (Bissell 1981).

Collectively, the abnormal biomarkers observed in fibroblasts from ACR patients describe the changing phenotype of cells undergoing neoplastic transformation (Table 1). Such cells presumably represent an initiated state that, for the first time, provides a means of characterizing cancer initiation in humans (Kopelovich 1988, 1989). These abnormal biomarkers are intrinsically linked to cancer, because all so-affected individuals eventually develop cancer. However, additional mutations are apparently necessary, with certain promoters acting to increase the probability for expression of the malignant phenotype. The probability of such a transition occurring spontaneously is extremely rare, since, for example, very few initiated cells, or adenomas for that matter, become tumorigenic even in the colon of ACR patients. This observation is consistent with in vitro studies as well (Kopelovich 1988, 1989).

SUSCEPTIBILITY MECHANISMS

The oncogene paradigm developed over the past decade has proved to be particularly helpful in generating insights into cancer at the molecular level. A simple model would identify protooncogenes, the antecedents of cellular oncogenes, with genetic targets the alteration of which defines distinct steps in multistep cellular transformation/neodifferentiation. In this view, the evolution of a tumor cell clone is provided by a series of oncogene activations, each of which would confer some of the phenotypes that in aggregate constitute a fully malignant behavior. Oncogenes were identified wherein each acting alone was unable to cause full transformation; however, two or possibly more oncogenes, working in collaboration, effected a full tumorigenic phenotype (Weinberg 1989).

The classification of oncogenes based on their collaborative potential in transformation assays was paralleled in a striking way by ordering them according to the intracellular localization of their respective gene products. For example, those oncogenes that function like ras encode cytoplasmic proteins, while those that function like myc specify nuclear proteins. Working in collaboration, nuclear oncoproteins and cytoplasmic proteins appear able to effect the tumorigenic phenotype (Weinberg 1989). Nuclear oncoproteins per se can also induce DNA synthesis and can affect transcription of particular target genes. In addition, some nuclear oncoproteins have properties or activities characteristic of transcription factors (Green 1989).

Recent findings, however, lead to the conjecture that diverse nuclear oncoproteins participate in transformation through a common mechanism; they inactivate specific cellular proteins that themselves control normal cell proliferation (Dyson et al., 1989; Green 1989; Weinberg 1989).

How instructive is this oncogene model in understanding multistep carcinogenesis as it occurs in humans? The scenario of tumor evolution drawn above echoes work that has been carried out on cultured human adult skin fibroblasts from ACR patients. The effects of an ACR mutation seen in such studies, in many instances do appear to run parallel with the broad concept of the collaborating oncogenes/antioncogenes paradigm. For example, the association between colorectal cancer and increased transformation by the ras-oncogene was first seen in skin fibroblasts from ACR patients (Kopelovich 1988). In this instance, however, no differences were found between normal and ACR cells at the level of DNA, RNA transcripts, or gene products of the ras gene family (Kopelovich L, and Ellis R., unpublished (1982)). DNA from ACR cells also lacked transforming activity in the NIH/3T3 transfection assay (Needleman et al., 1983). It was concluded that the increased sensitivity of ACR cells to transformation by the ras family of oncogenes is dissociated, at least in part, from the ability of such cells to express an altered c-ras protooncogene (Kopelovich 1989). How exactly the increased sensitivity of ACR cells to transformation by KiMSV and HaMSV might be related etiologically to an altered ras gene expression in colon adenomas and colon, lung, and breast adenocarcinomas (Vogelstein et al., 1989) has yet to be established.

An association between colorectal cancer and increased transformation by SV40 and Adeno 12-SV40 was subsequently demonstrated in skin fibroblasts from ACR patients. We also found increased expression of the transformation-associated p53 protein in ACR cells. Moreover, fibroblasts from clinically identifiable precursor states showed increasingly greater amounts of the p53 protein, suggesting a correlation with cancer progression as well (Kopelovich and DeLeo 1986,1990). The extent to which over-expression of the p53 protein in ACR cells is responsible for the initiated cell phenotype, and whether this over-expression represents a mutational activation in the promoter/enhancer elements (Tuck and Crawford 1989) or alterations in the p53 gene itself (Baker et al., 1989), is under investigation. The increased expression of the p53 protein in ACR cells prior to any alterations in expression, or to the transforming potential of the c-ras family of oncogenes, suggests that it is an early event associated with cancer predisposition. The localization of the p53 gene to human chromosome 17 (McBride et al., 1986) is of interest, since progression of colorectal cancer may also be associated with chromosome 17 (Vogelstein 1989).

Taken together, in a way yet unknown to us, the data on cultured ACR cells suggest a cooperative effect between the cytoplasmic ras oncogenes and several nuclear oncoproteins (e.g., Ela, large T, p53) that, in general, appears to conform to the oncogenes/antioncogenes paradigm (Weinberg 1989). In these interactions, the role of endogenous cellular sequences vis a vis viral proteins is unclear. These interactions may occur by gene activation, regulation through cis-or trans-acting mechanisms, and/or selective gene product associations which in several permutations are brought to bear, to confer a genotypic profile that is associated with cancer initiation.

The ACR mutation as seen through analysis of cultured ACR cells is able to effect many phenotypic changes simultaneously. Whether the ACR gene, if isolated, would represent a mechanism similar to that of the RB gene product is, in our view, not at all certain. Conceivably, the many questions that were applied to the RB protein would be applicable to a potential ACR gene product as well (Bernards et al., 1989). Is it a tumor suppressor gene? Does it complex with other oncogene products? What is the tissue and species distribution? If widely distributed, why would the ACR trait confine itself clinically to a limited number of tissues that are not always necessarily related developmentally, and why would the ACR trait limit itself clinically principally to humans?

GENETIC ALTERATIONS DURING COLORECTAL CANCER

The phenotypic progression, normal colon ⟶ hyperplastic epithelium ⟶ ⟶ adenoma stages I to III ⟶ carcinoma in situ, has been associated with a series of genetic changes, including DNA content, hypomethylation, the Ki-ras oncogene (early events), a mutation and subsequent deletion at the p53 locus, and loss of heterozygosity of RFLP alleles on chromosomes 5q, 17q and 18q (Vogelstein 1989). It has been suggested that high frequency of specific allelic losses in hyperploid tumors results from the clonal proliferation of a cell in which loss of chromosomal segments had taken place before or during the endomitosis leading to hyperploidy (Delattre et al, 1989). The ACR locus has presently been mapped to chromosome 5q (Bodmer et al., 1987; Leppert et al., 1987; Solomon et al., 1987). If the ACR gene is, in fact, located at chromosome 5, loss of heterozygosity on this chromosome might be identified as a major event leading to clinical progression in genetic and sporadic colorectal cancer. Presumably, it is the accumulation of these genetic alterations, rather than any specific progressive changes, that is important for the development of colorectal cancer.

Observations like these refocus attention on cell specimens derived from persons who are genetically predisposed to cancer. These early-passage cells have ostensibly undergone few, if any, changes in growth control mechanisms following explantation from the patient. They should, therefore, represent good models of cells that suffer transformation within living tissues. It is fair to assume that the abnormal expressions which are observed in clinically normal, early-passage fibroblasts from ACR patients represent the earliest events associated with the occurrence of occult cancer. These alterations are directly related to the etiology of clinical cancer (Kopelovich 1988, 1989), and together with changes found in clinical cancer (Vogelstein et al., 1989), can provide insight about the sequence of the events leading to genetic and sporadic forms of colorectal cancer. Stated differently, genetic changes that occur in adenomas and colon adenocarcinomas are rather late events. They would be more relevant to an understanding of mechanisms of cancer inception if they could be related to changes seen in clinically uninvolved tissues from ACR patients **(compare Table 1 and Vogelstein et al., 1989; Stanbridge 1989).**

TABLE 1: PHENOTYPIC PROFILE OF AN INITIATED CELL

A. Growth Parameters

1. Growth in nutrient-deprived environment
2. Loss of contact-inhibition
3. Increased cloning-efficiency
4. A partial loss of anchorage-sensitivity
5. Increased life-span[a]
6. Increased spontaneous transformation[b]
7. Decreased sensitivity to hydrocortisone-induced cell proliferation in monolayers and in agar

B. Cytogenetics

1. Increased tetraploidy/hyperploidy (Danes B.)
2. Increased cytogenetic aberrations (Danes B.)

C. Cytoskeletal Structures

1. Defective actin-containing cables
2. Lack of restoration of deformed cytoskeletal-actin by exogenous fibronectin/collagen
3. Normal organization of microtubules
4. Normal organization of intermediate filaments

D. Membrane-Associated Parameters

1. Increased 2-deoxyglucose uptake
2. Increased Con-A agglutination (in suspension and onto derivatized matrices)
3. Increased intra-and extracellular levels of plasminogen activator
4. Defective polymerization of collagen (tertiary structure)
5. Normal expression of fibronectin
6. Defective tac subunit chain of the interleukin-2 receptor (Azzarone B., and Kopelovich L., in preparation)
7. Decreased expression of a 52Kd cell-attachment glycoprotein, a serine-protease inhibitor (Higgins P., and Kopelovich L., in preparation)

E. Expression of Cellular Oncogenes

1. No apparent change in c-ras oncogenes
2. Increased expression of the transformation-associated, host-cell coded, p53 protein that is further amplified during cancer progression

F. Cytotoxic Effects by Chemical and Physical Agents

1. Apparently normal sensitivity to x-rays and uv-irradiation. Increased tolerance to x-rays and uv-irradiation during cancer progression
2. Decreased cytotoxic response to retinoic acid
3. Decreased cytotoxic response to 5-azacytidine that is further amplified during cancer progression
4. Decreased cytotoxic response to TPA that is bimodally expressed and becoming progressively hyperbolic during cancer development

G. Increased Sensitivity to Further Transformation by Oncogenic Viruses

1. Kirsten murine sarcoma virus; Harvey murine sarcoma virus (associated with an expression of a human fetal-like antigen)
2. SV40 (associated with an expression of a human placenta-like antigen)

H. Increased sensitivity to Further Transformation by Chemical and Physical Agents

1. TPA (also characterized by a marked increase in cell-ploidy and by expression of a human fetal-like antigen)
2. MNNG (also characterized by a marked increase in cell-ploidy)
3. X-rays (associated with a progressive increase in radiotolerance during cancer development)

I. Metabolic Parameters

1. Normal cholesterol feedback regulation (HMG-CoA reductase)
2. Normal methionine requirement[c]
3. Increased lactate production[c]
4. Decreased prostaglandins production [c]

J. Virus-Induced Transformation/Neodifferentiation

1. Adipocytic conversion by ras oncogenes in the presence of glucocorticosteroids
2. Histiocytic conversion by a fes oncogene in the presence of glucocorticosteroids

---

These results have been recently summarized in great detail (Kopelovich 1988, 1989) In general, the pattern of abnormal biomarkers found in initiated ACR cells becomes progressively amplified during cancer progression (Kopelovich 1988, 1989). In these studies no differences have ever been seen between ACR and its Gardner Syndrome variant.

[a] Proc. Natl. Acad. Sci. (USA) 86:2008-2012, 1989.

[b] Li-Fraumeni Syndrome, Lung cancer.

[c] Preliminary observations.

The following specific questions now emerge:

1. Does information imprinted in initiated ACR cells (and presumably all organs) represent a recapitulation of some or all events that are **sequentially** acquired upon inception of sporadic colorecatal cancer?
2. Does the increased tendency for endoreduplication seen in ACR cells mirror the rare events that occur in colonic mucosa cells undergoing neoplastic transformation, wherein endomitoses are presumably followed by loss of heterozygosity at critical loci which, through clonal selection/expansion, may lead to colon adenocarcinoma?
3. How is the decreased cytotoxic response by ACR cells to 5-azacytidine related to the hypomethylated state seen in early stage adenomas?
4. How is the increased sensitivity of ACR cells to transformation by the ras oncogene, with no change in the antecedent protooncogene, being brought about? How is it related to activation of the ras oncogene during clinical progression of colorectal cancer?

5. How is the increased sensitivity of ACR cells to transformation by SV40 and Adeno-12/SV40 being brought about?
6. Is the p53 protein an antioncogene? If so, why is it elevated in initiated ACR cells?
7. Do p53, large T, or Ela, and ras-related sequences/proteins work in concert with each other in ACR cells, as suggested by the collaborating oncogene paradigm?

These questions are only a few of the many examples that illustrate the relevance of biomarkers in initiated ACR cells to an understanding of the clinical progression of sporadic and genetic forms of colorectal cancer in man.

Reconsideration of the sequence of progression in genetic and sporadic forms of colorectal cancer can be viewed through the use of cultured cells from ACR patients. It would appear that such cells which themselves are clinically uninvolved, have recaptured, in principle, most or all of the events attributed to the progression of clinical cancer to date. Does this mean that the ACR gene has essentially programmed all cells to express the majority of changes associated with clinical cancer? What are the mechanisms in sporadic colorectal cancer that direct a sequence of such genetic-clinical events over time? It is conceivable, however, that in sporadic cancer as well, most relevant changes occur in a single cell, yet technically these changes can only be detected after sufficient cell expansion has taken place (e.g., hyperplasia, adenoma I-III). Yet in ACR, as well as in sporadic colorectal cancer, a second event, presumably, although by no means proven, a mutation, followed by clonal selection/expansion would be necessary to bring about cancer.

We must continue to try to define not only the inherited and acquired gene defects that initiate the neoplastic state, but also the subsequent genetic alterations involved in tumor progression. These genetic alterations are already proving useful in diagnosis and prognosis. The hope is that they may be useful for designing specific therapy.

VIRUS-INDUCED NEODIFFERENTIATION AND POTENTIAL THERAPEUTIC APPROACHES

As part of our study of mechanisms associated with transformation of human adult skin fibrobalsts by oncogenic viruses, we demonstrated the adipocytic conversion of human adult skin fibroblasts by the kirsten murine sarcoma virus (KiMSV), the Harvey murine sarcoma virus (HaMSV), and the Balb murine sarcoma virus (BaMSV) (Kopelovich et al., 1986, 1987a,b; Kopelovich and Fenyk 1988). This conversion occurred in the presence of dexamethasone (DX). The Moloney murine sarcoma virus (MoMSV), which bears no resemblance to the ras or balb family of oncogenes (Kopelovich and Fenyk 1988), also effected adipocytic conversion of HSF in the presence of DX. These findings suggest that the v-ras, v-balb, as well as the v-mos families of oncogenes, represent variations of two or more major genes which either are facilitators of fat-cell differentiation or are themselves specific fat-cell differentiation genes. An alternative molecular mechanism may involve the action of cis-acting sequences, or diffusable trans-acting factors on the expression of these oncogenes.
We have recently also described the role and specificity of the feline family of oncogenes in morphogenetic processes of human cells in vitro. Through the use of the ST:feline sarcoma virus (ST:(FeSV) and glucocorticosteroids, we showed the de novo conversion of human adult skin fibroblasts to histiocytes (also known as tissue macrophages) in a large fraction of virus-transformed foci (Kopelovich and Wang 1990).

Oncogenes have long been implicated in cancer causation (Bishop 1983; Varmus 1988; Weinberg 1989). In principle, however, reversal of the cancer cell phenotype or change in a normal cell phenotype (spontaneous or experimentally-induced), is possible through mechanisms similar to those caused by the v-ras, v-balb, v-mos, and the v-fes oncogenes (Kopelovich et al., 1988; Kopelovich and Wang 1990). Activation of protooncogenes may, in certain instances, represent a physiological process which ranges in quality from a reversible reaction to an essentially irreversible one in much the same way as enzymatic reactions occur. For example, the cellular homolog of ST:FeSV, upon activation, could give rise to histiocytes in mesenchyme-derived tissues as a means of increasing the number of such cells to counteract inflammatory diseases and immunodeficient states, including cancer. These data also suggest that increased production of histiocytes by an activated c-ST:fes oncogene is likely to be affected by the hormonal milieu in situ and/or administration of hormone therapy (Kopelovich and Wang 1990).

A novel concept is presented that (a), mesenchyme-derived tissues in vivo may serve as a reservoir of different cell phenotypes that are embryologically derived from the mesoblast, and (b), this reservoir can be modulated by physiological conditions in normal and diseased states. Thus mesenchyme-derived cells can exist in a "status quo", and if manipulated, may be recruited to perform new and specific functions. This recruitment process may occur spontaneously, or it may be experimentally induced. In the case of histiocytes, this phenomenon may also provide insight into the origin of tissue macrophage heterogeneity (Kopelovich and Wang 1990).

The following specific questions now appear relevant: (1) Can histiocytes arise in most or all mesenchyme-derived tissues de novo? (2) Would ST:FeSV-induced histiocytes be considered normal cells? (3) What is the potential for **therapy** by the fes protein through direct conversion of solid tumors of mesenchyme origin, and/or the de novo conversion of normal mesenchyme-derived cells to histiocytes, including their cytokines (self-derived), during local inflammatory episodes and in immunocompromised syndromes, HIV, and soft tissue cancers?

EPILOGUE

It is generally accepted that cancer is caused by a number of apparently unrelated environmental factors that interact with genetic components in susceptible individuals. Having worked on genetic mechanisms that might underlie colorectal cancer, I have held the firm belief over the years that DNA from certain bacteria through **integration** into the DNA of colonic mucosa cells within the digestive tract is likely to act as a powerful mutagen in the causation of colorectal cancer (Kopelovich 1987).

The amounts of DNA from lysed bacteria present in the gastrointestinal tract are enormous. The molecular genetic mechanisms that could be involved in the causation of colorectal cancer by bacteria may be analogous to those identified in plant tumors due to Agrobacterium tumefacieus (Stachel and Zambryski 1986) and, perhaps, nodulation of legumes by Rhizobium (Downie and Johnson 1986). These mechanisms include activation of gene expression in response to an external stimulus followed by recognition, attachment, and conjugative transfer of DNA from a donor to a susceptible recipient colonic ephitelial cells.

Other factors that would contribute to bacterial involvement may include alteration of cell membranes through secretion by certain bacteria (e.g., Clostridium, Streptococcus, Staphylococcus) of modifier proteins (Lennette et al., 1985), leading to increased uptake of colonic bacterial DNA. Insertion of DNA sequences from **anaerobic** bacteria into colonic mucosa cells can be of considerable consequence to our understanding of metabolic mechanisms that are involved in the etiology of colorectal cancer. Similarly, insertion of methylated base sequences that are unique to bacterial DNA may, directly or indirectly, contribute to mutational events that would lead to the development of colorectal cancer.

Increased injury to or fragility of certain colonic epithelial cells, as in plant tumors (Stachel and Zambryski 1986), would represent yet another factor contributing to colorectal cancer by bacterial DNA. Such occurrences could partially explain the presence of solitary or even multiple tumors in areas of the gastrointestinal tract that are subjected to mechanical insult and, thus, increased cell injury. We know that cell injury, in turn, will stimulate both DNA replication and cell proliferation which typically trigger recombination/repair processes, essential for bacterial DNA integration and for "relevant" rearrangements of target sequences. Incidentally, the α-toxin of C. perfringens is also a powerful lecithinase (Lennette et al., 1985) which generates diacylglycerol, a phorbol ester protagonist, and a potential tumor promoter (Rozengurt 1986).

The present hypothesis would have to reconcile some or all of the abnormal phenotypes that were observed in cells from individuals predisposed to colorectal cancer (this article). Conceivably, however, cancers of other organs may be caused by similar mechanisms. The extent to which bacterial DNA should be considered a risk factor in human cancer deserves to be a major focus of research activity.

ACKNOWLEDGEMENTS

The author would like to thank Joyce Ross for assistance in preparing the manuscript, and Mrs. Ana Mackino for typing same. This work was supported in part by grants from the Department of Veterans Affairs, Veterans Health Services and Research Administration.

REFERENCES

Akam M: Hox and HOM (1989) Homologous gene clusters in insects and vertebrates. Cell 57:347-349.

Antecol MH, Darveau A, Sonenberg N, Mukherjee BB (1986) Altered biochemical properties of actin in normal skin fibroblasts from individuals predisposed to dominantly inherited cancer. Cancer Res. 46:1867-1873.

Baker SJ, Fearson ER, Nigro JM, Hamilton SR, Preisinger AC, Jessup JM, van Tuinen P, Ledbetter DH, Barker, DF, Nakamura Y, White R, Vogelstein B (1989) Chromosome 17 deletions and p53 gene mutations in colorectal carcinomas. Science 244:217-221.

Bernards R, Schackleford GM, Gerber MR, Horowitz JM, Friend SH, Schartl M, Bogenmann E, Rapaport JM, McGee T, Dryja TP, Weinberg RA (1989) Structure and expression of the murine retinoblastoma gene and characterization of its encoded protein. Proc. Natl. Acad. Sci. (U.S.A.) 86:6474-6478.

Bishop JM (1983) Cellular oncogenes and retroviruses. Ann. Rev. Biochem. 52:350-354.

Bissell MJ (1981) The differential state of normal and malignant cells, or how to define a normal cell in culture. Intl. Rev. Cytol. 70:27-100.

Bodmer WF, Bailey CJ, Bodmer J, Bussey HJR, Ellis A, Gorman P, Lucibelo FC, Murday VA, Ryder SH, Scambler P, Sheer D, Solomon E, Spurr NK (1987) Localization of the gene for familial adenomatous polyposis on chromosome 5. Nature 328:614-616.

Buchkovich K, Duffy LA, Harlow E (1989) The retinoblastoma protein is phosphorylated during specific phases of the cell cycle. Cell 58:1097-1105.

Chou CC, Davis RC, Fuller ML, Slovin JP, Wing A, Wright J, Tania S, Shaked R, Gatti RA, Sasler WA (1987) Actin: unusual mRNA 3'-untranslated sequence conservation and amino acid substitutions that may be cancer related. Proc. Natl. Acad. Sci (U.S.A.) 84:2575-2579.

DeCaprio JA, Ludlow JW, Lynch D, Furukawa Y, Griffin J, Piwnica-Worms H, Huang C-M, Livingston DM (1989) The product of the retinoblastoma susceptibility gene has properties of a cell cycle regulatory element. Cell 58:1085-1095.

Delattre O, Law DJ, Remvikos Y, Sastre X, Feinberg AP, Olschwang S, Melot T, Salmon RJ, Validire P, Thomas G (1989) Multiple genetic alterations in distal and proximal colorectal cancer. The Lancet 2:353-355.

Downie JA, Johnson AWB (1986) Nodulation of legumes by Rhizobium: The recognized root? Cell 47:153-154.
Dynan WS (1989) Modularity in promoters and enhancers. Cell 58:1-4.
Dyson N, Buchkovich K, Whyte P, Harlow E (1989) The cellular 107K protein that binds to adenovirus ElA also associates with the large T antigens of SV40 and JC virus. Cell 58:249-255.
Friend SH, Dryja TP, Weinberg RA (1988) Oncogenes and tumor suppressing genes. New Engl. J. Med. 318:618-622.
Gardner EJ, Richards R (1953) Multiple cutaneous and subcutaneous lesions occurring simultaneously with hereditary polyposis and osteomatosis. Am. J. Human Genet. 5:139-148.
Gardner EJ, Rogers SW (1980) Growth properties of cells from Gardner's patients. Natl. Large Bowel Bulletin 3:10-15.
Green MR (1989) When the products of oncogenes and anti-oncogenes meet. Cell 56:1-3.
Higgins PJ, Ryan MP (1989) Biochemical localization of the transformation-sensitive 52Kd (p52) protein to the substratum contact regions of cultured rat fibroblasts. Biochem. J. 258:173-182.
Kakunaga T, Leavitt TJ, Hamada H (1984) A mutation in actin associated with neoplastic transformation. Fed. Proc. 43:2275-2279.
Knudson AG (1985) Hereditary cancer, oncogenes, and anti-oncogenes. Cancer Res. 45:1437-1443.
Kopelovich L (1985) Recent observations and considerations in hereditary adenomatosis of the colon and rectum, in: H.A. Guirgis and H.T. Lynch (Eds.), Biomarkers genetics and cancer, New York, Van Nostrand Reinhold, pp 50-80.
Kopelovich L (1987a) Tissue culture assays in familial polyposis coli: Observations and considerations, in: G.P. Murphy (Ed.), Seminars in Surgical Oncology, Alan A. Liss, New York 3:159-164.
Kopelovich L (1987b) 5-Azacytidine inhibits adipocytic conversion of human skin fibroblasts by acute oncornaviruses and dexamethasone. Exptl. Cell Biol. 56:276-280.
Kopelovich L (1988) The transformed (initiated) human cell phenotype: Study of cultured skin fibroblasts from individuals predisposed to cancer. Mutat. Res. 199:369-385.
Kopelovich L (1989) Tissue culture studies in familial polyposis coli: Biomarkers, genetics, and cancer. In: Herrera (ed), Familial Adenomatous Polyposis. New York, Alan R. Liss, pp 263-270.
Kopelovich L, Conlon S, Pollack R (1977) Defective organization of actin in cultured skin fibroblasts. Proc. Natl. Acad. Sci (U.S.A) 74:3019-3022.
Kopelovich L, DeLeo AB (1986) Increased levels of p53 antigen in cultured fibroblasts from patients with hereditary adenomatosis of the colon and rectum and its relevance to oncogenic mechanisms. J. Natl. Cancer Inst. 77:1241-1246.
Kopelovich L, DeLeo AB (1990) Increased levels of p53 antigen in cultured fibroblasts from preneoplastic lesions in neurofibromatosis patients. Cancer Genet. Cytogenet. (in press).
Kopelovich L, Fenyk J (1988) Transformation/neodifferentiation of human skin fibroblasts by acute oncornaviruses and dexamethasone. Exptl. Cell Biol. 56:311-320.
Kopelovich L, Lipkin M, Blattner WA, Fraumeni Jr. JF, Lynch HJ, Pollack RE (1980) Organization of cytoskeletal actin in cultured skin fibroblasts from individuals at high risk of colon cancer. Int. J. Cancer 26:301-307.
Kopelovich L, Murray CJ, Kleinman HK, Martin GR, Fukuda Y, Renard SJ (1985) Defective actin organization in cultured skin fibroblasts from individuals with inherited colon adenocarcinoma is not restored by addition of fibronectin. Exptl. Cell Biol. 50:314-321.
Kopelovich L, Rich R, Wallace A (1986) Hydrocortisone promotes the neodifferentiation of Kirsten murine sarcoma virus transformed human skin fibroblasts to adipose cells, Relevance to oncogenic mechanisms. Exptl. Cell Biol. 54:25-33.

Kopelovich L, Wallace A, Rich RF (1987) The kinetics of neodifferentiation of Kirsten murine sarcoma virus transformed human skin fibroblasts to adipose cells by hydrocortisone. Cancer Invest. 5:567-581.

Kopelovich L, Wang TY (1990) Histiocytic conversion of human adult skin fibroblasts by the Snyder-Theilen Feline Sarcoma Virus. Am. J. Pathol. (in press).

Lennette EH, Balows A, Hausler WJ, Jr, Shadomy HJ (eds): Manual of clinical microbiology, 4th Edition, Washington, DC Am. Soc. Microbiol 1-1270, 1985.

Leppert M, Dobbs M, Scambler P, O'Connel P, Nakamura Y, Stauffer D, Woodward S, Burt R, Hughes J, Gardner E, Lathrop M, Wasmuth J, Lalouel J-M, White R (1987) The gene for familial polyposis coli maps to the long arm of chromosome 5. Science 238:1411-1413.

Lynch HT, Guirgis HA (1985) (eds): Biomarkers, genetics, and cancer. New York Van Nostrand, Reinhold, Inc. pp 1-204.

McBride OW, Merry D, Givol D (1986) The gene for human p53 cellular tumor antigen is located on chromosome 17 short arm. Proc. Natl. Acad. Sci. (U.S.A) 83:130-134.

Morson BC, Bussey JR (1970) Predisposing causes of intestinal cancer. Curr. Probl. Surg. 6:1-46.

Needleman SW, Yuasa Y, Srivastava S, Aaronson SA (1983) Normal cells of patients with high cancer risk syndromes lack transforming activity in the NIH/3T3 transfection assay. Science 222:173-174.

Norberg R, Thorstensson R, Utter G, Fragraeus A (1979) F-actin depolymerizing activity of human serum. Eur. J. Biochem. 100:575-585.

Rozengurt E (1986) Early signals in the mitogenic response. Science 234:161-167.

Sandberg AA (1980) The chromosomes in human cancer and leukemia, New York, Elsevier pp 1-748.

Solomon E, Voss R, Hall V, Bodmer WF, Jass JR, Jeffreys AJ, Lucibelo FC, Patel I, Rider SH (1987) Chromosome 5 allele loss in human colorectal carcinomas Nature 328:616-619.

Stachel SE, Zambryski PC (1986) Agrobacterium tumefacieus and the susceptible plant cell: A novel adaptation of extracellular recognition and DNA conjugation. Cell 47:155-157.

Stanbridge EJ (1989) The reemergence of tumor suppression. Cancer Cells 1:31-33.

Tainsky MA, Zamaniyan F, Yim SO, Pathak S, Giovanella BC, Strong LC (1989) Normal fibroblasts derived from patients with Li-Fraumeni cancer syndrome spontaneously transform in vitro. Proc. Amer. Assoc. Cancer Res. 30:315(#1250).

Tuck SP, Crawford L (1989) Overexpression of normal human p53 in established fibroblasts leads to their tumorigenic conversion. Oncog. Res. 4:81-96.

Varmus H (1988) Retroviruses. Science 240:1427-1435.

Vogelstein B, Fearson ER, Kern SE, Hamiltin SR, Preisinger AC, Nakamura Y, White R (1989) Allelotype of colorectal carcinoma. Science 244:207-211.

Weinberg RA (1989) Oncogenes, antioncogenes, and the molecular bases of multistep carcinogenesis. Cancer Res. 49:3713-3721.

White R, Caskey CT (1988) The human as an experimental system in molecular genetics. Science 240:1483-1488.

Chapter 6

Cytomolecular Aspects of Polyposis

Summary of Chapter 6: Cytomolecular Aspects of Polyposis

P. MEERA KHAN

The well known adenoma-carcinoma sequence hypothesis implies that adenoma is a precursor to adenocarcinoma. The development of hundreds of adenomatous polyps in the colorectal epithelium is a cardinal feature of the dominantly inherited familial adenomatous polyposis (FAP) due to lesions in a putative gene designated as <u>adenomatous polyposis coli</u> (<u>APC</u>) in the chromosome 5q15-q22 region. Herrera's report on a deletion in 5q in a FAP patient with multiple congenital malformations gave the first clue on the chromosomal localization of <u>APC</u>.

Two sporadic cases of mental retardation with classical FAP complicated by adenocarcinoma in their forties were reported by Chiba. It was pointed out that in the past several cases with FAP and mental retardation were reported and suggested that mental retardation is probably an additional manifestation of the FAP gene. Their studies revealed no chromosomal abnormalities.

In situ hybridization studies using the already available DNA probes (see below), mapping close to the <u>APC</u> locus may help identifying submicroscopic deletions. If the condition is due to a deletion, the associated mental retardation can be explained by the possible involvement of a contiguous gene or genes maintaining normal mental development. This could as well be the explanation for the mental impairment observed in other cases including the one reported by Herrera and those mentioned by Solomon (see below) in which the deletions were microscopically visible. The developmental abnormalities associated with the later cases are probably due to more extensive deletions resulting in the so called contiguous gene deletion syndrome. Thus the observed clinical heterogeneity in FAP may be a reflection of heterogeneity in the lesions at the <u>APC</u> locus, whether microscopically detectable or not. The family reported by Ray White (see below) is probably another instance of this phenomenon. Desmoid tumors and other occassional extra colonic manifestations associated with FAP may be due to localized post zygotic somatic events; or alternatively, interactions with other independantly segregating unlinked genes.

Heterogeneity in the presentation of polyps in the patients with FAP is a frequent observation. The number, size and distribution of adenomas in polyposis is so variable that, at times, they raise questions regarding genetic homogeneity. Descrete polyp-proneness was thought to be a distinct genetic trait by Veale and others about two decades ago. Several genetic models were discussed to explain the pattern of their inheritance and a possiblility of the trait being allelic to FAP was not excluded.

Based upon their recent studies in Utah, Bishop and colleagues obtained a convincing genetic explanation for the familial occurrence of discrete adenomas. Results from pedigree analysis using likelihood theory suggested that a dominantly inherited susceptibility gene prevails in the general population with a frequency of 0.19 and that all the adenomas in such families are attributable to this allele; preliminary calculations suggested that the contribution by polygenic factors is small. If this suggestion gains support from direct molecular evidence by way of linked polymorphic

DNA markers and ultimately the susceptibility gene itself, it will have far reaching consequences in the prediction and prevention of colorectal cancer in the general population. Bishop estimated the probabilities of developing adenomas among the first degree relatives of the affected persons to be 0.11, 0.16, 0.23 and 0.31 when they are respectively less than 40 years, 40-49 years, 50-60 years and more than 60 years.

Linkage analysis by Petersen and collaborators in a 3 generation family segregating for juvenile polyposis coli (JPC) revealed an obligate recombinant between JPC and the polymorphic DNA marker EF5.44 (see below) mapping very close to the APC locus. This is interesting, especially in view of the observed close inkage between the APC-linked DNA markers and the gene determining an unusual "colorectal polyp/cancer susceptibility" trait dominantly inherited in a pedigree reported by Dr. Ray White at the Plenary Session I. Two clinically distinct genetic defects, familial polyposis coli (FPC) and Garner syndrome have been mapped earlier to the same locus designated as adenomatous polyposis coli (APC). In the family with the third APC-linked defect mentioned above the affected persons rarely present typical polyposis and the documented cases of colon carcinoma were not usually accompanied buy polyposis. White and his associates observed that a single adenomatous polyp in this family can be an indication of the defective gene. This observation calls for linkage studies in different families segregating for various types of HNPCC and polyp-proneness. The future availability of cloned sequences of the APC gene will offer the basis to investigate the nature of APC mutations involved in the observed clinical heterogeneity.

A number of polymorphic DNA markers closely linked to APC are already available for presymptomatic prediction of FAP in appropriate families. They include C11p11, Pi227, ECB28 and YN5.48 and other probes isolated by Nakamura (see below). A Dutch family with an obligate recombinant between YN5.48, the closest of the markers published by Nakamura, and APC gave the first direct evidence that APC is flanked by YN5.48 on one side and C11p11, Pi227, YN5.61 etc. on the other side within a genetic stretch of less than 10 centimorgans. If pairs of such closely linked bridging markers become informative the positive as well as negative risk estimates can raise to unity and thus, eliminate uncertainities in performing presymptomatic and prenatal diagnosis and in establishing genetic heterogeneity of FAP. The Dutch FAP family data and those from a panel of radiation hybrids presented by Tops have shown that also the probe M4 lies within measurable distance from APC and that the order of the markers around APC on the long arm of chromosome 5 is Cen-M4-Pi227-C11p11-APC-YN5.48-qter.

Petersen discussed problems related to genetic counselling in families with FAP and eventual screening recommandations for individuals at risk by presenting the pattern of segregation of the marker EF5.44 having 2% chance of recombination with APC in a typical FAP family.

Miyaki presented data showing that carcinomas in FAP patients undergo genetic alterations similar to those in sporadic cases. Most frequent losses were in alleles on 5q and 17p. K-ras mutation frequency in adenomas was significantly lower than that in carcinomas. It was concluded that the loss of alleles on chromosomes 5 and 17 are early events involved in the initiation and those on 6, 12, 18 and 22 together with the K-ras mutation are late events involved in the progression of tumors in the FAP patients. Results obtained by Miyaki and her collaborators in a family segregating for a DNA marker on 5q showed that the non-carrier parental allele was lost in the tumor of a patient with inherited FAP. This is the first direct demonstration that homozygous loss of APC function is probably involved in the initiation of colorectal cancer in the FAP patients.

In contrast to Miyaki, Wyllie et al. noticed the loss of APC-linked alleles to be low or absent in adenomas from FAP patients even when they are associated with aggressive histology and feautures of aneuploidy normally associated with the emergence of carcinoma.

The panel of reduced complexity hamster hybrids containing the human chromosome 5 fragments harbouring the APC locus described by Carli Tops will be of profit in constructing yeast artificial chromosome (YAC) and cosmid libraries to isolate probes to cover limited human sequences including APC.

Frischauf discussed strategies for cloning the APC gene, mainly by concentrating on the CpG islands in the 5q21 region known to contain the APC locus. They involve construction of (1) a library of human "BssHII end clones" from a hamster hybrid containing human chromosomes 4 and 5, (2) a NotI linking library from a sorted chromosome 5 library (3) EagI linking libraries from radiation hybrids with fragments of 5 containing the APC sequences, and (4) after identifying the probes mapping in the region of interest (see below), to use them to construct a complete long range restriction map of the region and look for sequences that are conserved between species to identify functional genes that may include APC.

Soloman obtained two sets of human-hamster somatic cell hybrids by fusing respect-ively with cells from two unrelated mentally retarded patients with constitutional interstitial deletions involving 5q15-q21. Hybrids containing the deleted 5 but not its normal counterpart and vice versa were used to map the BssHII end clones derived by Frischauf, to the deletions putatively including the APC locus. Two probes (ECB 27 and ECB 220) were found to map in both the deletions called PD and MD respectively.

Nakamura identified 8 polymorphic DNA markers that showed no recombination with the APC locus, all mapping within a physical map of about 5Mb. A constitutional heterozygous deletion that included one of these markers was identified in one of the 40 sporadic cases of FAP screened for the above markers. The authors concluded that the marker L5.79 should overlap APC. A family with an aberrant segregation of alleles at another marker EF5.44 mapping distal to but not overlapping with YN5.79 indicated that EF5.44 similarly overlaps APC.

The markers overlapping the PD/MD deletions investigated by Frischauf appear to map close to YN5.64 which is located about 2-3Mb proximal to the Nakamura deletions. If all these different deletions are proven to include the APC sequences the size of the FAP gene should turn out to be unusually large.

Sasazuki presented data on genetic and molecular analysis of FAP. He investigated adenomas and carcinomas from FAP patients for the expression of c-myc and c-fos, K-ras mutations and losses of alleles on chromosomes. A decrease in the c-fos expression was found in all the samples while an increase in the c-myc expression was noticed in 75% of carcinomas and 62% of adenomas. K-Ras mutations occurred in 12% of adenomas and 36% of carcinomas. Allele losses were low (<7%) in adenomas and high (upto 40%) in carcinomas. Sasazuki introduced total human chromosome 5 into a murine heptoma cell line and noted the suppression of tumor formation in the nude mice while its introduction into the colorectal cancer cell line SW620 with a 5q15-q31 deletion, suppressed its growth rate. These observations indicated the presence of tumor suppressor genes on chromosome 5 presumably in the APC region. These systems will be useful in eventual characterization of the APC gene sequences on their isolation in the future.

Two Cases of Familial Adenomatous Polyposis Associated with Mental Retardation

MITSURO CHIBA, RYO ITO, OSAMU MASAMUNE, TAKASHI WAGA, and SHINICHI SATO

ABSTRACTS

Two cases of familial adenomatous polyposis (FAP) with mental retardation, in a 40-year-old female and a 46-year-old male, are reported. Their IQs were 40 and 31, respectively. The cause of mental retardation, in both cases, was most likely to have been congenital. There have been six cases of FAP with mental retardation reported in the literature. Recent investigations have revealed an interstitial deletion of the long arm of chromosome 5 in FAP as well as in mental retardation. These case reports of FAP with mental retardation, and the cytogenetic studies, strongly suggest that mental retardation is a further feature of FAP.

Key words: familial adenomatous polyposis (familial polyposis coli, adenomatosis coli), mental retardation, complication

INTRODUCTION

Extra-colonic tumors among various organs (soft tissue, bone, teeth, stomach, duodenum) are known to be associated with familial adenomatous polyposis (FAP). There have also been several reports of FAP with mental retardation, but this retardation has not been recognized as a complication of FAP. This observed mental retardation may be extremely important as a possible complication of FAP, and as a phenotypic marker of a putative FAP gene (Bodmer 1987). In this paper, we describe two cases of FAP associated with mental retardation.

CASE 1.

A 40-year-old single female, who noticed bloody stool in January 1985, visited Yonaizawa General Hospital on March 13 and was referred to Akita University Hospital on April 13. She had had hystrectomy for myoma uteri at the age of 36. She was short in height (139 cm), with a body weight of 48 kg. She appeared retarded, and her IQ was 41. She had lived in a facility for the retarded for 20 years from the age of 20, when her IQ was 40. She needed an attendant of her family during the admission. A digital examination revealed a tumor in the lower rectum. Laboratory data on admission were unremarkable except for a slight increase in erythrocyte sedimentation rate and a mild anemia (Table 1).

Table 1. Laboratory data on admission (case 1)

Stool		TP	7.0 g/dl
occult blood (++)		Alb	4.3 g/dl
Urine	normal	GOT	19 U/L
ESR (1°)	23 mm	Bil(T)	0.4 mg/dl
Hb	11.9 g/dl	Fe	84 μg/dl
WBC	7200 /mm^3	CEA	2.7 ng/ml

Examination revealed more than one thousand adenomatous polyps in the large intestine, a moderately-differentiated adenocarcinoma (31 x 22 mm) in the lowest portion of the rectum (Figs. 1a, 1b), and fundic gland polyps in the stomach (Fig. 2). No abnormalities were found in the duodenum by X-ray studies with contrast medium. Panoramic radiographs of the mandible and upper jaw revealed increased shadows in the mandible and right upper jaw, suggesting osteoma. Studies into the possible causes of the mental retardation, including birth state, mother's toxemia during pregnancy, a history of trauma to the head, plain radiographs of the skull, EEG, and thyroid function (T3, T4, thyroid stimulating hormone, T3 uptake) were found to be normal. The family noticed that she looked retarded when she was around three years old. The cause of mental retardation is most likely to have been congenital.

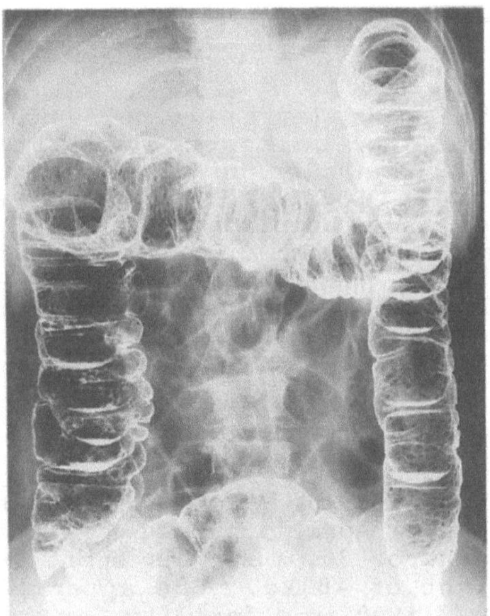

1a

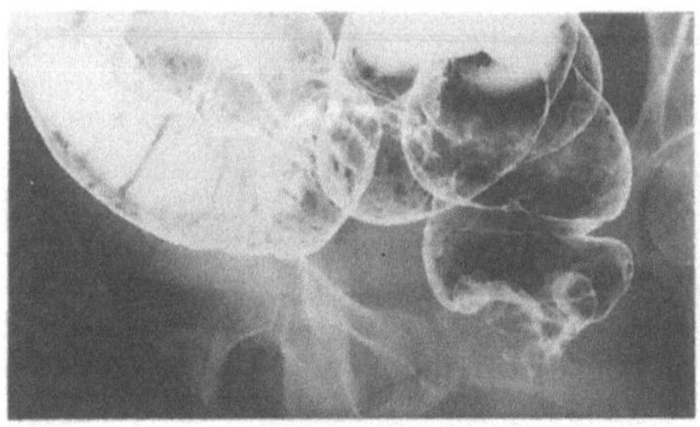

1b

Fig. 1: Barium enema examination demonstrated multiple polyps in the large intestine (1a) with a defect shadow in the lowest portion of the rectum (1b).

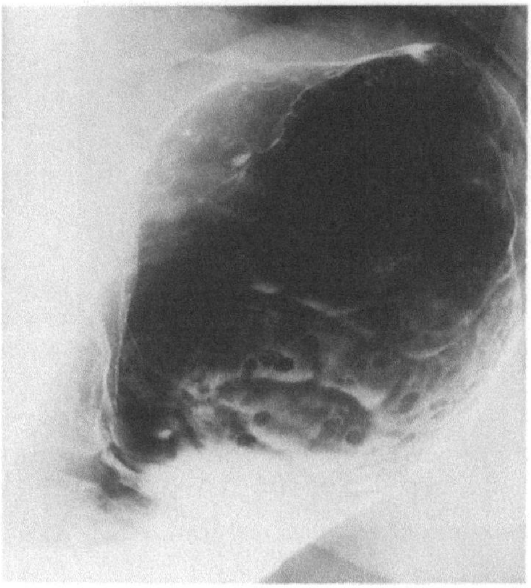

Fig. 2: Gastrofluoroscopy revealed polyps in the fundus.

There were no other cases of FAP or mental retardation among her 42 family members (2 siblings, 2 parents, 4 grandparents, 7 aunts and uncles, 8 nieces and nephews, and 18 cousins). She had proctocolectomy with ileostomy on June 12, 1985. The Dukes stage was C.

CASE 2.

A 46-year-old single male, was found to have anemia by a medical examination in February, 1986. He had had an operation for a bone fracture of the left femur at the age of 29. His height was 158 cm, and his body weight was 68 kg. He was restless and often unable to follow our directions. He could neither read nor write, and had an IQ of 31. He lived in a facility for the retarded for 7 years from the age of 39, when his IQ was 31. He had a habit of wandering from place to place and stealing, and had been guided by the police several times. Laboratory data, on admission, revealed moderate anemia with a low level of serum iron (Table 2).

Table 2. Laboratory data on admission (case 2)

Stool		TP	7.3 g/dl
occult blood	(+)	Alb	4.5 g/dl
Urine	normal	GOT	10 U/L
ESR (1°)	8 mm	Bil(T)	0.3 mg/dl
Hb	10.6 g/dl	Fe	35 μg/dl
WBC	8300 /mm^3	CEA	2.3 ng/ml

Examination revealed more than a hundred adenomatous polyps (Fig. 3a) with a well-differentiated adenocarcinoma (55 x 35 mm) in the hepatic flexure (Fig. 3b). No abnormalities were found in the upper gastrointestinal tract. Studies into the possible causes

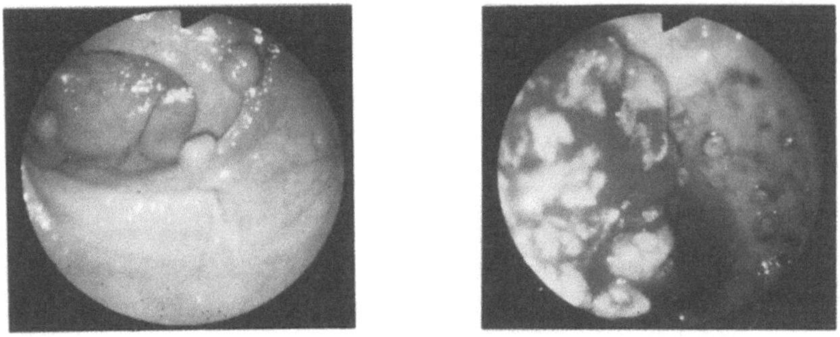

3a 3b

Fig. 3: Colonoscopy revealed multiple polyps in the large intestine (3a), with a Borrman 2 type tumor in the hepatic flexure (3b).

of the mental retardation, including a history of trauma to the head, plain radiographs of the skull and thyroid function, were found to be normal.

His family noticed that he looked retarded when he was around three years old. The cause of mental retardation is most likely to have been congenital. There were no cases of FAP or mental retardation among his 8 family members (4 siblings, 2 parents, and 2 grandparents). He had proctocolectomy with ileoproctostomy on May 1, 1986. The Dukes stage was C.

DISCUSSION

Up to August, 1986, 771 cases with FAP had been registered at the Japanese Polyposis Center. However, there were no registered cases of FAP with mental retardation. This does not exclude the possibility that there were such cases, since mental retardation has not been recognized as a possible complication in FAP, it is likely that mental retardation was not reported to the Center. We have been able to find six cases of FAP with mental retardation in the literature (Table 3).

All cases, including our two cases but excluding that of Sachatello were propositus. All these propositus cases, except that of Shimizu et al, had malignant changes (cancer) when the diagnosis 'FAP' was made. The frequency of developing malignant changes (85.7%, 6/7) in these propositus cases with mental retardation, is higher than that (60%) of the propositus cases reported by Bussey 1978. This is probably due to a lack of alert observations for symptoms and signs, and also inadequate complaint from the patients because of mental retardation.
Recent achievements in cytogenetics have been remarkable. Silengo (1981) demonstrated an interstitial deletion of the long arm (q) of chromosome 5 (del (5)(q13 q22) or (q15 q31)) in

Table 3. Cases of familial adenomatous polyposis with mental retardation

Authors	Age	Sex	Malignant change	IQ	Others
Heald 1967	35	f	Dukes Cl	n.d.	subaceous cysts, colostomy for intestinal obstruction
Sachatello 1970	17	m	absent	n.d.	Klinefelter syndrome (XXY)
Ohtsuka et al. 1973	41	m	Dukes A	64	soft tissue tumor (epidermal cysts, fibrous tumor)
Shimizu et al. 1975	17	m	absent	43	osteoma, soft tissue tumor, epididymus tumor (bil), nasal polyp, malformation of bone
Oiwa et al. 1978	36	m	Dukes C	n.d.	exostosis, gastric cancers (advanced, IIc), carcinoid of the stomach, duodenal adenoma
Herrera et al. 1986	42	m	Dukes A, B	n.d.	desmoid tumor, del(5)(q13 q15) or del(5)(q15 q22)
Present study	40	f	Dukes C	40	osteoma of the mandibular and the upper jaw
	46	m	Dukes C	31	

Abbreviations; n.d., not described

mentally retarded children. Herrera (1986) found a similar deletion on the same chromosome no.5 (del (5)(q13 q15) or (q15 q22)) in patients with FAP and mental retardation (Table 3). The deletion of the long arm of chromosome 5 in FAP was confirmed by Bodmer (1987). He referred to the gene as FAP, and suggested its location as 5q 21-22 by analysis of restriction fragment length polymorphisms. Chromosome 5 allele loss has been shown in at least 20 % of cases with sporadic colorectal cancer (Solomon 1987).

These cytogenetic studies, showing deletion of chromosome 5 in FAP as well as in mental retardation cases, together with the existence of case reports of FAP with mental retardation, strongly suggest that mental retardation is a further feature of FAP. The frequency of association of mental retardation with FAP is still to be established.

The authors thank Miss C. Igarashi for her skilful preparation of the manuscript.

REFERENCES

Bodmer WF, Bailey CJ, Bodmer J, Bussey HJR, Ellis A, Gorman P, Lucibello FC, Murday VA, Rider SH, Scambler P, Sheer D, Solomon E, Spurr NK (1987) Localization of the gene for familial adenomatous polyposis on chromosome 5. Nature 328:614-616

Bussey HJR (1978) Polyosis syndromes. In: Morson BC (ed). The pathogenesis of colorectal cancer. W.B. Saunders Company, Philadelphia, London, Toronto, pp81-94

Heald RJ (1967) Gardner's syndrome in association with two tumours in the ileum. Proc R Soc Med 60:914-915

Herrera L, Kakati S, Gibas L, Pietrzak E, Sandberg AA (1986) Garder syndrome in a man with an interstitial deletion of 5q. Am J Med Genet 25:473-476

Ito R, Chiba M, Masamune O, Waga T, Sato S (1987) Two cases of adenomatosis coli associated with mental retardation. Jpn J Gastroenterol 84:1457-1461 (in Jpn)

Ohtsuka H, Kamiishi H, Shinseki T, Ito M, Hara M, Shioya N, Fukushima T, Kikyo T, Hara M (1973) A case of Gardner's syndrome. Keiseigeka 16:240-250 (in Jpn)

Oiwa T, Watanabe H (1978) Report of a case of familial adenomatosis coli with gastric cancer. Stomach and Intestine 13:1105-1111 (in Jpn)

Sachatello RJ (1970) Familial polyposis of the colon: I. Leukocytic chromosome determination -Report of a patient with familial polyposis of the colon and Klinefelter's syndrome. Dis Col Rect 13:368-371

Shimizu M, Watanabe K, Yamada M (1975) A case of Gardner's syndrome with bilateral epididymis tumors, nasal polyp, bone anomalies and mental deficiency. J Jap Soc Intern Med 64: 1384-1390 (in Jpn)

Silengo MC, Luzpzaitti L, Centerwall WR, Costello JM, Parslow M (1981) Interstitial deletion of the long arm of chromosome no.5 in two unrelated children with congenital anomalies and mental retardation. Clin Genet 19:174-180

Solomon E, Voss R, Hall V, Bodmer WF, Jass JR, Jeffreys AJ, Lucibello FC, Patel I, Rider SH (1987) Chromosome 5 allele loss in human colorectal carcinomas. Nature 328:616-619

Pedigree Analysis of Susceptibility to Colonic Adenomas

D. TIMOTHY BISHOP, LISA A. CANNON-ALBRIGHT, RANDALL W. BURT, and MARK H. SKOLNICK

ABSTRACT

This paper details a study of colonic adenomas performed in Utah on families ascertained for colonic cancers and/or colonic adenomas in one or more probands. The relatives were studied using flexible proctosigmoidoscopy for the presence of polyps which were classified histologically. Statistical analysis showed an excess of adenomas among the relatives of probands as compared to population controls with a relative risk of between 2 and 3 depending on the age of the relatives. Pedigree analysis involving the oligogenic model suggested that susceptibility was inherited as a common autosomal dominant with incomplete penetrance.

Keywords: Adenomas, Pedigree Analysis, Colorectal Carcinoma, Likelihood Analysis

1. RATIONALE AND DESIGN OF STUDY

1.1 Rationale

Colon cancer has been reported to be familial by a number of investigators. Initially, Woolf (1958) examined death certificates for first degree relatives of cases of colorectal cancer diagnosed in Utah between 1931 and 1951. He found 26 cancers among 763 first degree relatives in the relatives of cases and 8 among the relatives of controls (Relative Odds for a family history = 3.25). Odds of this magnitude have been found in other more recent studies including Macklin (1960, relative risk = 3.20) and Lovett (1976, relative risk = 3.50) in studies similar to Woolf's initial study (1958). Studies which have examined colorectal cancer incidence as opposed to mortality have also found relative risks of the same magnitude.

With the recognition of the adenoma as a premalignant lesion, attention has focussed on the familial aggregation of adenomas, partly in attempts to explain the familial aggregation of colorectal cancer and partly as investigations of the biology of the adenoma itself. Various studies have examined the family history of colorectal cancer in the relatives of probands with adenomas but these are at least one stage removed from the definitive study which would involve screening the relatives of sets of probands for adenomas. This study is designed to investigate this aspect although limited because of ethical and practical considerations of using colonoscopy and obtaining information on polyps within the whole of the colon.

1.2 Design of this Study

The examination of the extent and causes of familial clustering of adenomas requires examination of members of pedigrees. We chose to examine the extended pedigrees available in Utah. Families were chosen from each of four ascertainment groups (1) multiple affected members with colorectal cancers, (2) a member with a large (greater than 5mm) or multiple adenomas, and (3) a member with an adenoma. Group 2 families were identified from the pathology files at the University of Utah Health Sciences Center and the Veterans Administration Medical Center in Salt Lake City. Group 3 families were identified from a member who married into one of the families collected in groups 1 and 2 and who was found to have an adenoma on examination. These individuals were sampled as population controls in the initial study. By comparison with the Group 2 probands, the adenomas were usually smaller, rarely multiple and never symptomatic. Families for Groups 2 and 3 were sampled independent of family history of adenomas or colorectal cancer unlike the Group 1 families. The Group 1 pedigrees are divided into two subgroups; the first includes a single pedigree (labelled Pedigree 1002) which was initially reported in Burt et al. (1985) while the second includes four families which were subsequently studied. Each of these five pedigrees contains minimally a pair of affected siblings.

A 60 cm. flexible proctosigmoidoscopy was used to examine the relatives in the families defined above. Examination was attempted to the splenic flexure. A medical examination was also included looking particularly for signs of the rare dominantly inherited polyposis syndromes but none were found.

1.3 Histology

Polyps were measured and all polyps and mucosa that appeared abnormal were biopsied. Adenomas and hyperplastic polyps were identified by standard histological methods.

1.4 The Method of Pedigree Analysis

Pedigree analysis involves the examination of the pattern of disease affection among the pedigree members. For instance, for a rare dominant fully penetrant disease, approximately one half of the offspring of an affected parent would be expected to be affected. Consistency between the expected number and distribution of affected children with a binomial random variable with parameter 0.5 would be supportive of this mode of inheritance. Pedigree analysis is more general in the sense that it includes complex modes of inheritance involving partial penetrance and allele frequency. The penetrance can be dependent on parameters and the allele frequency is a parameter, each of which can be estimated within the analysis. Usually maximum likelihood methods are employed to estimate these parameters while likelihood ratio tests are applied for hypothesis testing.

For these analyses, we assumed a single locus which determines susceptibility to adenomas and/or colorectal cancer. Individuals with colorectal cancer were classified as affected as were individuals found to have adenomas during our screening examination. Individuals studied and found not to have adenomas were classified as unaffected for pedigree analysis. Individuals not available for study and with no evidence of colorectal cancer were classified as being of unknown adenoma phenotype.

1.5 Other Family Studies

There have been a number of studies which have examined the family history of colorectal cancer among the relatives of incident cases of colorectal cancer (Kune et al, 1987, 1989; Duncan and Kyle, 1982; Bonelli et al, 1988; Ponz de Leon et al, 1987). The results have been quite consistent in terms of showing increased clustering among relatives (usually, first degree relatives) but inconsistent in terms of the magnitude of the increased rates with relative odds of a positive family history of between 1.8 (Kune et al, 1989) and 13.2 (Ponz de Leon et al, 1987). This variation is attributable to a number of causes, presumably, including varying diagnostic criteria and standards and methods of statistical analysis. The most recent study was performed by St. John et al. (1989) who found relative odds of 2.3. In this study of over 500 probands, the relative odds varied by age of onset of the proband but was not related to site or type of tumour.

There have been two reported studies which have looked at the family history of colorectal cancer in the families of probands with adenomatous polyps (Bonelli et al, 1988; Ponz de Leon, 1987). The relative odds of a positive family history in both these studies was 3.2.

Two studies have also examined relatives of colorectal cancer probands. The first (Rozen et al, 1987) studied first degree asymptomatic relatives using flexible sigmoidoscopy and fecal occult blood testing and found that 8.1% of relatives and 3.7% of controls had adenomas. Guillem et al (1989) using colonoscopy found 12% of relatives had adenomas as compared to 8% of controls.

2. RESULTS

2.1 Summary of Results

In all, 670 persons in 34 pedigrees were examined using flexible proctosigmoidoscopy. Only individuals aged 25 years and older were screened. Ninety five percent of relatives consented to be examined as did 90% of spouses. Eighteen relatives in the pedigrees and 4 spouses were found to have colorectal cancer although none were found during our screening.

2.2 Frequency tabulations

The prevalence of adenomas was found to be 19% (78 affected out of 407 examined) in relatives of probands and 12% (32 of 263) in controls. The relatives involve many differing degrees of genetic relationship. These percentages are statistically significantly different ($p < 0.02$). The average age of the relatives of cases was 51 years and of the controls was 52 years. There was no significant difference in the frequency of adenomas by sex ($p > 0.20$) in either relatives of cases or controls.

2.3 Results for First Degree Relatives

We examined the prevalence of adenomas in the first degree relatives of probands examined in this study. Since the rates were similar in both relatives of cancer probands as well as adenoma probands, we have combined these rates. The rates obtained are given in Table I.

The relative odds shown in Table I are similar to those given for colon cancer in other studies suggesting that the aggregation of polyps may explain the aggregation of colorectal cancers.

We examined the prevalence of adenomas in the first degree relatives of colorectal cancer cases, some of whom were probands, in the pedigrees as compared to all other individuals within the pedigrees. Increased rates of polyps might suggest differences between polyps that developed into colorectal cancer and those that did not on the basis that first degree relatives are likely to be more similar to their affected relative both in terms of genetic background and environmental exposure. Table II summarizes these results.

<u>TABLE I</u>: This table shows the frequency of adenomas among the family members as compared to controls. The figures for each cell are the number of adenomas identified (/ number of examinations performed). The relative odds report the frequency of adenomas in relatives compared to the rates in controls.

	AGE AT EXAMINATION		
GROUP	< 50 years	50-59 years	60+ years
Relatives	17/119 (14%)	19/71 (27%)	10/32 (31%)
Controls	3/50 (6%)	4/43 (9%)	5/39 (13%)
RELATIVE ODDS	2.4	2.9	2.4

TABLE II: This table shows the number of adenomas identified in first degree relatives of colorectal cases (/ number of examinations performed) as compared to all other individuals within the families.

	AGE OF RELATIVES		
	30-59 years	60+ years	TOTAL
TOTAL FIRST DEGREE	9/60 (15%)	11/26 (42%)	23%
ALL OTHER INDIVIDUALS	57/489 (12%)	48/182 (26%)	16%

These frequencies are statistically different between first degree relatives and other individuals; the results parallel those obtained from the study of probands alone.

2.4 Hyperplastic Polyps

The prevalence of hyperplastic polyps was found to be 30% in male relatives of probands (56 affected out of 185 examinations) and in male controls (44 out of 145); in females the prevalence was 23% (51 out of 222) in relatives of probands and 25% (29 out of 118) in controls. The sex differences and family/control rates were all non-significant.

2.5 Pedigree Analysis Results

Pedigree analysis was performed assuming that susceptibility to adenomas (and/or colorectal cancer) was determined by an autosomal locus with two alleles (A and a); we think of 'A' as being more associated with disease expression that 'a'. Penetrance is determined by a logistic function of age and genotype. Under this general model, each genotype is allowed to express an adenoma or cancer and the parameters relating the age and genotype to expression in addition to the allele frequency are estimated using maximum likelihood methods. We examined a general model where all genotypes are considered to have distinct probabilities of expression, a dominant model, a recessive model and a random model where each individual has a probability of expression which is only dependent on the age of the individual.

Sample sizes precluded a detailed study of each group of families separately and as the phenotypes frequencies and characteristics of the adenomas were similar in the groups, we combined the pedigrees for analysis. Since hyperplastic polyps showed no familial tendency, they were ignored for subsequent analyses.

Table III shows the likelihood results for these families.

TABLE III: Table of log likelihood differences (base 10) between the specified genetic model and the random model where the probability that each individual expresses a polyp depends only on the age of the individual (the 'sporadic' model).

MODE OF INHERITANCE	POPULATION FREQUENCY	PENETRANCE BY AGE 60	LOG LIKELIHOOD DIFFERENCE
DOMINANT			
Genotypes AA + Aa	0.34	0.41	+5.99
Genotype aa	0.66	0.00	
RECESSIVE			
Genotype AA	0.66	0.00	+5.99
Genotypes Aa, aa	0.34	0.41	
SPORADIC			
Genotypes AA + Aa + aa	1.00	0.14	0.00

The maximum likelihood dominant model implies that only individuals carrying the 'A' allele express adenomas and hence colorectal cancer and that for these individuals, the probability of an adenoma by age 60 is approximately 0.41. For the general population, approximately one third of all individuals are 'susceptible' to polyps while the remaining two thirds are not. The likelihood of the dominant model is almost one million times that of the sporadic model.

There is no recessive model of increased susceptibility compatible with the observations since the maximum likelihood recessive model is merely the dominant model with the alleles being reversed in role.

3. DISCUSSION

Our analysis shows that close relatives of colorectal cancer or adenoma probands have an increased frequency of adenomas over population controls. The magnitude of this increased frequency is consistent with the increased rate of colorectal cancer in either colorectal cancer or adenoma probands found in previous studies, although detailed analysis is difficult because of the ways these families were ascertained. In particular, since many of the families were chosen for multiple cases of colorectal cancer, it is not possible to estimate meaningfully the relative risk to siblings and the relative risks to offspring since many individuals are related in both these ways to colorectal cancer cases. This study therefore suggests that the aggregation of colorectal cancer within families may be explainable by aggregation of adenomas. Under this model, transition to carcinoma is determined by factors unrelated to adenoma formation.

These results together with the known biological relationship between adenomas and carcinoma suggest that joint analysis of the presence of adenomas and colorectal cancer should provide information on the inheritance of susceptibility. Likelihood analysis suggests that the increased rates of adenomas among relatives is best explained assuming a major gene model as an autosomal dominant susceptibility with a high population frequency. Further, the likelihood analysis suggests that susceptibility is due to this particular allele but expression involves many factors since the age dependent penetrance is considerably less than one. These factors could be either genetic or environmental. More detailed genetic modeling is in progress to examine the evidence for other genetic factors, such as polygenic inheritance but conclusive evidence for inheritance will only come from the mapping of this locus.

ACKNOWLEDGEMENTS

This research was supported by Public Health Service Awards CA-363632, CA-28854 and CA-40641.

REFERENCES

Bonelli L, Martines H, Conio M, Bruzzi P, Aste H (1988) Family history of colorectal cancer as a risk factor for benign and malignant tumours of the large bowel. A case-control study. Int J Cancer 41:513-517

Burt RW, Bishop DT, Cannon LA, Dowdle MA, Lee RG, Skolnick MH (1985) Dominant inheritance of adenomatous colonic polyps and colorectal cancer. NEJM 312:1540-1544

LA Cannon-Albright, MH Skolnick, DT Bishop, RG Lee, RW Burt (1988) Common inheritance of susceptibility to colonic adenomatous polyps and associated colorectal cancers. NEJM 319:533-537

Duncan JL, Kyle J (1982) Family incidence of carcinoma of the colon and rectum in north-east Scotland. Gut 23:169-171

Guillem JG, Forde KA, Treat MR, Neugut AI (1989) The colonoscopic detection of adenomas in asymptomatic first-degree relatives (FDR) of colon cancer patients: A controlled, prospective study. Abstract submitted to the Am Soc of Gastrointestinal Endoscopy Annual Meeting

Kune GA, Kune S, Watson LF (1987) The Melbourne Colorectal Cancer Study Characterization of Patients with a Family History of Colorectal Cancer. Dis Col & Rec 30:600-606

Kune GA, Kune S, Watson LF (1989) The role of heredity in the etiology of large bowel cancer: Data from the Melbourne Cancer Study. World J Surg 13:124-131

Lovett E (1976) Family studies in cancer of the colon and rectum. Brit J Surg 63:13-18

Macklin MT (1960) Inheritance of cancer of the stomach and large intestine in man. J Nat Cancer Inst 24:551-571

Ponz de Leon M, Antonioli A, Ascari A, Zanghieri G, Sacchetti C et al (1987) Incidence and Familial Occurrence of Colorectal Cancer and Polyps in a Health-Care District of Northern Italy. Cancer 60:2848-2859

Rozen P, Fireman ZVI, Figer A, Legum C, Ron E, Lynch HT (1987) Family history of colorectal cancer as a marker of potential malignancy within a screening program. Cancer 60:248-254.

St. John DJB, McDermott FT, Katrivessis H, Debney EA, Johnson WR, Hughes ESR (1989) Cancer Risk for Relatives of Patients With Sporadic Colorectal Cancer. Abstract presented at the 2nd International Conference on Colorectal Cancer, Jerusalem, Isreal.

Woolf CM (1958) A genetic study of carcinoma of the large intestine. Am J Hum Genet 10:42-52

Genetic Linkage Study of Juvenile Polyposis: Preliminary Analysis

GLORIA M. PETERSEN, JANE BROWN, XIANGDONG BU, ROBERT S. SPARKES, and YUSUKE NAKAMURA

ABSTRACT

We report initial linkage studies of a family in which three generations are affected with colonic polyps. We analyzed chromosome 5q (familial adenomatous polyposis) and phenotypic markers in this family. We could reject tight linkage for eight markers; it is of particular interest that this form of familial juvenile polyposis is not linked to the gene for familial adenomatous polyposis.

Keywords: genetic markers, lod scores

BACKGROUND AND DESCRIPTION OF FAMILY

Familial juvenile polyposis is a rare, and likely heterogeneous entity. Although the polyps found in this condition are classically hamartomas, there is some acknowledgment among gastroenterologists of

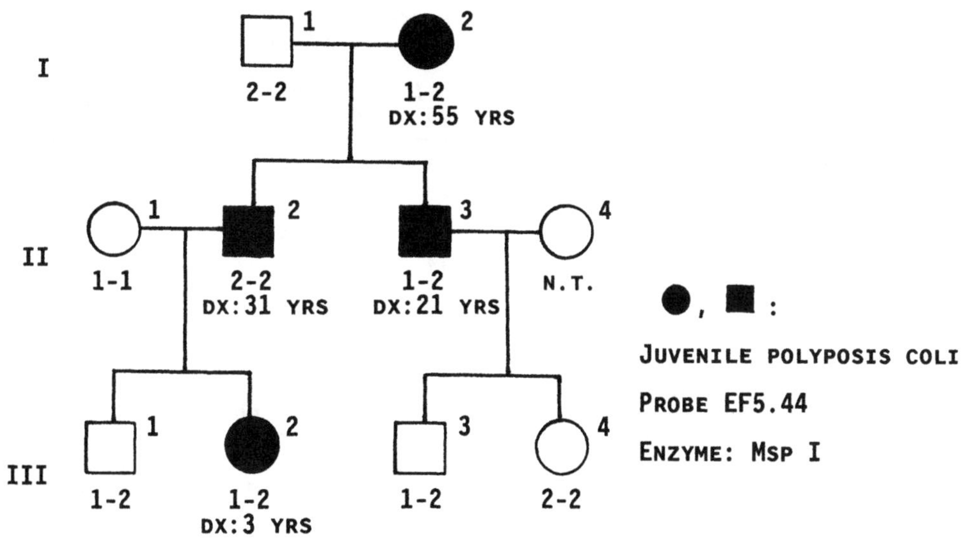

Fig. 1. Pedigree of family showing results for marker EF5.44, which is linked to FAP, but apparently not linked to juvenile polyposis in this family. Age at diagnosis (DX) of polyps is shown under symbol of each affected individual. N.T.=not tested.

an increased colon cancer risk. The inclusion of adenomas as part of its clinical spectrum underscores its etiologic heterogeneity as well.

We studied a family (See Fig. 1) in which three generations are affected with colonic polyps. The propositus (II-3) is a 29-year old male with an 8-year history of juvenile polyposis. He has had repeated episodes of rectal bleeding, and juvenile polyps have been consistently found on periodic colonoscopies. His asymptomatic mother (I-2) was screened at age 55 and was found also to have scattered colonic polyps (not adenomatous) on screening. Two large (7 cm and 5 cm) polypoid tumors were detected in her cecum, resulting in a hemicolectomy. His asymptomatic 31-year old brother (II-2) was screened and found to have 6 juvenile polyps. The daughter (III-2) of this brother presented at age 3 with juvenile polyps and her sigmoid colon was resected. All other members of this family shown in Figure 1 are asymptomatic.

LINKAGE ANALYSIS

A chromosome 5q region molecular marker (EF5.44) linked to familial adenomatous polyposis and biochemical phenotypic markers were evaluated in this family. The following markers were uninformative: amylase 2, transferrin, complement 3, E2, ABO, Duffy, Kell, KP, Lewis, P, adenylate kinase, 6-phosphogluconate dehydrogenase, phosphoglycollate phosphatase, galactose 1 phosphate uridyl transferase, esterase D, and glyoxalase 1.

We could reject tight linkage for Rhesus blood group (RH), group specific component (GC), familial adenomatous polyposis (FAP), properdin factor B (BF), glutamate pyruvate transaminase (GPT), alpha-1-antitrypsin (PI), haptoglobin (HP), and adenosine deaminase (ADA). In each case, there was evidence of a recombination event. See Table 1.

Table 1. Lod score results for markers not tightly linked to juvenile polyposis, under varying values of θ, the recombination fractions.

Locus	Chromosome Location	Lod Score θ=0.0	θ=0.05	θ=0.10	θ=0.20	θ=0.30
RH	1p36-p34	- ∞	-2.163	-1.331	- .581	- .227
GC	4q11-q13	- ∞	- .464	- .229	- .060	- .011
FAP	5q21-22	-3.375	- .724	- .430	- .158	- .033
BF	6p21.3	- ∞	- .863	- .533	- .212	- .065
GPT	8q24.2-qter	- ∞	- .444	- .195	- .011	- .038
PI	14q24-q32.1	- ∞	-1.454	- .897	- .394	- .155
HP	16q21-q22	- ∞	-1.672	-1.109	- .587	- .314
ADA	20q13.2-qter	- ∞	- .721	- .444	- .194	- .076

We could not reject tight linkage in the case of blood group MNSs (4q28-q31), phosphoglucomutase 1 (1p22.1), or acid phosphatase (2p25). Maximum lod scores occurred at θ=0.0 with values of .94, .602, and .300, respectively. However, the interpretation of these values must be treated with some caution, as individual II-4 has not been tested yet.

It is of particular interest that this form of familial juvenile polyposis is not linked to the gene for familial adenomatous polyposis on chromosome 5q.

Linkage Studies on Familial Adenomatous Polyposis in the Netherlands

CARLI M.J. TOPS, COR BREUKEL, JUUL TH. WIJNEN, HELEEN M. VD KLIFT, INGE S.J. V LEEUWEN-CORNELISSE, HANS F.A. VASEN, GERRIT GRIFFIOEN, FRIEDA C.A. DEN HARTOG JAGER, CORNELIS B.H.W. LAMERS, and P. MEERA KHAN

ABSTRACT

A number of polymorphic DNA markers on the long arm of chromosome 5, including C11p11, Pi227 and YN5.48, are known to be closely linked to the gene for familial adenomatous polyposis (FAP). C11p11 and Pi227 are localized centromeric to FAP. A critical Dutch pedigree revealed that YN5.48 is located on the other, telomeric, side of the FAP locus. This finding raises the reliability of presymptomatic diagnosis of FAP by linkage analysis to more than 99.9%. Genetic heterogeneity was considered to explain a small family in which the condition failed to segregate with C11p11.

Keywords: Familial adenomatous polyposis, diagnosis by linkage, presymptomatic and prenatal diagnosis, linked DNA markers, genetic heterogeneity.

1. INTRODUCTION

Familial adenomatous polyposis (FAP) is an autosomal dominant condition with complete penetrance (Bussey 1975). Carriers of the FAP gene develop hundreds or thousands of adenomatous polyps and eventually adenocarcinoma in the colorectal region, if the affected colon is not removed. Early detection of the carriers, at present, is based on constant surveillance including periodic sigmoidoscopic examinations, to see the appearance of polyps in the colorectal region. The age at clinical diagnosis is variable and all the first degree relatives of the affected have, a priori, a 50% risk of carrying the disease gene. Therefore, they need to be put under surveillance throughout a considerable span of their life (Bussey 1975, Bulow 1987). But, closely linked polymorphic markers would be helpful in the prenatal and presymptomatic diagnosis or the exclusion of FAP.

Family studies revealed that a DNA probe called C11p11, located on the long arm of chromosome 5, is closely linked to the FAP locus (Bodmer et al. 1987). In the initial studies, no recombinant was found between C11p11 and FAP in about 50 informative meioses in 8 families, yielding a combined maximum lod score of 6.6 at a recombination fraction of 0.00 (Bodmer et al. 1987, Leppert et al.

1987). Although the TaqI polymorphism of C11p11 was not informative in our Dutch polyposis families (Meera Khan et al. 1988), with the advent of a 4-base deletion polymorphism (Breukel et al. 1989) 8 families turned out to be informative for linkage between FAP and C11p11 (Tops et al. 1989a,c).
The polymorphic DNA markers so far reported to be closely linked to FAP are listed in Table 1. Using each of these markers it is possible to follow the inheritance of FAP through families. However, this approach has a serious limitation: a possible occurrence of

Table 1: Site-specific polymorphism information content (PIC values) and recombination fraction of DNA markers known to map close to FAP

Probe	Polymorphic site	PIC[A]	Recombination fraction[B]	References
C11p11	TaqI	0.17[C]	0.05	Bodmer et al (1987);
	DEL1	0.22		Leppert et al (1987);
				Dunlop et al (1989);
				Tops et al (1989c);
				Breukel et al (1989).
Pi227	BclI	0.56[C]	0.05	Meera Khan et al (1988);
	BstXI	0.37		Tops et al (1989a,b);
	PstI	0.23		Dunlop et al (1989).
	MboI	0.37		
YN5.64	PstI	0.36	0.06	Nakamura et al (1988).
	TaqI	0.22		
KK5.33	TaqI	0.37	0.07	Nakamura et al (1988).
	PstI	0.29		
YN5.48	TaqI	0.38	0.01	Nakamura et al (1989);
	MspI	0.37		Tops et al (1989b);
	EcoRI	0.44		pers.comm. Y.Nakamura.
MC5.61	MspI	0.37	0.04	Nakamura et al (1989).
	TaqI	0.37		
ECB27	BglII	0.36	0.05	Murday et al (1989).

[A] PIC: the polymorphic information content of a genetic marker indicates its relative usefulness in linkage studies.

[B] Updated estimations of recombination fractions between the markers and FAP, based on two point linkage analyses. The data are pooled when they are from more than one report.

[C] The TaqI-DEL1 haplotypes of C11p11, have a PIC of 0.40 (Breukel et al. 1989). The net PIC of Pi227, with BclI, BstXI and PstI is 0.75 (Tops et al. 1989a). The net PIC values for the other markers with more than one polymorphic site are not estimated yet.

recombination between a given marker and the FAP gene can not be identified. The availability and use of closely linked markers on either side of FAP would greatly increase the reliability of diagnosis by linkage. Their use would facilitate also the detection of genetic heterogeneity, which is another potential source of error in presymptomatic diagnosis by linkage. This paper deals with our observations on these aspects in the Dutch polyposis families.

2. METHODS AND MATERIAL

2.1 Families

All the persons included in our study are Dutch by descent. The patients and their families are systematically reviewed and registered at the Dutch Polyposis Registration Centre at Leiden. Registration routinely includes personal data, results of investigation, pathology reports and results of treatment of the patients as well as personal data and results of clinical screening of the at-risk family members (Vasen et al. 1989).

2.2 DNA polymorphism analysis

Samples of DNA were isolated from freshly collected peripheral venous 7blood. The routines for DNA isolation and polymorphism analyses were as described elsewhere (Hofker et al. 1985, Breukel et al. 1989). The DNA marker C11p11 recognizes a TaqI polymorphism (Bodmer et al. 1987) and a 4-base deletion polymorphism (DEL1) (Breukel et al. 1989). Both the polymorphisms were used in this study. In addition we screened the MspI polymorphism of YN5.48 (Y. Nakamura and R. White, personal communication, Nakamura et al. 1988) and the BclI, PstI and BstXI polymorphisms of Pi227 (Stewart et al. 1987, Meera Khan et al. 1988).

2.3 Linkage analysis

Lod scores were calculated using the program LINKAGE (Lathrop et al. 1984), modified by an age at diagnosis correction. Age dependent penetrance classification used in these calculations was based on the distribution of ages at which 58 Dutch call-up patients under the age of 30 were first diagnosed (Vasen et al. 1989; H. Vasen, personal communication). The penetrance was assigned as follows: 6.0% for ages 0 to 12, 32.5% for 13 to 17, 66.5% for 18 to 22, 89% for 23 to 27 years and 98% for ages 28 and over. The 95% confidence intervals were approximated with the minus 1-lod unit method as described by Conneally et al. (1985).

3. MARKERS CLOSELY LINKED TO FAP AND LINKAGE DATA IN THE DUTCH FAMILIES

We screened 21 Dutch polyposis families with 266 individuals for polymorphisms at C11p11, Pi227 and YN5.48 (Table 1.)

Eight families were informative for linkage between C11p11 and FAP, yielding a maximum lod score of 4.70 at a recombination fraction of 0.06 (95% confidence limits 0.005-0.180). We encountered only one obligate recombinant in 39 meioses (see section 6 for a detailed discussion on this recombinant).
Pi227 was found to be closely linked to FAP with a peak lod score of 15.18 at a recombination fraction of 0.04 (95% confidence limits 0.01-0.11) in 16 informative families. We found three obligate recombination events in 110 informative meioses (Tops et al. 1989b). Six families were informative for linkage with the MspI polymorphism of YN5.48. One obligate recombinant between YN5.48 and FAP was found among 22 meioses giving a peak lod score of 2.59 at a recombination fraction of 0.05 with 95% confidence interval of 0.002-0.200. The family with the recombinant was informative also for Pi227. In this family, 3 affected sibs recieved the YN5.48 allele B1 from the affected parent, while the affected recombinant sib inherited the allele B2, as did the two healthy sibs. However, all the 4 affected sibs recieved the allele A3 of Pi227, while the 2 healthy sibs (aged 39 and 46 years) recieved its A2 allele from their affected parent (Tops et al. 1989b).

4. MARKERS FLANKING ON EITHER SIDE OF THE FAP LOCUS AND THEIR SIGNIFICANCE IN PRESYMPTOMATIC DIAGNOSIS

Since the recombination fraction between Pi227 and FAP is considerably higher than that between YN5.48 and FAP (Table 1), the above described obligate recombinant between YN5.48 and FAP provides the first direct evidence that FAP is located between YN5.48 and Pi227 (Tops et al. 1989b). Other linkage data have indicated that C11p11 and Pi227 are located on the same side of FAP (Dunlop et al. 1989, Tops et al. 1989a). Our observations in a panel of recently derived reduced complexity somatic cell hybrids indicate that C11p11 is closer than Pi227 to YN5.48 (see Tops et al. abstract 67, this meeting). Results reported by Nakamura et al. (1988) suggest that C11p11 is located closer than YN5.48 to the centromer. Therefore the following gene order seems to be most likely: chromosome 5 Cen.--Pi227--C11p11--FAP--YN5.48--qter. This information, together with the data reported in the literature indicates that in addition to Pi227 and C11p11 the markers KK5.33 and YN5.64 map centromeric to FAP and YN5.61 maps beyond YN5.48 on the telomeric side. When the markers on either side of FAP are informative, recombinants which would otherwise escape detection and lead to wrong prediction, can be identified. The combined use of these markers, provides a powerful tool to discriminate the carriers of the FAP gene from the non-carriers among all the at risk relatives of FAP patients with more than 99.9% reliability (Tops et al. 1989b).

5. POLYMORPHISM INFORMATION CONTENTS (OR PIC VALUES) OF FLANKING MARKERS AND THEIR VALUE IN DIAGNOSTIC SCREENING

The polymorphism information content (PIC) of a genetic marker indicates the proportion of families that would be informative for linkage with a dominant trait. The PIC values of C11p11 and Pi227 were estimated to be 0.40 and 0.75 respectively, while that for the MspI polymorphism of YN5.48, located on the other side of the FAP locus, is 0.37 (Table 1.) The combined PIC value for C11p11 and Pi227 is estimated to be 0.85. The product of the PIC values of the flanking (sets of) markers will give a rough estimate of the fraction of families that would be informative for diagnostic tests by linkage, when these three polymorphisms are used; in the present case, this amounts to 0.31. In fact YN5.48 was found to possess two other restriction polymorphisms recognized by TaqI and EcoRI with PIC values of 0.38 (Nakamura et al. 1988) and 0.44 (Y.Nakamura and R.White, personal communication) respectively. Collectively, the markers listed in Table 1 present enough markers with reasonable degree of informativity on either side of the FAP locus, to make a majority of the families informative and amenable for diagnosis through linkage.

6. RELIABILITY OF DIAGNOSIS BY LINKAGE VERSUS GENETIC AS WELL AS CLINICAL HETEROGENEITY

As mentioned earlier, a potential source of error in the diagnosis of FAP through linked markers is genetic heterogeneity. There has been no indication of heterogeneity in about 25 FAP families reported from 4 countries (Bodmer et al. 1987, Meera Khan et al. 1988, Nakamura et al. 1988, Dunlop et al. 1989). An eventual family with an unexpected number of recombinants, with or without additional deviations, may suggest genetic heterogeneity. The linked gene marker approach is powerful in detecting genetic heterogeneity and helpful in avoiding errors in diagnosis.
Certain features encountered recently in a Dutch family, made it a case for discussion in terms of genetic heterogeneity (Tops et al. 1989c). In this odd nuclear family with two male sibs diagnosed clinically and established pathologically as patients with adenomatous polyposis of the colon and the rectum, there was an obligate recombinant between the disease allele and the FAP linked marker C11p11. There was a history of large bowel obstruction in their paternal grandmother, whose sister's grandson died of stomach cancer at the age of 24 years. Further details on them are not available since the hospital records of the grandmother were destroyed during the second world war and the grand-nephew was treated in a remote country. The father of the affected sibs was treated for rectal cancer and was said to have had adenomas (number unspecified). He had three older, apparently healthy, sibs. No other members of the family are known to have FAP. Further search is in

progress in this family (Tops et al. 1989c). The condition segregating in this family is apparently atypical and somewhat ambiguous. The FAP-linked markers would resolve this riddle. The marker C11p11 was informative for linkage studies in this family. The paternal grandparents were dead but their C11p11 (TaqI-DEL1) haplotypes could be derived. If the grandmother and the father were assumed to be carrying a gene different from FAP, but with FAP-like phenotypes occassionally forming parts of its pleiotropy, one of the affected sibs and one of the sibs of the father will be scored as recombinants with C11p11. On the other hand, it is possible that the father carried a de novo mutation at the FAP locus and that the gastrointestinal conditions in the relatives farther than their father are not relevant to the condition seen in the two affected brothers. Then, one of the sibs will be a recombinant between C11p11 and the FAP locus.
This dilemma of genetic and/or clinical hetrogeneity can be resolved, if markers closely flanking on either side of the putative FAP locus become informative for linkage. An independent segregation of the disease and the markers is an absolute indication of the involvement of a different gene. Unfortunately, YN5.48 is not informative in this family. In certain instances it may be possible that a rare allelic variant at FAP may result in atypical manifestations in its carriers. Such cases can be identified with equal ease also through the linkage approach (Tops et al. 1989c).

7. CONCLUSIONS

1. There are seven polymorphic DNA markers reported to be linked to the FAP locus. The recently obtained critical evidence in a Dutch family together with the available linkage data, localize two of them on one side and four on the other side of FAP.

2. Because of their moderately high polymorphism information contents, the above markers will facilitate presymptomatic diagnosis of FAP by linkage in a majority of families. They are powerful also in detecting genetic as well as clinical heterogeneity even in small families.

3. Future availability of the FAP gene seqeuences will offer a direct approach to the diagnosis of all the cases of FAP.

ACKNOWLEDGMENTS

We thank Sir Walter Bodmer (Imperial Cancer Research Fund Laboratories, London, U.K), Dr. N. Spurr (London, U.K.), Dr. G.D. Stewart (Ann Arbor, Michigan, U.S.A.), Dr. Y. Nakamura (Salt Lake City, Utah, U.S.A.) and Dr. R. White (Howard Hughes Medical Institute, Salt Lake City, Utah, U.S.A.) for probes, Dr. M. Dunlop (Medical Research Council Unit, Edinburgh, Scotland) for helpfull discussions, Dr. J.G. Goedhardt, Dr. J. Lens, Dr. G.J.D. Dorrepaal and Dr. A.L.J. van der Veer for providing some of the family samples, and all the members of the families, who volunteered to participate in this study. The study was supported by the Dutch Praeventiefonds.

REFERENCES

Bodmer WF, Baily CJ, Bodmer J, Bussey HJR, Ellis A, GormanP, Lucibello FC, Murday VA, Rider SH, Scambler P, Sheer D, Solomon E, Spurr NK (1987) Localization of the gene for familial adenomatous polyposis on chromosome 5. Nature 328: 614-616

Breukel C, Tops CMJ, Meera Khan P (1989) A 4-base-pair deletion polymorphism at D5S71 (C11p11) in the human chromosome 5q21-q22 region. (Submitted for publication)

Bussey HJR (1975) Familial polyposis coli. John Hopkins University Press, Baltimore

Bulow S (1987) Familial Adenomatous Polyposis. Danish Med. Bull. 34: 1-15

Conneally PM, Edwards JH, Kidd KK, Lalouel JM, Morton NE, Ott J, White R (1985) Report of the committee on methods of linkage and reporting. 8th Int. Workshop on Human Gene Mapping, Cytogenet Cell Genet 40: 356-359

Dunlop MG, Steel CM, Wyllie AH, Bird CC, Evans HJ (1989) Linkage analysis in familial adenomatous polyposis: Order of C11p11 (D5S71) and Pi227 (D5S37) loci at the apc gene. Genomics 5: 350-353

Hofker MH, Wapenaar MC, Goor N, Bakker E, van Ommen GJB, Pearson PL (1985) Isolation of probes detecting restriction fragment length polymorphisms from X chromosome-specific libraries: potential use for diagnosis of Duchenne muscular dystrophy. Hum Genet 70:148-156

Lathrop GM, Lalouel JM (1984) Easy calculations of lodscores and genetic risks on small computers. Am J Hum Genet 36: 460-465

Leppert M, Dobbs M, Scambler P, O'Connel P, Nakamura Y, Stauffer D, Woodward S, Burt R, Hughes J, Gardner E, Lathrop M, Wasmuth J, Lalouel M, White R (1987) The gene for familial polyposis coli maps to the long arm of chromosome 5. Science 238: 1411-1413

Meera Khan P, Tops CMJ, Broek Mvd, Breukel C, Wijnen JTh, Oldenburg M, Bos Jvd, Leeuwen-Cornelisse ISJv, Vasen HFA, Griffioen G, Verspaget HM, den Hartog Jager FCA, Lamers CBHW (1988) Close linkage of a highly polymorphic marker (D5S37) to familial adenomatous polyposis (FAP) and confirmation of FAP localization on chromosome 5q21-22. Hum Genet 79: 183-185

Murday V, Cottrell S, Bodmer WF, Sheer d, Jones TA, Varesco L, Frishauf AM, Thomas HJ, Solomon E, Hockey A, Dunlop MG, Steele CM (1989) Fine linkage map around the Adenomatous Poloyposis (APC) gene. 10th Int. Workshop on Human Gene Mapping, Cytogenet Cell Genet 51: 1049

Nakamura Y, Lathrop M, Leppert M, Dobbs M, Wasmuth J, Wolff E, Carlson M, Fujimoto E, Krapcho K, Sears T, Woodward S, Hughes J, Burt R, Gardner E, Lalouel JM, White R (1988) Localization of the genetic defect in familial adenomatous polyposis within a small region of chromosome 5. Am J Hum Genet 43: 638-644

Stewart GD, Bruns GAP, Wasmuth JJ, Kurnitt DM (1987) An anonymous DNA segment (Pi227) maps to the long arm of chromosome 5 and identifies a BstX I polymorphism (D5S37). Nucl Acid Res 15: 3939

Tops CMJ, Breukel C, Wijnen JTh, vd Klift HM, vd Broek MH, Oldenburg M, vd Bos J, v Leeuwen-Cornelisse ISJ, Vasen HFA, Griffioen G, Lamers CBHW, Meera Khan P (1989a) Linkage relationships between APC, D5S37 (Probe pi227) and D5S71 (probe C11p11) in the Dutch polyposis families. 10th Int. Workshop on Human Gene Mapping, Cytogenet Cell Genet 51: 1092

Tops CMJ, Griffioen G, Vasen HFA, Breukel C, Klift HMvd, Wijnen JTh, Leeuwen ISJv, den Hartog Jager FCA, Nagengast FM, Lamers CBHW, Meera Khan P (1989b) Presymptomatic Diagnosis of Familial Adenomatous Polyposis by Flanking Markers on Either Side. The Lancet (in press)
Tops CMJ, Breukel C, vd Klift HM, den Hartog Jager FCA, Vasen HFA, v Leeuwen-Cornelisse ISJ, Griffioen G, Lamers CBHW, Meera Khan P (1989c) Linkage studies with DEL1 polymorphism at D5S71 (probe C11p11) in the Dutch polyposis (FAP) families; report on a possible case of genetic heterogeneity (Submitted for publication)
Vasen HFA, Griffioen G, Offerhaus GJA, den Hartog Jager FCA, van Leeuwen-Cornelisse ISJ, Lamers CBHW, van Slooten EA (1989). The value of screening and central registration of families with familial adenomatous polyposis. Dis Colon and Rectum (in press)

Genetic Counseling for Familial Adenomatous Polyposis with Chromosome 5q Linkage Information

GLORIA M. PETERSEN, TAMAR SHOHAT, JANE BROWN, and YUSUKE NAKAMURA

ABSTRACT

Molecular genetic markers linked to familial adenomatous polyposis (FAP) in the chromosome 5q21-22 region now permit the clinical application of linkage information for premorbid diagnosis in at-risk individuals. While screening management for those found by linkage to have inherited FAP remains unchanged from established recommendations, we have developed new screening guidelines for individuals who most likely have not inherited FAP. We propose baseline flexible sigmoidoscopies at ages 11 and 12, with repeated screening every 3 years thereafter until age 35. For such relatives, the clinician can emphasize the positive aspects of screening management (i.e., longer screening intervals).

Keywords: genetic linkage, premorbid diagnosis, preventive screening

BACKGROUND

Familial adenomatous polyposis (or familial polyposis coli) is an autosomal dominant condition with high (>90%) penetrance. It is characterized by numerous (>100) adenomatous polyps in the colon, and there is virtually 100% risk of colon cancer in persons who inherit the gene and manifest the adenomatous polyps. Offspring of an affected individual are at 50% risk of inheriting the condition. Screening management of these at-risk relatives has consisted of annual colon examinations by endoscopy beginning at age 11 or 12 years. The objective of this regimen is early detection of those who have inherited the gene, to whom preventive colectomy is advised.

Reports by Bodmer et al. (1987) and Leppert et al. (1987) that the gene for familial adenomatous polyposis was localized to chromosome 5q21-22 opened the way to development of diagnostic linkage analysis in pedigrees where the disease was segregating. One of the considerations, however, in molecular diagnosis using linkage is the markers' "informativeness." This is dependent upon the number of alleles and their relative frequencies in the population. Subsequent work reported by Meera Khan et al. (1988) added additional markers; and Nakamura et al. (1988) developed numerous informative flanking markers in this region, additionally demonstrating that Gardner syndrome is allelic with familial adenomatous polyposis. Although combinations of markers can be analyzed to develop a molecular "haplotype" that is linked to the familial adenomatous polyposis, highly informative markers as developed by Nakamura may also yield a premorbid diagnosis. Certainly with the array of molecular probes now available, it is likely that most pedigrees in which familial adenomatous polyposis is segregating can be made informative.

LINKAGE ANALYSIS OF FAMILY

The development of such informative linked markers now permits the clinical application of linkage information for premorbid diagnosis in at-risk individuals. We have performed the first such diagnostic linkage analysis using probe EF5.44 with restriction enzyme Msp I. In the case of the EF5.44 marker, no recombination with the FAP locus has been observed in family studies. See Fig. 1. The proband, who has a positive family history of familial adenomatous polyposis, is a 36-year old father of four asymptomatic children, all under age 10.

Prior to linkage analysis, all children had a 50% risk of developing FAP. Screening protocols for all four children would have consisted of annual flexible sigmoidoscopies beginning at age 11. With the linkage information, we could counsel the family with > 98% confidence that the first three children did not inherit the polyposis gene and that the youngest child did inherit the condition, which is linked to allele 1.

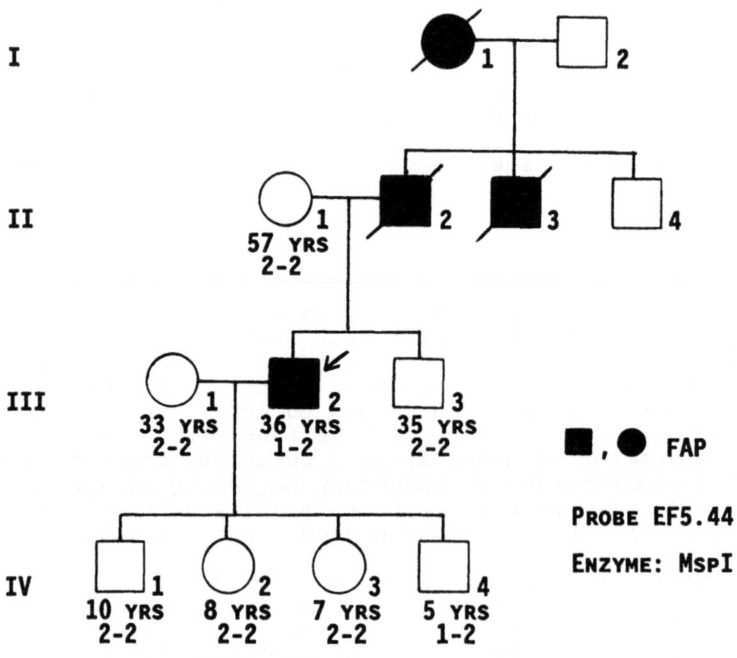

Fig. 1. With the linkage information, we could counsel the family with >98% confidence that the three oldest children were not at risk and the youngest child (IV-4) did inherit the polyposis gene. Allele 1 of the EF5.44 gene marker is segregating with the polyposis gene.

SCREENING RECOMMENDATIONS

There is now a need to modify the at-risk family member screening guidelines that were valid before the molecular genetic era. We have developed such recommendations for individuals who have received premorbid diagnosis for familial adenomatous polyposis using the linkage information. These recommendations were based upon the analyses of age at diagnosis reported by Bussey (1975) and Bussey et al. (1978) in two distinct groups of patients.

In his evaluation of the St. Mark's Hospital Polyposis Register data of 281 cases diagnosed by symptoms, Bussey (1975) found that there was a large range in the age at diagnosis of polyposis, from 4 to 73 years, with a mean age of 35.8 years. At 35 years of age, only around 50% of cases will have been diagnosed, and by age 50, there still remains an additional 10% of undiagnosed cases. In contrast, the age at diagnosis within the group of at-risk ("call-up") relatives has a distribution that is shifted to younger ages. It is this second study group that is of importance in developing estimates of age at risk for our families. Bussey et al. (1978) reported that the age range at diagnosis was 8 to 57 years, with an average of 23.8 years. Seventy-five percent of this group is diagnosed before age 30.

Using Bussey's published information, we have developed alternative screening recommendations for those relatives who most likely have <u>not</u> inherited FAP. In these cases, we propose baseline flexible sigmoidoscopies at ages 11 and 12, with repeated screening every 3 years thereafter until age 35. This latter recommendation decreases the number of times an individual would have to undergo the procedure, but still provides a margin of safety in the event of recombination or error (in our reported family, an estimated 2% chance). This modified screening recommendation can be presented as a positive improvement when the results are communicated by the clinician to the family members.

For those relatives who are found by linkage analysis to have inherited the polyposis gene, the screening management regimen will not differ from that which they would have had to undergo without the linkage information. It will be important in the future to study the psychosocial impact of the certainty of this information upon these at-risk relatives, and the effect of knowing at a younger age that they will develop polyposis.

Thus, we can summarize the differences in recommendations as follows:

1. Genetic counseling <u>WITHOUT</u> linkage information:

   - All offspring of affected parent are at 50% risk

   - Preventive screening should consist of flexible sigmoidoscopy of at-risk relatives beginning at age 11

   - If the relative is found to be affected, he or she should be counseled to consider prophylactic total colectomy to prevent colon cancer.

2. Genetic counseling <u>WITH</u> linkage information. If upon linkage analysis, the probability of the phenotype is:

   A. AFFECTED with familial adenomatous polyposis:

   - Annual flexible sigmoidoscopy examinations beginning at age 11

   - Counsel patient to consider prophylactic total colectomy to prevent colon cancer

B. NOT AFFECTED:

- Baseline flexible sigmoidoscopy examinations at ages 11 and 12
- Repeat flexible sigmoidoscopy examinations every three years until age 35.

CONCLUSIONS

Highly informative molecular markers linked to familial adenomatous polyposis can be used clinically in the premorbid diagnosis of this autosomal dominant condition. If on linkage analysis, an at-risk individual is found to have inherited the polyposis gene, there will be no change in the recommended screening regimen for this condition. However, if an at-risk individual is found to have inherited the normal gene, the clinician or genetic counselor can emphasize the positive aspects of screening management (i.e., longer screening intervals).

REFERENCES

Bodmer WF, Bailey CJ, Bodmer J, Bussey HJR, Ellis A, Gorman P, Lucibello FC, Murday VA, Rider SH, Scambler P, Sheer D, Solomon E, Spurr NK (1987) Localization of the gene for familial adenomatous polyposis on chromosome 5. Nature 328:614-616

Bussey HJR (1975) Familial polyposis coli. Family studies, histopathology, differential diagnosis, and results of treatment. Johns Hopkins University Press, Baltimore, MD

Bussey HJR, Veale AMO, Morson BC (1978) Genetics of gastrointestinal polyposis. Gastroenterology 74:1325-1330

Leppert M, Dobbs M, Scambler P, O'Connell P, Nakamura Y, Stauffer D, Woodward, Burt R, Hughes J, Gardner E, Lathrop M, Wasmuth J, Lalouel J-M, White R (1987) The gene for familial polyposis coli maps to the long arm of chromosome 5. Science 238:1411-1413

Meera Khan P, Tops CMJ, Broek MVD, Breukel C, Wijnen JT, Oldenburg M, Bos JVD, van Leeuwen-Cornelisse ISJ, Vasen HFA, Griffioen G, Verspaget HM, den Hartog Jager FCA, Lamers CBHW (1988) Close linkage of a highly polymorphic marker (D5S37) to familial adenomatous polyposis (FAP) and confirmation of FAP localization on chromosome 5q21-22. Hum Genet 79:183-185

Nakamura Y, Lathrop M, Leppert M, Dobbs M, Wasmuth J, Wolff E, Carlson M, Fujimoto E, Krapcho K, Sears T, Woodward S, Hughes J, Burt R, Gardner E, Lalouel J-M, White R (1988) Localization of the genetic defect in familial adenomatous polyposis within a small region of chromosome 5. Am J Hum Genet 43:638-644

Allele Loss and Kras Mutation Involved in the Development of Colorectal Tumors in Patients with Familial Adenomatous Polyposis

MICHIKO MIYAKI, MADOKA SEKI, MIEKO OKAMOTO, CHIEKO SATO, KIYOKO TANAKA, AKIYOSHI YAMANAKA, MORIO KOIKE, TAKEO MORI, JOJI UTSUNOMIYA, and TAKEO IWAMA

ABSTRACT To investigate the mechanism of colon carcinogenesis, the loss of heterozygosity and Kras mutation were analyzed in 24 advanced FAP carcinomas, 20 advanced non-FAP carcinomas, and 111 FAP polyps with distinct histopathological dysplasia. Allele loss was observed in advanced FAP carcinomas most frequently on chromosome 5q(38%), 17p(57%), 18(36%) and 22q(35%). Non-FAP carcinomas exhibited allele losses similar to those in the FAP carcinomas. The frequency of allele loss in polyps from FAP patients was low, but it was higher in more advanced polyps; the loss was observed on chromosome 5q(24%) in severe adenomas, and on chromosome 5q(25%) and 17p(30%) in intramucosal early carcinomas. Kras mutations were detected in 50% of the advanced FAP carcinomas. The mutation frequency in polyps was lower than that in advanced carcinomas, the frequency increasing with polyp size. The present results suggest, in addition to the FAP gene on chromosome 5q, a significant role of cumulative changes in multiple tumor suppressor genes and the Kras gene during the development of colon tumors.
KEY WORDS Familial adenomatous polyposis, Colorectal tumor, Loss of heterozygosity, Kras mutation, Tumor development

ALLELE LOSS ON CHROMOSOME 5q IN COLORECTAL TUMORS

Autosomal dominant trait familial adenomatous polyposis is inherited by heterozygous mutation in the FAP gene, a recessive oncogene. The FAP gene has been mapped to near C11p11(D5S71) on chromosome 5q21-22 (Bodmer et al. 1987; Leppert et al. 1987), and recently it has been demonstrated to be more close to YN5.48(D5S81) (Nakamura et al. 1988). The nature of the FAP gene as a tumor suppressor in colon carcinogenesis has been suggested by the loss of heterozygosity on chromosome 5q in colorectal tumors from both FAP and non-FAP patients (Solomon et al. 1987; Okamoto et al. 1988; Law et al. 1988; Vogelstein et al. 1988; Sasaki et al. 1989; Rees et al. 1989). However, rather low frequencies of 5q loss have been observed, and it has not been clear yet whether the normal allele or mutant allele is lost in colorectal tumors. In this study, a high frequency of allele loss on chromosome 5q was detected in advanced carcinomas from both FAP and non-FAP patients by using additional probes, including YN5.48. Moreover, loss of the normal allele of the FAP gene was observed in several tumors from FAP patients.
Figure 1A shows examples of allele loss on chromosome 5q in colon tumors. In FAP patient PLK42, the allele a2 of D543, which was assumed

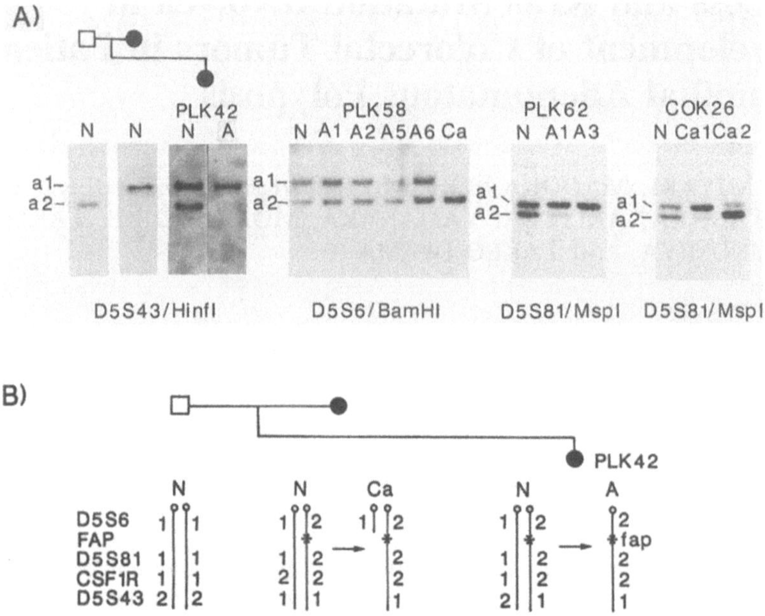

Fig. 1. Allele losses on chromosome 5q in colon tumors from FAP and non-FAP patients. A) Southern blot hybridization of DNA with RFLP probes. B) Loss of the 5q region carrying the normal FAP gene in colon tumors in an FAP family. N: normal tissue, A: adenoma, Ca: carcinoma, PLK: FAP patient, COK: non-FAP patient, FAP: normal FAP gene, fap: mutated FAP gene.

to exist in chromosome 5q carrying the normal FAP gene, was lost in a large advanced adenoma. Further analysis using other probes on chromosome 5q revealed that the normal allele of the FAP gene was lost and the chromosomal region including the mutated FAP gene was retained in this tumor. This chromosomal region was also retained in the advanced colon carcinoma after loss of heterozygosity on chromosome 5q in the affected mother of PLK42 (Fig. 1B) (Okamoto et al.,submitted). These results suggest that the FAP gene is recessively expressed in these tumors in FAP patients, as in the case of recessive expression of the RB gene in hereditary retinoblastoma. In other FAP patients, PLK58 and PLK62, the same allele was lost in two tumors from the same patient. In contrast to FAP, a non-FAP patient, COK26, showed a loss in different alleles in two carcinomas, Ca1 and Ca2 (Fig. 1B). Approximately 40% of advanced colon carcinomas and 12% of polyps from FAP patients, and 50% of advanced carcinomas from non-FAP patients exhibited allele loss on chromosome 5. The loss in both advanced carcinomas and polyps occurred most frequently in the region near the FAP gene, including the region for YN5.48 and C11p11 (Fig. 2). More than 86% of the tumor, which showed allele loss on chromosome 5, lost the region near the FAP gene. At more proximal (D5S6) and more distal region (CSF1R and D5S43), the frequency of loss was lower, and the short arm including D5S4 showed a minor loss.

Loss of the entire chromosome 5 was rare. A difference in the range of loss was not observed between carcinoma and adenoma, or between FAP and non-FAP. A similar high frequency of loss on chromosome 5q has recently been described in cases of sporadic colorectal tumors (Ashton-Rickardt et al., 1989). These results suggest that the loss of heterozygosity in the FAP gene is involved in colon carcinogenesis in both FAP and non-FAP patients, and that the loss leads to inactivation of the FAP gene.

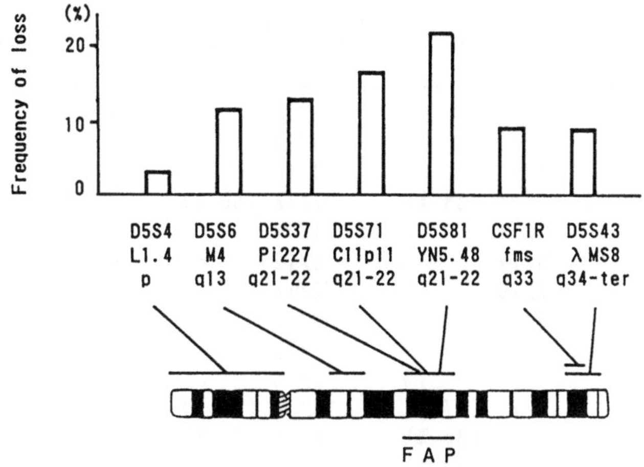

Fig. 2. Frequency of allele loss on chromosome 5 in colon tumors. Frequency was defined as the number of tumors that showed allele loss, divided by the number of informative cases in which DNA from the normal tissue exhibited heterozygosity for each RFLP probe. The frequencies were derived from analysis of 155 tumors, including 24 advanced colon carcinomas and 111 polyps from FAP patients, and 20 advanced carcinomas from non-FAP patients.

ALLELE LOSS ON MULTIPLE CHROMOSOMES IN ADVANCED COLORECTAL CARCINOMAS

Further examination of advanced carcinomas using 44 RFLP probes mapped on chromosomes 1 to 22 revealed frequent allele losses on several chromosomes other than 5q (Table I and Fig. 3). Allele loss was most frequently observed on chromosome 17p in advanced colon carcinomas from both FAP (13 of 23 informative cases, 57%) and non-FAP patients (13 of 16 informative cases, 81%). These high values were obtained from analysis by the VNTR probe YNZ22 (D17S30), mapped to 17p13.3, after digestion of DNAs with four kinds of restriction enzymes. The present results and those previously reported for sporadic cases (Fearon et al., 1987; Law et al., 1988; Monpezat et al.,1988; Vogelstein et al., 1988, 1989) indicate that allele loss on chromosome 17p is common in advanced colon carcinomas from both FAP and non-FAP patients. Allele loss on chromosome 18 was observed in 35% and 60% of FAP and non-FAP carcinomas, respectively. The high frequency of allele loss on chromosome 18 in previous studies (Monpezat et al., 1988; Law et al. 1988) and the present study suggests the existence of a tumor suppressor gene for colon carcinogenesis in this chromosome. The frequency of loss in chromosome 22q was also high in advanced FAP carcinomas (35%) and in non-FAP carcinomas (36%). In addition to the FAP gene, these results suggest that tumor suppressor genes on multiple chromosomes, 17p, 18, and 22q, may also play a critical role in colon carcinogenesis in both FAP and non-FAP patients.

Table I Allele losses and Kras mutations in colon tumors

Chromosome	Cases with allele loss/informative cases Ca (FAP)	Ca (non-FAP)	Polyp (FAP)
1	2/8	1/15	
2	0/9	0/12	
3	0/8	0/10	
5q	8/21 (38 %)	9/18 (50 %)	12/102 (12 %)
6p	2/14	4/19	
7	0/12	0/12	
11	0/10	0/14	
12	3/18	2/16	
14	0/10	3/12	
15	2/10	0/14	
17p	13/23 (57 %)	13/16 (81 %)	10/119 (8 %)
18	6/17 (35 %)	6/10 (60 %)	4/97 (4 %)
22q	8/23 (35 %)	5/14 (36 %)	2/87 (2 %)
Kras mutation	11/22 (50 %)	4/18 (22 %)	23/110 (21 %)

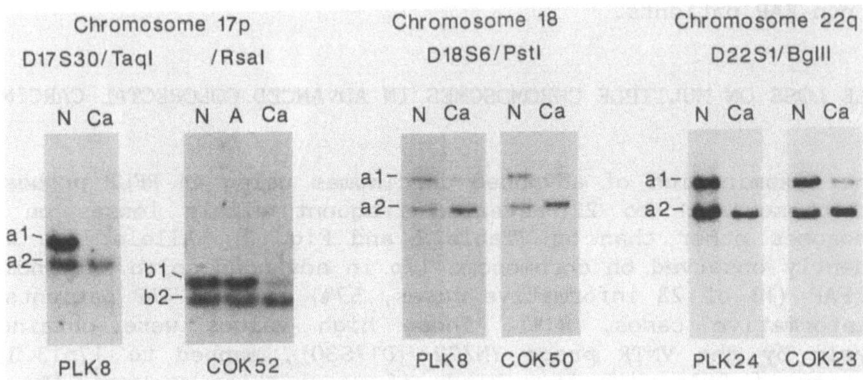

Fig. 3. Allele losses on chromosome 17p, 18 and 22q in colon tumors from FAP and non-FAP patients. N: normal tissue, Ca: carcinoma, A: adenoma, PLK: FAP patient, COK: non-FAP patient.

ALLELE LOSS AND KRAS MUTATION DURING THE DEVELOPMENT OF COLORECTAL TUMOR

The frequency of allele loss in polyps was low: 12% on chromosome 5, and 8%, 4%, and 2% on chromosomes, 17, 18, and 22, respectively. The low frequencies in polyps indicate that the allele loss is not involved in the polyp formation, but it is involved in carcinoma formation. We then classified these polyps into 5 groups according to the pathological diagnosis: moderate adenoma (54 samples), moderate-to-severe adenoma (12 samples), severe adenoma (22 samples), carcinoma in adenoma (7 samples), and intramucosal carcinoma (16 samples) (Fig. 4). In moderate adenomas allele loss was very low. In more advanced severe adenomas, including moderate-to-severe adenomas, a loss on chromosome 5q was detected with a frequency of 24%. Intramucosal carcinomas, including carcinomas in adenoma, exhibited a loss on both chromosomes 5q and 17p in 25% and 30%, respectively. This indicates that the malignant change from adenoma to carcinoma may be caused by additional loss on 17p. Advanced carcinomas showed high frequencies of loss on chromosomes 18 (35%) and 22 (35%) in addition to those on 5q and 17p, which indicates losses on 18 and 22 are involved in the progression of early carcinoma to advanced carcinoma. Kras mutation at codon 12 was detected in 11% of moderate adenomas and 38% of severe adenomas, which suggests a role of the activated Kras gene in the development of adenomas. The frequency of Kras mutation increased

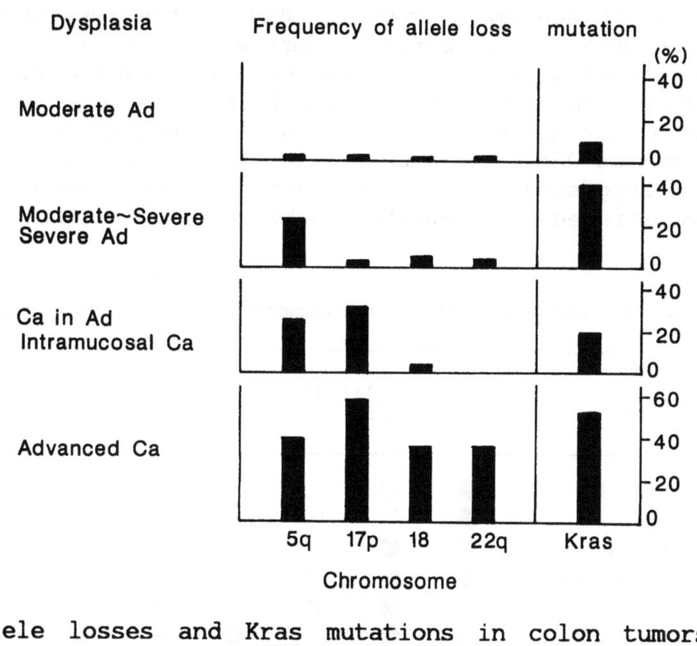

Fig. 4. Allele losses and Kras mutations in colon tumors from FAP patients. Analyses of allele loss and Kras mutation and pathological diagnosis were done independently, and the frequencies of loss and mutation were calculated for each group classified by histopathological dysplasia. Ad: adenoma, Ca: carcinoma

with an increase in the size of adenomas. However, the frequency of Kras mutation in intramucosal carcinomas was rather low, as only 18% contained the mutation. This indicates that Kras mutation had no relation to the conversion of adenoma to carcinoma. While the mutation seems to be involved in the progression from intramucosal carcinoma to advanced carcinoma, since the frequency was remarkably increased (50%) in advanced carcinomas. Moreover, the kind of mutation was not the same between adenoma and carcinoma. For example, adenomas contained mutations GGT(Gly) to GAT(Asp), GGT to TGT(Cys), GGT to GTT(Val), and GGT to GCT(Ala) at codon 12, while advanced carcinomas contained significantly higher GGT to GAT(Asp) mutation compared to other types.

Cumulative genetic changes were observed in more advanced colorectal tumors in FAP patients. Table II shows examples of tumors with allele losses and Kras mutations. Severe adenomas showed a loss only on chromosome 5q. Some intramucosal carcinomas had losses on two chromosomes, 5q and 17p. And many advanced carcinomas exhibited losses on multiple chromosomes, including 5q, 17p, 18, 22q, 6p, and 12p.

Vogelstein et al.(1988) have reported the accumulation of four molecular alterations, including allelic deletions of chromosomes 5q, 17p, and 18q, and ras mutations during the development of sporadic carcinomas, however they found no allelic deletions in adenomas from FAP patients. Class I adenomas from FAP patients in their study seem to be like the moderate dysplasia, which showed quite a low frequency of loss on 5q in this study. Severe adenomas from FAP patients exhibited allele loss on 5q at a frequency of 24%, which is comparable to the frequency in sporadic Class II adenomas. However, whether the remaining FAP allele was normal or mutated in sporadic adenoma is not clear, although the loss of the normal allele of the FAP gene was demonstrable in several tumors in FAP patients. A gene dosage effect of the FAP gene through the loss of one allele cannot be ruled out in sporadic benign tumors. In loss on chromosome 17p in sporadic colon carcinoma, the target gene has recently been suggested to be the p53 gene, and the remaining p53 allele has been demonstrated to be mutated (Baker et al., 1989).

Table II Examples of colon tumors with genetic changes

Tumor	Allele loss 5q	17p	18	22q	6p	12p	Kras mut
87A1 Severe Ad	●	○	○	○	—	—	—
62A1 Severe Ad	●	○	○	○	—	○	Val
58A5 Intramucosal Ca	●	●	○	○	○	—	—
72A2 Intramucosal Ca	●	●	○	○	—	—	Asp
4Ca Advanced Ca	●	●	●	—	●	●	Asp
24Ca Advanced Ca	●	●	—	●	●	●	—
87Ca Advanced Ca	●	●	○	●	—	—	Asp
32Ca Advanced Ca	●	—	—	●	●	●	Asp
8Ca Advanced Ca	○	●	●	○	○	●	Cys

● : loss of heterozygosity was observed, ○ : no loss,
— : not informative or without mutation, Ad: adenoma, Ca:carcinoma

CONCLUSION REMARKS

Our present results suggest a mechanism on developmemt from benign to malignant colorectal tumors in FAP patients as follows: 1) In FAP patients, colon adenomas are produced by an inherited heterozygous mutation in the FAP gene. 2) The loss of heterozygosity in the FAP gene causes the change from moderate to severe adenoma. 3) In addition, further allele loss on chromosome 17p results in the formation of intramucosal early carcinoma. 4) Furthermore, allele losses on multiple chromosomes, such as 18 and 22q, cause the progression of early carcinoma to advanced carcinoma. 5) Kras mutation may affect the growth of adenoma and the progression of carcinoma.
However, the mechanism of adenoma formation by the heterozygous mutation in the FAP gene is yet unclear. The normal FAP gene is assumed to function as a growth regulatory gene, and inactivation of one copy of two alleles gives rise to hyperproliferation in the colorectal mucosa through a threshold effect produced by fluctuating levels of gene product (Solomon et al., 1987). This effect may also be manifested in extracolonic tissues of FAP patients, since these patients have a high incidence of various tumors, such as gastric cancer, thyroid tumor, osteoma, and desmoid tumor. In a desmoid tumor we have detected the loss of heterozygosity at near the FAP gene on chromosome 5q. The heterozygous mutant FAP gene may also be expressed in cultured skin fibroblasts that have exhibited properties of hyperproliferation, such as high susceptibility to chemical and viral transformation in vitro (Miyaki et al., 1988). Investigation of the mechanism of growth abnormalities in these cultured cells may also be important to reveal the effect of the inherited heterozygous FAP gene.

MATERIALS AND METHODS

Twenty four advanced colon carcinomas and 111 polyps were obtained from 38 FAP patients, and 20 advanced colon carcinomas were from 19 non-FAP patients. A part of each specimen was diagnosed histopathologically. DNA was isolated from tumor specimens and the corresponding normal tissues, and hybridized with radiolabeled RFLP probes: MYCL, D1S57, D2S1, CRYG, D3S2, AFP, D5S1, D5S2, D5S4, D5S6, D5S37, D5S43, D5S71, D5S81, CSF1R, KRAS1P, MYB, HLADQ1A, HLADQ1B, COL1A2, D8S18, D9S14, HRAS1, KRAS2, D12S7, D12S8, D13S1, D13S2, D13S3, D14S1, D15S1, HBA, D17S1, D17S4, D17S30, D17S37, D18S1, D18S6, D22S1, D22S9, IGLC, IGLV, D22S1 and PDGFB. DNA samples were also analyzed for Kras mutations by hybridization with radiolabeled 19 mer probes containing normal (Gly) and mutated sequences (Ala, Arg, Asp, Cys, Ser, Val) at codon 12, and mutation (Asp) at codon 13, after amplification of 90 bp sequence of K-ras gene.

ACKNOWLEDGEMENTS

We are grateful to all of the surgeons that provided tumor specimens, to the scientists who provided probes, and to Dr.Y.Nakamura and Dr.R.White for providing YN5.48. Several probes were supplied by Japanese Cancer Research Resources Bank. This work was supported in part by Grants in Aid for Cancer Research from the Ministry of Education, Science and Culture of Japan and from the Ministry of Health and Welfare of Japan.

REFERENCES

Ashton-Rickardt PG, Dunlop MG, Nakamura Y, Morris RG, Purdie CA, Steel CM, Evans HJ, Bird CC, Wyllie AH (1989) High frequency of APC loss in sporadic colorectal carcinoma due to breaks clustered in 5q21-22. Oncogene 4: 1169-1174

Baker SJ, Fearon ER, Nigro JM, Hamilton SR, Preisinger AC, Jessup M, vanTuinen P, Lederbetter DH, Barker DF, Nakamura Y, White R, Vogelstein B (1989) Crromosome 17 deletions and p53 gene mutations in colorectal carcinomas. Science 244: 217-221

Bodmer WF, Bailey CJ, Bodmer J, Bussey HJR, Ellis A, Gorman P, Lucibello FC, Murday VA, Rider SH, Scambler P, Sheer D, Solomon E, Spurr NK (1987) Localization of the gene for familial adenomatous polyposis on chromosome 5. Nature 328: 614-616

Fearon ER, Hamilton SR, Vogelstein B (1987) Clonal analysis of human colorectal tumors. Science 238: 193-197

Law DJ, Olschwang S, Monpezat J-P, Lefrancois D, Jagelman D, Petrelli N, Thomas G, Feinberg AP (1988) Concerted nonsyntenic allelic loss in human colorectal carcinoma. Science 241: 961-965

Leppert M, Dobbs M, Scamber P, O'Connell P, Nakamura Y, Stauffer D, Woodward S, Burt R, Hughes J, Gardner E, Lathrop M, Wasmuth J, Lalouel JM, White R (1987) The gene for familial polyposis coli maps to the long arm of chromosome 5. Science 238: 1411-1413

Miyaki M, Akamatsu N, Sato C, Utsunomiya J (1988) Chemical and viral transformation of cultured skin fibroblasts from patients with familial polyposis coli. Mutation Research 199: 399-414

Monpezat J-P, Delattre O, Bernard A, Grunwald D, Remvikos Y, Muleris M, Salmon RJ, Frelat G, Dutrillaux B, Thomas G (1988) Loss of alleles on chromosome 18 and on the short arm of chromosome 17 in polyploid colorectal carcinomas. Int. J. Cancer 41: 404-408

Nakamura Y, Lathrop M, Leppert M, Dobbs M, Wasmuth J, Wolff E, Carlson M, Fujimoto E, Krapcho K, Sears,T, Woodward S, Hughes J, Burt R, Gardner E, Lalouel J-M, White R (1989) Localization of the genetic defect in familial adenomatous polyposis within a small region of chromosome 5. Am. J. Hum. Genet. 43: 638-644

Okamoto M, Sasaki M, Sugio K, Sato C, Iwama T, Ikeuchi T, Tonomura A, Sasazuki T, Miyaki M (1988) Loss of constitutional heterozygosity in colon carcinoma from patients with FPC. Nature 331: 273-277

Okamoto M, Sato C, Kohno Y, Mori T, Iwama T, Tonomura A, Miki Y, Utsunomiya J, Nakamura Y, White R, Miyaki M. Loss of alleles on 5q in colorectal and desmoid tumors from patients with FAP (submitted)

Rees M, Leigh SEA, Delhanty JDA, Jass JR (1989) Chromosome 5 allele loss in familial and sporadic colorectal adenomas. Br.J. Cancer 59:361-365

Sasaki M, Okamoto M, Sato C, Sugio K, Soejima J, Iwama T, Ikeuchi T, Tonomura A, Miyaki M, Sasazuki T (1989) Loss of heterozygosity in colon tumors from patients with FAP non-FPC. Cancer Res. 49: 4402-4406

Solomon E, Voss R, Hall V, Bodmer WF, Jass JR, Jeffreys AJ, Lucibello FC, Patel I, Rider SH (1987) Chromosome 5 allele loss in human colorectal carcinomas. Nature 328: 616-619

Vogelstein B, Fearon ER, Hamilton SR, Kern SE, Preisinger AC, Leppert M, Nakamura Y, White R, Smith AMM, Bos JL (1988) Genetic alterations during colorectal-tumor development. New Engl. J. Med. 319: 525-532

Vogelstein B, Fearon ER, Kern SE, Hamilton SR, Preisinger AC, Nakamura Y White R. (1989) Allotype of colorectal carcinoms. Science 244: 207-211

Status of the APC Gene in Familial and Sporadic Colorectal Tumours as Determined by Closely Flanking Markers

A.H. WYLLIE, P. ASHTON-RICKARDT, M.G. DUNLOP, Y. NAKAMURA, J. PIRIS, C. PURDIE, C.M. STEEL, and C.C. BIRD

ABSTRACT

Using polymorphic close-flanking markers, allele deletion in the vicinity of APC was detected in the majority of sporadic colorectal cancers in a large unselected series. Deletion was due to interstitial deletion or mitotic recombination, but seldom to whole chromosome loss. Mitotic recombination affecting APC was associated with smaller tumours than interstitial deletion. Sporadic adenomas showed a slightly lesser frequency of allele loss, but no such loss was observed in 28 adenomas from 4 cases of familial polyposis.

INTRODUCTION

This paper presents new data on the incidence of deletion of the APC (Familial Polyposis) gene in human colorectal tumours. Accurate measurement of this incidence provides the only firm clues at present available to the functional significance of APC. In previous work, incidence of allelic deletion involving chromosome 5q is variously reported between 20% and 40% in sporadic colorectal carcinomas (Solomon et al 1987; Vogelstein et al 1988; Law et al 1989) in around 30% sporadic adenomas (Vogelstein et al 1988; Rees et al 1989), and in few if any adenomas of patients suffering from polyposis coli. Only one group has presented convincing data on the status of 5q alleles in carcinomas from polyposis patients, allele loss being observed in around 24% (Okamoto et al 1988; Sasaki et al 1989). In all of these studies, however, the analysis of 5q alleles was based on relatively few, dispersed loci. In this paper we describe a large series of sporadic carcinomas, and substantial numbers of sporadic and familial adenomas, using a group of probes detecting polymorphic sequences tightly clustered around APC.

A CLUSTER OF PROBES LINKED TO APC

Maximum lod scores and the corresponding recombination fractions are shown for five probes tightly linked to APC as tested in nine Scottish polyposis kindreds involving more than 90 meioses (Table 1). Critical recombinations indicated that π227 and C11P11 are on the same side of APC,(Dunlop et al 1989), whereas YN5.48 is on the opposite side. Physical maps suggest that the probes lie in the order: cen-π227-C11P11-L5.62-EF5.44-YN5.44-MC5.61-ter.

LOSS OF APC ALLELES IN SPORADIC COLORECTAL CARCINOMA

π227, YN5.48 and MC5.61 detect highly polymorphic sequences, so that the majority of patients studied are informative. EF5.44 and L5.62 are less informative. Accordingly, we initially studied a series of 146 sporadic colorectal carcinomas with π227, C11P11, YN5.48 and MC5.61 to determine the frequency of allele loss close to APC

TABLE 1

APC LINKAGE DATA DERIVED FROM STUDY OF 9 SCOTTISH POLYPOSIS KINDREDS.

probe tested with APC	max. lod score (Z)	recombination at Z (θ)	95% probability limits (θ)
π227	4.40	0.11	(0.035-0.235)
C11P11	5.45	0.09	(0.025-0.21)
L5.62	13.31	0.02	(0.005-0.095)
EF5.44	3.50	0.00	(0.00-0.16)
YN5.48	7.00	0.00	(0.00-0.07)

(Ashton-Rickardt et al 1989). 53% of the 85 tumours informative on both sides of APC showed loss of the centromeric or telomeric flanking markers, or both. We then focussed on those tumours in which the first four polymorphic flanking markers had failed to detect allelic losses. Of the 40 tumours in this category, 22 were informative at the L5.62 or EF5.44 loci, and 5 showed allele loss. Hence the true overall frequency of APC-linked allele loss detected by these probes is 53% + (47% x 5/22), i.e. 63%. This frequency can only rise further as probes closer to APC are employed. Hence APC joins the putative anti-oncogene loci on 17p and 18q (Fearon et al 1987; Vogelstein et al 1988; Monpezat et al 1988; Lothe et al 1988) in showing allele loss in the majority (and perhaps being abnormal in all) of sporadic colorectal carcinomas.

THE CHROMOSOMAL LESIONS RESPONSIBLE FOR APC LOSS

Use of the probes listed above, together with probes hybridising to more distant loci on both long and short arms of chromosome 5 permitted description of the chromosomal lesions most commonly involved in APC allele loss. There were three major findings.

Firstly, whole chromosome loss is rare. Hence 5q allele loss in colorectal cancers can seldom be the result of chromosomal nondisjunction, although this accounts for much of the aneuploidy of such tumours, as judged from the reported karyotypes (Reichmann et al 1981). Aneuploidy appears in the course of tumour progression, being rare in adenomas, but present in at least 60% of carcinomas (Goh & Jass, 1986; Quirke et al 1987). APC loss therefore appears to precede this stage of tumour progression, and this is confirmed by the observation that 5q allele loss was found in equal frequency in DNA-diploid and DNA-aneuploid carcinomas (Ashton-Rickardt et al 1989). Anecdotal evidence from other groups confirms this view (Remvikos et al 1988).

Secondly, the common causes of APC-linked allele loss are interstitial deletion and mitotic recombination (or conceivably partial chromosomal arm loss, which is not distinguished by this method of analysis). Many interstitial deletions are relatively small. Amongst the tumours in which APC-linked alleles are lost by interstitial deletions, the site most commonly involved (in informative tumours) is that detected by EF5.44. This completely accords with the suggestion from linkage and physical mapping data that this genomic sequence lies close to APC.

Thirdly, and quite unexpectedly, tumours in which APC alleles are lost through mitotic recombination are significantly smaller than tumours in which the allele loss results from interstitial deletion. This difference persists after excluding from the analysis all right-sided colonic carcinomas, which may tend to present later than those in the rectosigmoid. This finding underlines the importance of the status of APC in colorectal tumour growth, and may result from a gene dosage effect.

APC ALLELE LOSS IN ADENOMAS

In a series of 63 sporadic adenomas from 40 patients informative at some site on 5q, we identified 19 (30.2%) with allelic deletion. The analysis of these adenomas has not involved as many loci as in the carcinomas, but comparison of the incidence of allele loss at three polymorphic loci confirmed the trend that adenomas show less allelic deletion than carcinomas. Differences in incidence of allele loss between carcinomas and adenomas were significant when tumours with informative flanking markers on both sides of APC are compared. In contrast, none of 28 adenomas from four patients with polyposis showed allele loss. Although many of these were smaller than the sporadic adenomas, several showed features normally regarded as signifying aggressive behaviour: aneuploidy and severely dysplastic histology.

CONCLUSIONS

The data support the view that allele loss at the APC locus is a highly significant and common event in human colorectal carcinogenesis. Single allele abnormality (as in polyposis adenomas) appears to be adequate to permit development of adenomas, presumably in conjunction with some additional event, acquired during exposure to carcinogens in the gut lumen. The majority of carcinomas have demonstrable allele loss (and presumably point mutations in the residual allele) at APC. Similar abnormalities frequently occur in sporadic adenomas, and may permit their progression to carcinoma. These findings, and also the observation that major tumour aneuploidy develops after 5q allele loss in many sporadic carcinomas, show that APC abnormalities affect colorectal mucosal epithelium at an early stage in carcinogenesis. The mechanism whereby the alleles are lost, however, appears to influence the subsequent growth pattern of the tumour.

REFERENCES

Ashton-Rickardt PG, Dunlop MG, Nakamura Y, Morris RG, Purdie CA, Steel CM, Evans HJ, Bird CC and Wyllie AH. (1989) High Frequency of APC loss in sporadic colorectal carcinoma due to breaks clustered in 5q21-22. Oncogene, 4:1169-1174.

Dunlop MG, Steel CM, Wyllie AH, Bird CC, and Evans HJ. (1989) Linkage analysis in Familial Adenomatous Polyposis: order of C11P11 (D5S71) and pi227 (D5S37) loci at the apc gene. Genomics, 5:350-353.

Fearon ER, Hamilton SR, Vogelstein B. (1987) Clonal analysis of human colorectal tumours. Science 238:193-197.

Goh HS, Jass JR. (1986) DNA content and the adenoma-carcinoma sequence in the colorectum. J. Clin. Pathol. 39:387-392.

Law DJ, Olschwang S, Monpezat JP, Lefrancois D, Jagelman D, Petrelli NJ, Thomas G, Feinberg AP. (1988) Concerted nonsyntenic allelic loss in human colorectal carcinoma. Science 241:961-965.

Lothe RA, Nakamura Y, Woodward S, Gedde-Dahl T, White R. (1988) VNTR (variable number of tandem repeats) markers show loss of chromosome 17p sequences in human colorectal carcinomas. Cyto-genet. Cell Genet. 48:167-169.

Monpezat J-Ph, Delattre O, Bernard A, Grunwald D, Remvikos Y, Muleris M, Salmon RJ, Frelat G, Dutrillaux B, Thomas G (1988) Loss of alleles on chromosome 18 and on the short arm of chromosome 17 in polypoid colorectal carcinomas. Int. J. Cancer 41:404-408.

Okamoto M, Sasaki M, Sugio K, Sato C, Iwama T, Ikeuchi T, Tonomura A, Sasazuki T, Miyaki M. (1988) Loss of constitutional heterozygosity in colon carcinoma from patients with familial polyposis coli. Nature 331:273-277.

Quirke P, Dixon MF, Clayden AD, Durdey P, Dyson JED, Williams NS, and Bird CC. (1987) Prognostic Significance of DNA aneuploidy and cell proliferation in rectal adenocarcinomas. J. Pathol. 151:285-291.

Rees M, Leigh SEA, Delhanty JDA, Jass JR. (1989) Chromosome 5 allele loss in familial and sporadic colorectal adenomas. Brit. J. Cancer 59:361-365.

Reichmann A, Martin P, Levin B. (1981) Chromosomal banding patterns in human large bowel cancer. Int. J. Cancer 28:431-440.

Remvikos Y, Muleris M, Vielh P, Salmon RJ, Dutrillaux B. (1988) DNA content and genetic evolution of human colorectal adeno-carcinoma. A study by flow cytometry and cytogenetic analysis. Int. J. Cancer 42:539-543.

Sasaki M, Okamoto M, Sato C, Sugio K, Soejima J, Iwama T, Ikeuchi T, Tonomura A, Miyaki M, Sasazuki T (1989) Loss of constitutional heterozygosity in colorectal tumours from patients with familial polyposis coli and those with nonpolyposis colorectal carcinoma. Cancer Res. 49:4402-4406.

Solomon E, Voss R, Hall V, Bodmer WF, Jass JR, Jeffreys AJ, Lucibello FC, Patel I, Rider SH. (1987) Chromosome 5 allele loss in human colorectal carcinomas. Nature 328:616-619.

Vogelstein B, Fearon ER, Hamilton SR, Kern SF, Preisinger AC, Leppert M, Nakamura Y, White R, Smits AMM, Bos JL. (1988) Genetic alterations during colorectal-tumour development. New Eng. J. Med. 319:525-532.

Strategies for Cloning the Gene for Adenomatous Polyposis Coli

LILIANA VARESCO, HUW THOMAS, J.R. TRISTAN WARD,
ELLEN SOLOMON, and ANNA-MARIA FRISCHAUF

ABSTRACT
To search for the gene for adenomatous poylposis coli (APC) we have concentrated on cloning sequences from CpG rich undermethylated islands from the 5q21 region known to contain the APC mutation. We have constructed a library of endclones from 0.5-2Mb BssHII fragments. These clones were mapped on hybrids containing deletions in the region of the APC gene. The clones allow the construction of a partial long range restriction map of the region and identify some conserved sequences.

Keywords: Adenomatous polyposis coli, CpG islands, long range restriction map, gene isolation

1. GENERAL CONSIDERATIONS

Many genes are known to be associated with CpG rich undermethylated islands (Bird 1987). These islands contain the majority of cutting sites for methylation sensitive enzymes that contain one or more CpG dinucleotides in their recognition sequence and therefore cut rarely in mammalian DNA. To physically identify and clone a disease gene that has been localised by genetic analysis it is necessary to construct a long range restriction map around the disease gene to search for coding sequences in this region. An approach that revolves around CpG island sequences should therefore provide an efficient route to both map construction and the isolation of candidate genes.

The gene responsible for adenomatous polyposis coli (APC) has been mapped by linkage analysis (Bodmer 1987, Leppert 1987) to 5q15-q21. In choosing a strategy for isolating the gene we wanted to minimise the number of DNA markers to be mapped and characterised. We therefore concentrated on cloning sequences flanking rare cutting restriction sites. One possible approach involves the construction of linking libraries.(Poustka 1986). This is especially advantageous if desired wanted gene is situated in a region very rich in CpG islands since in this case a large percentage of the clones comes from the region of the gene (Pohl 1988). The APC gene seems to lie in a region that looks exactly the opposite. Pulsed Field gel analysis of the DNA hybridising to C11P11 (D5S71), a marker linked to APC (Bodmer 1987, Leppert 1987) showed a highly methylated region with CpG islands spaced at long distances. We therefore decided to derive new DNA markers specifically from the ends of long BssHII fragments (Varesco in press). This should exclude clones from regions with closely spaced CpG islands and result in a small number of clones that would , however, be derived from the islands of the overall highly methylated regions.

2. BssHII ENDCLONES

To obtain clones from the ends of long BssHII fragments (Michiels 1987) high molecular weight DNA from H64 (MacDonald 1987), a hamster hybrid cell line containing the human chromosomes 4 and 5 was digested in agarose blocks with BssHII, and size fractionated on an inverted field gel. DNA in the 0.5-2Mb size range was eluted, cut with MboI to 10-20kb average size and cloned into EMBL7, a lambda vector with a BamHI and a BssHII compatible MluI cloning site (Frischauf 1987). In this way only the ends of the fragments are cloned resulting in a library of relatively low complexity. Human clones were identified by hybridisation to labelled total human DNA.
The human BssHII endclones were then mapped using a panel of hamster hybrids including two lines containing human chromosomes 5 with deletions of 5q15-q21 (Varesco in press, Thomas 1989). PD/TS-1 is derived from a patient with APC (Hockey 1989), MD/TS-1 from an individual of unknown status. It was therefore possible to assign clones to the region of the APC gene. Of 154 clones characterised, 94 clones mapped to chromosome 5, of these 2 were absent in the deletion chromosomes PD and MD, and a further 2 were absent in MD only. Table 1 shows a summary of these results.

Table 1: Mapping of BssHII endclones

Clone	chr.5	PD	MD
ECB27	+	-	-
ECB220	+	-	-
ECB134	+	+	-
ECB362	+	+	-

Since the BssHII endclones contain the flanking sequences on one side of the BssHII sites only, short chromosome walks were made from ECB27 (D5S98) and ECB220 to cross the restriction site and allow significant extension of the long range restriction map. Genomic human lambda libraries were screened and the clones ECB27F1 and ECB220F1 isolated and used for pulsed field gel analysis.

THE LONG RANGE RESTRICTION MAP AROUND THE MARKER CLONES

To establish the extent of the deletions in PD and MD and to determine accurately their overlap, we constructed a partial restriction map of the region concentrating on the fragments created by the enzymes BssHII and MluI. In the region around the APC gene these enzymes cut the DNA into fragments <5Mb that can be well resolved under our PFG conditions. Table 2 shows the approximate fragment sizes for the probes tested. Most of the BssHII are in a similar size range but inspection of the film shows that they cannot be identical.

Table 2: Restriction fragments in GM1416B DNA

Clone	BssHII	MluI
ECB27	800kb	2300kb, 2700kb
ECB27F1	800kb	2200kb
ECB220	<800kb, 1300kb	1100kb, 2700kb
ECB220F1	1500kb	1100kb, 2700kb
ECB134	1000kb	2400kb, 2900kb
ECB362	n.t.	n.t.
C11P11	<800kb, 1500kb	2800kb, 3000kb, 4000kb

All fragment sizes are derived from a single gel. Overlaps can therefore be excluded for fragments of only slightly different mobilities. Sizes are approximate only and bands below 800kb were not well resolved.

The order of the clones within the deletions has not yet been established. It is therefore not possible to say whether MD extends further in both directions than PD or whether the two markers that are not deleted in PD are both located on the same side. Mapping of the clones in radiation hybrids (Thomas 1989) and genetic mapping may resolve this question even before a complete physical map has been established. It appears, however, that though the two deletions are cytologically equivalent they seem to differ significantly at the molecular level. Additional markers will be necessary to delineate exactly the deletion breakpoints and show the length of the deletions. Markers from the region obtained by others (Nakamura 1988) should contribute additional information.

FURTHER APPROACHES

The availability of radiation hybrids containing fragments of chromosome 5 (Thomas 1989) permits the application of strategies that would be too laborious if applied to hybrids like H64 (MacDonald 1987) containing chromosomes 4 and 5, or PN/TS-1 (Varesco in press) containing chromosome 5 only. We have started to characterise clones from EagI linking libraries made from one of the hybrids containing the ECB27 marker (Thomas 1989). With only small amounts of human DNA present in the hybrid cell lines it should be possible to avoid isolating clones predominantly from CpG rich undermethylated regions even without size fractionating the DNA that has been cut with rare cutting enzymes. This makes the characterisation of linking libraries easier and avoids the less efficient procedure of endcloning.

As we continue isolating markers from CpG rich islands we are testing them for the presence of sequences that are conserved between different species. Such sequences have been identified in ECB27 and in ECB220F1 (data not shown). This provides the opportunity to screen for cDNA clones which then may be tested as candidates for the disease gene.

In summary, the strategy of concentrating on CpG island sequences seems to be as efficient as predicted in terms of long range restriction mapping and the identification of coding regions with a small number of markers. As the region becomes completely mapped and the localisation of the gene more closely defined it will be necessary to go to a more laborious approach of cloning long stretches of DNA for a more detailed analysis.

REFERENCES

Bird AP (1987) CpG islands as gene markers in the vertebrate nucleus. Trends Genet. 3: 342-347

Bodmer WF, Bailey CJ, Bodmer J, Bussey HJR, Ellis A, Gorman P, Lucibello FC, Murday VA, Rider SH, Scambler P, Sheer D, Solomon E.& Spurr NK (1987) Localization of the gene for familial adenomatous polyposis on chromosome 5. Nature 328: 614-616

Frischauf A-M, Murray N, Lehrach H (1987) Lambda phage vectors- EMBL series Methods Enzymol. 153: 103-115

Hockey, KA, Mulcahy MT, Montgomery P, Levit S (1989) Deletion of chromosome 5q and familial adenomatous polyposis. J. Med. Genet. 26: 61-68

Leppert M, Dobbs M, Scambler P, O'Connell P, Nakamura Y, Stauffer D, Woodward S, Burt R, Hughes J, Gardner E, Lathrop M, Wasmuth J, Lalouel J-M, White R (1987) The Gene for Familial Polyposis Coli Maps to the Long Arm of Chromosome 5. Science 238: 1411-1413

MacDonald ME, Anderson MA, Gilliam TC, Tranebjaerg L, Carpenter NJ, Magenis E, Hayden MR, Healey ST, Bonner TI, Gusella JF (1987) A Somatic Cell Hybrid Panel for Localizing DNA Segments near the Huntington's Disease Gene. Genomics 1: 29-34

Michiels F, Burmeister M, Lehrach H (1987) Derivation of Clones Close to met by Preparative Field Inversion Gel Electrophoresis. Science 236: 1305-1307

Nakamura Y, Lathrop M, Leppert M, Dobbs M, Wasmuth J, Wolff E, Carlson M, Fujimoto E, Krapcho K, Sears T, Woodward S, Hughes J, Burt R, Gardner J, Lalouel JM, White R (1988) Localization of the Genetic Defect in Familial Adenomatous Polyposis within a Small Region of Chromosome 5. Am.J.Hum.Genet. 43: 638-644

Pohl TM, Zimmer M, MacDonald ME., Smith B, Bucan M, Poustka A, Volinia S, Searle S, Zehetner G, Wasmuth JJ, Gusella J, Lehrach H, Frischauf A-M (1988) Construction of a NotI linking library and isolation of new markers close to the Huntington's disease gene. Nucl. Acids Res. 16: 9185-9198

Poustka A & Lehrach H (1986) Jumping libraries and linking libraries: the next generation of molecular tools in mammalian genetics. Trends Genet. 2: 174-179

Thomas H, Varesco L, Frischauf A-M and Solomon E (1989) Chromosome 5 Deletions and Colorectal Cancer. these proceedings

Varesco L, Thomas H, Cottrell S, Murday V, Fennell SJ, Williams S, Sheer D, Bodmer WF, Frischauf A-M, Solomon E CpG island clones from a deletion encompassing the gene for Adenomatous Polyposis Coli. Proc.Natl Acad.Sci, in press

Genetic and Molecular Analysis of Familial Polyposis Coli

TAKEHIKO SASAZUKI, KENJI SUGIO, MASAYUKI SASAKI, YUCHIO YANAGAWA, and KAZUNORI URABE

ABSTRACT

Molecular and genetic analysis of familial polyposis coli (FPC) paves the way toward a better understanding of the mechanism of tumorigenesis in the colon and rectum. We examined events related to tumorigenesis by activation of oncogenes and inactivation of tumor suppressor genes. Evidence was obtained for an increased expression of the c-*myc* gene and a decreased expression of the c-*fos* gene, and point mutations in the K-*ras* gene. Frequent loss of heterozygosity was also evident on chromosomes 5, 14, 17, 18, and 22. These results suggest that in addition to the mutated FPC gene, various genetic events are involved in colorectal tumorigenesis of FPC.

Keywords: familial polyposis coli, oncogenes, tumor suppressor genes, loss of heterozygosity, genetic events

Familial polyposis coli is an autosomal dominant genetic trait characterized by numerous colorectal adenomatous polyps. The risk for colorectal carcinoma in these patients is high. Adenomatous polyps seem to be the major premalignant regions in the colon and rectum, hence an analysis of molecular mechanisms involved in the tumorigenesis of FPC[2] should provide information on tumor progression in colorectal cancers. The major gene for FPC was mapped to chromosome 5q21-22 by linkage analysis (Bodmer et al., 198; Leppert et al., 1987; Nakamura et al., 1988) and the mutated FPC gene is thought to play a critical role in tumorigenesis in the colon and rectum. Frequent mutations in the *ras* gene (Bos et al., 1987; Vogelstein et al., 1988), deregulated expression of the c-*myc* gene (Erissman et al., 1985), and loss of heterozygosity on several chromosomes (Fearon et al., 1987; Solomon et al., 1987; Law et al., 1988; Vogelstein et al., 1988) have been noted in sporadic colorectal carcinomas. Therefore, multiple steps are involved in the colorectal tumorigenesis.

In investigations on the molecular mechanism of colorectal carcinogenesis in patients with FPC, an analysis was made of the sporadic colorectal carcinomas. To elucidate the mechanism of colorectal tumorigenesis, we examined colorectal tumors in patients with FPC or NPCC and notes various kinds of genetic events occuring at the molecular level.

T. Sasazuki, K. Sugio, M. Sasaki, Y. Yanagawa, K. Urabe are in the Department of Genetics, Medical Institute of Bioregulation, Kyushu University, 3-1-1 Maidashi, Higashi-ku, Fukuoka 812, Japan.

[1] To whom correspondence should be addressed.

[2] Abbreviations used are: FPC, familial polyposis coli; NPCC, nonpolyposis colorectal carcinoma.

1. ONCOGENES

Deregulated expression of c-*myc* gene and c-*fos* gene

The level of expression of oncogenes (c-*myc*, c-*fos*,) was examined in 13 adenomatous polyps, 8 adenocarcinomas, and 15 normal colonic mucosa derived from 15 patients with FPC. In Northern blot analysis, 8 of 13 adenomas showed a moderately elevated expression (more than 1.5-fold) of the c-*myc* gene, compared with the corresponding normal colonic mucosa. Four of 8 carcinomas showed a moderately elevated expression (1.5-4-fold), and two carcinomas had a marked elevated expression (more than 9-fold). Thus, the expression of the c-*myc* gene was most elevated in the carcinoma and was moderately elevated in the adenoma (Fig. 1). The c-*myc* gene was amplified about 16-fold in one carcinoma and was not amplified in either the normal colonic mucosa or the adenoma, of the same patient.

On the contrary, the c-*fos* gene transcript in the normal colonic mucosa showed a remarkable decrease in expression in both adenomas and carcinomas. Levels of the c-*fos* transcript in adenomas varied from 4 to 89% and from 4 to 63% in cases of carcinoma, compared with findings in the normal colonic mucosa of the same patients (Fig. 1).

We also examined expression of these genes in cases of NPCC. In 5 patients with NPCC, expression of the c-*myc* gene was elevated in cases of carcinoma compared with findings in the corresponding colonic mucosa, whereas expression of the c-*fos* gene was markedly decreased in cases of carcinoma. These data suggest that there is a common pattern of the expression of c-*myc* and c-*fos* genes, in both hereditary and nonhereditary colon carcinoma.

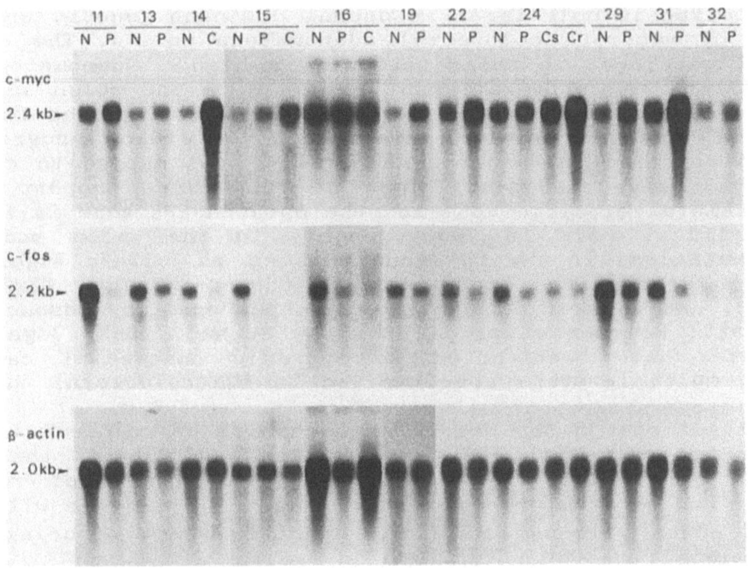

Figure 1. Northern blot analysis of transcripts related to c-*myc* (top), c-*fos* (middle), and β-actin (bottom) genes from colon tissues from patients with FPC. The hybridizations with the β-actin probe were performed as controls of the amount of RNA present and reacting on each lane. N, normal colonic mucosa; P, adenomatous polyp; C, adenocarcinoma; Cs, adenocarcinoma of sigmoid; Cr, adenocarcinoma of rectum (from Sugio et al., 1988).

Table 1. K-*ras* activation in colorectal tumors from FPC patients.

	Mutation*				
codon	nucleotide	amino acid	Adenoma	Carcinoma	Line
12	GGT-GAT	Gly-Asp	3	3	0
	GGT-AGT	Gly-Ser	0	2	0
	GGT-TGT	Gly-Cys	0	1	1
	GGT-GTT	Gly-Val	1	0	0
13	GGC-GAC	Gly-Asp	2	1	0
	Total number of tumors with mutation		6	7	1
	Total number of tumors		51	20	2
	Percent of tumors with mutation		12%	35%	50%

*For each mutation, the nucleotide and amino acid sequence of the codon present in the corresponding proto-oncogene is listed on the left, and the sequence present in the tumor is listed on the right (from Sasaki et al., 1990).

Our observations showed that the expression of c-*myc* gene was most elevated in carcinoma and moderately elevated in adenoma, compared with findings in the corresponding normal colonic mucosa. These results suggest that elevated expression of the c-*myc* gene in the adenoma reflects proliferative activity. Amplification of the c-*myc* gene may be a late event in the carcinogenesis and play an important role in tumor progression. On the other hand, we found that expression of the c-*fos* gene was markedly decreased in all samples of adenoma and carcinoma. Thus, the level of expression of the c-*fos* gene in the normal colonic mucosa may reflect the state of terminal differentiation and the c-*fos* gene might be a prerequsite to stabilize the state of terminal differentiation of colonic epithelial cells.

Mutations in K-*ras* gene

K-*ras* gene mutation in colorectal tumors from patients with FPC was investigated using oligonucleotide probes specific for a mutation at codon 12, 13 or 61 of K-*ras* gene. We examined 22 colorectal carcinomas and 51 colorectal adenomas from 41 FPC patients, and observed mutations at codon 12 and 13 in 8 out of 22 colorectal carcinomas (36%) and 6 out of 51 colorectal adenomas (12%) from these patients. These results are summarized in Table 1.

In case of NPCC, K-*ras* gene mutation was detected in 40% (38 out of 92 cases) (Vogelstein et al., 1988) and in 37% (10 out of 27 cases) (Bos et al., 1987). Our findings are not significantly different with regard to sporadic colorectal tumors, and types of mutations were similar. K-*ras* gene mutation in colorectal carcinomas and may not be the first genetic alteration which occurs during colorectal tumorigenesis.

2. TUMOR SUPPRESSOR GENES

Loss of heterozygosity in colorectal carcinomas

We examined loss of heterozygosity in 49 adenomatous polyps, 21 adenocarcinomas, and 39 normal tissues from 39 patients with FPC. Loss of heterozygosity in colorectal tumors from patients with FPC was observed on 15 different chromosomes (Table 2). In the carcinomas, frequency of loss of heterozygosity ranged from 8% to 40%.

Frequent loss was observed on chromosomes 5 (24%), 14 (20%), 17 (31%), 18 (40%), and 22 (35%). In the adenomas, the loss of heterozygosity was observed on 9 chromosomes and the frequencies were less than 7%. On the other hand, the loss of heterozygosity in carcinomas from patients with NPCC was observed on 8 chromosomes (Table 2), the frequency ranging from 11% to 32%. This loss in colorectal carcinomas from NPCC patients was frequent on chromosomes 5 (32%), 14 (30%), 17 (27%), 18 (20%), and 22 (19%).

The tumor suppressor genes for colorectal carcinogenesis may locate on chromosomes 5, 14, 17, 18, and 22, and alteration of these genes may commonly affect both FPC and NPCC patients. As the FPC gene has been mapped on chromosome 5 (Bodmer et al., 1987; Leppert et al., 1987), it might act as a tumor suppressor gene for colorectal carcinoma (refer to Knudson's hypothesis; Knudson, 1971). D5S71, one of the markers on chromosome 5, was reported to be linked to FPC (Bodmer et al., 1987). We observed that the frequency of the loss of heterozygosity on this locus was extremely high in carcinomas from both FPC and NPCC patients. These results supported the possibility that the FPC gene was tumor suppressor gene.

However, the loss of heterozygosity on chromosome 5 in colorectal carcinoma was not specific event; rather, it was less frequent than on chromosomes 17, 18 and 22. This would suggest that the mechanism of colorectal carcinogenesis in FPC cannot be explained by a one-locus model for the FPC gene and that chromosome 5 is the locating of the tumor suppressor gene.

Table 2. Number of tumors which showed a loss of heterozygosity

	FPC		
Chromosome	Adenoma	Carcinoma	NPCC
1	1/38 (3%)	2/13 (15%)	0/15
2	0/24	1/13 (8%)	0/13
3	0/19	0/8	0/10
4	0/26	0/6	0/5
5	1/42 (2%)	4/17 (24%)	7/22 (32%)
6	1/37 (3%)	2/14 (14%)	2/15 (13%)
7	0/18	0/12	0/11
8	0/23	0/6	1/4 (25%)
9	0/28	1/8 (13%)	0/6
10	0/7	0/3	0/3
11	0/21	1/10 (10%)	0/10
12	1/39 (3%)	3/18 (17%)	2/18 (11%)
13	0/21	0/10	0/11
14	1/38 (3%)	2/10 (20%)	3/10 (30%)
15	0/7	1/3 (33%)	0/8
16	0/25	1/6 (17%)	0/8
17	3/44 (7%)	5/16 (31%)	6/22 (27%)
18	2/31 (7%)	4/10 (40%)	3/15 (20%)
19	0/24	0/5	0/6
20	0/12	1/5 (20%)	0/3
21	1/22 (5%)	1/7 (14%)	0/6
22	1/38 (3%)	6/17 (35%)	4/21 (19%)

The number of cases in which the normal tissue was found to be heterozygous for at least one of the DNA markers for each chromosome is shown as a denominator. The number of informative cases in which the loss of heterozygosity was seen in colorectal tumors is shown as a numerator (from Sasaki et al., 1989).

Mutations in p53 gene
All tumors that showed a loss of heterozygosity on at least one marker on chromosome 17 commonly lost heterozygosity for the D17S5 locus on the short arm of chromosome 17. It was reported that the p53 gene was likely to be the target of deletions of the short arm of chromosome 17 in several tumors containing sporadic colorectal carcinomas (Barker et al., 1989; Nigro et al., 1989; Takahashi et al., 1989). We observed a frequent loss of heterozygosity for the p53 gene in 3 adenomas (14%) and 5 carcinomas (56%) from FPC patients and 3 carcinomas (43%) from NPCC patients. Mutations of the remaining p53 gene were also identified in two adenomas (13bp deletion in one adenoma and a point mutation in the other) and one carcinoma (point mutation) from FPC patients. These results suggest that the inactivation of p53 gene might be involved in the tumorigenesis of FPC.

Tumor suppressive activity of human chromosome 5
To identify the existence of tumor suppressor gene, we introduced by microcell fusion a human chromosome 5 derived from a normal human fibroblast into the colon carcinoma cell line SW620, which has a deletion of long arm of chromosome 5. The human chromosome 5 suppressed the growth rate of SW620.

3. GENETIC EVENTS DURING COLORECTAL TUMOR PROGRESSION IN FPC

Multiple genetic events are believed to be required to achieve the malignant phenotype. To examine these genetic events during colorectal tumor progression, we asked whether such mutations occurred in colorectal tumors in patients with FPC or NPCC. It seems most probable that the mutated FPC gene on chromosome 5q initiates the development of the adenoma. We found that in colonic mucosa tumor-associated antigens, sialylated Le^x and sialylated Le^x-i antigens were expressed to a greater extent in patients with FPC than in non-hereditary sporadic cases (Soejima et al., unpublished). These results suggest that colonic tissues from patients with FPC differ from those from patients with a non-hereditary sporadic form of the disease. We speculate that the normal-appearing mucosa of FPC has already undergone preneoplastic change at areas between the true normal mucosa and adenomas. According to the multistep theory in tumorigenesis, there has to be additional events promoting the transition from a normal mucosa in FPC to adenomas or carcinomas. Here,

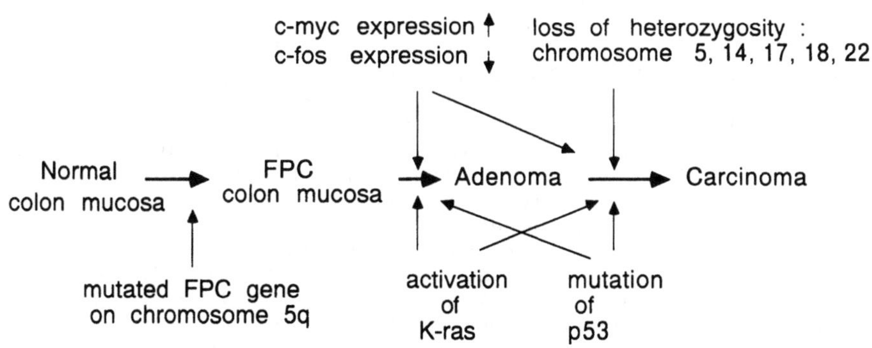

Figure 2. Genetic events during colorectal tumor progression in familial polyposis coli.

point mutations in the *ras* gene, deregulated expression of c-*myc* gene and c-*fos* gene, and mutations of p53 gene are involved. Furthermore, the loss of heterozygosity on chromosomes 5, 14, 17, 18, and 22 and amplification of c-*myc* gene play an important role in the transition from adenomas to colorectal carcinomas.

In conclusion, during the course of colorectal tumorigenesis in FPC patients, several genetic events at DNA and/or chromosomal levels are operative in addition to the mutated FPC gene, including activation of the *ras* and c-*myc* genes, inactivation of the c-*fos* gene and putative tumor suppressor genes on chromosomes 5, 14, 17, 18, and 22.

ACKNOWLEDGMENTS

We thank Professors F. Nakayama, K. Sugimachi, M. Fujishima, and other doctors who provided surgical specimens. We also thank Dr. R. White, Dr. Y. Nakamura, Dr. P.L. Pearson, Dr. W.K. Cavenee, Dr. A.J. Jeffrey, and Dr. A.E. Retief for DNA probes. We are very grateful to Dr. M. Ohara for critical reading of the manuscript.

REFFERENCES

Barker SJ, Fearon ER, Nigro JM, Hamilton SR, Preisinger AC, Jessup JM, vanTuinen P, Ledbetter DH, Barker DF, Nakamura Y, White R, Vogelstein B (1989) Chromosome 17 deletions and p53 gene mutations in colorectal carcinomas. Science 244:217-221.

Bodmer WF, Bailey CJ, Bodmer J, Bussey HJR, Ellis A, Gorman P, Lucibello FC, Murday VA, Rider SH, Scambler P, Sheer D, Solomon E, Spurr NK (1987) Localization of the gene for familial adenomatous polyposis on chromosome 5. Nature 328:614-616.

Bos JL, Fearon ER, Hamilton SR, Verlaan-de Vries M, van Boom JH, van der Eb AJ, Vogelstein B. (1987) Prevalence of ras gene mutations in human colorectal cancers. Nature 327: 293-297.

Erisman MD, Rothberg PG, Diehl RE, Morse CC, Spandorfer JM, Astrin SM (1985) Deregulation of c-*myc* gene expression in human colon carcinoma is not accompanied by amplification or rearrangement of the gene. Mol. Cell. Biol. 5:1969-1974.

Fearon ER, Hamilton SR, Vogelstein B (1987) Clonal analysis of human colorectal carcinomas. Nature 328:616-619.

Law DJ, Olschwang S, Monpezat JP, Lefrancois D, Jagelman D, Petrelli NJ, Thomas G, Feinberg AP (1988) Concerted nonsynthenic allelic loss in human colorectal carcinoma. Science 241: 961-965.

Knudson AG (1971) Mutation and Cancer: statistical study of retinoblastoma. Proc. Natl. Acad. Sci. USA, 68:820-823.

Leppert M, Dobbs M, Scambler P, O'Coneell P, Nakamura Y, Stautfer D, Woodward S, Burt R, Hughes J, Gardner E, Lathrop M, Wasmuth J, Lalouel JM, White R (1987) The gene for familial polyposis coli maps to the long arm of chromosome 5. Science 238:1411-1413.

Nakamura Y, Lathrop M, Leppert M. Dobbs M, Wasmuth J, Wolff E, Carlson M, Fujimoto E, Krapcho K, Sears T, Woodward S, Hughes J, Burt R, Gardner E, Lalouel J, White R (1988) Localization of the genetic defects in familial adenomatous polyposis with a small region of chromosome 5. Am. J. Hum. Genet. 43:638-644.

Nigro JM, Baker SJ, Preeisinger AC, Jessup JM, Hostetter R, Cleary K, Bigner SH, Davidson N, Baylin S, Devilee P, Glover T, Collins FS, Weston A, Modali R, Harris CC, Vogelstein B (1989) Mutations in p53 gene occur in diverse human tumor types. Nature 342:705-708.

Sasaki M, Okamoto M, Sato C, Sugio K, Soejima J, Iwama T, Ikeuchi T, Tonomura A, Miyaki M, Sasazuki T (1989) Loss of constitutional heterozygosity in colorectal tumors from patients with familial polyposis coli and those with nonpolyposis colorectal carcinoma. Cancer Res. 49:4402-4406.

Sasaki M, Sugio K, Sasazuki T (1990) K-*ras* activation in colorectal carcinomas from patients with familial polyposis coli. Cancer in press

Solomon E, Voss R, Hall V, Bodmer WF, Jass JR, Jeffreys AJ, Licibello FC, Patel I, Rider SH (1987) Chromosome 5 allele loss in human colorectal carcinomas. Nature 328:616-619.

Sugio K, Kurata S, Sasaki M, Soejima J, Sasazuki T (1988) Differential expression of c-*myc* gene and c-*fos* gene in premalignant and malignant tissues from patients with familial polyposis coli. Cancer Res. 48:4855-4861.

Takahashi T, Nau MM, Chiba I, Birrer MJ, Rosenberg RK, Vinocour M, Levitt M, Pass H, Gazdar AF, Minna JD (1989) A freqent target for genetic abnormalities in lung cancer. Science 246:491-494.

Vogelstein B, Fearon ER, Hamilton SR, Kern SE, Preisinger AC, Leppert M, Nakamura Y, White R, Smits AMM, Bos JL (1988) Genetic alterations during colorectal tumor development. N. Engl. J. Med. 319:525-532.

Searching the Gene Responsible to Familial Polyposis Coli (FAP)

YUSUKE NAKAMURA, JOHN WASMUTH, and RAY WHITE

Colorectal cancer is one of the common cancers in the world. Interestingly, the incidence of colon cancer in Japan has increased sharply in the last 10 years, probably due to the change in diet as Japan has been westernized. Although this malignancy is curable if a cancer is detected at an early stage, many cancers are still found at an advanced or incurable stage. We do not understand the changes occuring at a molecular genetic level in colon cancers. However, as a result of the recent developments in molecular biology, alterations in DNA or chromosomal changes in colorectal cancer cells have been discovered (1,2).

Colon cancer is of interest in the study of carcinogenesis. Although de novo type of colon cancers have been reported recently, there is no doubt that some of adenomatous polyps found in the colon are precancerous tumors and will develop into cancers if left untreated. Adenomatous polyps in the colon are relatively common in the general population over 40 years old; the frequency is estimated at 10-15%. In the majority of cases, we see one or a few polyps are found, but in some cases (1/10,000-50,000) patients develop hundreds to thousands of adenomatous polyps in their teens or twenties. 50-80% of such cases have a family history in their parents or relatives and follow an autosomal dominant inheritance. This type of hereditary colon polyp syndrome is called Adenomatous Polyposis Coli (APC).

Two forms of APC have been reported. One from (Familial Adenomatous Polyposis = FAP) only shows the development of colon polyps. The other form, which is called Gardner syndrome, shows the development of colon polyps as well as multiple osteomas, severe dental abnormalities, desmoid tumors and/or benign soft tissue tumors. Both FAP and Gardner syndrome also exhibit gastric, duodenal or small intestinal polyps relatively frequently.

The gene responsible for APC was mapped to the long arm of chromosome 5 in 1987 as a result of the tight linkage between the phenotypes (affected or unaffected) in the APC families and the genotypes of the DNA marker D5S71 (pC11P11), which had been mapped to 5q21-22 (3,4).

The mutation at this region is not peculiar to in APC, but has also been observed as a somatic mutation in non-familial colon cancers and in benign adenomas where it is detected using RFLP markers as the loss of one chromosome. This evidence support the idea that the mutation in the APC gene is one of the significant causes of sporadic colon adenoma and cancer. Hence, the isolation of the APC gene is very important for an understanding of the mechanism of transformation of a normal colon mucosal cell into a cancer cell.

Using an approach based on reverse genetic in order to identify the gene responsible for APC, we have developed a high resolution map of the distal long arm of chromosome 5 (5). First, we constructed a cosmid library using DNA isolated from a somatic hybrid cell line (HHW141) which contains two thirds of the long arm of human chromosome 5 as the only human chromosome (6). The cosmid clones which contain human DNA insert were selected by colony hybridization with 32P-labeled total human DNA as a probe.

DNAs from one thousand cosmid clones were isolated and tested for RFLPs with 6 restriction enzymes (MspI, TaqI, RsaI, BglII, PstI, PvuII). Nearly 400 cosmid clones have shown RFLPs with one or more enzymes. 98 clones out of 400 RFLP clones have been mapped between C11P11 and the telomere by linkage analysis using 60 three generations CEPH reference families (822 individuals)(7).

We have chosen 6 cosmid clones (YN5.120, YN5.64, KK5.33, YN5.48, MC5.61, EW5.5) close to D5S71 for further analysis and made a linkage map with these. The result is shown in Fig.1.

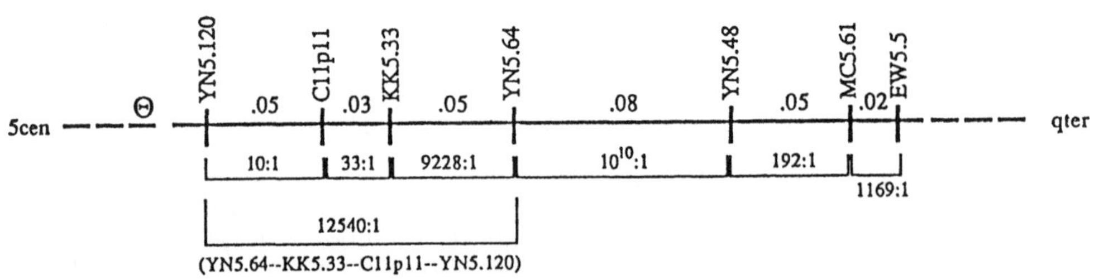

Fig.1
Map of Markers on a short region of chromosome 5. Odds against inversion of adjacent loci are indicated in brackets. Odds are 12,540:1 against reversing the orientation of the subgroup containing the proximal four loci.

This continuous linkage map covers nearly 30CM. The results of linkage analysis using FAP families ed as shown in tables 1 and 2.

Table 1.
Lod-Score Tables of Markers with FAP

	Recombination Fraction								
Locus	.00	.05	.10	.15	.20	.30	.40	0	Zmax
C11p11.......	3.32	2.99	2.64	2.27	1.88	1.10	.37	.00	3.32
YN5.48.......	8.25	7.41	6.55	5.67	4.75	2.83	1.03	.00	8.25
YN5.64.......	-	5.61	5.53	5.13	4.57	3.15	1.45	.06	5.64
YN5.120......	-	1.69	2.00	1.96	1.74	1.08	.04	.11	2.01
MC5.61.......	-	8.03	7.59	6.83	5.91	3.79	1.55	.04	8.05
KK5.33.......	-	7.66	7.69	7.16	6.36	4.26	1.84	.07	7.80
EW5.5........	-	1.92	2.27	2.21	1.98	1.25	.47	.11	2.28

Note. -A dash(-)= significantly negative.

Table 2
Lod Scores in Families Informative for Locus YN5.48

Family	Recombination Fraction .00	.05	.10	.15
FPC:				
415..................	.54	.50	.46	.42
1452.................	1.29	1.14	.97	.81
1441.................	1.67	1.48	1.31	1.14
Total................	3.50	3.12	2.74	2.37
GS:				
1498.................	1.11	1.00	.98	.77
1507.................	.90	.81	.72	.62
109..................	2.74	2.47	2.20	1.92
Total................	4.75	4.28	3.81	3.31
Combined total......	8.25	7.40	6.55	5.68

From these results, two important conclusions can be reached. The first is that there is no genetic heterogeneity between simple FAP and GS; the difference between phenotypes is probably due to a different of mutation in the gene causing these byndromes, like that between the Duchenne type and Becker type of muscular dystrophies. Alternatively GS patients may have larger deletions or rearrangements which involve more than one gene. The second is that the APC gene is 10-15CM distal to D5S74 (pC11P11), the marker which first showed linkage to APC, although the linkage data reported from two groups showed no recombination with D5S74.

For the fine localization of the APC gene, we have constructed a cosmid library from a somatic hybrid cell line 1021 which contains ~30CM of human chromosome5 and which was derived from HHW141. Cosmid clones which contain human DNA were isolated as described above. These cosmid clones were characterized by linkage analysis or by mapping using somatic hybrid cell lines. 40 clones selected as mapping within a deletion in one of the cell lines have been further characterized by pulsed-field gel analysis. The sizes of bands from digestion with 8 enzymes (Not I, Sfi I, Sac II, Sal I, Mlu I, Nru I, BssH II, Cla I) and which hybridise to the selected clones have been determined. Identity of bands has been confirmed by using the same blots repeatedly. The results obtained is shown in table 3.

Linkage analysis has also been done with some clones which have show RFLPs. L5.62 is the most proximal probe which detected a recombinant and KK5.97 is the most distal probe which detected a recombinant. The cosmid clones between KK5.97 and L5.62 have not shown any recombinants and have a lod score of between 2.5-12.4. By multipoint analysis, the possibility that the APC gene is between L5.62 and KK5.97 is more than 10 times higher than it being located outside of L5.62 or KK5.97.

We have constructed a 5,000kb of the physical map of the region which contains the gene responsible for APC and are now looking for a specific mutation in the APC patients.

Table 3
The sizes of fragments obtained by pulsed-field gel electrophoresis. (kb)

	ClaI	NotI	SfiI	SacII	BssHII	NruI	MluI	SalI
L5.62	240		690	1500	1500	>2000	640	480
15A6	640		750	440	440	>1500	>2000	470
L5.71	360	1500	430	640	450	1500	830	410
N5.46	360	1500	430	640	450	1500	830	410
L5.79	360	1500	430	640	450	1500	830	410
EF5.44	120	<100	290	780	760	550	830	470
E5.50				810	810	1500		
L5.69	300	1000	470		810	1500		
YN5.48	270	1000	470		810	1500	>2000	660
LS5.3	190	270	470	370	540		280	420
KK5.97	200	520	370	200	550	360	420	

References:

1. B.Vogelstein,E.Fearon,S.Kern,S.Hamilton,A.Preisinger, Y.Nakamura,R.White. 1989. Allelotype of colorectal carcinomas. Science 244:207-211.
2. S.Baker,E.Fearon,J.Nigro,S.Hamilton,A.Preisinger,J.Jessup, P.vanTuinen,D.Ledbetter,D.Barker,Y.Nakamura,R.White,B.Vogelstein. 1989. Chromosome 17 deletions and p53 gene mutations in colorectal carcinomas. Science 244:217-221.
3. M.Leppert,M.Dobbs,P.Scambler,P.O'Connell,Y.Nakamura, D.Stauffer,S.Woodward,R.Burt,J.Hughes,R.White.1987. The gene for familial polyposis coli maps to the long arm of chromosome 5. Science 238:1411-1413.
4. W.Bodmer,C.Bailey,J.Bodmer,H.Bussey,A.Ellis,P.Gorman, F.Lucibell,V.Murday,S.Rider,P.Scambler,D.Sheer,E.Solomon, N.Spurr.1987. Localization of the gene for familial adenomatous poluposis on chromosome5. Nature 328:614-616.
5. Y.Nakamura,M.Lathrop,M.Leppert,M.Dobbs,J.Wasmuth,E.Wolff, M.Carlson,E.Fujimoto,K.Krapcho,T.Sears,S.Woodward,J.Hughes,R.B urt,E.GardnerJ.Lalouel,R.White. 1988. Localization of the genetic defect in familial adenomatous polyposis within a small region of chromosome 5. Am.J.Hum.Genet. 43:638-644.
6. R.Cirullo,S.Dana,J.Wasmuth.1983. Efficient procedure for transferring specific human genes into Chinese hamster cell mutants:interspecific transfer of the human genes encoding leucyl-and asparaginyl-tRNA synthetases. Mol.Cell.Biol. 3:892-902.

Chapter 7

Cytomolecular Aspects of Colorectal Cancer

Summary of Chapter 7: Cytomolecular Aspects of Colorectal Cancer

YUSUKE NAKAMURA and RAYMOND L. WHITE

In session C3, many interesting observations in familial and no-familial colon cancers have been reported.

First, Dr. Agnantis presented the immunohistochemical in colon. The ras oncogene product p21 and c-myc oncogene product p21 and c-myc oncogene product p62 were analyzed by monoclonal antibodies. Increased expression of these proteins have been shown in both adenomas and carcinomas and the amount of oncogene products have been associated with the grade of pathological malignancy.

Dr. Boman reported the overexpression of the retinoblastoma (Rb) gene in colorectal carcinomas. Although no loss of heterozygosity of chromosome 13 has been detected, 75% of colorectal carcinomas expressed 2-5 fold of 4.7kb normal size of Rb mRNA and 25% of them expressed at the normal level and none of them decreased the expression of the Rb gene.

This overexpression of the Rb gene is very interesting and these may reflect the gain of additional chromosome 13 in carcinomas or may be due to the loss of supressor oncogenes located on the other chromosome. The role or significance of this overexpression during tumorgenesis is not yet known.

Dr. Paraskeva reported the karyotype analysis of epithelial cell lines from both hereditary (FPC) and sporadic colorectal adenomas. By extensive analysis, he suggested the significance of loss of the short arm of chromosome 1 in in vitro immortalization.

His group is now attempting a study of the adenoma carcinoma sequence in vitro by using established cell lines.

Dr. Hamilton reported the difference of molecular genetic alterations betweem left-sided carcinomas and right-sided carcinomas. Deletion of 17p was more common in left-sided carcinomas (93%) than right-sided carcinomas (60%) with p-value of 0.04.

17p and 18p loss were more common in non-mucin producing carcinomas than much producing carcinomas.

Furthermore, the deletion of 17p has seen common in carcinomas with patients who have family history.

He has also suggested the possibility of the usefulness of 17p and 18p deletions or fractional allelic loss (FAL), which is defined as the number of chromosomal arms lost divided by the number of evaluable chromosomal arms, for prognosis or metastasic potentiality tumors.

Dr. Thomas presented the loss of heterozygosity of chromosome 5 (39%), 17 (63%) and 18 (62%) in colorectal carcinomas. He also reported the difference between left-sided and right-sided carcinomas. DNA content of right-sided carcinoma was equal to that of normal cells but DNA content of left-sided

carcinoma was increased to nearly 2 fold of that of normal cells.
The majority of colorectal tumors which has no loss of chromosome 5, 17 or 18 were located at the proximal side of colon.

Dr. Hamilton's and Dr. Thomas's papers suggested that carcinogenesis of right-sided and left-sided colon might be different.

The second session of Workshop C3 developed the themes of tumor cytogenetics and cell culture. Dr. Suresh Jhanwer reported his examination of a series of 57 tumors with both cytogenetic and RFLP analysis. He found that there was significant information to be obtained from cytogenetic analysis in addition to the RFLP analysis. He found that, in addition to the expected anomalies of chromosomes 5, 17 and 18, the cytogenetic analysis revealed trisomies of two chromosomes, 1 and 7, that were not revealed by RFLPs. Cell cultures were initiated from 15 tumors, forming a stable resource for further characterization.

Dr.Ikeuchi reviewed his examination of the cytogenetics of both adenomas and carcinomas from FAP patients. This work is especially important to test the hypothesis that carcinomas in FAP 5 carcinomas revealed the same losses of chromosome 17 and 18 genetic etiology. In addition, examination of 17 adenomas revealed a high frequency of increased numbers of chromosome 7 (trisomies) and 13 (tri-pentasomies). The chromosome 7 finding supports the previous report and the chromosome 13 finding extends the report earlier in the workshop by Boman of enhanced activity of the Rb gene.

Dr. Boman reported the characterization of a carcinoma cell line developed from a Gardner patient. The cell line has been characterized with respect to a number of biological and cytogenetic parameters, but the most striking finding was the production of TGF-alpha and a high level of EGF-receptor activity. The high level of EGF-receptor could be traced to amplification of the gene in double minute chromosomes. The finding supports the hypothesis of an autocrine growth simulation for this tumor cell line.

Dr. Macrae described his cytogenetic findings from a colon cancer cell line derived from a patient with HNPCC. The findings were somewhat surprising in that the karyotype was almost normal diploid, the only exception being a translocation of the distal segment of a chromosome 1 to 13p. The origin of the translocated bit in chromosome 1 was confirmed by in situ hybridization with a chromosome 1 DNA probe.

Dr. Friedman reported her studies on a comparison of growth stimulation in primary cultures of adenoma cells versus cultures of normal colonocytes. Her initial finding was that the tumor promoter TPA significantly increased the percentage of cycling cells in the adenoma cells, but not colonocytes. She reasoned that perhaps the TPA might be acting at the same stage as diacylglycerol and if so, there might be an adequate level of diglycerides in fecal material to provide growth stimulation to adenomas in vivo. She and her collaborators were able to establish that the concentration of fecal diglycerides was adequately high to serve as a growth promoter of adenoma cells. Furthermore, in her serum free primary culture cells she was able to directly demonstrate a growth stimulatory effect of DAG comparable in magnitude to that obtained with TPA.

It seems quite clear that cytogenetics and cell culture will continue to have important roles in the study of the fundamental mechanisms of colon carcinogenesis.

Genetic Alterations in Colorectal Tumors

KATHLEEN R. CHO and BERT VOGELSTEIN

ABSTRACT:

Tumors of the colorectum provide an excellent system in which to study the genetic alterations responsible for tumorigenesis. Molecular genetic studies have revealed several such alterations, including DNA hypomethylation, ras gene mutation, and allelic loss and/or mutation of specific chromosomal regions (5q, 17p, and 18q) presumed to harbor tumor suppressor genes. The accumulation of these genetic lesions accompanies, and is likely to be responsible for, tumor initiation and progression.

Keywords: Tumor suppressor genes, allelic loss, genetic alterations, p53, RAS.

The notion that genetic damage might be responsible for cancer is not new; hereditary predispositions to cancer, cancer family syndromes, damaged chromosomes in cancer cells, and DNA damage mediated by chemical carcinogens have long been recognized. As the mechanisms underlying tumorigenesis are revealed, it is becoming clear that these genetic alterations are manifold, including amplification, point mutation, rearrangement and deletion of particular genes. Epithelial tumors of the colorectum provide an excellent system in which to study such genetic alterations and the manner in which they affect tumor progression.

It is widely accepted that colorectal tumors progress through a series of easily recognizable clinicopathologic stages. Tumorigenesis may be preceded by widespread hyperproliferation of colonic epithelial cells which can be detected by in situ DNA labelling techniques (Lipkin 1988). One or a few of these hyperproliferating cells may then undergo clonal expansion (Fearon et al. 1987) to form a small benign neoplasm known as a tubular adenoma. Usually pedunculated, these tumors are more commonly known as polyps. Progression of the adenoma is marked by gradual increase in tumor size, acquisition of cytologic atypia, and development of a villous or fingerlike growth pattern and a sessile base. Once an adenoma cell develops the capacity to overgrow its sister cells and invade the basement membrane, the tumor is by definition, a carcinoma. Unlike many other types of human solid tumors, colon carcinomas are often histologically recognized in a clinical lesion containing an adenoma, its benign precursor. Progression of the carcinoma is manifest by the capacity for metastasis to regional lymph nodes and distant sites such as the liver or lungs. The progression is gradual and usually slow, taking decades for culmination.

Several genetic changes accompany this tumor progression and may at least in part, be responsible for it. Some of these alterations may be present in the germline, while others are acquired somatically. One of the earliest recognizable changes in colorectal tumorigenesis is a significant loss of methyl groups in DNA (Goelz et al. 1985). Using restriction endonuclease analysis, substantial hypomethylation was found in both adenomas and carcinomas when compared to normal mucosa. The role of this hypomethylation in tumorigenesis is unclear, but we have postulated that hypomethylated DNA may inhibit chromosome condensation during mitosis and that these undercondensed regions may stick to one another during anaphase, leading to aneuploidy. Mitotic chromosomal abnormalities have been shown to result from areas of chromosome decondensation created by experimentally induced hypomethylation (Schmid et al. 1983).

RAS gene mutations as detected by hybridization to oligonucleotide probes are present in approximately 50% of colorectal carcinomas (Bos et al. 1987, Forrester et al. 1987) and in a similar percentage of intermediate and late stage adenomas (Vogelstein et al. 1988). The great majority of these mutations are in the K-RAS gene. In several of the tumors studied, the same mutation was found in both the adenomatous and carcinomatous portions of the same clinical lesion, suggesting that the mutation preceded the emergence of the malignant phenotype. In contrast, RAS gene mutations are present in less than 10% of small (<1 cm) adenomas. There are at least two possible explanations for these findings. RAS gene mutations may be the initiating event in a subset of colorectal tumors, and adenomas with these mutations may be more likely to progress than adenomas without them. Alternatively, RAS gene mutations may be responsible, in part, for conversion of a small adenoma to a larger, more dysplastic one. While the full effects of mutated RAS genes are not yet known, mutated RAS genes have been shown to transform immortalized cell lines and to cooperate with other oncogenes to transform primary cells in culture (Land et al. 1983, Ruley 1983, Newbold and Overrell 1983). Some of the same RAS mutations have been identified in the RAS genes of RNA tumor viruses and in the cellular RAS homologues of animal tumors induced by carcinogens (Land et al. 1983, Barbacid 1986). It is interesting that RAS gene mutations occur at very similar frequencies in the colorectal tumors of patients with and without familial adenomatous polyposis. This suggests that some of the molecular genetic events responsible for tumor progression are identical in both groups of patients.

Allelic loss of specific chromosomal regions, presumably harboring tumor suppressor genes, are yet another type of genetic alteration identified in colorectal neoplasia. Using polymorphic DNA probes, the extent and nature of allelic loss events were evaluated in 56 pairs of colorectal carcinomas and adjacent normal mucosa (Vogelstein et al. 1989). Termed "allelotyping," this analysis showed that allelic deletions were extremely common and that eight chromosomal regions were each affected in more than 25% of the carcinomas studied. A median of four to six allelic losses were observed in individual carcinomas. Some of these losses may be "passengers," that is, they may have coincidentally occurred in the same mitosis as another genetic alteration which provided a selective growth advantage. However, we believe it is likely that many of these changes reflect the presence of suppressor genes in the deleted regions. Since each allelic loss is presumably accompanied by mutation of the residual suppressor gene allele, these data suggest that a large number of independent genetic alterations (8-12) are commonly associated with colorectal tumorigenesis. Although this number seems large in comparison to the few that are required to transform rodent fibroblasts in vitro, it should be noted that carcinomas have acquired many properties in addition to those associated with in vitro transformation (for example, the ability to invade surrounding tissues and to metastasize to different sites). The large number of genetic alterations required for cancer formation is also emphasized by the study of colonic adenomas. We have observed large adenomas, which by definition have not acquired the ability to invade or metastasize, yet have already each suffered allelic loss of chromosomes 5,17, and 18, and a RAS gene mutation. Thus, these genetic alterations alone are clearly insufficient for cancer formation.

Allelic deletions on chromosome 5q have been noted in nearly 40% of carcinomas studied (Solomon et al. 1987, Vogelstein et al. 1988). The gene responsible for familial adenomatous polyposis (FAP) has been mapped to this region (Bodmer et al. 1987, Leppert et al. 1987). Further studies have shown that while allelic deletions of 5q were identified in 36% of sporadically acquired intermediate and late stage adenomas, they were absent from early stage adenomas from FAP patients (Vogelstein et al. 1988). Knudson has proposed a model of tumorigenesis in which defective genes involved in inherited neoplastic syndromes such as FAP, normally function as tumor suppressor genes (Knudson 1985). At the cellular level, these genes function in a recessive manner, such that both alleles must be inactivated to allow tumor growth. The recent cloning and characterization of the retinoblastoma (RB) gene provide support for Knudson's hypothesis (Friend et al. 1986, Dunn et al. 1988). If the FAP gene is also a tumor suppressor gene and the target of the 5q allelic loss events, how then might the absence of 5q allelic deletions in FAP adenomas be explained? We have hypothesized that the FAP gene product normally functions to control epithelial proliferation. If one allele is inactivated by mutation, the resultant decrease in gene expression could lead to inefficient control of cellular proliferation even in the presence of a functional wild-type allele. This could lead to the hyperproliferative state previously noted to characterize the epithelium of FAP patients (Lipkin 1988). Such mutations could be inherited in the germline or acquired somatically. There must then be a second event which promotes the transition from hyperproliferative epithelium to an actual neoplasm (the adenoma), and this event does not appear to be loss of the wild type allele. Candidates for such second events include mutational activation of RAS oncogenes, DNA hypomethylation, or the inactivation of suppressor genes on other chromosomes. Inactivation of wild type FAP genes could lead to further tumor progression, but would not be required for initial adenoma formation.

Deletions on the short arm of chromosome 17 are very common, occurring in over 75% of colorectal carcinomas. While RAS gene mutations, DNA hypomethylation, and 5q alterations appear to occur early in colorectal tumorigenesis, 17p deletions appear to be relatively late events associated with the transition from the benign adenoma to malignant carcinoma. Using 20 polymorphic chromosome 17p markers, the common region of deletion in the carcinomas was localized to a region centered at 17p13 (Baker et al. 1989). The gene encoding the transformation associated protein p53 is contained within this region (van Tuinen et al. 1987). p53 was originally considered to be an oncogene, based on its ability to immortalize primary rodent cells and cooperate with RAS for transformation (Jenkins et al. 1984, Eliyahu et al. 1984, Parada et al. 1984, Rovinski and Benchimol 1988). Recent evidence has shown, however, that the p53 derivatives used in these experiments were mutants, and that normal p53 may function as a tumor suppressor gene rather than an oncogene (Finlay et al. 1989, Eliyahu et al. 1989). Southern and Northern blot analysis provided no evidence for gross alterations of the p53 gene or of its surrounding sequences in over 80 colorectal tumors studied. Although such Southern and Northern blot analyses suggested that p53 might not be the "target" of the allelic loss events, we felt that it was important to more rigorously test this possibility before discarding it. We thus examined in detail the p53 coding region of two colon carcinomas. Both tumors had sustained loss of one p53 allele and expressed considerable p53 message from the remaining allele. Mutations in highly conserved regions of the p53 gene were found in both tumors (Baker et al. 1989). Further studies have found p53 gene mutations in each of 10 additional colon carcinomas which had sustained 17p allelic deletion (Nigro et al. unpublished data). Furthermore, in a carcinoma which had retained two parental 17p alleles, we found that one allele contained a point mutation, and that both the wild type and mutant alleles were expressed at equal levels. Such findings have led us to speculate that a mutated p53 gene in colorectal carcinomas can provide a selective growth advantage promoting tumor progression even in the presence of a normal p53 allele. Deletion of the remaining allele amplifies the growth advantage and leads to further progression, often manifest as the transition from the benign to the malignant state. p53 alterations may play a role in several other human solid tumors exhibiting high frequency of 17p allelic loss. p53 mutations have already been identified in several gliomas, a neurofibrosarcoma, and in breast, bladder, and lung carcinomas (Nigro et al. unpublished data). Thus, p53 gene mutations appear to play a prominent role in the development of many, if not most, common human malignancies.

Allelic loss events on chromosome 18q are also extremely common, occurring in approximately 75% of colorectal carcinomas. Deletions are also seen in 47% of large adenomas, but in less than 10% of small and intermediate stage adenomas, suggesting that 18q loss events occur relatively late in colorectal tumor progression. We have recently sought to identify the "target" gene of the 18q deletions, as summarized below.

Previous studies have localized the common region of deletion to 18q21-qter (Vogelstein et al. 1988). Genes which have been mapped to this region include the BCL-2 gene (Tsujimoto et al. 1984), the gastrin releasing peptide gene (Spindel et al. 1984), and the cellular homologue of the YES-1 oncogene (Semba et al. 1985). Southern blot analyses demonstrated no gross alterations of these genes in DNA samples from several colorectal carcinomas.

A chromosomal walking strategy was used to identify another gene in this region, termed DCC, for deleted in colorectal carcinomas. To date, approximately 3 kb of contiguous cDNA from this locus has been cloned and sequenced, including a putative translation start site and sequence encoding over 750 amino acids. Using polymerase chain reaction techniques we have been able to detect expression of the DCC gene in normal brain and colon tissue. Fifteen of seventeen colon cancer cell lines showed absent or negligible expression. Using this cDNA as a probe on Southern blots, we have detected somatic alterations of the gene in five primary colorectal tumors, two colon carcinoma xenografts, and five colon carcinoma cell lines. These alterations include one tumor with homozygous loss of both alleles, one tumor with a point mutation creating a potential new splice acceptor site, and several tumors with insertions within a 170bp XbaI-Eco0109 intron fragment just distal to an exon. Further characterization of these mutations and how they might affect gene transcription are currently in progress.

In studying the genetic alterations occurring in colorectal tumorigenesis, several pertinent points have become evident. First, it appears that the accumulation rather than the order of genetic changes is most important. While DNA hypomethylation, RAS gene mutation and 5q allelic loss tend to occur relatively early in tumor progression, and 17p/18q loss relatively late, the sequence of events is by no means absolute. For example, 17p allelic deletions are occasionally seen in very small adenomas, and from amongst several cases where it was possible to examine different stages of neoplasia in the same tumor specimen, there were cases in which 17p deletion preceded 18q loss and 18q deletion preceded RAS gene mutation. Second, genetic alterations probably continue to accumulate once carcinomas have developed and this accumulation may parallel clinical progression. As noted above, most colonic carcinomas contain 4-6 identifiable genetic alterations. Patients with tumors having more than the median percentage of allelic loss have been shown to have a considerably worse prognosis than patients with fewer loss events despite comparable size and stage of the primary tumors (Kern et al. 1989). Thus "allelotyping" tumors may provide a molecular adjunct with which to improve prediction of prognosis in patients with colorectal carcinoma. This multiplicity of genetic changes must be considered in any model of the genetic origin of human neoplasia and should prompt caution in overinterpreting the significance of any single alteration. Third, colorectal carcinogenesis is a complex process in molecular terms. Although 5q, 17p, and 18q deletions occur most often, deletions of other chromosomes do occur frequently in the same tumors with 5,17, and 18 loss. These regions may contain tumor suppressor genes in addition to the ones which we have studied. The complexity of genetic changes in human neoplasia is quite likely reflected in the biologic heterogeneity of these tumors.

In summary, the findings suggest a model of colorectal tumorigenesis in which mutational activation of a dominantly acting oncogene acts in concert with alteration of several tumor suppressor genes to bring about tumor progression. Further studies should provide a more complete understanding of the molecular pathogenesis of this common human disease.

ACKNOWLEDGEMENTS

The authors acknowledge our many colleagues at Johns Hopkins, the University of Utah and the University of Leiden, who have been instrumental in the studies described above. Our work was supported by the Clayton Fund, the McAshan Fund, The Stetler Fund, and National Institutes of Health grant CA 35494.

REFERENCES

Baker S, Fearon E, Nigro J, Hamilton S, Preisinger A, Jessup J, vanTuinen P, Ledbetter D, Barker D, Nakamura Y, White R, Vogelstein B (1989) chromosome 17 deletions and p53 gene mutations in colorectal carcinomas. Science 244:217-221

Barbacid M (1986) Mutations, oncogenes and cancer. Trends Genet 2:188-192

Bodmer W, Bailey C, Bodmer J, Bussey H, Ellis A, Gorman P, Lucibello F, Murday V, Rider S, Scambler P, Sheer D, Solomon E, Spurr N (1987) Localization of the gene for familial adenomatous polyposis on chromosome 5. Nature 328:614-619

Bos J, Fearon E, Hamilton S, Verlaan-de Vries M, van Boom J, van der Eb A, Vogelstein B (1987) Prevalence of ras gene mutations in human colorectal cancers. Nature 327:293-297

Dunn J, Phillips R, Becker A, Gallie B (1988) Identification of germline and somatic mutations affecting the retinoblastoma gene. Science 241:1797-1800

Eliyahu D, Raz a, Gruss P, Givol D, Oren M (1984) Participation of p53 cellular tumour antigen in transformation of normal embryonic cells. Nature 312:646-649

Eliyahu D et al. (1989) PNAS (in press)

Fearon E, Hamilton S, Vogelstein B (1987) Clonal analysis of human colorectal tumors. Science 238:193-197.

Finlay C, Hinds P, Levine A (1989) The p53 proto-oncogene can act as a suppressor of transformation. Cell 57:1083-1093

Forrester K, Almoguera C, Han K, Grizzle W, Perucho M (1987) Detection of high incidence of K-ras oncogenes during human colon tumorigenesis. Nature 327:298-303

Friend S, Bernards R, Rogelj S, Weinberg R, Rapaport J, Albert D, Dryja T (1986) A human DNA segment with porperties of the gene that predisposes to retinoblastoma and osteosarcoma. Nature 323:643-646

Goelz S, Vogelstein B, Hamilton S, Feinberg A (1985) Hypomethylation of DNA from benign and malignant human colon neoplasms. Science 228:187-190

Jenkins J, Rudge K, Currie G (1984) Cellular immortalization by a cDNA clone encoding the transformation-associated phosphoprotein p53. Nature 312:651-654

Kern S, Fearon E, Tersmett W, Enterline J, Leppert M, Nakamura Y, White R, Vogelstein B, Hamilton S (1989) Allelic loss in colorectal carcinoma. JAMA 261:3099-3103

Knudson A (1985) Hereditary cancer, oncogenes and antioncogenes. Cancer Res 45:1437-1443

Land H, Parada L, Weinberg R (1983) Tumorigenic conversion of primary embryo fibroblasts requires at least two cooperating oncogenes. Nature 304:596-601

Land H, Parada L, Weinberg R (1983) Cellular oncogenes and multistep carcinogenesis. Science 222:771-778

Leppert M, Dobbs M, Scambler P, O'Connell P, Nakamura Y, Stauffer D, Woodward S, Burt R, Hughes J, Gardner E, Lathrop M, Wasmuth J, Lalouel J-M, White R (1987) The gene for familial polyposis coli maps to the long arm of chromosome 5. Science 238:1411-1413

Lipkin M (1988) Biomarkers of increased susceptibility to gastrointestinal cancer: New application to studies of cancer prevention in human subjects (1988) Cancer Res 48:235-245

Newbold R, Overell R (1983) Fibroblast immortality is a prerequisite for transformation by EJ c-Ha-ras oncogene. Nature 304:648-651

Nigro J, Baker S, Preisinger A, Jessup J, Hostetter R, Bigner S, Davidson N, Baylin S, Fearon E, Devilee P, Glover T, Collins F, Westin A, Harris C, Vogelstein, B (1989) p53 gene mutations occur in diverse human tumor types. Submitted for publication

Parada L, Land H, Weinberg R, Wolf D, Rotter V (1984) Cooperation between gene encoding p53 tumour antigen and ras in cellular transformation. Nature 312:649-651

Rovinski B, Benchimol S (1988) Immortalization of rat embryo fibroblasts by the cellular p53 oncogene. Oncogene 2:445-452

Ruley H (1983) Adenovirus early region 1A enables viral and cellular transforming genes to transform primary cells in culture. Nature 304:602-606

Schmid M, Grunert D, Haaf T, Engel W (1983) A direct demonstration of somatically paired heterochromatin of human chromosomes. Cytogenet Cell Genet 36:554-561

Semba K, Yamanashi Y, Hishizawa M, Sukegawa J, Yoshida M, Sasaki M, Yamamoto T, Toyoshima K (1984) Locations of the c-yes gene on the human chromosome and its expression in various tissues. Science 227:1038-1040

Solomon E, Voss R, Hall V, Bodmer, W, Jeffreys, A, Lucibello, F, Patel, I, Rider, (1987) Chromosome 5 allele loss in human colorectal carcinomas. Nature 328:616-619

Spindel E, Chin W, Price J, Rees L, Besser G, Habener J (1984) Cloning and characterization of cDNAs encoding human gastrin-releasing peptide. PNAS 81:5699-5703

Tsujimoto Y, Finger L, Yunis J, Nowell P, Croce C (1984) Cloning of the chromosome breakpoint of neoplastic B cells with the t(14;18) chromosome translocation. Science 226:1097-1099

Van Tuinen P, Rich D, Summers K, Ledbetter D (1987) Regional mapping panel for human chromosome 17: application to neurofibromatosis type I. Genomics 1:374-381

Vogelstein B, Fearon E, Hamilton S, Kern S, Preisinger A, Leppert M, Nakamura Y, White R, Smits A, Bos J (1988) Genetic alterations during colorectal tumor development. NEJM 319:525-532

Vogelstein B, Fearon E, Kern S, Hamilton S, Preisinger A, Nakamura Y, White R (1989) Allelotype of colorectal carcinomas. Science 244:207-211

Ras and c-*myc* Oncoprotein Expression in Human Colorectal Tumors

NIKI J. AGNANTIS and DEMETRIOS A. SPANDIDOS

ABSTRACT

We review our results on the use of monoclonal antibodies (M. Abs) Y13 259 and MYC1 9E10 to the ras p21 and c-myc p62 oncoproteins respectively in human tumors and tumor-like conditions of the colorectum. A total of 78 tissue sections were analysed immunohistochemically and comprised the following: 42 adenocarcinomas with 8 normal mucosae neighbouring the tumor, 25 adenomas (with or without dysplasia and with in situ carcinoma) and 3 hyperplastic polyps. The main conclusions were the following: 1. All but one adenocarcinomas expressed both ras and myc oncoproteins at high levels. 2. All adenomas showed higher expression for the ras p21 when compared with the respective sections of c-myc p62. 3. All normal intestinal mucosae and the 3 benign hyperplastic polyps were negative.

Key-words: ras, c-myc, oncoproteins, human colorectal tumors.

INTRODUCTION

It is well known that the survival of large bowel cancer patients has not changed the last 30 years, in spite of the use of the fiberoptic colonoscope and the current advances in surgical manipulations. In most of the Pathology Departments different immunohistochemical tumor markers are examined for the differential diagnosis of problematic cases. The use of monoclonal antibodies against oncogene products makes feasible the study of these genes from the action of their proteins. Using molecular hybridization (Spandidos and Kerr 1984; Spandidos and Agnantis 1984; Field and Spandidos 1987) and immunohistochemical analysis (Williams et.al. 1985; Agnantis et.al. 1986a; Agnantis et.al. 1986b; Spandidos et.al.,1987; Agnantis et.al. 1988; Agnantis et.al. 1989) we have studied the expression of the ras and myc oncoproteins in a variety of humans tumors. We have employed the M.Ab. Y13 259 to the ras p21 (Furth et.al. 1982) and the M.Ab. MYC1 9E10 to the c-myc p62 (Evan et.al. 1985) oncoproteins. We found that these oncoproteins are expressed mainly in epithelial cells which have benign hyperplastic, borderline or malignant phenotype. The normal epithelial component rarely shows a very low or mild expresion of ras and myc proteins (Agnantis et. al. 1986a, Spandidos et. al. 1987; Agnantis et. al. 1988). Nevertheless, one should always take into consideration the effects after formalin fixation and paraffin embedding for the evaluation of the subcellular distribution of the two oncoproteins (Stewart et. al. 1986, Going et. al. 1988; Loke et.al. 1988).

In the present study we review our results on the expression of ras and myc oncoproteins in lesions of the human large bowel (Agnantis et. al. in preparation).

MATERIAL AND METHODS

Seventy eight tissue sections were analysed for the ras p21 using the M. Ab. Y13 259. Another 78 parallel sections were additionally studied for the c-myc p62. The expression of ras and myc oncoproteins was compared. Each group of sections comprised the following: 42 adenocarcinomas (with 8 normal mucosae neighbouring the tumor) 25 adenomas (associated or not with dysplasia or with coexistent in situ Ca) and 3 benign hyperplastic polyps.

The immunohistochemical technique used was streptavidin-biotin peroxidase as previously described (Agnantis et. al. 1986a, Spandidos et. al. 1987). The M.Ab. Y13 259 was generated by Furth et. al. (1982). It is a rat derived monoclonal and reacts with both the mutated and the unaltered forms of ras p21 of the human, rat and mouse. As controls for the ras p21 were used two Chinese Hamster Lung (CHL) cell lines. The negative control was the early passage CHL cells and the positive the same cells transformed with the human T24 bladder carcinoma Harvey-ras1 oncogene (Spandidos and Wilkie, 1984).

The M. Ab. MYC1 9E10 has been previously described by Evan et. al. (1985). The ability of the M.Ab. MYC1 9E10 to detect the c-myc oncoprotein was confirmed with the following controls: The negative control with human embryo fibroblasts and the positive control with human HL60 promyelocytic leukemic cell line which overexpresses the c-myc gene (Spandidos et. al. 1987).

The staining intensity of the positive control was used as an indicator for the strong expression of both oncoproteins and corresponded with +++. Consequently the moderate expression was indicated with ++ and the mild one with +. The negative staining agreed with the negative control and was labeled with -/+.

All slides were reviewed and scored in blind faschion by two experienced Pathologists. The method applied to evaluate the results has been described previously (Efremidis et. al. 1989).

RESULTS

After reviewing the results, of 156 tissue sections from human large bowel lesions, we made the following observations:

1. All but one adenocarcinomas expressed both ras and myc oncoproteins, most of them being strongly positive.
2. All adenomas (either tubular, tubulovillous or villous) showed elevated expression of both oncoproteins, but the ras p21 was expressed at higher levels. An interesting point was that the degree of staining intensity was increased according to the

degree of dysplasia and/or the presence of in situ carcinoma.
3. All normal intestinal mucosae neibouring the primary tumor and the 3 benign hyperplastic polyps didn't show any reactivity with both ras and myc monoclonals.

DISCUSSION

Up to now a variety of tumor markers has been assesed with the hope to contribute in the prevention, early diagnosis and postoperative follow-up of colon cancer patients. Unfortunately none of them proved to be beneficial in practice. Most recently analysis of oncogenes and their products hold a promise that they may be useful as prognostic indicators of cancer. Amplification of several oncogenes (such as H-ras, K-ras, c-myc, N-myc, c-erbB and c-myb) have been reported in a variety of human tumors ana cancer cell lines (Yokota et. al., 1986). On the other hand the immunohistochemical analysis of oncoprotein expression at the cellular level may provide new tools in the field of tumor markers.

The role of ras p21 in normal tissues remains unclear. Several reports suggest that the degree of differentiation plays an important role in the expression of these proteins in non growing cells (Furth et. al. 1987).

Expression of c-myc p62 in normal tissues showed marked differences in its intracellular distribution and possible relationship of this oncoprotein with cell division is still a matter of further investigation (Jack et.al. 1986).

Our results reinforce the hypothesis that when both oncoproteins are overexpressed, especially in premalignant conditions, could indicate their malignant potential and therefore contribute in the prevention of the disease (Agnantis et. al. 1986, Spandidos et. al. 1987, Agnantis et. al. 1988).

Similar studies, using the same M.Abs, showed that both oncoproteins are overexpressed in the premalignant group of colon lesions and in well differentiated colonic adenocarcinomas, while only low levels of expression were observed in the undiferentiated tumors (Gallick et.al. 1985, Williams et.al. 1985, Stewart et.al. 1986, Sikora et.al. 1987). Our material comprised mainly well and moderately differentiated adenocarcinomas and we believe this may be the reason why we didn't find any stricking difference in expression of ras and myc gene products.

We suggest that the group of oncogene products should be included in the armory of tumor markers for determining the bioligical behavior and for the guidance of treatment.

REFERENCES

Agnantis, N.J., Petraki, C., Markoulatos, P. and Spandidos D.A. (1986a). Immunohistochemical study of the ras oncogene expression in human breast lesions. Anticancer Res. 6, 1157-1160.

Agnantis, N.J., Parissi, P., Anagnostakis, D. and Spandidos D.A. (1986b). Comparative study of Harvey ras oncogene expression with conventional clinopathologic parameters of breast cancer. Oncology 43,366-369

Agnantis, N.J., Spandidos, D.A., Mahera, H., Parissi, P., Kakkanas, A., Pintzas, A. and Papacharalampous, N.X. (1988). Immunohistochemical study of ras oncogene expression in endometrial and cervical human lesions. European Journal of Gynaecological Oncology. 9, 360-365.

Agnantis, N.J., Constantinidou, A., Poulios, C., Pintzas, A., Kakkanas, A., and Spandidos, D.A. (1989). Immunohistochemical study of the ras oncogene expression in human bladder endoscopy specimens. Eur. J. Surg. Onc. In Press.

Efremidis, A.P., Agnantis, N.J., Patra, F., Papadopoulou, C. and Spandidos, D.A. (1989). Clinical significance of elevated p21 ras oncogene expression in breast cancer patients. Cancer Journal 2, 288-291.

Evan, G.I., Lewis, G.K., Ramsay G. and Bischop, J.M. (1985) Isolation of monoclonal antibodies specific for human c-myc proto-oncogene product. Mol. Cell. Biol. 5, 3610-3616.

Field J.K. and Spandidos, D.A. (1987). Expression of oncogenes in human tumors with special reference to the head and neck region. J. Oral Path. 16, 97-107.

Furth, M.E., Davis, L.J., Fleurdelys B. and Scolnick, E.M. (1982). Monoclonal antobodies to the p21 products of the transforming gene of Harvey murine carcinoma virus and of the cellular ras gene family. J. Virol. 43, 294-304.

Furth, M.E., Aldrich T.H. and Cordon-Cardo, C. (1987). Expression of protooncogene proteins in normal human tissues. Oncogene 1, 47-58

Gallick, G.E., Kurzock, R., Kloetzer, W.S., Arlinghaus, R.B. and Gutterman, J.V. (1985). Expression of p21 ras in fresh primary and metastatic human colorectal tumors. Proc. Natl. Acad. Sci. USA 82, 1795-1799.

Going J.J., Williams A.R.W., Wyllie A.H., Anderson T.J., and Piris, J. (1988). Optimal preservation of p21 ras immunoreactivity and morphology in paraffin-embedded tissue. J. Pathol. 155, 185-190.

Jack, A.S., Kerr, I.B., Evan, G., Lee, F.D. (1986). The distribution of the c-myc oncogene product in malignant lymphomas and various normal tissues as demonstrated by immunocytochemistry. Br. J. Cancer 53, 713-719.

Loke, S. L., Neckers, L.M., Schwab, G. and Jaffe, E.S. (1988). c-myc protein in normal tissue. Effects of fixation on its apparent subcellular distribution. Am. J. Path. 131, 29-37.

Sikora, K., Chan, S., Evan, G., Gabra, H., Markham, N., Stewart J. and Watson, J. (1987). c-myc oncogene expression in colorectal cancer. Cancer, 59, 1289-1295.

Spandidos D.A. and Kerr, I.B. (1984). Elevated expression of the human ras oncogene family in premalignant tumors of the colorectum. Br. J. Cancer 49, 681-688.

Spandidos, D.A. and Agnantis N.J. (1984). Human malignant tumors of the breast, as compared to their respective normal tissue, have elevated expression of the Harvey ras oncogene. Anticancer Res. 4, 269-272.

Spandidos D.A. and Wilkie N.M. (1984). Malignant transformation of early passage rodent cells by a single mutated human oncogene. Nature 310, 469-475.

Spandidos D.A., Pintzas, A., Kakkanas, A. Yiagnisis, M., Mahera, H., Patra, E. and Agnantis, N.J. (1987). Elevated expression of the myc gene in human benign and malignant breast lesions compared to normal tissue. Anticancer Res. 7, 1299-1304.

Stewart, J., Evan, G., Watson J. and Sikora, K. (1986). Detection of the c-myc oncogene product in colonic polyps and carcinomas. Br. J. Cancer 53, 1-6.

Williams, A.R.W., Piris, J., Spandidos, D.A. and Wyllie, A.H. (1985). Immunohistochemical detection of the ras oncogene p21 product in an experimental tumor and in human colorectal neoplasms. Brit. J. Cancer 52 687-693.

Yokota, J., Tsunetsugu-Yokota, Y., Battifora, H., Le Fevre, C., Cline, J.N. (1986). Alterations of myc, myb and ras Ha proto-oncogenes in cancers are frequent and show clinical correlations. Science 231, 261-265.

Molecular Analysis of the Retinoblastoma (Rb) Gene in Human Colorectal Carcinomas

RAJALAKSHMI GOPE, MARK A. CHRISTENSEN, ALAN THORSON, HENRY T. LYNCH, THOMAS SMYRK, MOHAN L. GOPE, and BRUCE M. BOMAN

ABSTRACT

We have examined the structure and expression of the Rb gene on chromosome 13 in matched pairs of normal and malignant colonic tissues from 68 patients. Northern blots showed a normal size 4.7 kb transcript in the 33 normal mucosal tissues and 38 colorectal carcinomas examined. However, increased expression of the Rb gene (2-5 fold) was detected in approximately 70% of colorectal carcinomas relative to normal colonic mucosa. The remaining malignant tissues showed an equal level of Rb specific RNA as compared to normal colonic mucosa and none showed a decrease in hybridization signal. Southern blot analysis of DNA from 45 colorectal carcinomas showed an increase in hydridization intensity (at least two fold) in 20 tumors in comparison to normal mucosa. These results coupled with previous reports of nonrandom chromosome 13 gains in approximately 50% of colorectal carcinomas suggest that an increase in Rb gene copy number occurs frequently in these tumors. Southern blot analysis also shows that none of the colorectal cancers examined had allelic loss at the Rb locus. These results suggest that the Rb gene is not lost or transcriptionally inactivated in colorectal cancers.

INTRODUCTION

The first clue to the chromosome location of the Rb gene locus was the observation of constitutional deletions in the chromosomal region 13q14 of retinoblastoma patients (reviewed in Murphree and Benedict, 1984). Chromosome 13 allelic loss in hereditary and nonhereditary retinoblastomas provided further evidence supporting the location of the Rb gene to this chromosome region (Cavenee, 1983). The Rb gene was then mapped to chromosome 13q14 by linkage analysis of retinoblastoma pedigrees (Sparkes, 1983). Recent cloning of the Rb gene has provided the opportunity to analyze the Rb gene structure and expression in retinoblastomas. Rb gene structural changes and absent or truncated Rb transcripts have been found in hereditary and nonhereditary retinoblastomas (Friend et al., 1986; Fung et al., 1987; Lee et al., 1987; Benedict et al., 1988; Lee et al., 1988a; Bookstein et al., 1988). Results from these studies indicate that inactivation of both alleles of the Rb gene is necessary for tumorigenesis in the retina and possibly at other anatomic sites.

The observation that hereditary retinoblastoma patients have an increased risk for developing other cancers such as osteosarcomas, fibrosarcomas, and soft tissue sarcomas suggested that some non-ocular cancers might arise as a consequence of mutations in the Rb gene (Draper et al., 1986; Abramson, et al., 1984). Tumor-specific allele loss at loci on chromosome 13 was also observed in osteosarcomas (Hansen et al., 1985; Dryja et al., 1986). Rb gene structural changes and absent or altered RNA transcripts have now been reported to occur in osteosarcomas (Friend et al., 1986; Fung et al., 1987; Weichselbaum et al., 1988; Toguchida et al., 1988).

The increased risk for breast cancer in mothers of children with osteosarcoma and the familial aggregation of sarcomas of soft tissue and bone, breast cancer, and lung cancer in young people seen with the Li-Fraumeni syndrome suggested that other malignancies may have a similar genetic etiology (Hartley et al., 1986; Li and Fraumeni, 1969; Li and Fraumeni, 1982; Li, 1988). Chromosome 13 allele loss has been observed by others in small cell lung cancer (SCLC) and breast cancer (Lundberg et al., 1987; Yokota et al., 1987). Recently, both SCLC and breast cancer have been reported to have internal structural changes in the Rb gene and abnormalities in Rb gene expression (Harbour et al., 1988; T'Ang et al., 1988; Lee et al., 1988b). In addition, the absence of the Rb protein has been observed frequently in SCLC when no abnormalities in DNA and RNA could be detected (Yokota, et al., 1988).

Breast cancer has also been described as occurring in association with colon cancer in some families with Lynch syndrome II (Lynch et al., 1972; Lynch et al 1988). Whether this is due to a single pleiotropic gene with a variable tumor-inducing spectrum or transmission of two or more different cancer-predisposing genes in these families remains elusive.

Colorectal carcinomas have also been tested for tumor-specific loss of alleles on chromosome 13 and found to have infrequent loss of heterozygosity (Solomon et al., 1987; Fearon et al., 1987; Vogelstein et al., 1989; reviewed in Boman, 1988). Karyotypic studies have shown that non-random gains of chromosome 13, including trisomy and tetrasomy, occur in a significant proportion (48-55%) of colorectal carcinomas (Reichmann et al., 1981; Muleris et al., 1987). This suggests that the Rb gene is probably not lost or deleted in colorectal carcinomas. Our study reported here was designed to directly examine the structure and expression of the Rb gene in colorectal cancer.

MATERIALS AND METHODS

<u>Samples Used:</u> Fresh tumor samples were obtained immediately following surgery from 68 patients with colorectal carcinoma at the Creighton University Cancer Center and The University of Texas M.D. Anderson Cancer Center (Wildrick and Boman, 1988). One patient (No. 21) had confirmed familial adenomatous polyposis (FAP). All tumors were histopathologically confirmed as primary adenocarcinomas of the colon. Any gross contaminating normal stromal tissue was completely dissected away from each tumor specimen. Normal mucosa was obtained from the wide margin of resection of 63 of the surgical specimens by blunt dissection of the colonic mucosa away from the underlying submucosa.

The DiFi carcinoma cell line was established from the malignant ascitic fluid of another FAP patient (No. 10) with rectal cancer (see chapter by Boman et al.). The HT-29, SW620, and SW480 were obtained from the American Type Culture Collection (Rockville, MD). These cell lines were grown in RPMI 1640: L-15 (50:50 for DiFi), DMEM (HT-29) or L-15 (SW620, SW480) media containing 10% FBS.

Detailed family histories were obtained on the two FAP patients (Nos. 10, 21, see Table 1), one of whom (No. 10) had extracolonic manifestations typical of the Gardner Syndrome (see chapter by

Boman et al.). The remainder of cases were classified as sporadic because a positive family history was not reported in the patient's clinical records.

Table 1. Expression of Rb message in human colon tissue

NO.	PATIENT/ CELL LINE	SITE	NORMAL	TUMOR
1	MDA7	rc	+	++
2	MDA8	s	+	+++
3	MDA9	r	+	++
4	MDA12	s	ND	++
5	MDA14	rs	++	++
6	MDA15	lc	++	++++
7	MDA17	rs	+	++
8	MDA18	lc	ND	+++
9	MDA19	c	ND	++
10*	DiFi	r′	ND	++++
11	CCC3	c	+	+++
12	CCC5	r	++	++
13	CCC8	c	+	++++
14	CCC9	r	+	++
15	CCC11	s	+	++
16	CCC13	c	+	+++
17	CCC14	lc	+	++
18	CCC15	tc	++	++
19	CCC16	c	+	+++
20	CCC17	m	+	++
21*	CCC19	c	+	++
22	CCC25	r	+	++
23	CCC28	r	+	++++
24	CCC29	r	+	+++++
25	CCC30	c	++	++
26	CCC34	r	+	+++
27	CCC35	s	+	+++
28	CCC36	s	+	+
29	CCC58	c	ND	+++
30	CCC60	r	++	+++
31	CCC61	r	ND	++
32	CCC63	c	+	+
33	CCC64	lc	+	+++
34	CCC65	s	+	+++
35	CCC66	lc	++	++
36	CCC67	rc	++	+++
37	CCC69	c	+	+
38	CCC70	rc	+	+
39	CCC71	s	++	+++
40	HT-29	c′	ND	+++
41	SW620	c′	ND	++
42	SW480	c′	ND	+++

*Patients had confirmed FAP

Abbreviations: rs, rectosigmoid carcinoma; s, sigmoid carcinoma; lc, left colonic carcinoma; rc, right colonic carcinoma; r, rectal carcinoma; tc, transverse colonic carcinoma; c, colonic carcinoma site unknown; m, locally metastatic colonic carcinoma; r′, cell line derived from a rectal carcinoma of an FAP patient (see Chapter by Boman et al.); c′, established colon carcinoma cell lines; ND, not determined, + to +++++, low to high levels of hybridization intensity.

<u>cDNA Probes:</u> The Rb 3.8 probe for the Rb gene is a cDNA subclone, pG 3.8M, encoding the 3′ region of the 4.73-kb Rb cDNA (kindly provided by Yuen-Kai Fung; Fung et al., 1987). The cDNA probes for beta-actin (Cleveland et al., 1980) and GAPDH (Dugaiczyk et al. 1983) were used for the controls in northern and Southern blots respectively. The probe p6NRO.5 (kindly provided by Eva Y.-H.P. Lee; Bookstein et al., 1988) for the first intron of the Rb gene was used to analyze allelic loss at this locus.

<u>Northern and Southern Blot Analysis:</u> The isolation of RNA and DNA as well as the hybridization conditions for northern and Southern blots were performed as described previously (Maniatis, 1982; Wildrick and Boman, 1988; Siegel and Bresnick, 1986).

RESULTS

We examined total RNA isolated from primary colorectal carcinomas of 38 patients and adjacent normal-appearing colonic mucosa from 33 of these patients for Rb gene expression using the Rb cDNA probe 3.8. The normal size 4.7-kb transcript was observed in RNA from all normal mucosa tissues and primary colorectal carcinomas analyzed. However, an increased level of hybridization intensity was detected in 24 of 33 carcinomas where normal mucosa was available for comparison (Table 1). The degree of increased hybridization signal varied from two- to fivefold (Table 1). None of the malignant tissues showed a decrease in hybridization signal, and nine cases showed equal hybridization intensity as compared to their normal mucosa.

The majority of normal tissues showed relatively low levels (+ or ++) of hybridization intensity on northern blot analysis (see Table 1). Seventeen of the thirty-eight tumor samples analyzed showed a level of hybridization intensity (+++ to +++++) that was higher than the range of hybridization signal observed for normal samples (Table 1). Hybridization with the beta-actin probe was performed as a control to verify the amounts of RNA loaded in each lane. The Rb message was also found to be expressed in four colorectal carcinoma cell lines (nos. 10, 40-42; Table 1).

Southern blot analysis was performed using DNA from 45 colorectal carcinomas and adjacent normal mucosa. All of the normal and tumor tissue samples showed normal size <u>Bam</u>HI fragments (Lee et al., 1988b) using the Rb 3.8 probe for the 3′ region of the gene. An increase in the hybridization intensity (at least twofold) was observed in the DNA from 20 of the 45 colorectal carcinomas analyzed glyceraldehyde-3-phosphate dehydrogenase (GAPDH) probe was performed as a control to verify the amounts of DNA loaded.

The 45 normal/tumor DNA pairs were also examined for tumor-specific allele loss at the <u>Bam</u>HI RFLP of the Rb locus using the p6NRO.5 probe. Twenty-two patients were heterozygous at the Rb locus and none showed allelic loss in the tumor (Table 2).

Table 2. SOUTHERN BLOT ANALYSIS OF NORMAL AND MALIGNANT COLON TISSUES

NUMBER	PATIENT	FOLD INCREASE	Alleles at the Rb Locus NORMAL	TUMOR
11	CCC 3	1	2/1	2/1
12	CCC 5	2	-	-
13	CCC 6	1	-	-
14	CCC 7	2	-	-
15	CCC 8	1	-	-
17	CCC 9	1	-	-
18	CCC 11	1	-	-
19	CCC 14	2	2/1	2/1
21	CCC 15	1	-	-
23	CCC 16	2	2/1	2/1
24	CCC 19	1	-	-
25	CCC 21	2	-	-
26	CCC 28	3	-	-
27	CCC 29	2.5	2/1	2/1
28	CCC 30	1	2/1	2/1
43	CCC 34	1	2/1	2/1
44	CCC 35	1	2/1	2/1
45	CCC 36	1	2/1	2/1
46	CCC 37	2	-	-
47	CCC 39	1.5	-	-
48	CCC 40	1	-	-
49	CCC 42	1	-	-
50	CCC 44	2	-	-
51	CCC 45	2	2/1	2/1
52	CCC 46	1	-	-
53	CCC 50	1.5	2/1	2/1
54	CCC 52	1	2/1	2/1
55	CCC 55	3	2/1	2/1
56	CCC 56	3	2/1	2/1
57	CCC 57	2	2/1	2/1
58	CCC 58	1	2/1	2/1
59	CCC 60	2	2/1	2/1
60	CCC 61	1	2/1	2/1
61	CCC 62	2	-	-
62	CCC 63	3	2/1	2/1
63	CCC 64	2.5	-	-
64	CCC 65	2.5	-	-
65	CCC 66	2	-	-
66	CCC 67	1	-	-
67	CCC 69	1.5	2/1	2/1
68	CCC 70	2	2/1	2/1
69	CCC 71	1	2/1	2/1
70	CCC 79	1	-	-
71	CCC 85	1	2/1	2/1
72	CCC 88	1	-	-

DNA from colorectal cancer patients was hybridized with the Rb 3.8 probe to analyze Rb gene copy number and with the p6NR0.5 probe to analyze for allelic loss in tumors versus normal mucosa. The fold increase in tumors relative to normal mucosa was determined by densitometry (BioRad Model 620 densitometer). Rb is biallelic in DNA digested with BamHI using the p6NR0.5 probe that reveals fragments of 4.5 kb (G1) and 2.2 kb (G2). "2/1" indicates heterozygosity and a "-" indicates uninformative.

DISCUSSION

The observed increase in Rb gene expression in colorectal carcinomas might result from one of several possible mechanisms: 1. Increased Rb gene dosage due to gains of chromosome 13, 2. Rb gene amplification, 3. Increased rate of Rb gene transcription, or 4. Decreased rate of Rb mRNA turnover.

Our data show that at least 44% of colorectal cancers have an increase in Rb gene copy number that is characterized by an increase in the hybridization signal in tumor DNA as compared to normal DNA. This is consistent with reports of non-random gains of chromosome 13 in approximately 50% of colorectal cancers (Reichmann et al., 1981; Muleris et al., 1987). In some tumors with non-random gains of chromosome 13, it may not be possible to detect an increase in Rb gene copy number by Southern analysis because of the technical limitation in detecting an increase of just one or two extra copies of the Rb gene and because these tumors are often polyploid leading to an overall increase in total genomic DNA content. A recent study on the chromosomal evolution of colorectal tumors shows that gains of chromosome 13 occurs early in the carcinogenetic process (Muleris et al., 1988). Our observation of an increased Rb gene copy number in 44% of colorectal carcinomas coupled with reports of non-random gains of chromosome 13 in 50% of these tumors suggests that an increase in Rb gene dosage is very common in colorectal cancer.

This study reveals that colorectal cancers have equal or increased levels of the Rb transcript as compared to normal colonic mucosa and that the Rb transcript is of normal size in these tumors. Our study also shows that none of the colorectal cancers analyzed had allelic loss at the Rb locus. These data suggest that the Rb gene is not lost or transcriptionally inactivated in colorectal cancers. Preliminary studies have also shown that a normal size Rb protein product is present in DiFi colorectal carcinoma cells (Hong-Ji Xu, personal communication). Thus it appears that the Rb message is normally translated in malignant colonic epithelial cells. The possibility that the Rb protein product might be inactive in colorectal cancers due to a point mutation in the Rb gene leading to an altered amino acid sequence of the protein cannot be ruled out.

It has been proposed that the Rb gene normally has a suppressor function (Murphree and Benedict, 1984). If the Rb protein retains its normal function in the colorectal carcinomas, it may be functioning as a growth suppressor-gene in terms of proliferation kinetics. For example, cellular kinetic studies on the doubling time of colorectal carcinomas indicate that the proliferation of this tumor is relatively slow compared to normal epithelial cells in the colon (Deschner and Lipkin, 1978).

ACKNOWLEDGEMENTS

We thank Barbara Lorimor for secretarial assistance in the preparation of this manuscript. This work was supported by Health Future Foundation Funds.

REFERENCES

Abramson DH, Ellsworth RM, Kitchin FD, Tung G (1984) Second nonocular tumors in retinoblastoma survivors. Opthalmology 91:1351-1355

Benedict WF, Fung Y-KT, Murphree AL (1988) The gene responsible for the development of retinoblastoma and osteosarcoma Cancer 62: 1691-1694
Boman BM (1988) Biomolecular genetics of cancer. In: Lynch T and Hirayama T (ed) Genetic Epidemiology of Cancer. CRC Press, Inc. Boca Raton, FL, pp 343-349
Bookstein R, Lee EY-HP, To H, Young LJ, Sery TW, Hayes RC, Friedmann T, Lee W-H (1988) Human retinoblastoma susceptibility gene: genomic organization and analysis of heterozygous intragenic deletion mutants. Proc. Natl. Acad. Sci. USA 85:2210-2214
Cavenee WK, Dryja TP, Phillips RA, Benedict WF, Godbout R, Gallie BL, Murphree AL, Strong LC and White RL (1983) Expression of recessive alleles by chromosomal mechanisms in retinoblastoma. Nature 305:779-783
Cleveland DN, Lopata MA, MacDonald RJ, Cowan NJ, Rutter WJ, Kirschner MW (1980) Number and evolutionary conservation of alpha- and beta- tubulin and cytoplasmic beta- and gamma-actin genes using specific cloned cDNA probes. Cell 20:95-105
Deschner EE, Lipkin M (1978) Proliferation and differentiation of Gastrointestinal Cells in Health and Disease. In: Lipkin M and Good RA (ed)Gastrointestional Tract Cancer. Plenum Publishing Corp., New York, NY
Draper GJ, Sanders BM, Kingston JE (1986) Second primary neoplasms in patients with retinoblastoma. Br. J. Cancer 53:661-671
Dryja TP, Rapaport JM, Epstein J, Goorin AM, Weichselbaum R, Koufos A, Cavenee WK (1986) Chromosome 13 homozygosity in osteosarcoma with retinoblastoma. Am. J. Hum. Genet. 38:59-66
Dugaiczyk A, Haron JA, Stone EM, et al (1983) Cloning and sequencing of a deoxyribonucleic acid copy of glyceraldehyde-3-phosphate dehydrogenase messenger ribonucleic acid isolated from chicken muscle Biochemistry 22:1605-1613
Fearon ER, Hamilton SR, Vogelstein B (1987) Clonal analysis of human colorectal tumors. Science 238:193-197
Friend SH, Bernards R, Rogelj S, Weinberg RA, Rapaport JM, Albert DM, Dryja TP (1986) A human DNA segment with properties of the gene that predisposes to retinoblastoma and osteosarcoma. Nature 323:643-646
Fung Y-KT, Murphree AL, T'Ang A, Qian J, Hinrichs SH, Benedict WF (1987) Structural evidence for the authenticity of the human retinoblastoma gene. Science 236:1657-1661
Hansen MF, Koufos A, Gallie BL, Phillips RA, Fodstad O, Brogger A, Gedde-Dahl T, Cavenee WK (1985) Osteosarcoma and retinoblaqstoma: a shared chromosomal mechanism revealing recessive predisposition. Proc. Natl. Acad. Sci. USA 82:6216-6220
Harbour JW, Lai S-L, Whang-Peng J, Gazdar AF, Minna JD, Kaye FJ (1988) Abnormalities in structure and expression of the human retinoblastoma gene in SCLC. Science 241:353-357
Hartley AL, Birch JM, Marsden HB, Harris M (1986) Breast cancer risk in mothers of children with osteosarcoma and chondrosarcoma. Br. J. Cancer 54:819-823
Lee WH, Bookstein R, Hong F, Young LJ, Shew J-Y, Lee EY-H (1987) Human retinoblastoma susceptibility gene: cloning, identification, and sequence. Science 235:1394-1399
Lee EY-HP, Bookstein R, Young LJ, Lin CJ, Rosenfeld MG, Lee WH (1988a) Molecular mechanism of retinoblastoma gene inactivation in retinoblastoma cell line Y79. Proc. Natl. Acad. Sci. USA 85:6017-6021
Lee EY-HP, To H, Shew J-Y, et al. (1988b) Inactivation of the retinoblastoma susceptibility gene in human breast cancers. Science 241:281-221
Li FP, Fraumeni JF, Jr. (1969) Soft-tissue sarcomas, breast cancer, and other neoplasms a familial syndrome? Ann Intern Med 71:747-752

Li FP, Fraumeni JF, Jr. (1982) Prospective Study of a family cancer syndrome. JAMA 247:2692-2694

Li FP (1988) Cancer families: Human models of susceptibility to neoplasia-The Richard and Hinda Rosenthal Foundation Award Lecture. Cancer 48:5381-5386

Lundberg C, Skoog L, Cavenee WK, Nordenskjold M (1987) Loss of heterozygosity in human ductal breast tumors indicates a recessive mutation on chromosome 13. Proc. Natl. Acad. Sci. USA 84:2372-2376

Lynch HT, Krush AJ, Lemon HM, Kaplan AR, Condit PT, Bottomley RH (1972) Tumor variation in families with breast cancer. JAMA 222:1631-1635

Lynch HT, Ens J, Lynch JF, Watson P (1988) Tumor variation in three extended Lynch syndrome II kindreds. Am. J. Gastroenterol 83:741-747

Maniatis T, Fritsch EF, Sambrook J (1982) Molecular cloning: A laboratory manual, Cold Spring Harbor Laboratory, Cold Spring Harbor, New York

Muleris M, Salmon R-J, Dutrillaux A-M, Vielh P, Zafrani B, Girodet J, Dutrillaux B (1987) Characteristic chromosomal imbalances in 18 near-diploid colorectal tumors. Cancer Genet. Cytogenet. 29:289-301

Muleris M, Salmon RJ, Dutrillaux B (1988) Existence of two distinct processes of chromosomal evolution in near-diploid colorectal tumors Cancer Genet. Cytogenet. 32:43-50

Murphree AL, Benedict WF (1984) Retinoblastoma: Clues to human oncogenesis. Science 223:1028-1033

Reichmann A, Martin P, Levin B (1981) Chromosomal banding patterns in human large bowel cancer. Int. J. Cancer 28:431-440

Siegel LI, Bresnick E (1986) Northern hybridization analysis of RNA using diethylpyrocarbonate-treated nonfat milk. Anal. Biochem. 159:82-87

Solomon E, Voss R, Hall V, Bodmer WF, Jass JR, Jeffreys AJ, Lucibello FC, Patel I, Rider SH (1987) Chromosome 5 allele loss in human colorectal carcinomas. Nature 328:616-619

Sparkes RS, Murphree AL, Lingua R, Sparkes MC, Field LL, Funderburk SJ, Benedict WF (1983) Gene for hereditary retinoblastoma assigned to human chromosome 13 by linkage to esterase D. Science 219:971-973

T'Ang A, Varley JM, Chakraborty S, et al. (1988) Structural rearrangement of the retinoblastoma gene in human breast carcinoma. Science 242:263-266

Toguchida J, Ishizaki K, Sasaki MS, Ikenaga M, Sugimoto M, Kotoura Y, Yamamuro T (1988) Chromosomal reorganization for the expression of recessive mutation of retinoblastoma susceptibility gene in the development of osteosarcoma. Cancer 48:3939-3943

Vogelstein B, Fearon ER, Kearn SE, et al. (1989) Allelotype of colorectal carcinomas. Science 244:207-211

Weichselbaum RR, Beckett M, Diamond A (1988) Some retinoblastomas, osteosarcomas, and soft tissue sarcomas may share a common etiology. Proc. Natl. Acad. Sci. USA 85:2106-2109

Wildrick DM, Boman BM (1988) Chromosome 5 allele loss at the glucocorticoid receptor locus in human colorectal carcinomas. Biochem. Biophys. Res. Commun. 150:591-598

Yokota J, Wada M, Shimosata Y, et al. (1987) Loss of heterozygosity on chromosome 3, 13, and 17 in small-cell carcinoma and on chromosome 3 in adenocarcinoma of the lung. Proc. Natl. Acad. Sci. 84:9252-9256

Yokota J, Akiyama T, Fung Y-KT, Benedict WF, Namba Y, Hanaoka M, Wada M, Terasaki T, Shimosato Y, Sugimura T, Terada M (1988) Altered expression of the retinoblastoma (Rb) gene in small-cell

Cellular and Molecular Events Involved in Tumour Progression in Colorectal Carcinogenesis: A Study of the Adenoma Carcinoma Sequence In Vitro

CHRISTOS PARASKEVA, SUSAN FINERTY, SARA HARPER, and ANN C. WILLIAMS

ABSTRACT

Epithelial cell lines from hereditary and sporadic adenomas have been isolated with abnormalities of chromosomes 1, 7, 14, 17, 18 and 22. Chromosome 1 may be involved in *in vitro* immortalization. Several stages have been described in the transformation of an adenoma cell line to anchorage independence and a possible role for sodium butyrate in tumour promotion discussed. *In vitro* immortality, aneuploidy, clonogenicity, resistance to sodium butyrate, *ras* gene activation and production of active proteinases are potential markers of tumour progression. A role for a constitutively produced tumour promoter(s) in colorectal carcinogenesis is discussed together with a possible different mechanism for adenoma formation in sporadic versus hereditary cancer patients.

Keywords: **adenoma**, **culture**, **aneuploidy**, **promotion**, **transformation**

INTRODUCTION

The development of colorectal cancer is an excellent example of the multistage process of carcinogenesis. A clear premalignant stage, the adenoma, has been recognised and most colorectal cancers develop from adenomas. The premalignant stage is, however, complicated by there being several histological states of adenomas representing different malignant potentials. In general, small tubular adenomas of less than 1cm in diameter have a low malignant potential whereas large villous adenomas have a high malignant potential. Tubular villous adenomas fall between the other two types in malignant potential (Muto et al., 1975). An analysis of these precancer stages is essential to understand the complex initiation and promotional events involved in the development of the adenomas and their progression and conversion to malignancy. To study colorectal carcinogenesis we have isolated epithelial cell lines from small and large sporadic and familial polyposis coli (FPC) adenomas (Paraskeva et al., 1984, 1989a) with the following objectives: (i) To develop *in vitro* parameters to distinguish the different premalignant adenoma stages. (ii) To investigate the biology of the precancer states and whether specitic chromosome abnormalities and oncogene activation occurs during the precancer stages. (iii) To examine the possible role of dietary factors such as sodium butyrate in tumour promotion. (iv) To examine sequential changes as adenomas progress towards the malignant phenotype *in vitro*. This work is described in this paper.

MATERIALS AND METHODS

Medium and Standard Culture Conditions

Growth medium and all cell culture techniques have been described (Paraskeva et al., 1984). Briefly, most adenoma cell cultures cannot be passaged by routine trypsinization since they only grow from clumps of cells and not from single cells. Instead dispase prepared in growth medium was used. Dispase solution was added to cell monolayers and removed the epithelium as sheets of cells and not as single cells (Paraskeva et al., 1984).

Carcinogen Treatment. AA/C1 and AA/C1/SB cells (both at passage 64) were seeded at 10^6 cells/T25 flask and allowed to grow until 60-80% confluent (8-10 days). The cells were then treated with the following N-Methyl-N-Nitro-N-Nitrosoguanidine (MNG) concentrations, 0(DMSO control), 0.1, 1.0 and 10.0 ug/ml for 24 hours. Two of each of the treatment flasks were then trypsinized, and counted to determine the inhibitory effect of the treatment. These same cell suspensions were used to determine the effect of the carcinogen treatment on the colony forming efficiency (C.F.E.). The remaining treatment flasks were allowed to recover under standard growth conditions.

RESULTS AND DISCUSSION

Tumour Progression and Acquisition of *in vitro* Immortality

We have raised the question whether adenoma derived cell lines give rise to immortal cell lines. The acquisition of *in vitro* immortality and the significance of this parameter to the different stages in carcinogenesis have attracted a great deal of interest. Of fifteen independently derived cultures from colorectal adenomas of FPC patients, three, PC/AA, PC/FF and PC/BH, grew extensively although only PC/AA has become immortal *in vitro* without going through a crisis (Paraskeva et al., 1988). PC/AA was derived from a large tubular adenoma with mild dysplasia 3-4cm in diameter whereas the majority of adenomas from which the original 15 cultures were derived (including PC/BH and PC/FF) were small tubular adenomas less than 1cm in diameter.

Of sixteen independently derived primary cultures from sporadic adenomas, four designated S/AN, S/BR, S/RG and S/RR have reached passages 28, 10, 23 and 14 respectively. All four except S/RR were derived from relatively large adenomas of greater than 1cm in diameter (Table 1). S/AN and S/RG show no signs of senescence and S/BR and S/RR are still under test. The majority of small adenomas (< 1cm in diameter) whether sporadic or hereditary did not give rise to immortal cell lines. Therefore, whatever event(s) are involved in the development of small adenomas these are generally insufficient for the immortal phenotype. However, the acquisition of *in vitro* immortality could be associated with a pre-cancerous stage, but at a relatively late stage when the adenomas are large, or villous or display severe levels of dysplasia. In support of this the continuous epithelial cell line VACO 235 reported by Willson et al. (1987) was derived from a villous adenoma.

Escape from senescence as a marker of tumour progression. An aneuploid variant was isolated from the PC/BH cell line which normally senesces between passages 16 and 20 (Paraskeva et al., 1988). This variant is currently at passage 26 and shows no signs of senescence. (Paraskeva - unpublished results). The acquisition of *in vitro* immortality and the ability to escape senescence can therefore be used as a marker of tumour progression by adenoma cells *in vitro*.

Table 1: Biology of Colorectal Adenoma Cell Lines

Familial (FPC)	**Adenoma[1,2] Histology**	**Mucin[3]**	**Passage Reached[4]**	**Clonogenic[5]**	**Karyotype**
PC/AA	T (3-4)	+	>80 (80)	-	Diploid
PC/FF	T (<1)	+	18-22(24)	-	Diploid
PC/BH	T (<1)	+	16-20(21)	-	Diploid
Sporadic					
S/AN	V (1-2)	+	>28 (38)	-	Aneuploid
S/RG	T (1-2)	+	>23 (23)	+	Aneuploid
S/BR	T/V(3-4)	+	>10 (10)	+	Aneuploid
S/RR	T/V (<1)	+	>14 (21)	-	In progress
S/WG	T/V(1-2)	ND	>3 (8)	ND	In progress

[1] T = Tubular, T/V = Tubular Villous, V = Villous Adenoma, [2] Figure in brackets refers to size of adenoma in cm from which cell line isolated, [3] Mucin detected by EM and Histological stains, [4] Figure in brackets refers to time in culture in months, [5] Refers to ability to grow after trypsinization to single cells. All adenoma lines are non-tumorigenic in nude mice and are positive with keratin antibodies LE61, LE65 and LP34 (Lane 1982).

Specific Chromosome Abnormalities in Adenoma Cell Lines

Karyotypic analysis of adenoma cell lines is important for several reasons: (i) chromosome changes can be monitored as adenoma cells progress *in vitro* to the malignant phenotype (ii) chromosome abnormalities can give a clue to the location of oncogenes and tumour suppressor genes (iii) chromosome analysis with determining loss of heterozygosity can identify which cells to use as targets when reinserting genes implicated in colorectal carcinogenesis.

Familial Polyposis Coli Adenoma and Carcinoma Cell Lines. The adenoma cell line PC/AA at early passage was normal diploid with no detectable chromosome abnormalities. PC/FF and PC/BH at early passage had a low rate of division and were therefore impossible to karyotype fully. However, both cell lines had chromosome numbers in the diploid range (Paraskeva et al., 1984 and unpublished results). The karyotype of the FPC carcinoma cell line PC/JW has an isochromosome 1(q), an abnormality of chromosome 17 and other markers (Paraskeva et al., 1984).

Sporadic Adenoma Cell Lines. Every cell examined of the adenoma line S/AN has a deletion on the short arm of chromosome 1 and one normal copy of chromosome 1. S/AN is also monosomic for chromosome 18. The majority of cells of S/RG only have one normal copy of chromosomes 6,7,14,17,18 and 22. Although aneuploid S/AN and S/RG are non-tumorigenic in athymic nude mice. The common abnormality for S/AN and S/RG is monosomy for chromosome 18. The villous adenoma-derived cell line VACO 235, (Willson et al., 1987) has a deleted chromosome 18. Monosomy for chromosome 18 therefore appears to be an important and central step in the sequential development of colorectal cancer (Paraskeva et al., 1989a). The VACO 235 cell line also had other abnormalities including a deletion of the short arm of chromosome 1 and an isochromosome 1 (q). The adenoma cell line S/BR is also aneuploid and is currently being karyotyped.

Chromosome 1, Tumour Progression and *in vitro* Immortalization

PC/AA at early passage was diploid and at late passage (passage 50-60), after subculture in the presence of 3T3 feeders, became aneuploid (Paraskeva et al., 1988). Each late-passage PC/AA had an isochromosome 1(q) and led us to propose that abnormalities involving chromosome 1 may be involved in tumour progression (Paraskeva et al., 1988). To further study tumour progression *in vitro*, one of our aims was to isolate from early passage diploid PC/AA variants with a higher malignant potential. A 3T3 feeder independent variant of PC/AA, designated PC/AA/FI, was therefore isolated. PC/AA/FI while remaining non-tumorigenic, acquired several characteristics normally associated with colorectal cancers, notably *in vitro* immortality, aneuploidy, 3T3 feeder independence and the ability to grow at clonal density (Paraskeva et al., 1989b). Each cell of PC/AA/FI has an isochromosome 1(q) like the late passage PC/AA (Paraskeva et al., 1988). However, with PC/AA/FI it is the other chromosome 1 of the homologous pair (distinguishable by C-banding) which is involved in the formation of the isochromosome 1(q). With the late-passage PC/AA (grown with 3T3 feeders) the homologue with the large C-band has given rise to an isochromosome 1(q) whereas with PC/AA/FI it is the homologue with the smaller C-band which has given rise to this isochromosome.

After extended *in vitro* growth either with or without 3T3 feeders, parental diploid PC/AA has given rise to immortal variants, both of which are aneuploid. The common abnormality is isochromosome 1(q). The fact that different homologues of chromosome 1 are involved shows that they have independent abnormalities involving chromosome 1. These results indicate that chromosome 1 may be involved in extended *in vitro* growth and/or *in vitro* immortalization (Paraskeva et al., 1988, 1989a). It is also of interest that the adenoma cell line S/AN, which has an extended *in vitro* growth capacity has a deletion on the short arm of chromosome 1 (Paraskeva et al., 1989a) and the established villous adenoma line VACO 235 has chromosome 1 abnormalities (Willson et al., 1987).

Ras Mutations, Colonic Adenomas and Immortality

Previous reports have shown a prevalence of codon 12 k-*ras* gene mutations in sporadic colorectal cancers (Bos et al., 1987, Forrester et al., 1987) and in adenoma tissue with a high malignant potential associated with these cancers. We have reported the presence of a mutation in codon 12 of the k-*ras* gene in 5 of 75 individual polyp specimens from 29 FPC patients (Farr et al., 1988). Those FPC polyps with the *ras* mutations represented in general large polyps or dysplastic polyps with a relatively high malignant potential. An activated k-*ras* gene was also detected in the adenoma cell line S/AN, which was isolated from a sporadic villous adenoma (1-2cm in diameter). Thus activated *ras* occurs infrequently in adenomas and generally in those with a high malignant potential. These data are consistent with the hypothesis that *ras* gene mutations are not necessary for adenoma formation but that adenomas which acquire *ras* mutations have a high probability of malignant progression.

K-*ras* codon 12 mutations were also detected in the FPC cell line PC/AA derived from a large tubular adenoma (3-4cm) and the FPC carcinoma cell line PC/JW. *Ras* mutations were not detected in the FPC adenoma line PC/BH or the sporadic S/RG (Farr et al., 1988). PC/BH was derived from multiple tubular adenomas all less than 5mm in diameter (Paraskeva et al., 1984). These results provide further support that there are common molecular events involved in sporadic and hereditary colorectal carcinogenesis and that k-*ras* mutations can precede the development of malignancy.

PC/AA is immortal *in vitro* and contains an activated k-*ras* gene. To our knowledge PC/AA is the first reported example of a human cell line bearing the mutant *ras* gene which is not tumorigenic and shows that the presence of an activated *ras* gene even in immortal human cell lines is insufficient for malignancy. The new adenoma line S/RR derived from a small sporadic adenoma (< 1cm in diameter) also has a codon 12 *ras* gene mutation (Farr - unpublished results). This is the first case of a cell line from a small adenoma containing such a mutation and this adenoma may represent the relatively rare case of small adenoma which progress towards the malignant phenotype.

Cysteine Proteinases and their Specific Inhibitors in Tumour Invasion and Colorectal Carcinogenesis

One of the important biological and clinically significant differences between benign and malignant colorectal tumours is the ability of the latter to invade surrounding tissue and metastasize. The secretion and/or plasma membrane association of proteinases from tumour cells has been implicated in tumour invasion since invasion by tumour cells requires the local dissolution of the basement membrane. Adenoma and carcinoma cell lines both secreted precursor forms of the 2 cysteine proteinases, cathepsins B and L (Maciewicz et al., 1989). The adenoma cell line PC/AA secreted as much, or more of both cathepsin B and L precursors as did the carcinoma line PC/JW/FI, PC/JW/FI being a 3T3 feeder independent variant of PC/JW (Maciewicz et al., 1989). However, mature forms of cathepsins B and L were detected in the culture media of only the carcinoma-derived cell line. Thus indicating that the invasive potential of a tumour may be related to its ability to process extracellularly the secreted precursor enzyme to a mature and consequently active enzyme, rather than to the amount of proteinase synthesized and/or secreted (Maciewicz et al., 1989). However, it is the balance between active proteinases and their specific inhibitors that is of importance in the events leading to tumour invasion.

Transformation of the Adenoma Cell Line PC/AA to Anchorage Independence by the Carcinogen MNG (Fig 1)

One of our objectives is to study *in vitro* the sequential changes involved in the progression of adenomas to carcinomas. PC/AA was continuously passaged *in vitro* and at late passage (passage 50-60) became aneuploid but remained non-tumorigenic and retained a very poor cloning ability after single cell trypsinization (Paraskeva et al., 1988). Taking advantage of our previous observation that colorectal cancer cell lines will grow clonally (after single cell trypsinization) but the majority of adenoma cultures will not grow clonally, we isolated a clonogenic variant of late passage PC/AA designated AA/C1. We argued that a clonogenic variant of late passage PC/AA may represent a later stage in tumour progression and that the adenoma cells are acquiring certain characteristics of cancer cells. AA/C1 however remained non anchorage independent and non tumorigenic.

PC/AA adenoma cells are more sensitive to the inhibitory effects of sodium butyrate than the carcinoma cell lines HT29 and PC/JW (Berry and Paraskeva, 1988). In an attempt to further select for adenoma cells with an increased malignant potential AA/C1 cells were treated with sodium butyrate (1mM for fourteen days) which resulted in a population of cells designated AA/C1/SB with an increased C.F.E. but again these cells remained non anchorage independent and non tumorigenic. Because the conversion of premalignant cells to malignant cells may require a further genetic change we treated both AA/C1 and AA/C1/SB with a range of concentrations (0.1 to 10.0 ug/ml) of the carcinogen MNG. From AA/C1/SB cells treated with 10 ug/ml of MNG we isolated an anchorage independent cell line designated AA/C1/SB/10 (Williams et al., manuscript in preparation). AA/C1/SB treated with lower concentrations of MNG were not anchorage independent. Under the same conditions of treatment with MNG even at 10 ug/ml the AA/C1 cells were not anchorage independent. Although the reason(s) for this are unclear it is interesting to postulate that the sodium butyrate treatment of AA/C1 has made them more susceptible to transformation by MNG. This is the first report of the transformation of human adenoma cells to the anchorage independent phenotype. On continuous *in vitro* passage the C.F.E. of AA/C1/SB/10 has increased from 0.16% in agar to 18%.

Sodium Butyrate as a Possible Promoter of Colorectal Carcinogenesis

Butyric acid is a naturally occurring four-carbon fatty acid and is an important energy source for colorectal epithelial cells. We reported that the diploid PC/AA adenoma cells were more sensitive to the growth inhibitory effects of sodium butyrate than the two colorectal cancer cell lines HT29 and PC/JW (Berry and Paraskeva, 1988). The differential growth response of these cell lines to sodium butyrate could have important implications for the emergence of malignant cells from the normal and pre-malignant epithelium of the human colon. This agent may select for cells with an increased malignant potential by a process analogous to the proposed mechanism of TPA induced carcinogenesis in mouse skin (Parkinson, 1985). If sodium butyrate is important in the control of cellular differentiation of the colonic epithelium, any cell that could escape that signal may be able to proliferate unchecked. We therefore argued that sodium butyrate may act as a tumour promoter in the human colon by selecting for epithelial cells which have acquired a reduced response to terminal differentiation signals as a result of initiation and/or promotion by dietary or environmental carcinogenesis (Berry and Paraskeva, 1988). If this is the case it might be possible to model colorectal tumour progression *in vitro* by treating pre-malignant adenoma cell lines with sodium butyrate to select for resistant populations with an increased malignant potential. Resistance to the inhibitory effects of sodium butyrate could also be used as an *in vitro* marker of tumour progression. To test this AA/C1 was treated with 1mM sodium butyrate and the variant cell line AA/C1/SB obtained (see transformation section above). Furthermore, AA/C1/SB was insensitive to the inhibitory effects of further treatment with the same concentrations of sodium butyrate (1mM) and less sensitive to higher concentrations of sodium butyrate (Williams et al., manuscript in preparation).

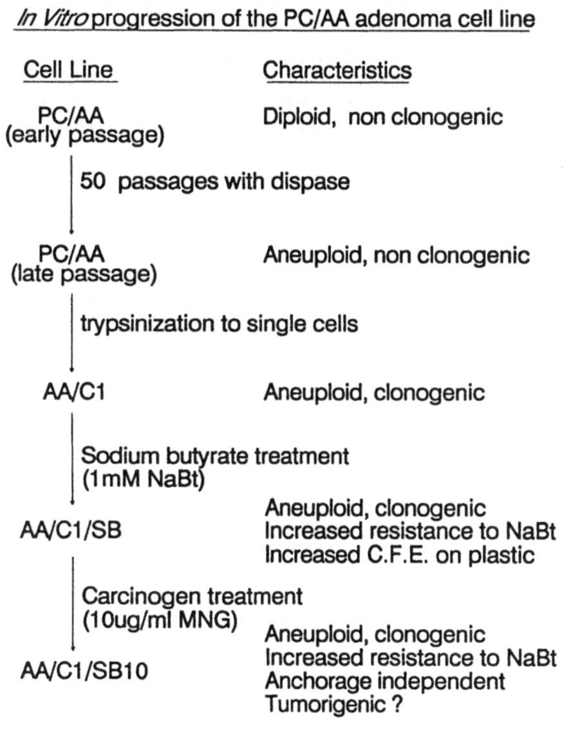

Fig. 1

CONCLUSIONS AND FUTURE PERSPECTIVES

There have been major developments in the molecular biology of colorectal cancer, in particular the mapping of the FPC gene to chromosome 5 (Bodmer et al., 1987), the realization that both activation of dominantly acting oncogenes and loss of tumour suppressor genes are involved (Solomon et al., 1987; Vogelstein et al., 1988). However, many important questions remain and some of these can be answered by a study of the biology of colorectal precancer. To analyse the multistage process of carcinogenesis it is necessary to have *in vitro* and *in vivo* markers (parameters) to distinguish the intermediate stages of cancer development. Potential markers to study tumour progression *in vitro* include: escape from senescence (*in vitro* immortalization), aneuploidy, clonogenicity, resistance to the inhibitory effects of the 'differentiation agent' sodium butyrate, anchorage independent growth, *ras* gene activation, production of mature (active) forms of proteinases and tumorigenicity in athymic nude mice. We have used some of these markers in our transformation of the diploid adenoma cell line to an aneuploid anchorage independent phenotype. This result is of particular interest and the PC/AA cells representing the different stages in progression (Figure 1) with a common genetic background should be invaluable to study genetic changes in tumour progression in relationship to the biology of the intermediate cells. The fact that it has taken approximately seven years and a series of insults for the PC/AA cells to progress to the anchorage independent phenotype emphasizes the remarkable stability of human cells.

Some of the remaining important questions are what events are involved in the development of colorectal adenomas, and are there different events involved in the formation of hereditary versus sporadic polyps? Although chromosome 5 allele loss has been reported in some FPC adenomas (Rees et al., 1989) most FPC adenomas do not show this loss of heterozygosity, however, chromosome 5 allele loss occurred relatively commonly (29%) in adenomas from patients without polyposis (Vogelstein et al., 1988). This implies that the development of adenomas, both hereditary and sporadic, but more commonly in hereditary adenomas, can occur even in the presence of one wild type FPC allele, i.e. when the polyps are heterozygous at the FPC locus. This is in contrast to the classical 2 mutation hypothesis of Knudson where in the event of 1 mutation occurring in one allele no tumour develops and only when the second allele is mutant or absent does the tumour occur. How does the heterozygous state therefore lead to the development of the polyps. One possibility is through a threshold effect involving for example negative control over the production of growth factors (Bodmer et al., 1987,) or that in the heterozygous state a mutant suppressor gene product (e.g. p53) may complex with the normal wild type gene product and inactivate it (Finlay et al., 1989).

If (as seems to be the case) all FPC patients develop many polyps, is the development of the polyps dependent simply on the loss of a single allele of the FPC gene or are other events involved? For example, in the classical mouse-skin 2 stage model of carcinogenesis there is evidence that *ras* gene mutations represent the initiation event but this is insufficient for the formation of the benign papilloma tumours and the application, after the initiation event, of the tumour promoter TPA is necessary for the development of the papilloma. If the initiation event (genetic) is insufficient for the development of a papilloma in mouse skin carcinogenesis, and it is quite clear that rodent cells are much less stable than human cells, then it may be that the development of a colorectal adenoma may require more than a simple loss of one FPC allele. If this is correct then the development of an adenoma may require the presence of a colonic tumour promoter. This would imply that the putative promoter of colonic carcinogenesis at least to the stage of the formation of an FPC adenoma is a compound found in every human intestine since all FPC patients regardless of diet and geography produce many polyps. This constitutively produced promoter could be a common physiological/dietary factor such as the bile/fatty acids. It is of course possible that the mouse-skin model is not an appropriate analogy for colorectal carcinogenesis and that a different mechanism is required for the formation of an adenoma such as a second mutation but in a different locus to the FPC.

However, when considering the development of adenomas and carcinomas in hereditary FPC patients it is important to remember that every cell in the colon (indeed in the body) is heterozygous at the FPC locus. Because each cell is heterozygous this has led to the belief that simply by chance there is an increased risk of the development of an adenoma because of the high number of "initiated" or altered target cells. Thus, making it inevitable that at least one or more of these "initiated" cells will acquire the remaining hit(s) necessary for tumour formation. This would be the case whether a further genetic change (although not at the same locus) or promotion is necessary for the development of the benign tumour. However, another possibly important factor is that in hereditary patients each cell as well as being heterozygous at the FPC locus is surrounded by heterozygous cells. In this situation there are no surrounding normal cells to restrain or suppress the growth of the FPC cells. In the case of sporadic patients rare somatic mutations giving rise to heterozygosity at the FPC locus or any other putative locus will result in altered cells which are surrounded by normal cells. Even in the possible situation where there is only one stem cell per crypt the initiated/altered cell in the sporadic patients may be suppressed by surrounding normal cells such as the muscularis mucosa/pericryptal cells or epithelial cells from surrounding crypts. In this case the surrounding influence of the normal cells may make it less likely for the sporadic heterozygous cell to progress to an adenoma. In this sporadic situation the action of a tumour promoter to allow clonal expansion of the altered cell may be necessary or another genetic event. This would imply that the local environment within the colon of an FPC patient is more amenable to the growth of the heterozygous cells than the local environment surrounding a heterozygous sporadic cell in a normal colon. Under these conditions therefore it is possible that in the FPC patients the development of the adenomas may not require either a further genetic change or tumour promoters whereas in sporadic patients one or more of these other events is necessary. This is consistent with the report of Vogelstein et al. (1988) that chromosome 5 allele loss occurs relatively commonly in patients without polyposis but not in polyposis patients.

With our isolation of sporadic and hereditary adenoma cell lines, some with *ras* and some without *ras* gene mutations, we may be able to investigate some of these possibilities. By doing reconstruction experiments involving mixing cells of different malignant potentials *in vitro* and determining whether the recovery of the more malignantly advanced cells depended on the presence of putative tumour promoters and/or whether the cells carried a *ras* gene mutation. One area which needs further work is the development of culture conditions for the long term *in vitro* growth of normal colonic epithelium. The response of normal colonic cells together with adenoma and carcinoma cells to putative promoters and growth factors such as Transforming Growth Factor ß could lead to important developments in understanding the control of growth and differentiation of both normal and neoplastic colonic epithelium. Cultured normal colonic epithelium could also be used in the reconstruction experiments involving adenoma and carcinoma cells described above.

ACKNOWLEDGEMENTS

This work was supported by the Cancer Research Campaign.

REFERENCES

Berry RD and Paraskeva C (1988) Expression of carcino-embryonic antigen by adenoma and carcinoma derived cell lines: possible marker of tumour progression and modulation of expression by sodium butyrate. Carcinogenesis 9: 447-450

Bodmer WF, Bailey CJ, Bodmer J and six others (1987) The gene for Familial Adenomatous Polyposis is on chromosome 5. Nature (Lond) 328: 614-616

Bos JL, Fearon ER, Hamilton SR, Verlaan de Vries M, van Boom JH , Van der Eb, AJ. and Vogelstein B (1987) Prevalence of *ras* gene mutations in human colorectal cancers. Nature 327: 293-297

Bussey HJR (1982) Colorectal Cancer: genetic factors. Rec. Res. Cancer Res. 83: 45-58

Farr CJ, Marshall CJ, Easty DJ, Wright NA, Powell SC, Paraskeva C (1988) A study of *ras* gene mutations in colonic adenomas from familial polyposis coli patients. Oncogene 3: 673-678

Finlay CA, Hinds PW, Levine A (1989) The p53 proto-oncogene can act as a suppressor of transformation. Cell 57: 1083-1093

Forrester K, Almoguera C, Han K, Grizzle WE, Pepucho M (1987) Detection of high incidence of K-*ras* oncogenes during human colon tumorigenesis. Nature (Lond) 327: 298-303

Lane EB (1982) Monoclonal antibodies provide specific intramolecular markers for the study of epithelial tonofilament organization. J. Cell. Biol. 92: 665-673

Maciewicz RA, Wardale RJ, Etherington DJ, Paraskeva C (1989) Immunodetection of cathepsins B and L present in and secreted from human pre-malignant and malignant colorectal tumour cell lines. Int J Cancer 43: 478-486

Muto T, Bussey HJR, Morson BC (1975) The evolution of cancer of the colon and rectum. Cancer 36: 2251-2270

Paraskeva C, Buckle BG, Sheer D, Wigley CB (1984) The isolation and characterization of colorectal epithelial cell lines at different stages in malignant transformation from familial polyposis coli patients. Int. J. Cancer 34: 49-56

Paraskeva C, Finerty S, Mountford RA, Powell SC (1989a) Specific cytogenetic abnormalities in two new human colorectal adenoma-derived epithelial cell lines. Cancer Res. 49: 1282-1286

Paraskeva C, Finerty S, Powell SC (1988) Immortalization of a human colorectal adenoma cell line by continuous *in vitro* passage: possible involvement of chromosome 1 in tumour progression. Int. J. Cancer 41: 908-912

Paraskeva C, Harvey A, Finerty S, Powell SC (1989b) Possible involvement of chromosome 1 in *in vitro* immortalization: evidence from progression of a human adenoma-derived cell line *in vitro*. Int. J. Cancer 43: 743-746

Parkinson EK (1985) Defective response of transformed keratinocytes to terminal differentiation stimuli. Their role in epidermal tumour promotion by phorbol esters and by deep skin wounding. Br. J. Cancer 52: 479-493

Rees M, Leigh SEA, Delhanty JDA, Jass JR (1989) Chromosome 5 allele loss in familial and sporadic colorectal adenomas. Br J Cancer 59: 361-365

Solomon E, Voss R, Hall V, Bodmer WF, Jass JR, Jeffreys AJ, Lucibello FC, Patel I, Rider SH (1987) Chromosome 5 allele loss in colorectal carcinomas. Nature (Lond) 328: 616-619

Vogelstein B, Fearon ER, Hamilton SR and seven others (1988). Genetic alterations during colorectal-tumour development. N. Engl. J. Med. 319: 525-532

Willson JKV, Bittner GN, Oberley TD, Meisner LF, Weese JL (1987) Cell culture of human colon adenomas and carcinomas. Cancer Res. 47: 2704-2713

Genetic Alterations in Colorectal Cancers in Correlation to Clinical Parameters

MANFRED SCHWAB, SILKE BRÜDERLEIN, KAI VAN DER BOSCH, ANDREAS WEITH, ILONA LEISTER, CELINA CZIEPLUCH, LUKAS AMLER, and PETER SCHLAG

ABSTRACT

Genetic alterations resulting in oncogenic activation of certain cellular genes or in deletion of tumor suppressor genes may play an important role in colorectal cancers. Cytogenetic and molecular genetic approaches led to the identification of non–random genetic alterations including mutational activation of *RAS* genes, and deletion of genetic material from various chromosomal loci. Our own systematic study of the chromosomal status of colorectal cancer cells has more recently uncovered cytogenetic evidence for DNA amplification. Our data raise the suspicion that amplification is mainly associated with an advanced or metastatic tumor stage (Dukes C or D). The study of other cancers had made evident that DNA amplification is a useful predictor for clinical outcome. Once the molecular identity of the amplified DNA in colorectal cancer is defined it should be possible to find out if amplified molecular probes may be useful for predicting the clinical behaviour of colorectal cancers.

Keywords: chromosomes; double minutes (DMs); homogeneously staining regions (HSRs); progression of tumors; deletion of DNA; oncogenes; tumor suppressor genes

1. ALLELIC LOSS AND MUTATIONAL CHANGE

1.1 Allelic loss

First indication for genetic changes in of colorectal cancer cells emerged from cytogenetic studies that had provided evidence for various chromosomal abnormalities. Because of the often bizarre complexity of chromosomal structures the significance of chromosomal abnormalities has remained enigmatic for long. Most of the chromosomal abnormalities found included complex translocations with generation of marker chromosomes of frequently unidentifyable genetic composition. A significant contribution was the observation of an interstitial deletion in chromosome 5 (5q13–22) in peripheral blood cells of a patient with Gardner's syndrome (Herrera et al., 1986). This finding would indicate loss of genetic material.

By application of molecular and cytogenetic techniques an increasing number of genetic changes of colorectal cancers is identified (Table 1). A number of investigators have surveyed colorectal cancers in order to find out whether loss of genetic material is a frequent genetic change in this malignancy. Interestingly, by using a polymorphic minisatellite probe, at least 20% of a heterogeneous set of tumors analyzed had lost genetic material from the 5q region (Solomon et al., 1987). Loss of genetic material in this region may be an important factor contributing to colorectal tumors and at the same time could point to a relationship between spontaneous colorectal tumors and familial adenomatous polyposis (FAP) for which the gene has also been localized by linkage analyses to the 5q region (Bodmer et al., 1987; Leppert et al., 1987; Meera Khan, 1988). The matter does become more complicated, though, considering the observation by Okamoto et al. (1988). They found loss of genetic material from colon carcinoma of patients with FAP not only in chromosome 5q but also in chromsome 22, with some additional losses in chromosomes 5, 6, 12q and 15.

Table 1. Genetic changes in colorectal cancers

Change	Chromosome	Reference
Deletion	5q	Herrera et al., 1986; Solomon et al., 1987 Okamoto et al., 1988
	22, 6, 5, 12q, 15	Okamoto et al., 1988
	1p	I. Leister et al. (unpublished data)
Mutation (*KRAS*)		Forrester et al., 1987 Bos et al., 1987
Amplification	DMs	Reichmann et al., 1981 Tal et al., 1988 S. Brüderlein et al. (unpublished data)

Loss of genetic material from chromsome 17 is a feature of more than 75% of colorectal cancers (Fearon et al., 1987; Vogelstein et al., 1989). Cells having lost genetic material from chromosome 17 have retained only one allele of the gene encoding the transformation associated protein p53, which has been identified to have tumor suppressing activity. In two of the analyzed tumors the remaining p53 allele had undergone a mutational change that converts the suppressor gene into an activated cellular oncogene (Baker et al., 1989). It is possible, therefore, that p53 mutations are involved in colorectal cancers, perhaps through inactivation of a tumor suppressor function of the wild-type 53 allele. Allelotyping of colorectal carcinomas has revealed additional chromosomal regions with allelic loss (Vogelstein et al., 1989).

Our own studies have detected an up to 50% incidence of allelic loss of the distal region of chromosome 1p (Leister et al., manuscript in preparation). This observation is particularly interesting in view of the fact that the distal 1p region is deleted in a major proportion of advanced stage neuroblastomas (Weith et al., 1989), in melanomas (Dracopoli et al., 1989), and in ductal carcinoma of the breast (Genuardi et al., 1989). It is possible that deletions of the chromosome 1p region play a role in a broad spectrum of tumors. Our preliminary data of 25 tumors suggest that 1p deletion was correlated to the histological grade of colorectal carcinoma and was most frequently observed in undifferentiated tumors of grade 3 (Table 2; Leister et al., manuscript in preparation).

Table 2. Deletion chromosome 1p and grading*

	GRADE		
	I	II	III
deletion (–)	3 (100%)	7 (70%)	5 (42%)
deletion (+)	0 (0%)	3 (30%)	7 (58%)

*Ilona Leister et al., manuscript in preparation

1.2 Mutational change

Additional genetic changes are associated with colorectal cancers, as shown in studies by Bos et al. (1987) and Forrester et al. (1987). A total of 93 colorectal tumors of various types was analyzed for mutational activation of *RAS* genes. Roughly 40% of the tumors were found to contain a mutationally activated *KRAS* oncogene. No significant difference was found between mutation frequency and degree of differentiation or tumor stage. A high incidence of mutated *KRAS* was found in tumors originating in villous adenomas. The mutations were specific for tumors and were not detected in normal surrounding colon tissue. Interestingly, in few cases both mutated *KRAS* and mutated *NRAS* coexisted in the same tumor (Forrester et al., 1987), although the investigators failed to show that the two mutated *RAS* genes were present in the same cell.

2. AMPLIFICATION OF CELLULAR ONCOGENES

Among the chromsomal abnormalities indicating genetic changes in cells of colorectal cancers "double minutes" (DMs) appear to be frequent. DMs indicate the presence of amplified cellular DNA. With the exception of metabolically specialized drug resistant cells, the DMs in cancer cells are indicators for amplified cellular oncogenes (for details see Schwab, 1985, 1990).

The term gene amplification refers to the selective increase of the gene copy number and is better designated as DNA amplification. It should not be confused with elevated gene expression, although amplification generally does result in enhanced levels of the products encoded by the amplified gene. Amplification is one of the mechanisms by which cells can meet the demand for synthesis of specific gene products in amounts exceeding the transcriptional capacity of a single copy gene.

2.1 Amplification in colorectal cancers

Colorectal cancers represent an interesting group of tumors in which cytogenetic evidence for amplification has been obtained but in which the identity of the amplified DNA is not known for most cases. Earlier studies of two cell lines had revealed amplification of *MYC* in line COLO 320 (Alitalo et al., 1983) and of *MYB* in line COLO 201/205 (Alitalo et al., 1984). These two lines presumably represent nontypical cases, because COLO 320 cells possess neuroendocrine properties and are of unknown provenience, and COLO 201/205 cells lack cytogenetic evidence for amplification. Amplification of *MYC* has also been reported for two of 12 primary tumors (Finley et al., 1989). The degree of amplification was only 3–4 fold, however, and did not correlate with expression. It is difficult, in the absence of cytogenetic data, to exclude the possibility of aneuploidy. In a recent study by Tal et al. (1988) amplification in the range of 20-fold of the *ERB*B2 gene was found in two of 45 patients with colon cancer and in one of four patients with rectal cancer.

In an effort to understand the role that gene amplification might have for the development of colorectal cancer we established a combined cytogenetic and molecular genetic program. At this point we have collected tumor material from more than 150 colorectal cancer patients and have established a series of cell lines, for cytogenetic and molecular analyses. We have identified 15 cases out of a series of 27 tumor cell lines analyzed in which cytogenetic evidence for gene amplification is evident. Usually DMs are easily detectable; in one case DMs were apparently replaced by an HSR during long-term culture. While we could identify amplification of the *ERB*B2 oncogene in four tumors out of 150 tested, most of the tumors that showed cytogenetic evidence for gene amplification were negative for amplification of *ERB*B2 or of several other oncogenes like *MYC* or *RAS* (Kai van der Bosch, unpublished data). Additionally, we did not detect amplification of a known oncogene in several cell lines obtained from another laboratory (Park et al., 1987). We assume that in many cases tumor cells showing cytogenetic evidence carry amplification of an as yet unidentified cellular oncogene.

In an attempt to define the identity of the genetic information in DMs, we are isolating amplified DNA. There are several strategies that can be used for isolation of amplified DNA in those cases in which molecular probes for identification are not yet available. One of the procedures involves isolation of DMs directly by micromanipulation procedures. We have collected under microscopic inspection DMs from metaphases of colon cancer cells with a fine needle. The DNA was isolated using micromanipulation, and was molecularly cloned. Future studies should inform us about the genetic nature and chromosomal origin of the amplified DNA, resulting in further understanding of the significance of gene amplification in colorectal cancer.

3. THE POSSIBLE ROLE OF DNA AMPLIFICATION IN TUMORIGENESIS

Amplification gained for the first time significance as a genetic change associated with tumorigenesis when it was discovered that human neuroblastomas frequently contain an amplified oncogene *MYCN* localized in DMs or HSRs (Schwab et al., 1983). *MYCN* is a member of a gene family referred to as *MYC*-box genes (Schwab, 1988). Neuroblastomas have been classified into Evans stages I-IV, with stage IV being the most advanced. In studies of more than 400 tumors, nearly all of the amplifications detected were present in the more advanced tumors of stage III and IV (Brodeur et al., 1984; Seeger et al., 1985). The progression-free survival over a period of 18 months of standardized therapy was 70% for patients whose tumors lacked amplification and decreased to 30% in cases with 3-10 copies and to 5% in cases with more than 10 copies (Seeger et al., 1985). *MYCN* copy number is a useful marker for assessing prognosis of neuroblastoma and may be useful for devising therapy.

Similar principles of a correlation between amplification of oncogenes and tumor progression have been found in other types of tumors, such as lung cancer (Brooks et al., 1987) and breast cancer (Slamon et al., 1987). In breast cancer the amplification of the *ERB*B2 oncogene has been frequently encountered. The *ERB*B2 gene has been found to be amplified between 2- and 20-fold in roughly 30% of breast cancer cells (Slamon et al., 1987; 1989). A positive correlation of *ERB*B2 amplification with involved lymph nodes was noted (Slamon et al., 1987), indicating a role of amplification in disease progression. In the same study a strong association between *ERB*B2 amplification and relapsefree and overallsurvival was detected. This clearly makes *ERB*B2 amplification a valuable parameter for assessment of prognosis. Altogether *ERB*B2 amplification in breast cancer provides a case in which amplification of an oncogene might contribute to tumor progression.

In the case of colorectal cancers the frequency of DNA amplification at this moment can only be assessed by cytogenetic inspections, due to the lack of informative molecular probes in most instances. The trend that has emerged from 27 tumors for which the cytogenetic analysis was successful is that amplification significantly correlates with high tumor stage (Dukes C or D; Table 3). This observation appears to be consistent with the idea of a contribution of amplification to tumor progression.

Table 3. Amplification and tumor stage*

	DUKES STAGE			
	A	B	C	D
Amplification (−)	5 (83%)	3 (75%)	3 (37%)	1 (11%)
Amplification (+)	1 (17%)	1 (25%)	5 (63%)	8 (89%)

* Silke Brüderlein et al., manuscript in preparation

4. CONCLUSIONS

Various genetic changes have been found in colorectal cancer. As fas as we know, there is no single genetic change that alone is associated with colorectal cancer. Progression to malignancy presumably results from a combination of various types of genetic changes on different chromosomes. Of particular significance appear to be three types of genetic changes: 1.) allelic loss of genetic material; 2.) mutations of *RAS* genes; and 3.) amplification of DNA. Whatever the role of each of these genetic alterations might be, their multiplicity indicates that several alterations are associated with the evolution of the normal to the malignant cell. Individual changes presumably represent single components of this evolutionary process with amplification apparently contributing to metastatic stages of colorectal cancers. Our present results suggest that amplification significantly correlates to advanced Dukes stage, while chromosme 1p deletion is prominent in high grade tumors consisting mainly of poorly differentiated cells. The observations indicate that knowledge about individual genetic changes, such as amplification of DNA, may provide us with useful tools to predict the clinical behaviour of colorectal cancers.

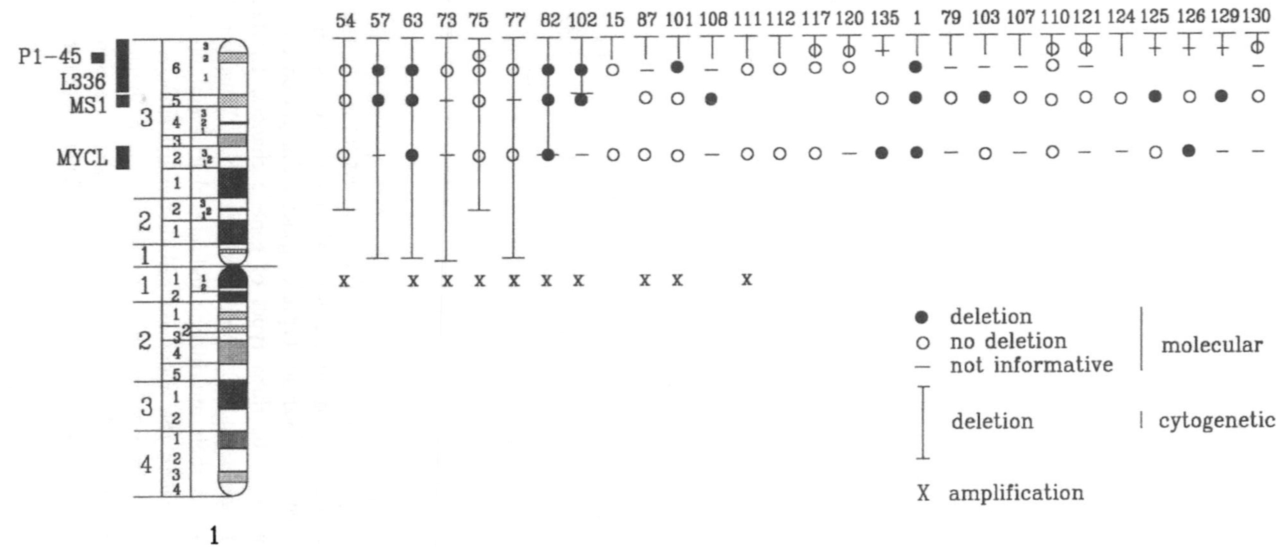

DNA-amplification (x) and chromosome 1p deletion (•) in colorectal cancers

REFERENCES

Alitalo K, Schwab M, Lin CC, Varmus HE, Bishop JM (1983) Homogeneously staining chromosomal regions contain amplified copies of an abundantly expressed cellular oncogene *MYC* in malignant neuroendocrine cells from a human colon carcinoma. Proc Natl Acad Sci USA 80:1707–1711

Alitalo K, Winqvist R, Lin CC, de la Chapelle A, Schwab M, Bishop JM (1984) Aberrant expression of an amplified c–myb oncogene in two cell lines from a colon carcinoma. Proc Natl Acad Sci USA 81:4534–4538

Baker S, Fearon ER, Nigro JM, Hamilton SR, Preisinger AC, Jessup JM, van Tuinen P, Ledbetter DH, Barker DF, Nakamura Y, White R, Vogelstein BC (1989) Chromosome 17 deletions and p53 gene mutations in colorectal carcinomas. Science 244:217–221

Bodmer WF, Bailey CJ, Bodmer J, Bussey HJR, Ellis A, Gorman P, Lubicello FC, Murday VA, Rider SH, Scambler P, Sheer D, Solomon E, Spurr NK (1987) Localization of the gene for familial adenomatous polyposis on chromosome 5. Nature 328:614–616

Bos J, Fearon E, Hamilton S, de Vries M, van Boom J, van der Eb A, Vogelstein B (1987) Prevalence of ras gene mutations in human colorectal cancers. Nature 327:293–297

Brodeur J, Seeger RC, Schwab M, Varmus HE, Bishop JM (1984). Amplification of *NMYC* in untreated human neuroblastoma correlates with advanced disease stage. Science 224 1121–1124

Brooks B, Battey J, Nau MM, Gazdar A, Minna J (1987). Amplification and expression of the myc gene in small cell lung cancer. Adv Viral Oncol 7:155–172

Dracopoli NC, Harnett P, Bale S, Stanger BZ, Tucker MA, Housman DE, Kefford RF (1989) Loss of alleles from the distal short arm of chromosome 1 occurs late in melanoma tumor progression. Proc Natl Acad Sci USA 86:4614–4618

Fearon ER, Hamilton SR, Vogelstein B (1987) Clonal analysis of human colorectal tumors. Science 238:193–197

Finley GG, Schulz NT, Hill SA, Geiser JR, Pipas JM, Meisler AI (1989) Expression of the *MYC* family in different stages of human colorectal cancer. Oncogene 4:963–971

Forrester K, Almoguere C, Han K, Grizzle W, Perucho M (1987) Detection of high incidence of K–ras oncogenes during human colon tumorigenesis. Nature 327:298–303

Genuardi M, Tsihir H, Anderson DEE, Saunders GF (1989) Distal deletion of chromosome 1p in ductal carcinoma of the breast. Am J Hum Genet 45:73–82

Herrera L, Kakati S, Gibas L, Pietrzak E, Sandberg AA (1986) Brief clinical Report: Gardner Syndrome in a man with an interstitial deletion of 5q. Am J Med Genet 25:473–476

Leppert M, Dobbs M, Scambler P, O'Conell P, Makamura Y, Stauffer D, Woodward S, Burt R, Hughes J, Gardner E, Lathrop M, Wasmuth J, Lalouel J–M, White R (1987) The gene for familial polyposis coli maps to the long arm of chromosome 5. Science 328:1411–1413

Meera Khan P, Tops CMJ, Broek M, Breukel C, Wignen JT, Oldenburg M, Bos J, Leeuwen–Cornelisse ISJ, Vasen HFA, Griffioen G, Verspaget HM, Hartog Jager FCA, Lamers CBHW (1988) Close linkage of highly polymorphic marker (D5S37) to familial adenomatous polyposis (FAP) and confirmation of FAP localization on chromosome 5q21–22. Hum Genet 79:183–185

Okamoto M, Sasaki M, Sugio K, Sato C, Iwama T, Ikeuchi T, Tonomura A, Sasazuki T, Miyaki M (1988) Loss of constitutional heterozygosity in colon carcinoma from patients with familial polyposis coli. Nature 331:273–277

Park JG, Oie HK, Sugarbaker PH, Henslee J, Chen T–R, Johnson BE, Gazdar AF (1987) Characteristics of cell lines established from human colorectal carcinoma. Cancer Res 47:6710–6718

Reichmann A, Martin P, Levin B (1981) Chromosomal banding pattern in human large bowel cancer. Int J Cancer 28:431–440

Schwab M, Alitalo K, Klempnauer KH, Varmus HE, Bishop JM, Gilbert F, Brodeur G, Goldstein M, Trent J (1983). Amplified DNA with limited homology to MYC cellular oncogene is shared by human neuroblastoma cell lines and a neuroblastoma tumor. Nature 305:245–248

Schwab M (1985). Amplification of N–myc in human neuroblastomas. Trends Genet 1:271–275

Schwab M (1988) The MYC–box oncogenes. In: Reddy P, Skalka AM, Curran T (eds) The Oncogene Handbook. Elsevier Science Publishers, pp 381–391

Schwab M, Schlag P, Brüderlein S, van der Bosch K (1989) Oncogene amplification in colorectal cancer. In: Herrera L (ed) Familial Adenomatous Polyposis. Alan Liss, pp 343–352

Schwab M (1990) Amplification of cellular oncogenes: A predictor for clinical outcome of some human malignancies. Genes, Chromosomes and Cancer (in press)

Seeger RC., Brodeur GM, Sather H, Dalton A, Siegel SE, Wong KY, Hammond D (1985). Association of multiple copies of the N–myc oncogene with rapid progression of neuroblastomas. N Engl J Med 313:1111–1116

Slamon DJ, Clark GM, Wong GS, Levin WJ, Ullrich A, McGuire WL (1987) Human breast cancer: Correlation of relapse and survival with amplification of the HER–2/neu oncogene. Science 235:177–182

Slamon D, Godolphin W, Jones LA, Holt JA, Wong SG, Keith DΓ, Levin WJ, Stuart SG, Udove J, Ullrich A, Press MF (1989) Studies of the HER–2/neu proto–oncogene in human breast and ovarian cancer. Science 244:707–712

Solomon E, Voss R, Hall V, Bodmer WF, Jass JR, Jeffreys AF, Lucibello FC, Patel I, Rider SH (1987) Chromosome 5 allele loss in human colorectal carcinomas. Nature 328:616–619

Tal M, Wetzler M, Josefberg Z, Deutch A, Gutmann M, Assaf D, Kris R, Shiloh Y, Girol D, Schlessinger J (1988) Sporadic amplification of the HER2/neu protooncogene in adenocarcinomas of various tissues. Cancer Res 48:1517–1520

Vogelstein B, Fearon ER, Kern SE, Hamilton SR, Preisinger AC, Nakamura Y, White R (1989) Allelotype of colorectal carcinoma. Science 244:207–211

Weith A, Martinsson T, Cziepluch C, Brüderlein S, Amler L, Berthold F, Schwab M (1989) Neuroblastoma consensus deletion maps to chromosome 1p36.1–2. Genes, Chromosomes and Cancer 1:81–88

Clinical and Pathological Associations with Molecular Genetic Alterations in Colorectal Carcinoma

STANLEY R. HAMILTON and SCOTT E. KERN

Abstract

Our collaborative group has studied molecular genetic alterations in colorectal neoplasms including ras gene mutations, allelic deletions on chromosomes 5, 17, and 18, and extent of allelic loss on non-acrocentric autosomal arms. These alterations were compared to the clinical and pathologic features of the carcinomas. Our findings suggest that: (1) "Familial" colorectal carcinoma may differ in pathogenesis from "sporadic" tumors, or familial factors may increase the tendancy of an established tumor to tolerate or promote the accumulation of clonal genetic abnormalities. (2) Right-sided as compared with left-sided carcinomas have different molecular genetic alterations, possibly related to different pathogenetic factors. (3) Deletions of 17p and 18q and extensive allelic deletions which include other sites are associated with poorer prognosis.

Key words: Colonic neoplasms, rectal neoplasms, oncogenes, chromosome deletions, prognosis.

Our collaborative group has studied molecular genetic alterations which occur during the development of colorectal neoplasms (Vogelstein 1988). Based on nonrandom cytogenetic abnormalities reported for colorectal carcinoma, we studied allelic deletions on chromosomes 17 and 18. We have now identified the gene for p53, a nuclear phosphoprotein, as the target of the chromosome 17p deletions (Baker 1989). We investigated genetic probes on the long arm of chromosome 5 which have been linked to adenomatous polyposis syndrome. We also studied mutation of the ras genes which encode for proteins involved in signal transduction across the cell membrane, due to their importance in carcinogenesis.

Our studies of the clinical and pathological associations with molecular genetic alterations in colorectal carcinomas shed light on the etiology and prognosis of these tumors (Kern 1989). To examine the extent and variation of allelic loss in this common tumor, we studied polymorphic DNA markers from every nonacrocentric autosomal arm in 56 pairs of specimens with colorectal carcinoma and adjacent grossly normal colonic mucosa (Vogelstein 1989). The result of this analysis was termed "allelotype", by analogy with karyotype. We found that allelic losses were remarkably common, as one of the alleles of each polymorphic marker tested was lost in at least some carcinomas, and some tumors lost more than half of their parental alleles. In addition to allelic deletions, new DNA fragments not present in grossly normal mucosa were identified in five carcinomas. These new fragments contained repeated sequences of the variable number of tandem repeat type.

As regards the etiology of colorectal cancer, patients with a family history of cancer in a first degree relative had a mean fractional allelic loss (FAL, defined as the number of chromosomal arms lost divided by the number of evaluable chromosomal arms) which was twice that of patients without a positive family history (0.296 vs. 0.150, p = .0002). When the specific deletions were assessed, a positive family history was associated with deletions of 17p, the site of p53. 17p deletion was more common in left-sided colorectal carcinomas than in right-sided tumors (93% of left-sided tumors vs. 60% of right-sided tumors, p= .004). Allelic deletions of 17p and of 18q were less common in mucin-producing carcinomas than in non-mucin producing tumors (17p deletion in 44% of mucin-producing carcinomas vs. 88% of non-mucin producing tumors; 18q deletion in 47% vs. 85%). These findings suggest that familial colorectal carcinoma, as opposed to "sporadic" tumors, may differ in pathogenesis or that familial factors may increase the tendency of an established tumor to tolerate or promote the accumulation of clonal genetic abnormalities. The differences in molecular genetics of right- vs. left-sided carcinomas is of interest due to the epidemiologic evidence suggesting different pathogenetic factors and the recent historical trend toward a higher proportion of right-sided tumors in the USA.

Molecular genetic alterations also appear to relate to prognosis. We found that the presence of distant metastases was significantly associated with high fractional allelic loss and with deletions of 17p and 18q. Among those patients with Dukes' B and C carcinomas who were without clinical metastases at the time of resection, 6 of 18 patients with 17p deletion were found to have metastases during follow-up, but all 10 patients without 17p deletion remained clinically free of metastasis. Although mutations of ras proto-oncogenes occurred in nearly half of the cancers and deletions of 5q in about 1/3, these genetic alterations had no prognostic importance. It remains uncertain whether the alterations of 17p and 18q are causally associated with metastatic potential or only represent sensitive markers of generalized chromosomal changes accounting for tumor aggressiveness. The relative importance of specific as opposed to general measures of allelic loss is not yet known.

Clinical documentation of metastatic disease remains as the single best predictor of poor prognosis in colorectal cancer. A major goal of studies of the cell biology of primary tumors is to explain the occurrence of the metastatic phenotype, i.e. the characteristics that lead to the development of metastases. Additional studies are clearly needed, but identification of molecular clues to aid in prognostication among patients without initial evidence of disseminated disease may be at hand.

REFERENCES

Baker SJ, Fearon ER, Nigro JM, Hamilton SR, Preisinger AC, Jessup JM, Vatuinen P, Ledbetter DH, Barker DF, Nakamura Y, White R, Vogelstein B (1989) Chromosome 17 deletions and p53 gene mutations in colorectal carcinomas. Science 244:217-221

Kern SE, Fearon ER, Tersmette KWF, Enterline JP, Leppert M, Nakamura Y, White R, Vogelstien B, Hamilton SR (1989) Allelic loss in colorectal carcinoma. JAMA 261:3099-3103

Vogelstein B, Fearon ER, Hamilton SR, Kern SE, Preisinger AC, Leppert M, Nakamura Y, White R, Smits AMM, Bos JL (1988) Genetic alterations during colorectal tumor development. N Engl J Med 319:525-532

Vogelstein B, Fearon ER, Kern SE, Hamilton SR, Preisinger AC, Nakamura Y, White R (1989) Allelotype of colorectal carcinomas. Science 244:207-211

A Subset of Genetic Alterations Distinguish Distal from Proximal Colorectal Cancer

S. Olschwang, O. Delattre, H. Leroy, Y. Remvikos, T. Melot, D.J. Law, A.P. Feinberg, and G. Thomas

ABSTRACT

The site distribution of colorectal carcinoma along the colorectum in Adenomatous Polyposis Coli syndrome differs from that observed in Hereditary Non-Polyposis Colorectal Cancer syndromes (Lynch syndromes). In the latter case most tumors appear in proximal colon and are not usually preceded by the development of polyps. A study of a set of acquired genetic alterations performed in more than one hundred sporadic colorectal adenocarcinomas has shown a nonrandom association of deletions and mitotic abnormalities by site, with both types of alterations occuring significantly more frequently in distal tumors. In contrast, the frequency of c-Ki-ras mutations and the Dukes'stage did not differ significantly between proximal and distal cancers. In accord with the study of familial predispositions to colorectal cancer, these data provide support to the hypothesis that proximal and distal colon carcinomas might differ in the genetic mechanisms involved in their initiation and/or progression.

KEY WORDS : Allelic Loss, DNA Index, Adenomatous Polyposis Coli, Lynch Syndromes, Tumor Initiation /Progression

INTRODUCTION

Three lines of evidence have suggested that adenocarcinomas from the proximal colon might differ both in their initiation and in their evolution from those of the rest of the colorectum. First epidemiological studies in western countries have reported over the last decades an increase in the incidence of the proximal tumors compared to that of distal tumors (Snyder 1978, Mamazza 1982, Beart 1983). This difference does not seem to be due to the advent of better diagnostic techniques (Beart 1983). Significant differences were also observed in the relative frequency of proximal and distal tumors in different populations (Johnson 1986). Second, familial studies have suggested that at least some genes involved in colorectal carcinogenesis might be different. In familial Adenomatous Polyposis Coli patients, numerous adenomatous polyps usually occur and degenerate to carcinoma in the distal part of the colorectum (Bussey 1975). In hereditary non-polyposis colorectal cancers (Lynch syndromes) most tumors appear in proximal colon and are not preceded by the development of multiple polyps (Lynch 1985). Third, proximal and distal tumors show difference in the expression of cellular oncogene such as c-myc (Rothberg 1985). The basis of these differences has not yet been explained from our present knowledge of colorectal carcinogenesis.

Three general types of genetic alterations are acquired in colorectal cancer. The first type is a change in the DNA content of the malignant cells which can be monitored by flow cytometry (Remvikos 1988). The second type of alterations is a loss of genetic material which is investigated either by cytogenetics or by looking for loss of alleles using RFLP probes. Although almost any part of the genome has been shown to be potent site for loss of alleles (Vogelstein 1989), the most frequent losses have been shown to occur on the short arm of chromosome 17 and on chromosome 18. Since the gene for Familial Adenomatous Polyposis Coli syndrome was mapped to the long arm of chromosome 5, it was found using RFLPs that alleles on 5q were lost in approximately one third to a half of carcinomas (Solomon 1987, Law 1988, Vogelstein 1988, Okamoto 1988, Wildrick 1988, Ashton-Rickardt 1989). The third frequent type of alteration is the mutation of specific genes. In nearly 40% of tumors, the activation by point mutation of a Ki-ras cellular oncogene has been observed (Bos 1987, Forrester 1987, Vogelstein 1988). This activation almost always occurs by altering the coding properties of the 12th or the 13th codon.

We have examined a large number of patients for each type of alteration and have tested the possible relationship of each of these alterations with tumor location.

MATERIALS AND METHODS

Fresh tissues were obtained from patients referred to the Curie Institute, the Johns Hopkins Hospital, the University of Michigan Hospital, the Roswell Park Memorial Institute, and the Cleveland Clinic from 1981 to 1988. The tumors were categorized into anatonomical subgroups : proximal (from caecum to splenic flexure), distal (from splenic flexure to end of sigmoid) and rectal. Tumors were classified according to modified Dukes'stage (Dukes 1932). Our series is representative of the colorectal carcinomas found in western countries with respect to site of tumor, age of patients at diagnosis and staging. However, in our series, tumors from female patients amounted to 60% of the total tumors studied. Sex does not appear to influence distribution of cancer by site or Dukes' stage (Eisenberg 1982). In this work, no heterogeneity was observed between sexes with respect to the occurence of genetic alterations. We have excluded from this study carcinomas which occurred in Adenomatous Polyposis Coli patients.

All but 20 tumor DNAs were extracted from surgical specimens which were cryostat-sectioned as had been described (Vogelstein 1988). In five cases, the tumor DNA was extracted from flow sorted hyperploid nuclei, and in fifteen cases, from first or second passage of tumors grafted on nude mice. In the nine cases in which it was possible to compare the karyotype of the primary tumor to that of its grafted homologue, only minor variations, which did not involve chromosome 5, 17 or 18, were observed (Lefrançois, in press). The probes used (and their chromosomal location) were : D17S28 (17p13.3), D17S30 (17p13.3), D17S1 (7p13), MYH2(17p13.1), D17S67 (17P12), D17S68 (17P13), D18S7 (18q11), D18S8 (18q21.3), D18S5 (18q21.3-qter), D18S3 (18p11.3), D5S71 (5q21-22), D5S52 (5q21-22), D5S49 (5q21-22), D5S58 (5q21-22) (Kidd 1988). Some of the data obtained on this series of patients have been previously reported (Monpezat 1988, Law 1988, Delattre 1989). Allelic typing of constitutional and tumor DNA was performed using slight modifications of Southern technique previously described (Monpezat 1988).

C-Ki-ras mutations were investigated on DNAs amplified with the Taq polymerase according to the method of Bos (1987) using the same amplimers. The detection of the mutations was performed by sequential hybridization to 12 oligonuclotides each specific for one of the twelve possible single point mutations that would substitute glycine at the 12th and 13th position of the peptide sequence.

Flow cytometry measurements were performed as previously described (Remvikos 1988). The ratio of the DNA content of malignant cells to that of normal cells is called the DNA index of the tumor and is here termed

n. When two proliferating clones with different DNA indexes were observed in a same tumor, the larger DNA index was used. Two by two tables were analysed by chi-square test with Yates' correction. Multiple regression analysis was performed with the statistical package SSPS/PC+.

RESULTS

1.Dependence of DNA Index Distribution on Tumor Site.

Figure 1 shows the histogram for the distribution of the DNA index of the cancerous cells of colorectal carcinomas as measured by flow cytometry and classified according to their site of occurence in the colorectum. All surgical specimens used for the preparation of the nuclei

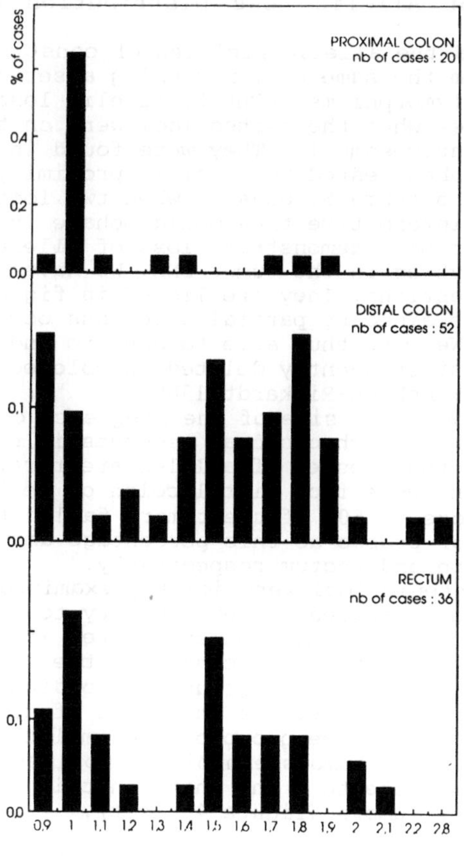

Figure 1: **Distribution of DNA indexes according to tumor site.** The nuclei of 108 colorectal adenocarcinomas were analyzed by flow-cytometry and their DNA index scored according to materials and methods. The data were grouped according to the site of occurence of the tumors along the colorectum.

to be analysed contained invariably exactly diploid cells (n=1) and most of the time a clearly aneuploid population whose DNA index was used to compile the figure. When the specimen exhibited only an exactly diploid population of cells, we ascertained the presence within this population of actively proliferating cancerous cells by checking for the presence in the flow cytogram of large populations in the S phase and the G2 phase which were never observed in preparations from non cancerous fragments of colorectal mucosae. It appeared that tumors from distal colon and rectum have a very wide distribution of DNA indexes which can schematically be divided into two groups : the tumors that have a DNA index smaller that 1.3 which were termed paradiploid and those that have a DNA index greater or equal to 1.3 which were termed hyperploid. At variance, cancer cells of most proximal colon carcinomas have an exactly diploid content of DNA (n=1) and the hyperploid tumors are hardly represented.

2.Dependence of Allelic Loss Distribution on Tumor Site

We next compared the allelic profiles of constitutional DNA and that of tumor DNA from the same patients using a set of probes detecting restriction length polymorphisms (RFLPs). Allelic losses were found in two thirds of the cases when the tested loci were on the short arm of chromosome 17 or on chromosome 18. They were found in close to 40% of the cases when the probes tested for loci in proximity to the APC locus on the long arm of chromosome 5. Usually when two loci on the same chromosomal arm were informative they would behave in a similar manner i.e. they would either both demonstrate loss of alleles or would both show retained heterozyties in the tumor DNA. We have however encountered a small number of exceptions. They are listed in fig 2. These exceptions can most simply be explained by partial deletions occuring in the tested chromosomal segment. We were thus able to confirm and further restrict the common regions most frequently deleted in colorectal carcinomas (Vogelstein 1988,1989; Ashton-Rickardt 1989).

The dependence on tumor site of the frequency of the loss of alleles on the three tested chromosomal segments is presented on figure 3. It clearly appears that losses of alleles are rarer in tumors from proximal colon than in those from distal colon or rectum.
In proximal colon, close to 60% of the tumors failed to exhibit loss of alleles with our set of probes as this percentage amounted to only 3% and 14% in distal colon and rectum respectively.

When two non syntenic loci were jointly examined it appeared that the loss of one allele increased the probability to observe a loss on the other non syntenic chromosomal segment tested (figure 4,right). This correlation was statistically significant when the tumors from all sites were included. When the tumors were grouped according to site, statistical significance was lost for the group of distal or rectal tumors but remained true for the group of proximal tumors.

We also observed that tumors exhibiting no loss of alleles on 17p and 18 had a DNA index close to 1 and that, in this series, none were in the hyperploid group of tumors (figure 4, left).

3.Dependence of the Distribution of Dukes' Stage and Frequency of Ki-ras Mutations According to Tumor Site

The distribution of Dukes'stage and the frequency of Ki-ras mutations is shown on figure 3. Although small differences were observed among subgroups, none reached statistical significance.

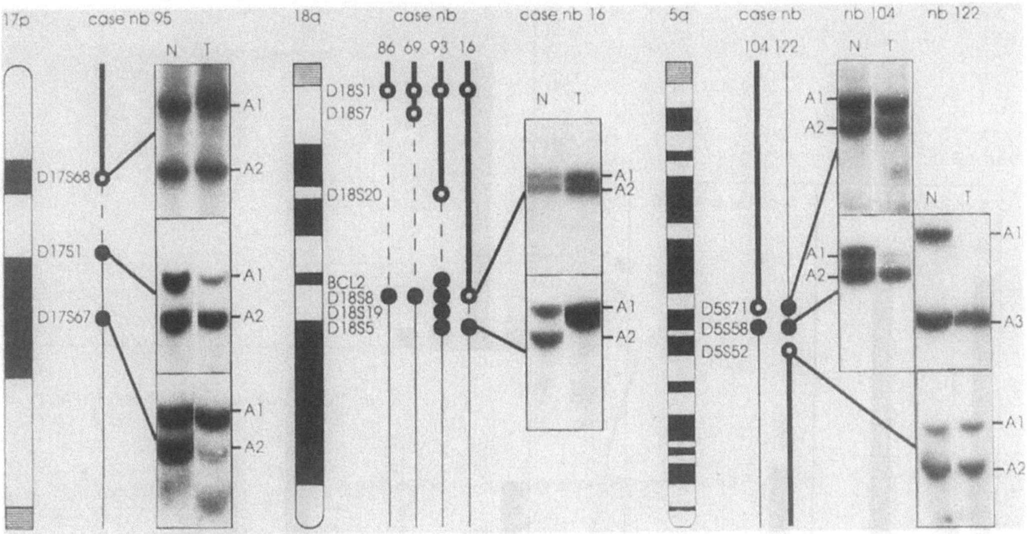

Figure 2: **Partial deletions of 17p, 18q and 5q in colorectal carcinomas.**The banding pattern of the three investigated segments is schematically shown. For each tumor, the open circles and closed circles represent sites where heterozygosity has been maintained and lost respectively. The regions most probably maintained diploid in the tumor and those being hemizigously present in the tumor cells are shown as a thick and a thin line respectively..Autoradiograms of the most interesting cases are also included.

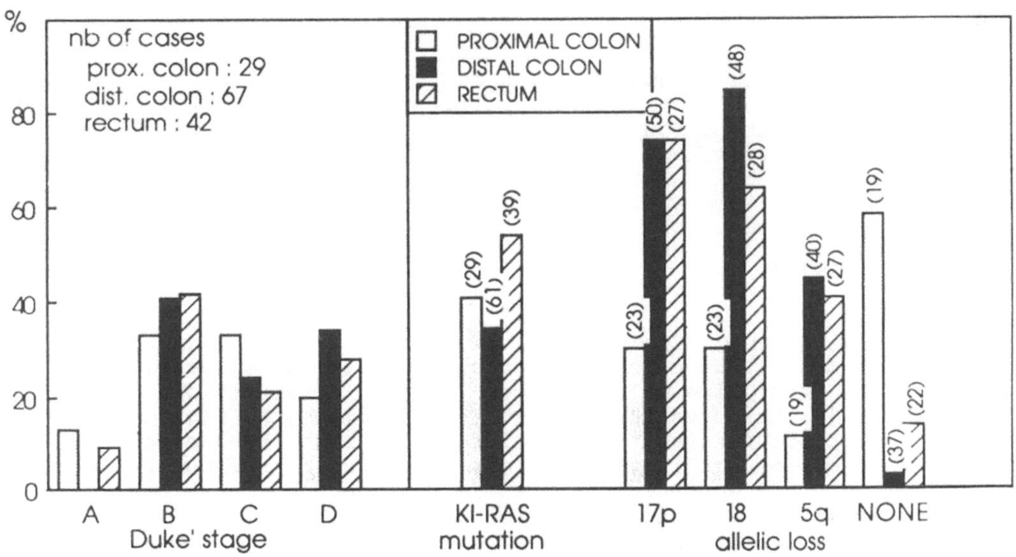

Figure 3: **Dependence according to site of occurence of Dukes'stage distribution and of Ki-ras mutation and allelic loss frequency.**On the left is shown the histogram distribution of Dukes'stage in our series.On the right, is displayed the frequency of allelic losses and of Ki-ras mutations. The number in parenthesis is the number of informative tumors from which these percentages were computed.

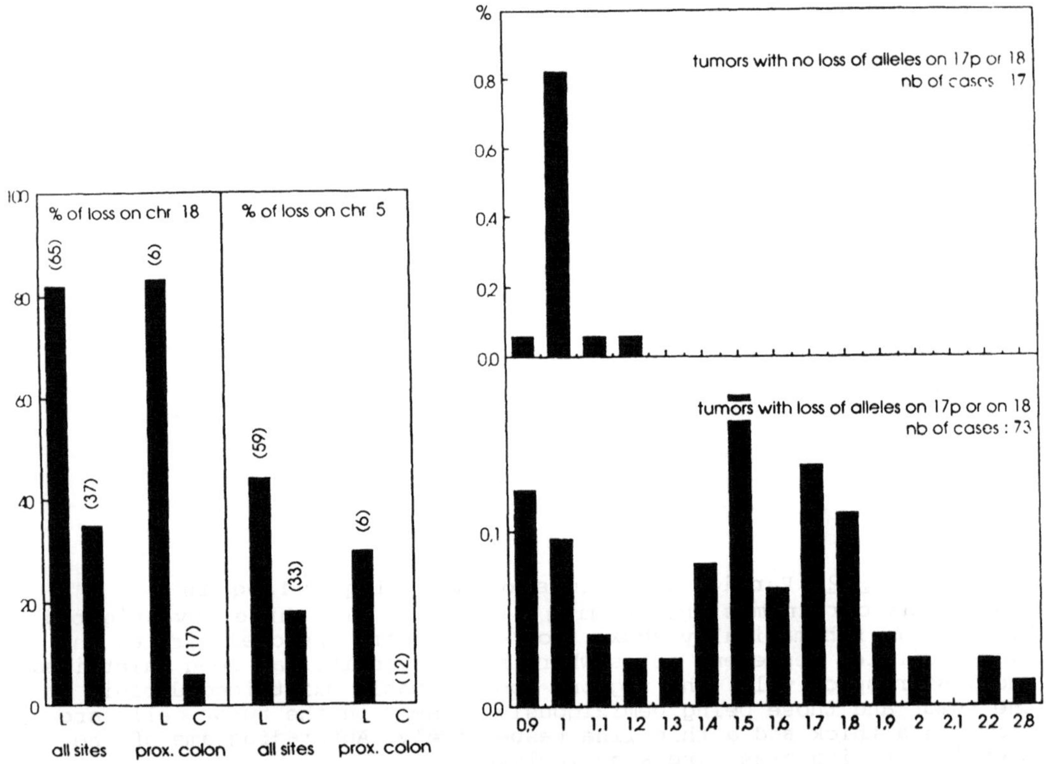

Figure 4: **Correlations between genetic alterations.** The percentage of informative tumors that lose at least one allele on chromosome 18 and 5q while demonstrating no (C) or at least one (L) loss of allele on 17p is shown on the left part of the figure. These frequencies are either shown for all tumors tested(all sites) or only for those tumors that occured in proximal colon. On the right is shown the DNA index distribution of tumors that have demonstrated no (top) or at least one (bottom) loss of allele on 17p or 18.

DISCUSSION

We have shown differences in the distribution of genetic alterations among subgroups of colorectal carcinomas classified according to their site of occurence. The lack of significant differences in the Dukes' stage distribution among the groups does not support the hypothesis that these differences might be due to a significant difference in the progression status of the tumors among the three subgroups. However, these differences might be the consequence of differences in the carcinogenetic mechanism itself.

The group of distal colon tumors appeared to behave homogeneously as being prone to random loss of chromosomal segments. These tumors are thus expected to demonstrate loss of alleles for almost any region of the human karyotype (Vogelstein 1989). The most frequently encountered losses are possibly those which would provide to the cancer cells the best selective advantage in terms of growth rate. Such advantage could be brought about by a two steps loss of an anti-oncogene activity (initiated by a localized mutation of one allele and achieved by the loss of the other allele) as amply discussed in the case of the retinoblastoma gene. Such tumor suppressor genes could be more precisely located in the common regions of deletion. Potential candidates of such gene are the FAP gene on chromosome 5q (Solomon 1987)and p53 on chromosome 17p (Baker 1989).

The observations that most hyperploid tumors have frequent loss of alleles suggest the following mechanism for tumor progression: sequential loss of chromosomal segments progressively deplete the cell in DNA content thus giving rise to tumors with a DNA index measurably smaller than one. Such tumors might have lost several functional tumor suppressor genes but would also be hemizygous for growth promoting genes located in the vicinity of the hemizygous mutated tumor suppressor genes.They would thus benefit from an endoreduplication which would double their DNA index and in one step restore a diploid set of these growth promoting genes

In contrast, the group of proximal colon tumors appeared heterogeneous. A minority of tumors would behave in a manner similar to that of the distal colon tumors. However the majority of tumors failed to demonstrate loss of alleles and kept a DNA index close to 1. These tumors therefore appear to differ from those of the distal colon and might constitute a group in which carcinogenesis has involved a different genetic pathway. The existence of such distinct processes in the course of tumor progression has already been suggested by the study of chromosomal evolution of colorectal carcinomas (Muleris 1988)

The profile of genetic alterations in rectal tumors is not statistically different from that of distal colon tumors. With the exception of the Ki-ras mutation frequency which is highest in rectum, the frequency of the other alterations in rectum is intermediate between those of the proximal colon and those of the distal colon.

The basis for the differences observed here between proximal and distal colon tumors is not known. At least three factors could be involved. The first factor is the chemical composition of microenvironment of the colonic epithelium : it differs in proximal and distal colon. Diet which has a clear influence on this microenvironment has been shown by epidemiological and experimental studies to influence the incidence of colorectal cancer. Second, it is possible although less documented that epithelial cells of the proximal colon differs in their susceptibility to this microenvironment. This difference might be related to differences in gene expression such as those revealed by lectin binding (Bresalier 1985) or expression of blood group substances (Cooper 1978). Finaly, it is possible that a large portion of colorectal carcinomas occurs in predisposed individuals. Patients with tumors which do not lose alleles might be differently predisposed than those who have tumors with numerous allelic losses.

Aknowledgements : We thank Dr. B. Dutrillaux for continued interest and help and Drs B. Weiffenbach, D. Barker, R. White, Y. Nakamura and B. Vogelstein for providing RFLP probes. This work has been supported by grants from the INSERM and the Ligue Nationale Contre le Cancer to G.T. and from H.H.M.I. to A.P.F.. O.D. is recipient of a grant from the L.N.C.C. comité de l'Yonne.

REFERENCES

Ashton-Rickardt PG, Dunlop MG, Nakamura Y, Morris RG, Purdie CA,Steel CM, Evans HJ, Bird CC ,Willie AH, High frequency of APC loss in sporadic colorectalcarcinoma due to breaks clustered in 5q21-22. *Oncogene* 1989 ; **4** : 1169-1174

Baker SJ, Fearon ER, Nigro JM, Hamilton SR, Preisinger AC, Jessup JM, VanTuinen P, Ledbetter DH, Barker DF et al. Chromosome 17 deletion and p53 gene mutation in colorectal carcinoma. *Science* 1989 ; **244** : 217-221.

Beart RW, Melton LJ, Maruta M, Dockerty MB, Frydenberg HB, O'Fallon WM. Trends in right and left-sided colon cancer. *Dis Col & Rect* 1983 ; **26** : 393-398.

Bos JL, Fearon ER, Hamilton SR et al. Prevalence of ras gene mutations in human colorectal cancer. *Nature* 1987 ; **327** : 293-297.

Bresalier HS, Boland CR, Kim YS. Regional differences in normal and cancer associated glycoconjugate of the human colon *J Natll Cancer Inst.*1985 ; 75 : 249-260

Bussey HJR. Familial polyposis coli. The Johns Hopkins University press, Baltimore, Maryland 1975.

Cooper HS, Haesler WE. Blood group substances as tumor antigens in the distal colon *Am J Clin Pathol* 1978 ; **69** : 594-598

Delattre O, Olschwang S, Law DJ, Melot T, Remvikos Y,Salmon RJ, Sastre X, Validire P, Feinberg AP, Thomas G Multiple genetic alterations in distal and proximal colorectal cancer *The Lancet* 353-356 (1989)

Dukes CE. Classification of cancer of the rectum. *J Pathol Bacteriol* 1932; 35 : 323-332.

Eisenberg B, Decosse JJ, Harford F, Michalek J. Carcinoma of the colon and rectum: the natural history reviewed in 1704 patients. *Cancer* 1982 ; **49**: 1131-1134.

Fearon ER, Hamilton SR, Vogelstein B. Clonal analysis of human colorectal tumors. *Science* 1987; **238** : 193-197.

Forrester K, Almoguera C, Han K, Grizzle WE, Perucho M. Detection of high incidence of K-ras oncogenes during human colon tumorigenesis. *Nature* 1987 ; **327** : 298-303.

Johnson H, Carstens R. Anatomical distribution of colonic carcinomas. *Cancer* 1986 ; **58**: 997-1000.

Kidd KK, Bowcock AM, Pearson PL, Schmidtke J, Willard HF, Track RK, Riciutti F. Human gene mapping 9.5. *Cytogenet Cell Genet* 1988 ; **49** : 132-218.

Law DJ, Olschwang S, Monpezat JP, Lefrançois D, Jagelman D, Petrelli NJ, Thomas G, Feinberg AP. Concerted nonsyntenic allelic loss in human colorectal carcinoma. *Science* 1988 ; **241** : 961-965.

Lynch HT, Lynch JF. Genetics and colorectal cancer. *Familial Cancer*, Müller HJ and Weber W (Eds Karger, Basel) 1985 : 72-77.

Mamazza J, Gordon PH. The changing distribution of large intestinal cancer. *Dis Col & Rect* 1982 ; **25** : 558-562.

Monpezat JP, Delattre O, Bernard A, Grunwald D, Remvikos Y, Muleris M, Salmon RJ, Frelat G, Dutrillaux B, Thomas G. Loss of alleles on chromosome 18 and on the short arm of chromosome 17 in polyploid colorectal carcinomas. *Int J Cancer* 1988 ; **41** : 404-408.

Muleris M, Salmon RJ, Dutrillaux AM, Vielh P, Zafrani B, Girodet J, Dutrillaux B. Characteristic chromosomal imbalances in 18 near-diploid colorectal tumors. *Cancer Genet Cytogenet* 1987 ; **29** : 289-302.

Muleris M, Salmon RJ, Dutrillaux B. Existence of two distinct processes of chromosomal evolution in near-diploid colorectal tumors. *Cancer genet Cytogenet* 1988 ; **32** : 43-50.

Muleris M, Salmon RJ, Zafrani B, Girodet J, Dutrillaux B. Consistent deficiencies of chromosome 18 and of the short arm of chromosome 17 in eleven cases of human large bowel cancer: a possible recessive determinism. *Ann Genet* 1985 ; **28** : 206-213.

Okamoto M, Sasaki M, Sugio K, Sato C, Iwama T, Ikeuchi T, Tonomura A, Sasazuki T, Miyaki M. Loss of constitutional heterozygosity in colon carcinoma from patients with familial polyposis coli. *Nature* 1988 ; **331**: 273-277.

Remvikos Y, Muleris M, Vielh P, Salmon RJ, Dutrillaux B. DNA content and genetic evolution of human colorectal adenocarcinoma. A study by flow cytometry and cytogenetic analysis. *Int J Cancer* 1988 ; **42** : 539-543.

Rothberg PG, Spanforder JM, Erisman MD, Staroscik RN, Sears HF, Peterson RO, Astrin SM. Evidence that c-myc expression defines two genetically distinct forms of colorectal carcinoma. *Br J Cancer* 1985 ; **52** : 629-632.

Snyder DN, Heston JF, Meigs JW, Flannery JT. Changes in site distribution of colorectal carcinoma in Connecticut, 1940-1973. *Dig Dis* 1977 ; **22** : 791-797.

Solomon E, Voss R, Hall V, Bodmer WF, Jass JR, Jeffrey AJ, Lucibello FC, Patel I, Rider SH. Chromosome 5 allele loss in human colorectal carcinomas. *Nature* 1987 ; **328** : 616-619.

Vogelstein B, Fearon ER, Hamilton SR, Kern SE, Preisinger AC, Leppert M, Nakamura Y, White R, Smits AM, Bos JL. Genetic alterations during colorectal-tumor development. *New Engl J Med* 1988 ; **319** : 525-532.

Vogelstein B, Fearon ER, Kern SE, Hamilton SR, Preisinger AC, Nakamura Y, White R Allelotype of colorectal carcinomas *Science* 1989 ; **244** : 207-210

Wildrick DM, Boman B. Chromosome 5 allele loss at the Glucocorticoid receptor locus in human Colorectal carcinomas. *Biochem Biophys Res Commun* 1988 ; **150** : 591-598.

Chromosome 5 Deletions as a Means of Defining the APC Region

HUW THOMAS, LILIANA VARESCO, ANNA-MARIA FRISCHAUF, and ELLEN SOLOMON

ABSTRACT

To define the region of the APC gene we have created a mapping panel from individuals with deletions around this gene. Libraries have been constructed from irradiation hybrids containing small fragments of chromosome 5 containing the APC region, and are being used to saturate the deleted region with probes.

Keywords: Adenomatous polyposis coli, chromosome deletions, irradiation hybrids

DELETIONS

The original clue as to the location of the Adenomatous Polyposis Coli (APC) gene came from a case report in which an individual with mental retardation, developmental anomalies and APC carried a constitutional deletion described as 5q13-q15 or 5q15-q22 (Herrera 1986). Since then we have obtained material from other individuals with similar deletions. The first of these is a girl of 12 (M) with mildly dysmorphic features and mild developmental delay, carrying a deletion of 5q13-q15 or 5q15-q22. As yet she is too young to have been screened for APC (Varesco 1989). The second and third individuals are brothers (P and N) both of whom are mentally retarded with developmental abnormalities and APC. Both carry a constitutional deletion, again of 5q13-q15 or 5q15-q22. Their mother died of inoperable carcinoma of the colon arising from APC (Hockey 1989) We now know from in situ annealing studies using probes linked to APC that in all of these cases the deletion is most likely to be of band 5q21 (Varesco 1989).

SOMATIC CELL HYBRID PANEL

Lymphocytes from patients M, P and N were transformed by EBV and permanent lymphoblastoid lines established. These were fused with the temperature-sensitive Chinese hamster cell line tsH1 (Thompson 1973). This line contains a temperature-sensitive gene for leucyl tRNA synthetase and the line does not grow at the non-permissive temperature of 39°C. The human leucyl tRNA synthetase gene maps to chromosome 5 at 5cen-q11. When the fusion products are grown at 39°C only hybrids containing human 5 will survive. The human lymphoid line is selected against with oubain. With this protocol we have produced the following somatic cell hybrids: PN/TS-1, containing a normal 5 from patient P and no other detectable human material; PD/TS-1, containing the deleted 5 from patient P and some further human chromosomes but not the normal 5; and MD/TS-1, containing the deleted 5 from patient M and no other detectable human material. These hybrids serve as a panel for the mapping of clones from this region of chromosome 5 (Varesco these proceedings; Varesco 1989). As several clones are not deleted in P but are in M it is clear that the M deletion extends further, but as yet it is not known whether these clones are on the same or opposite sides of the P deletion. Using our own clones (Varesco these proceedings) and some provided by Dr Y. Nakamura, we now know that patient M is deleted for clones that flank the APC gene. This suggests that she almost certainly has a deletion for one copy of the APC gene and that she is highly likely to develop the disease. This represents one of the first cases of premorbid diagnosis of this disease using DNA markers.

IRRADIATION HYBRIDS

Having established a panel with which to map clones in the APC region, our next step is to saturate this region with probes. To this end we established a panel of hybrids containing small fragments of 5. This was done by X-irradiation of the 5 only hybrid PN/TS-1, with 50,000 rads, followed by fusion with A23, a TK-Chinese hamster cell line (Cox 1989). One hundred and fifty colonies were picked and shown to contain human DNA. Table 1 shows the percentage of positive clones for a set of markers on the long arm of 5. These are each roughly 10%, suggesting that each irradiation hybrid contains about 10% of chromosome 5. In situ annealing experiments with fluorescence-labelled human DNA on metaphase spreads of a few of the hybrids revealed that each of these had retained several different fragments (S. Williams, unpublished). Results of a more detailed analysis of the APC region are shown in Table 2. Hybrids positive for ECB27 (Varesco 1989) were further tested for adjacent markers. The APC gene lies between ECB27 and YN5.48. The order of markers at the top of the Table was determined from the irradiation hybrids, assuming no interstitial deletions, and is compatable with that generated by a combination of in situ, genetic linkage, and deletion mapping. The order of YN5.48 and ECB27 is not known.

TABLE 1

Chromosome 5 Irradiation Hybrids

Marker	Location	% Positive Hybrids
p105/153[a]	(5q13)	13
C11P11[b]	(5q21)	9.8
YN5.64[c]	(5q21)	10.4
ECB27[d]	(5q21)	10.5
YN5.48[c]	(5q21)	9.2
λMS8[e]	(5q35)	7.7

[a] from JJ Wasmuth
[b] Bodmer 1987
[c] Nakamura 1988
[d] Varesco 1989
[e] Solomon 1987

TABLE 2

ECB27 positive irradiation hybrids

Hybrid	P105/153	Π227[a]	C11P11	YN5.64	ECB27	YN5.48	p3.1[b]	MS8
4	0	0	0	0	+	0	0	+
12	+	+	+	+	+	+	+	0
13	0	0	0	+	+	+	0	0
14	+	0	0	+	+	0		
20	0	0	0		+	0	0	
31	0	0	0		+	0	0	
32	0	+	+	+	+	+	0	
58	0	0	0		+	0	0	
59	0	0	0	0	+	0	0	0
78	0	0	0	+	+	0	0	0
87	0	0	0	0	+	0	0	+
144	0	0	0		+	0	0	
158	0	0	0		+	+	0	

[a] Bodmer 1987
[b] Spurr

CURRENT RESEARCH

These hybrids have been used to construct a cosmid library (hybrid number 158), EagI-linking libraries (hybrids 12 and 158) (J.R.T. Ward, unpublished) and several lambda libraries. Human colonies are being screened on the deletion panel and clones within the deletions will be used to create a physical map of the APC region. As each clone is isolated and placed within the map, it will be tested on pulsed-field gel electrophoresis (PFGE) blots of DNA from APC patients. As 30-40% of the APC mutations are estimated to be new ones, it is expected that a wide range of mutational types would exist for APC. The use of markers close to the APC gene on PGFE should therefore reveal those mutations resulting from gross chromosome changes such as submicroscopic deletions and rearrangements, and point to the precise location of the APC gene.

REFERENCES

Bodmer WF, Bailey CJ, Bodmer J, Bussey HJR, Ellis A, Gorman P, Lucibello FC, Murday VA, Rider SH, Scambler P, Sheer D, Solomon E, Spurr NK (1987) Localisation of the gene for familial adenomatous polyposis is on chromosome 5. Nature 328: 614-616

Cox DR, Pritchard CA, Uglum E, Casher D, Kobori J, Myers RM (1989) Segregation of the Huntington Disease region of human chromosome 4 in a somatic cell hybrid. Genomics 4: 397-407

Herrera L, Kakati L, Gibas E, Pietrzak E, Sandberg AA (1986) Brief Clinical Report: Gardner Syndrome in a man with an interstitial deletion of 5q. Am.J.Med.Genet. 25: 473-476

Hockey KA, Mulcahy MT, Montgomery P, Levitt S (1989) Deletion of chromosome 5q and familial adenomatous polyposis. J.Med.Genet. 26: 61-68

Nakamura Y, Lathrop M, Leppert M, Dobbs M, Wasmuth J, Wolff E, Carlson M, Fujimoto E, Krapcho K, Sears T, Woodward S, Hughes J, Burt R, Gardner J, Lalouel JM, White R (1988) Localization of the genetic defect in familial adenomatous polyposis within a small region of chromosome 5. Am.J.Hum.Genet. 43: 638-644

Solomon E, Voss R, Hall V, Bodmer WF, Jass JR, Jeffreys AJ, Lucibello FC, Patel I, Rider SH (1987) Chromosome 5 allele loss in human colorectal carcinomas. Nature 328: 616-619

Spurr NK, Rooke L, Miles C, Feder J, Bowcock AM, Cavalli-Sforza LL (1989) Assignment of anonymous DNA segments detecting RFLPs at moderate frequencies. Cytogenetics and Cell Genetics 51: 1089

Thompson LH, Harkins JL, Stanners CP (1973) A mammalian cell mutant with a temperature-sensitive leucyl-transfer RNA synthetase. Proc.Natl.Acad.Sci. USA 70: 3094-3098

Varesco L, Thomas H, Cottrell S, Murday V, Fennell SJ, Williams S, Sheer D, Bodmer WF, Frischauf A-M, Solomon E (In press). CpG island clones from a deletion encompassing the gene for Adenomatous Polyposis Coli. Proc.Natl.Acad.Sci.USA in press.

Cytogenetic Studies on Colon Carcinomas and Adenomas from Patients with Familial Polyposis Coli

TATSURO IKEUCHI, MITSUAKI A. YOSHIDA, TAKEO IWAMA, MICHIKO MIYAKI, ISAO OKAYASU, and AKIRA TONOMURA

ABSTRACT

Chromosome studies were performed on colonic or duodenal carcinomas of 5 patients with familial polyposis coli (FPC) and on multiple adenomatous polyps from 17 FPC patients. Among the various clonal chromosome abnormalities in cultures of carcinomas, recurrent losses of chromosomes 17p and 18 were prominent. Chromosome analyses in adenomas using short-term primary cultures revealed that the most frequent changes were gains of chromosomes 7 and 13. Structural changes were rather rare, but it was of interest that partial losses of chromosomes 1p, 5q, 10q and 17p were found as clonal changes in some small-sized individual polyps (<3mm in diameter).

Keywords: familial polyposis coli, colon carcinomas, colon adenomas, chromosome 5, chromosome 7, chromosome 13

1. INTRODUCTION

There have been several reports of chromosome analyses in sporadic colon carcinomas (Reichmann et al., 1981, 1984, 1985; Ochi et al.,1983), and recently special attention has been drawn to recurrent losses of chromosomes 17p and 18 (Muleris et al., 1985, 1987, 1988). However, there have been very few and only fragmentary chromosome studies on tumors of patients with familial polyposis coli (FPC) (cf. Muleris et al., 1989).

During the past two years, we have successfully analyzed chromosome abnormalities in both colon adenocarcinomas and adenomatous polyps from FPC patients, and the results will be presented in this report. Because adenomatous polyps are considered to be precancerous lesions, they are invaluable specimens for elucidating multi-step genetic alterations during the course of tumorigenesis in FPC patients.

2. MATERIALS AND METHODS

Chromosomes in carcinomas were analyzed using short-term cultures from fresh samples, or cultured cells taken from nude mouse-transplantable tumors, or both. In the case of adenoma specimens, short-term primary cultures were exclusively used for chromosome studies. In some of the tumors, a portion of the tissue was fixed and processed for histopathological examination.

Table 1. Results of chromosome analyses in carcinomas from 5 FPC patients

Case No.	Tumor origin*	No. cells analyzed	Modal chrom. no. (range)	Clonal chromosome abnormalities		
				Structural	Gain	Loss
1	P N	43 6	46 (42-85) 42 (41-84)	t(6;7)(p12,q36) t(8;13)(p21;q12) der(15),t(15;17)(p11;q11) del(6)(q21), DMs** 10p+, 19q+, 13p+ other markers	-	3, 8, 10, 17, 18, 20, 22, Y
2	P N	2 6	- 89 (72-92)	i(13q), i(17q) other markers	6, 13	5, 17, 18, 22, X
3	N	21	46 (41-53)	-	-	-
4	N	10	46 (43-100)	1p-, 7p+, 12p+	13 (pentasomy)	12, 17, 18, 20
5	P	17	46 (35-48)	-	7	-

* P: primary tumors obtained from patients.
N: tumors from nude mice after transplantation of primary tumors.

** DMs: double minutes.

The tumor specimens were washed thoroughly for 2 hours in Hanks' solution containing 5 antibiotics in concentrations 3-times as high as those used in standard culture media (penicillin 300 U/ml, kanamycin 300 μg/ml, streptomycin 300 μg/ml, gentamycin 300 μg/ml, fungizone 10 μg/ml). The specimens were then minced with scissors as finely as possible, and treated with 0.8% collagenase for 30 minutes at 37°C. After washing 3 times in Hanks' solution by centrifugation, the cells were suspended in RPMI 1640 medium supplemented with 20% fetal calf serum and the above antibiotics in the usual concentrations, and incubated in 10% carbon dioxide in air in an incubator.

The cells were harvested for chromosome analyses within 10 days after initial culture when the typical epithelial cells had started to grow in the absence of normal fibroblasts growing together. Chromosome preparations were made as described elsewhere (Yoshida et al., 1988), and Q-banding was performed for detailed chromosome analyses. Chromosome abnormalities were considered to be clonal, when at least 2 cells exhibited an identical structural change or when at least 3 cells had gained or lost the same chromosome.

3. RESULTS AND DISCUSSION

3.1 Carcinomas

The present specimens consisted of 4 colon carcinomas (Cases 1, 2, 4 and 5) and one duodenal carcinoma (Case 3). The results of chromosome analyses of specimens from 5 FPC patients are summarized in Table 1. Modal chromosome numbers were in the diploid range in 4 cases and one case was hypotetraploid with a modal chromosome number of 89.

There were various kinds of chromosome abnormalities, but only clonal abnormalities are presented in Table 1. Of these, chromosomes 17 and 18 were most frequently affected. In Case 1, all the cells analyzed had an unbalanced translocation between chromosomes 15 and 17 which resulted in partial monosomy for the 17pter-q11 region. Case 2 had an isochromosome for the long arm of chromosome 17, i(17q), leading to a loss of 17p. A whole chromosome 17 was lost in Case 4. In Cases 1, 2 and 4, one chromosome 18 was consistently lost. In Cases 3 and 5, there were numerous chromosome abnormalities, all of which were nonclonal except for trisomy 7 in Case 5.

It is well-known that in sporadic colon carcinomas the most frequent changes are losses of chromosomes 17q and 18 (Muleris et al., 1985, 1987, 1988), and these two deficiencies have been further confirmed by DNA analysis as revealed by a loss of heterozygosity (LOH)(Monpezat et al., 1988; Vogelstein et al., 1988; Law et al., 1988; Sasaki et al., 1989). Thus, the present findings in FPC colon carcinomas, though the number of specimens examined in this study is still limited, seems to be essentially similar to the findings in sporadic colon carcinomas.

Recently, the FPC gene has been localized to the long arm of chromosome 5 (5q21-q22 region) (Bodmer et al. 1987; Leppert et al. 1987), and 5q deletions, as revealed by chromosomal and LOH analyses, have frequently been observed in sporadic or FPC colon cancers (Reichmann et al., 1981; Solomon et al., 1987; Muleris et al., 1988; Okamoto et al., 1988; Vogelstein et al., 1988; Sasaki et al., 1989). However, as far as the present cancer specimens are concerned, there is no evidence of structural change in the long arm of chromosome 5.

3.2 Adenomatous polyps

When the polyps were large enough in size (>3mm in diameter), single polyps were cultured individually, and the smaller polyps from the same patients were mixed together and cultured for chromosome studies. In this manner, the chromosomes of a total of 43 cultured specimens derived from 17 FPC patients were examined. All the specimens were found to be in the diploid or near-diploid range.

Table 2 demonstrates the results of chromosome analyses in cultures of single or mixed polyps which were derived from 4 FPC patients as examples. In general, cells with a normal karyotype were predominant in each culture, but numerical chromosome changes were frequently observed. In particular, trisomy of chromosome 7 was repeatedly found with varied frequencies. An excess of chromosome 13 was also noted (Table 2). A representative aberrant karyotype is shown in Fig. 1.

The numerical and structural chromosome changes in the 43 polyp specimens are summarized in Figs. 2 and 3, respectively. As shown in Fig. 2, the most frequent numerical change was trisomy 7, and the other trisomies involved chromosomes 12, 13 and 20. The gains of these chromosomes were also recurrent in non-clonal abnormalities. In addition, monosomy of chromosome 10 was found as clonal changes in 8 cultured specimens. It seems unlikely that the monosomy 10 was due to a technical loss during chromosome preparation. Gains of chromosomes 7 and 13 were also found in the present specimens of carcinomas (Table 1), as have been reported in sporadic cases (Reichmann et al., 1985). Thus, these numerical changes may play certain significant roles in the development of colonic adenomas and carcinomas.

Compared with the numerical chromosome changes, structural abnormalities were very rare in polyp cells, but partial losses of chromosomes 1p and 5q were observed as clonal changes in 4 different cultured specimens. A partial loss of chromosome 10q was observed in 2 specimens (Fig. 3). In one cultured specimen (case FPC232 in Table 2), about 70%

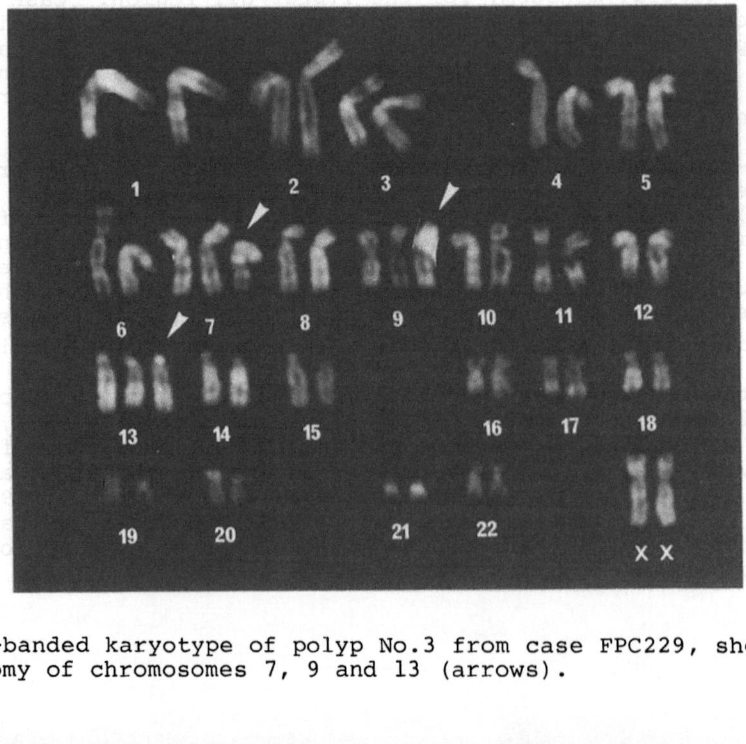

Fig. 1. Q-banded karyotype of polyp No.3 from case FPC229, showing trisomy of chromosomes 7, 9 and 13 (arrows).

Table 2. Results of chromosome analyses in polyps from 4 FPC patients

Case No.	Polyp No.	No. cells analyzed	Karyotypes	No. of cells
FPC228	mixed	18	46,XY	11
			92,XXYY	2
			45,X	1
			45,XY,-18	1
			45,XY,-21	1
			42,XY,-3,+7,-11,-13,-15,-16,-20, +mar	1
			57,XY,+3,+7,-8,-10,+12,+13,-15, +17,-18,+21,+ 9 markers	1
FPC229	1	25	46,XX	21
			47,XX,+7	1
			44,X ,+7,-12,-16	1
			44,XX,-19,-22	1
			45,XX,-5	1
	2	11	46,XX	9
			46,XX,-17	1
			46,XX,-18	1
	3	11	49,XX,+7,+9,+13 (Fig. 1)	7
			48,XX,+7,+13	1
			47,XX,+7,+9,+13,-20,-21	1
			45,XX,-10,+13,-14	1
			46,XX	1
FPC230	1	14	46,XX	7
			48,XX,+7,+20	2
			47,XX,+7	1
			46,XX,+7,-16	1
			46,XX,+7,+13,-6,-18	1
			47,XX,+20	1
			45,XX,-15	1
	mixed	10	49,XX,+7,+13,+20	3
			48,XX,+7,+13	2
			48,XX,+7,-13,-15,+mar,3q+	1
			47,XX,+7,+13,-6	1
			46,XX,+7,-10	1
			44,XX,+7,-8,-13,-13	1
			46,XX,10q-	1
FPC232	9	13	48,XX,+13,+13	3
			48,XX,+13,+13,-17,+i(17q)	3
			47,XX,+13,-17,+i(17q)	2
			48,XX,+13,+13,+13,-14,+i(17q)	1
			47,XX,+13,+13,-17,-19,+i(17q)	1
			46,XX,+13,-17,-22,+i(17q)	1
			46,X ,+13,-17,+i(17q)	1
			49,XX,+7,+13,+13	1

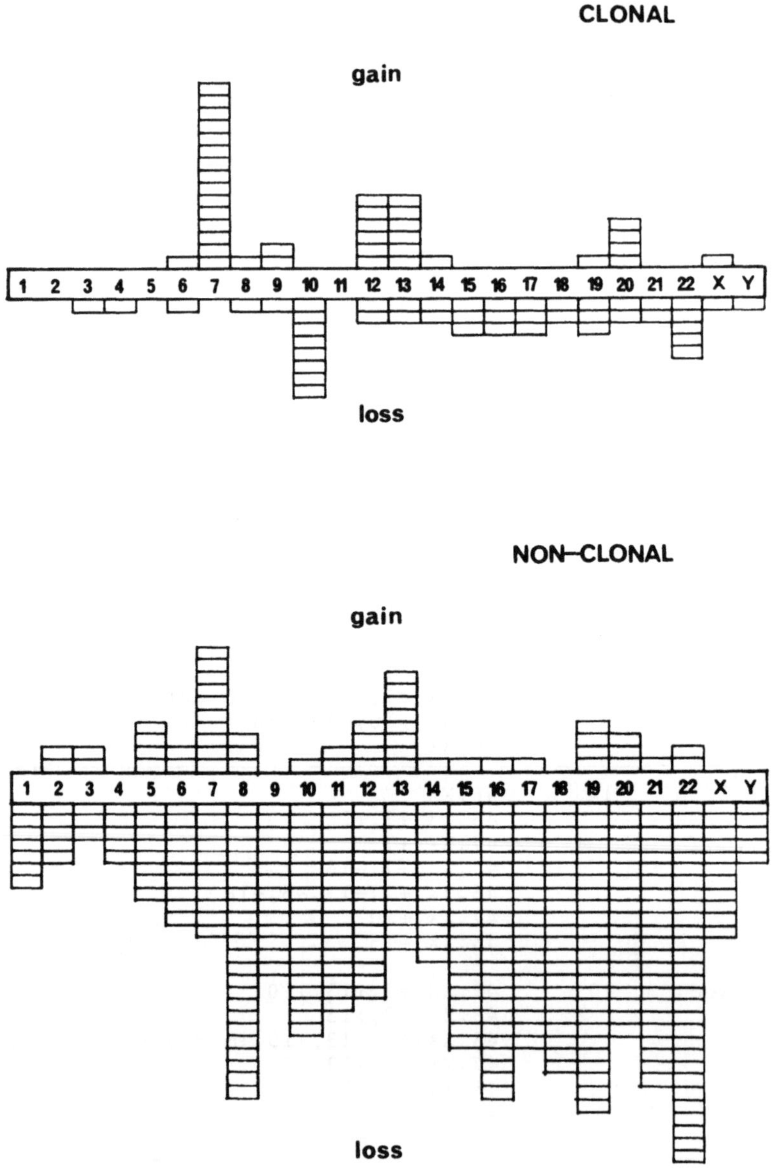

Fig. 2. Frequencies of involvement of individual chromosomes in numerical abnormalities (gains and losses) in 43 cultures from adenomatous polyps. Each block represents one polyp specimen.

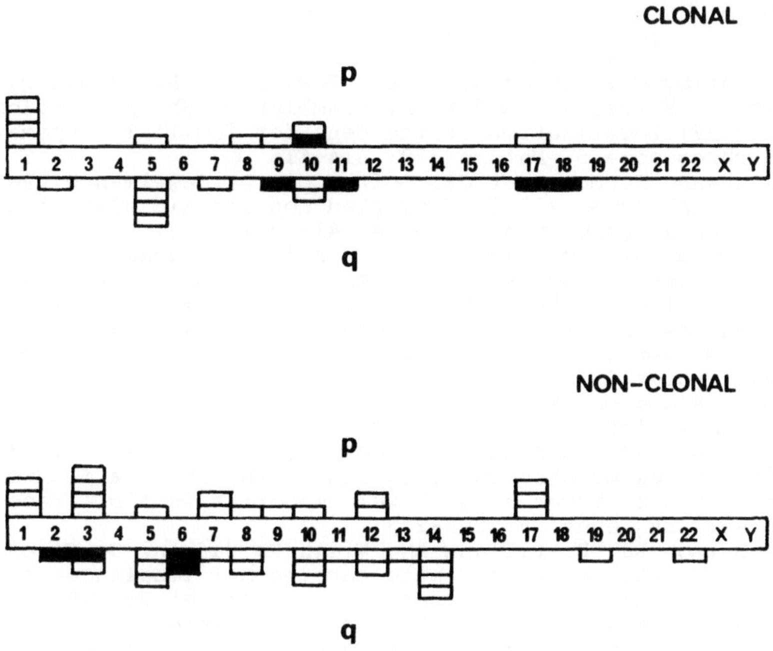

Fig. 3. Frequencies of involvement of chromosome arms (short and long arms) in structural abnormalities (clonal and non-clonal) in 43 adenomatous polyp specimens. Each block represents one polyp specimen. Opened block: a simple partial deletion. Filled block: a reciprocal translocation.

of cells analyzed were found to have an isochromosome for the long arm of chromosome 17 resulting in a loss of its short arm. Of special importance was the finding that the above structural chromosome changes were found in relatively small-sized polyps. In fact, partial losses of 1p, 5q and the i(17q) were found in polyps with mild or moderate dysplasia less than 3mm in diameter.

Though abnormalities of chromosome 10 have not been referred to in previous studies, frequent observation of 1p deletion has been reported in sporadic colon carcinomas (Muleris et al. 1987). Partial losses of 17p and 5q are recurrent changes in colon carcinomas as described above. Recent molecular studies have shown that allelic losses on chromosomes 5q and 17p are found in some adenomas with relatively advanced dysplasia (Vogelstein et al., 1988, 1989; Rees et al., 1989). The present chromosomal findings in small-sized adenomatous polyps suggest that the appearance of these structural changes might be much earlier events in tumorigenesis than currently considered.

Thus, further accumulation of chromosomal data on colon tumors from FPC patients in association with detailed histopathological findings is required, especially in adenomatous polyps in various stages of tumorigenesis.

4. REFERENCES

Bodmer WF, Bailey CJ, Bodmer J, Bussey HJR, Ellis A, Gorman P, Lucibello FC, Murday VA, Rider SH, Scambler P, Sheer D, Solomon E, Spurr NK (187) Localization of the gene for familial adenomatous polyposis on chromosome 5. Nature 328: 614-616

Law DJ, Olschwang S, Monpezat JP, Lefrançois D, Jagelman D, Petrelli NJ, Thomas G, Feinberg AP (1988) Concerted nonsyntenic allelic loss in human colorectal carcinoma. Science 241: 961-965

Leppert M, Dobbs M, Scambler P, O'Connell P, Nakamura Y, Stauffer D, Woodward S, Burt R, Hughes J, Gardner E, Lathrop M, Wasmuth J, Lalouel JM, White R (1987) The gene for familial polyposis coli maps to the long arm of chromosome 5. Science 238: 1411-1413

Monpezat JP, Delattre O, Bernard A, Grunwald D, Remvikos Y, Muleris M, Salmon RJ, Frelat G, Dutrillaux B, Thomas G (1988) Loss of alleles on chromosome 18 and on the short arm chromosome 17 in polyploid colorectal carcinomas. Int J Cancer 41: 404-408

Muleris M, Salmon RJ, Zafrani B, Girodet J, Dutrillaux B (1985) Consistent deficiencies of chromosome 18 and of the short arm chromosome 17 in eleven cases of human large bowel cancer: a possible recessive determinism. Ann Génét 28: 206-213

Muleris M, Salmon RJ, Dutrillaux AM, Vielh P, Zafrani B, Girodet J, Dutrillaux B (1987) Characteristic chromosomal imbalances in 18 near-diploid colorectal tumors. Cancer Genet Cytogenet 29: 289-301

Muleris M, Salmon RJ, Dutrillaux B (1988) Existence of two distinct processes of chromosomal evolution in near-diploid colorectal tumors. Cancer Genet Cytogenet 32: 43-50

Muleris M, Nordlinger B, Dutrillaux B (1989) Cytogenetic characterization of a colon adenocarcinoma from a familial polyposis coli patient. Cancer Genet Cytogenet 38: 249-253

Ochi H, Takeuchi J, Holyoke D, Sandberg AA (1983) Possible specific chromosome changes in large bowel cancer. Cancer Genet Cytogenet 10: 121-122

Okamoto M, Sasaki M, Sugio K, Sato C, Iwama T, Ikeuchi T, Tonomura A, Sasazuki T, Miyaki M (1988) Loss of constitutional heterozygosity in colon carcinoma from patients with familial polyposis coli. Nature 331: 273-277

Rees M, Leigh SEA, Delhanty JDA, Jass JR (1989) Chromosome 5 allele loss in familial and sporadic colorectal adenomas. Brit J Cancer 59: 361-365

Reichmann A, Martin P, Levin B (1981) Chromosome banding patterns in human large bowel cancer. Int J Cancer 28: 431-440

Reichmann A, Martin P, Levin B (1984) Chromosomes in human large bowel tumors. A study of chromosome #1. Cancer Genet Cytogenet 12: 295-301

Reichmann A, Martin P, Levin B (1985) Marker chromosomes in direct preparations of human bowel tumors. Cancer Genet Cytogenet 16: 229-233

Sasaki M, Okamoto M, Sato C, Sugio K, Soejima J, Iwama T, Ikeuchi T, Tonomura A, Miyaki M, Sasazuki T (1989) Loss of constitutional heterozygosity in colorectal tumors from patients with familial polyposis coli and those with nonpolyposis colorectal carcinoma. Cancer Res 49: 4402-4406

Solomon E, Voss R, Hall V, Bodmer WF, Jass JR, Jeffreys AJ, Lucibello FC, Patel I, Rider SH (1987) Chromosome 5 allele loss in human colorectal carcinomas. Nature 328: 616-619

Vogelstein B, Fearson ER, Hamilton SR, Kern SE, Preisinger AC, Leppert M, Nakamura Y, White R, Smits, AMM, Bos JL (1988) Genetic alterations during colorectal-tumor development. New Engl J Med 319: 525-532

Vogelstein B, Fearson E, Kern S, Hamilton SR, Preisinger AC, Nakamura, Y, White R (1989) Allelotype of colorectal carcinomas. Science 244: 207-211

Yoshida MA, Ikeuchi T, Tachibana Y, Takagi K, Moriyama M, Tonomura A (1988) Rearrangements of chromosome 3 in nonfamilial renal cell carcinomas from Japanese patients. Jpn J Cancer Res (Gann) 79: 600-607

The DiFi Rectal Carcinoma Cell Line from a Familial Adenomatous Polyposis Patient: An In Vitro Model System to Study Genetic Changes in Colorectal Cancer

BRUCE M. BOMAN, MATILDE OLIVE, SEEMA UNTAWALE, MARK BLICK, SUSAN NORTH, GARY GALLICK, GAUDENZ DOLF, MICHAEL J. SICILIANO, LEOR D. ROUBEIN, HERBERT FRITCHE, GILLES THOMAS, SEN PATHAK, DAVID M. WILDRICK, and BERNARD LEVIN

ABSTRACT

A new human colorectal cancer cell line (DiFi) has been established from a patient with the Gardner Syndrome. Characterization studies have shown that DiFi cells secrete carcinoembryonic antigen (CEA) and CA 19-9, are tumorigenic in nude mice, have a tetraploid karyotype, and possess an isozyme pattern characteristic of colorectal cancer cell lines. Southern blot analysis shows that DiFi cells have allelic loss on chromosomes 17p and 18, plus amplification of the EGF receptor gene. Northern blot analysis reveals that transforming growth factor (TGF)-alpha, c-myc, and p53 transcripts are clearly expressed in these cells. The significance of these molecular changes in relation to mechanisms leading to a selective growth advantage in DiFi cells will be discussed.

INTRODUCTION

Familial adenomatous polyposis (FAP) is a Mendelian disorder that includes two phenotypes, familial polyposis coli (FPC) and Gardner syndrome (GS). The classification of GS as a genetic entity distinct from FPC has been controversial (Gardner, 1983; Lynch et al., 1988a). Bulow (1987) argued against maintaining GS as a separate clinical entity because the great majority of FPC patients demonstrate mandibular osteomas or gastroduodenal polyps. In addition, a recent linkage analysis of families having the FPC versus GS phenotype revealed no evidence of genetic heterogeneity between the two phenotypes (Nakamura et al., 1988). Both phenotypes have an identical clinical course regarding the development of adenomatous polyps and high risk for colorectal cancer (reviewed in Boman and Levin, 1986 and Lynch et al., 1988b). When the FAP gene is isolated, its role in expressivity of extracolonic lesions and in the development of colorectal cancer will be better understood.

We report here the establishment and characterization of the DiFi colorectal carcinoma cell line which represents one of the first such cell lines from a Gardner syndrome patient. Colorectal cancer cell lines have been established from FPC patients (Paraskeva et al, 1984 ; Namba et al, 1983) and from a hereditary nonpolyposis colorectal cancer patient (Whitehead et al, 1985). We used the DiFi colorectal carcinoma cell line as an in vitro model system to study molecular and cellular changes associated with hereditary colorectal cancer.

CELL CULTURE AND BIOLOGY

DiFi cells from malignant ascitic fluid were isolated from a rectal cancer patient with the Gardner syndrome and initiated to grow in culture. The patient was a 46 year-old female with multiple adenomatous polyps of the colon and extracolonic manifestations characteristic of the disease including mesenteric fibromatosis, osteomas and congenital hypertrophy of the retinal pigment epithelium. Her serum CEA level was significantly elevated (Table 1).

DiFi cells are grown in L-15:RPMI 1640 (50:50) culture medium containing 10% fetal bovine serum in standard plastic tissue culture flasks without collagen. The cells have been maintained in culture for 3 years (90 passages). Analysis for mycoplasma was negative by the Hoechst stain. Immunochemical analysis showed DiFi cells to secrete the mucin CA 19-9 and CEA into the conditioned culture medium (Table 2).

Subcutaneous injection of DiFi cells into athymic mice resulted in the production of tumors in two of four mice. Immunocytochemical analysis showed these tumors to stain positively for keratin, CEA, and colon-specific mucin (Table 3).

Table 1. RADIOIMMUNOASSAY OF THE PATIENT'S SERUM

ANTIGEN	SERUM LEVEL	NORMAL
CEA	76.1 ng/ml	(0 - 3.0)
HCG	1.1 mIU/ml	(0 - 3.0)

Table 2. RADIOIMMUNOASSAY OF MEDIUM CONDITIONED BY DIFI COLON CARCINOMA CELLS

ANTIGEN	CULTURE MEDIUM	LYSED CELLS	CONTROL*
CEA	150 ng/ml	--	<1.5 ng/ml
HCG	1.2 mIU/ml	--	<1.0 mIU/ml
Alkaline phosphotase	7.0 mU/ml	<13 U/ml	<8.0 U/ml
Alk phos Isoenzyme	0 mU/ml	0 mU/ml	0.1 mU/ml
CA 19-9	552 U/ml	--	0 U/ml
CA 15-3	0 U/ml	--	0 U/ml

* Non-conditioned culture medium

Table 3. IMMUNOHISTOCHEMISTRY OF DIFI COLON CANCER

STAIN	PRIMARY TUMOR	NUDE MOUSE TUMOR
CEA	+	+
HCG	-	-
Colon Specific Mucin	NT	+
Keratin	NT	+

ISOZYMES

Determination of the genetic signature using eleven different isozymes showed a pattern having a frequency of 0.01 in Caucasian populations (Table 4). Several aspects of the isozyme profile were characteristic of other colon cancer cell lines such as strong expression of esterases and creatine kinase B. (Rutzky and Siciliano, 1982).

Table 4. - GENETIC SIGNATURE OF DIFI COLON CANCER LINE

ENZYME	LOCUS	CHROMOSOME	PHENOTYPE	FREQUENCY*
Acid phosphatase	ACP1	2	AB	0.43
Phosphoglucomutase	PGM1 PGM3	1 6	12	0.36
Adenylate kinase	AK1	9	1	0.90
Glyoxylase	GL01	6	2	0.31
Glutamate-oxaloacetate transaminase	GOT2	16	1	0.96
Adenosine deaminase	ADA	20	NR	
6-Phosphogluconate dehydrogenase	PGD	1	a	0.96
Esterase	ESD	13	1	0.82
Malic enzyme (mitochondrial)	ME2	6	1	0.48
Phosphoglycolic acid phosphatase	PGP	16	1	0.68
Glucose-6-phosphate dehydrogenase**	G6PD	X	B	0.99
		GENETIC SIGNATURE:		0.010653238

* in Caucasians ** Used to determine HeLa contamination

KARYOTYPE

The majority of the cells were near tetraploid and displayed a large number of marker chromosomes (Table 5). Chromosomes 5, 9, 18, 19, 21, and X had losses in chromosome number and no involvement in the formation of marker chromosomes. Gains in chromosome number occurred with chromosomes 6, 19, and 20, each of which had one too many copies. In addition, the DiFi line demonstrated a fairly high frequency of double minute chromosomes.

Table 5. Karyotype of DiFi Cells

Description	Numerical	Structural
85,XX	-X,-X,-1,-1,-1,-4,-4, -5,+6,-8,-8,-9,-10, -10,-12,-12,-12,-13, -13,-13,-13,-14, -14,-15,-15,-15,-15, -16,-17,-17,-17,-18, -18,+19,+20,-21 der(8)t(8;?)(p22;?)	m1:t(1;15)(q11;q26) m2:t(4;19;?) m3:i(7q) m4:der(2)t(2;15)(q13;q15) 2 copies m5:der(16)t(1;16)(p13;q13) m6:der(10)t(10;13)(p11;q12) m7:der(12)t(12;13)(p12;q11) 3 copies m8:der(15)t(15;?)(p12;?) m9:del(1)(q32) m10:i(14q) m11:i(8q) m12:der(13)t(13;?) m13:der(13) m14:der(17)t(17;?)(q25.1;?) 2 copies m15:i(16q) m16:del(12)(q14) 2 copies m17:der(20)t(20;?) um:two unidentified markers

ONCOGENES

The expression of five different oncogenes has been determined by northern (RNA) hybridization analysis (Table 6). The k-ras and c-fos signals were present faintly. The c-myb transcript was clearly expressed and the p53 and c-myc genes appear to have slightly increased levels of expression. DiFi cells did not show single point mutations on codon 12 and 13 of k-ras.

Table 6. LEVEL OF ONCOGENE EXPRESSION IN DIFI CELLS*

Oncogene	DiFi Cells
k-*ras*	+/-
p53	++
c-*myc*	++
c-*myb*	+
c-*fos*	+/-

* + to ++++, low to high levels of hybridization intensity

AUTOCRINE GROWTH FACTORS

The expression of autocrine growth factors and their receptors was analyzed (Table 7). Northern (RNA) hybridization studies showed that the mRNA for TGF alpha was clearly expressed in DiFi cells. Northern blot analysis also revealed significantly elevated EGF receptor gene mRNA levels. Immunocytochemical analysis showed markedly enhanced expression of EGF receptors on cultured DiFi cells. The level of EGF receptor tyrosine specific protein kinase activity in DiFi cells was also found to be increased approximately fifty-fold by immune complex kinase assay.

DNA dot- and Southern blot analysis showed amplification of the EGF receptor gene with more than 100 copies per cell. In situ hybridization revealed the amplified EGF receptor genes to be present in the double minutes.

Table 7. AUTOCRINE GROWTH FACTORS IN DIFI CELLS

TGF	alpha	mRNA	+
EGF	receptor	gene	>100 copies/cell
EGF	receptor	mRNA	50 x
EGF	receptor	protein	++++
EGF	receptor	kinase	50 x

ALLELIC LOSS

We examined normal versus tumor DNA from this patient for tumor specific allele loss on chromosomes 2, 5, 6, 12, 17, 18, and 19 (Table 8; Wildrick and Boman, 1988; Boman et al, 1988a). DiFi carcinoma cells show a loss of alleles on chromosomes 17p and 18. No allelic loss was observed on chromosomes 2, 6, or 19. Allelic markers on chromosomes 5 and 12 were non-informative.

Table 8. ALLELIC LOSS IN DIFI CELLS*

Chromosome	Locus	Normal	Tumor
2p	D2S5	1/2	1/2
2q	D2S6	1/2	1/2
5q	GRL	--	--
6	CGA	1/2	1/2
6q	MYB	1/2	1/2
12p	KRAS	--	--
12q	PAH	--	--
17p	D17S28	1/2	1/
18	D18S6	1/2	/2
19p	INSR	1/2	1/2
19q	CYP1	--	--

* "1/2" indicates heterozygosity and "1/ " or " /2" indicates homozygosity

DISCUSSION

The study of molecular and cellular alterations in DiFi cells should help us understand mechanisms by which colorectal carcinoma cells gain a selective growth advantage (Boman et al, 1988b).
One possibility is the loss of cellular mechanisms that normally function in growth-inhibition or suppression. The FAP gene has been proposed to be a growth suppressor gene (Vogelstein et al, 1988). DiFi cells contain a mutant FAP gene because they were derived from an FAP patient. It has not been determined whether DiFi cells have loss of the normal homologue of the FAP gene because normal DNA lacked heterozygosity at chromosome 5 loci (Wildrick and Boman, 1988). However, karyotypic analysis revealed that DiFi cells are tetraploid with loss of one copy of chromosome 5. This may represent loss of the wild-type chromosome 5 through non-disjunction and reduplication of the mutant chromosome, as described to occur with chromosome 13 in retinoblastoma (Cavenee et al, 1983; Murphree and Benedict 1984).

DiFi cells may also have loss of a different growth suppressor gene located on chromosome 18 because our study shows chromosome 18 loss on karyotypic analysis and allelic loss on chromosome 18 by Southern blot analysis. Recent studies revealing frequent allelic loss on chromosome 18 in colorectal cancers (Vogelstein et al., 1988; Law et al., 1988; Monpezat et al., 1988; Boman et al, 1988a) coupled with the tentative assignment of Lynch syndrome II to chromosome 18 (Boman et al., 1988c, Lynch et al., 1985) suggests that a growth suppressor gene may be located on this chromosome.

Our results also show chromosome 17p allelic loss. The p53 gene on chromosome 17p, another putative cancer gene, may be involved because Vogelstein et al (1989) showed that chromosome 17 deletions and p53 mutations occur frequently in colorectal carcinomas. Our results showing increased expression of the p53 gene in DiFi cells is consistent with Vogelsteins study showing that tumors with allelic deletions of chromosome 17 had expression of considerable amounts of p53 messenger RNA from the remaining mutant allele. Perhaps, loss of one p53 allele and mutation of other allele leads to increased cell proliferation which in turn might induce up-regulation of its mutant p53 gene expression through a feedback mechanism.

Autocrine growth factor production is another mechanism that probably gives DiFi cells a selective growth advantage because these cells produce TGF alpha and have amplification/increased expression of the EGF receptor gene. TGF-alpha production and overproduction of the EGF receptor have previously been reported to occur in colorectal carcinoma cells (Bradley et al., 1986; Wan et al., 1988). However, to our knowledge, DiFi represents the first colorectal cancer reported to have amplification of the EGF receptor gene.

Increased expression or mutational activation of oncogenes was also investigated in DiFi cells. Ras gene mutations have previously been reported in nearly 50% of colorectal adenomas and carcinomas (Bos et al., 1987; Forrester et al., 1987; Vogelstein et al, 1988). DiFi cells did not have mutation on codon 12 or 13 of k-ras. However DiFi cells did have increased expression of c-myc, which is consistent with previous reports of increased expression of this oncogene in colorectal cancers from FAP and sporadic cases (Sugio et al., 1988). Our finding of increased c-myc expression in a colorectal cancer from a FAP patient is also consistent with the recent study by Erisman (1989) showing that increased c-myc expression correlates with chromosome 5 allelic loss in sporadic colorectal cancers and with colorectal cancers in FAP patients.

In conclusion, our study on the DiFi colorectal carcinoma cell line from a FAP patient has identified several molecular alterations that probably give these cells a selective growth advantage. The isolation of growth suppressor genes should provide the opportunity to clearly define which growth suppressor genes are lost or inactivated in DiFi cells. These cells should be useful in studies to determine how inactivation of growth-suppressor genes alters normal cellular function and leads to malignant transformation.

ACKNOWLEDGEMENTS

We thank Barbara Lorimor for secretarial assistance in the preparation of this manuscript. This work was supported by the University of Texas Cancer Center New Program Funds and Health Future Foundation Funds.

REFERENCES

Boman BM and Levin B (1986) Familial polyposis. Hosp Pract 21:155-170

Boman BM, Wildrick DM, Alfaro SR (1988a) Chromosome 18 allele loss at the D18S6 locus in human colorectal carcinomas. Biochem. Biophys. Res. Commun. 155:463-469

Boman BM, Wildrick DM and Lointier P (1988b) Growth factors and colon cancer. In: Gastrointestinal Cancer: Current Approaches to Diagnosis and Treatment, University of Texas Press, Austin pp 71-86

Boman BM, Lynch HT, Kimberling WJ, et al. (1988c) Reassignment of a cancer family syndrome gene to chromosome 18. Cancer Genet. Cytogenet 34:153-154

Bos JL, Fearon ER, Hamilton SR, Verlaan-deVries M, van Boom JH, van der Eb AJ, and Vogelstein B (1987) Prevalence of ras gene mutations in human colorectal cancers. Nature 327:293-297

Bradley SJ, Garfinkle G, Walker E, Salem, RR, Bleday R, Chen LB, and Steele GD (1986) Increased epidermal growth factor receptor on human colon carcinoma cells without gene amplification. Arch. Surg. 121:1242-1247

Bulow, S. (1987) Familial polyposis coli. Dan. Med. Bull. 34:1-15

Cavenee WK, Dryja TP, Phillips RA, Benedict WF, Godbout R, Gallie BL, Murphree AL, Strong LC and White RL (1983) Expression of recessive alleles by chromosomal mechanisms in retinoblastoma. Nature 305:779-783

Erisman MD, Scott JK, Astrin SM (1989) Evidence that the familial adenomatous polyposis gene is involved in a subset of colon cancers with a complementable defect in c-myc regulation. Proc. Natl. Acad. Sci. 86:4264-4268

Forrester K, Almoguera C, Han K, Grizzle WE, and Perucho M (1987) Detection of high incidence of K-ras oncogenes during human colon tumorigenesis. Nature 327:298-303

Gardner, EJ, (1983) Familial polyposis coli and Gardner syndrome--is there a difference? JRF Ingall and AJ Mastromarino (ed) In: Prevention of Hereditary Large Bowel Cancer, AR Liss, Inc., New York pp 39-60

Law DJ, Olschwang S, Monpezat JP, Lefrancois D, Jagelman D, Petrelli NJ, Thomas G, and Feinberg, AP (1988) Concerted nonsyntenic allelic loss in human colorectal carcinoma. Science 241:961-965

Lynch HT, Boman BM, Lanspa S, Smyrk T, Lynch J. (1988a) Heritage of colon polyps. L Herrera (ed) In: Familial Adenomatous Polyposis. AR Liss Inc., New York (in press)

Lynch HT, Boman BM, Fitzgibbons RJ (1988b) Familial polyposis coli: genetics surveillance and treatment. Nebr. Med. J. 73: 329-334

Lynch HT, Schuelke GS, Kimberling WJ, et al. (1985) Hereditary nonpolyposis colorectal cancer (Lynch syndromes I and II):II. Biomarker Studies. Cancer 56:939-951

Monpezat J-PH, Delattre O, Bernard A, Grunwald D, Remvikos Y, Muleris M, Salmon RJ, Frelat G, Dutrillaux B and Thomas G (1988) Loss of alleles on chromosome 18 and on the short arm of chromosome 17 in polyploid colorectal carcinomas. Int. J. Cancer 41:404-408

Murphree AL, Benedict WF (1984) Retinoblastoma: clues to human oncogenesis. Science 223:1028-1033

Nakamura Y, Lathrop M, Leppert M, Dobbs M, Wasmuth J, Wolff E, Carlson M, Fujimoto E, Krapcho K, Sears T, Woodward S, Hughes J, Burt R, Gardner E, Lalouel J-M, and White R (1988) Localization of the genetic defect in familial adenomatous polyposis within a small region of chromosome 5. Am. J. Hum. Genet. 43:638-644

Namba M, Miyamoto K, Hyodoh F, Iwama T, Utsunomiya J, Fukushima F and Kimoto T (1983) Establishment and characterization of a human colon carcinoma cell line (KMS-4) from a patient with hereditary adenomatosis of the colon and rectum. Int. J. Cancer 32:697-702

Paraskeva C, Buckle BG, Sheer D and Wigley CB (1984) The isolation and characterization of colorectal epithelial cell lines at different stages in malignant transformation from familial polyposis coli patients. Int. J. Cancer 34:49-56

Rutzky, LP and Siciliano MJ, (1982) Various isozyme gene expression patterns among human colorectal adenocarcinoma cell lines and tissues. JNCI 68:81-90

Sugio K, Kurata S-I, Sasaki M, Soejima J-I, and Sasazuki T (1988) Differential expression of c-myc gene and c-fos gene in premalignant and malignant tissues from patients with familial polyposis coli. Cancer Research 48:4855-4861

Vogelstein B, Fearon ER, Hamilton SR, Kern SE, Preisinger AC, Leppert M, Nakamura Y, White R, Smits AMM, and Bos JL (1988) Genetic alterations during colorectal-tumor development. N. Engl. J. Med. 319:525-532

Vogelstein B, Fearon ER, Kearn SE, et al. (1989) Allelotype of colorectal carcinomas. Science 244:207-211

Wan, C-W, McKnight MK, Brattain DE, Brattain MG and Yeoman LC (1988) Different epidermal growth factor responses and receptor levels in human colon carcinoma cell lines. C Cancer Lett. 43:139-143

Whitehead RH, Macrae FA, St. John DJ, Ma J (1985) A colon cancer cell line (LIM1215) derived from a patient with inherited nonpolyposis colorectal cancer JNCI 74:759-765

Wildrick DM and Boman BM (1988) Chromosome 5 allele loss at the glucocorticoid receptor locus in human colorectal carcinomas. Biochem. Biophys. Res. Commun. 150:591-598

Dietary Fat Diglycerides Activate by Tyrosine Phosphorylation a pp63 Membrane Protein Only in Colon Tumors and not in Normal Colonocytes, Leading to Selective Biological Effects

EILEEN A. FRIEDMAN

ABSTRACT

Long-chain diglycerides, found in the colon at high concentrations, are mitogens selective for colon tumor cells, having no detectable effect on normal colonocytes. This selective mitogenic effect parallels the tyrosine phosphorylation of a pp63 membrane protein only in adenomas and carcinomas, but not normal colonocytes.

Keywords: tyrosine phosphorylation, primary culture

1. BACKGROUND

Normal colonocytes are converted into preneoplastic cells, then into more advanced premalignant cells, and finally to malignant cells by a series of genetic changes including loss of tumor suppressor genes on chromosomes 5, 17 and 18, (Bodmer et al, 1987; Baker et al, 1989; Vogelstein et al, 1989) and activation of ras oncogenes (Bos et al, 1987; Forrester et al, 1987). We had observed in earlier studies (Friedman, 1981; Friedman et al, 1984a and b), that adenomas of different histopathology or carcinomas, and preneoplastic cells from many, but not all, familial polyposis patients, exhibited responses to the phorbol ester tumor promoter TPA, including mitogenesis and enhanced secretion of the proteolytic enzyme, urokinase. Normal colonocytes were unaffected by TPA. This indicated that transformation of normal human colonocytes into adenomas, into carcinomas, or into the preneoplastic cell type found in patients symptomatic with familial polyposis, makes these genetically altered cells sensitive to new growth regulatory signals. More recently, data from Weinberg's lab (Dotto et al, 1985) showed that primary rat embryo fibroblasts containing a transfected, activated ras gene are strongly stimulated to grow by tumor promoters, while control fibroblasts containing only the retroviral carrier, but no oncogene, displayed no mitogenic response to TPA. It is tempting to speculate that activation of ras genes in adenomas leads to the selective mitogenic effects of TPA on these cells. However, only 30-40% of adenomas and carcinomas contain an activated ras oncogene, and all adenomas and carcinomas we have tested responded to TPA, either by mitogenesis or enhanced urokinase secretion (Friedman et al, 1984a) so the actual mechanism inducing TPA sensitivity in colon tumor cells may involve other genetic changes in addition to ras mutation.

2. FECAL DIGLYCERIDES FOUND IN COLON AT HIGH CONCENTRATIONS

A prominant, broad diglyceride (DG) band was found when fecal extracts from each of eight volunteers, on unrestricted diets, were analyzed by thin-layer chromatography (Friedman et al, 1989). The DGs were hydrolyzed to release their constitutive fatty acids, which were then identified and quantified by gas chromatography and mass spectrometry. Fecal DGs were mixed chain, composed of nonidentical fatty acid residues: oleic, stearic, palmitic and myristic. A broad range from 28 to 1324 um was found, with mean ranges of 185 to 447 uM, except for myristic acid, which was found at less than 22 uM, and in only five of the eight fecal samples. Since both 1,2- and 2,3-DGs could have been present on thin-layer chromatography, and only the 1,2-DG would activate protein kinase C, the TPA receptor in cells (Nishizuka, 1986), the active DG concentrations might be lower than the measured levels. This would dependent on the ratio of 1,2- and 2,3-DG forms the lipases active in the small intestine on triglycerides left uncleaved, and the generation of DGs from shed colonocyte membranes and bacterial membranes within the colon. It is likely that dietary triglyerides are a major source of the fecal DGs, as the major fatty acids found in the fecal DGs are identical to the three most common fatty acids found in fecal triglycerides : stearic, palmitic and oleic. In addition, no arachidonic acid residues were found which would have suggested a colonocyte membrane source of fecal DGs, and no fatty acids with odd-numbered carbon chains or branched chains, suggestive of bacterial membrane sources of fecal DGs were identified. Alternatively, DGs of such structures might have been evolved in the proximal colon, been active at those sites, but been further degraded and lost during the time of fecal transit.

3. DIGLYCERIDES INDUCE MITOGENESIS OF PREMALIGNANT CELLS

Adenomas, carcinomas, and normal colonic mucosal samples were partially digested to epithelial organoids and primary cultured in highly supplemented serum-free Dulbecco's modified Eagle's medium, as described (Schroy et al, 1988). The cultured cells were judged epithelial by the presence of cytokeratins, junctional complexes, and brush borders. Mitogenic activity on these cells was studied by measuring the growth fraction, obtained by culturing the cells with 5 uCi/ml ^{3}H-thymidine until the fraction of labeled cells reached a plateau value, 48-72 hr for adenomas and carcinomas, and 30 hr for normal cells, as determined by autoradiography <u>in situ</u>.

The putative endogenous tumor promoters, the fecal DGs, were tested for mitogenic activity on premalignant cells in primary culture using a detergent-micelle delivery system (Friedman et al, 1989). Dose-response curves on three adenomas showed a gradient of activity for DGs composed of saturated chain fatty acids, of 16 > 14 > 12 > 10 > 8 >>18, at 100 uM, the optimum concentration. Thus DGs composed of any two of the three saturated fatty acids found endogenously would be active if the fatty acids were either palmitic ($C_{16:0}$) or myristic ($C_{14:0}$). DGs containing an oleic acid residue (unsaturated fatty acid, chain length 18, one double bond, $C_{18:1}$), mixed with either another oleic acid or a palmitic acid residue were among the most active. Distearin exhibited very little activity and even the presence of one stearic acid residue in a DG decreased or eliminated its mitogenic activity.

The mitogenic activity of dimyristin, the DG closest in structure to TPA, phorbol myristic acetate, was studied in a survey of 10 adenomas. Three tubular, five villotubular and two villous adenomas were assayed in primary culture with dimyristin concentrations of 25 to 200 uM. The optimal concentration was 100 uM in seven adenomas, including all of the tubular, and 50 uM in three adenomas, including one villous and two villotubular adenomas. The DG induced mitogenesis in each adenoma of the ten assayed, approximately doubling the growth fraction. Mitogenesis experiments were performed with four primary cultured carcinomas, with dimyristin concentrations of 50 to 500 uM. Enhanced proliferation 46% above control values was found in two carcinomas.

4. DIMYRISTIN DOES NOT INDUCE MITOGENESIS OF NORMAL COLONOCYTES

Since dimyristin was among the most potent of the DGs tested on adenoma cells, and had been used in the survey, it was used to assay for possible mitogenic effects on normal colonocytes from seven subjects. Dimyristin at 25 to 500 uM induced no detectable mitogenesis in any of the normal cultures (Friedman et al, 1989). In contrast, addition of 5-10 mM of sodium propionate induced proliferation 140%, while 5 mM sodium butyrate inhibited proliferation 60% (Friedman et al, 1988), showing that normal colonocytes in primary culture can respond to proliferative signals.

5. MITOGENESIS INDUCED BY DIGLYCERIDES USES TYROSINE PHOSPHORYLATION OF A MEMBRANE PROTEIN AS A MECHANISM OF SIGNAL TRANSDUCTION

The mitogenic DG dimyristin induced basal phosphorylation levels 3 to 5 fold in adenoma cells, 1-2 fold in carcinoma cells, but not in normal cells, in initial experiments (Marian et al, 1989). These phosphorylation studies paralleled the pattern of biological effects of DGs. Basal phosphorylation levels were 8-fold higher in resected carcinomas than normal specimens. These data suggested that a protein(s) constitutively phosphorylated in carcinomas, but not in normal cells, might be further phosphorylated with DG treatment. In a survey of nine resected carcinomas, several proteins were found constitutively phosphorylated in NP40 lysates, which had been dialyzed to remove NP40 and cyclic nucleotides, and then supplemented with gamma-labeled ^{32}P-ATP, Ca++ and Mg++. A broad band at 60-64 kd on SDS-polyacrylamide gels, was found in each of the nine carcinomas, but not in any of the normal specimens analyzed. We expected that this protein(s) found only in tumor cells would be a protein kinase C substrate, and so be phosphorylated on threonine or serine residues, and thus be sensitive to alkali-treatment. To our surprise the 60-64 kd band was alkali-resistant, indicating the protein was phosphorylated on tyrosine. Phosphorylation of proteins on tyrosine characterizes several growth factor receptors and oncogene products (Sefton and Hunter, 1984). If colon tumor cell growth is mediated by a transient activation of tyrosine kinases after exposure to DGs, transient phosphorylation of a substrate in the signal pathway would then occur. This data suggested a tyrosine kinase substrate was in the 60-64 kd band. We then proceeded to use a more sensitive immunological assay for this substrate.

6. DIGLYCERIDE MITOGEN INDUCES TYROSINE PHOSPHORYLATION OF 63,000 kd MEMBRANE-BOUND CARCINOMA AND ADENOMA PROTEIN

HI-1 cells, a subclone of the HT29 colon carcinoma cell line, which was TPA and diglyceride sensitive, was used as the model system. The in vivo phosphorylation system described above showed that HI-1 cells constitutively express a 60,000-64,000 kd group of dimyristin-enhanced, alkali-resistant phosphoproteins, again implicating phosphorylation on tyrosine (Marian et al, 1989). Using immunoblotting with an antiphosphotyrosine monoclonal antibody developed by Glenney (1988), a doublet at 63,000 kd was observed, whose intensity was enhanced by a 2 minute pre-treatment of cells with dimyristin. Cellular fraction studies showed a 6-fold increase in tyrosine phosphorylation occurring only in the membrane-bound form of this protein, termed pp63, while no increase was seen in the cytoplasmic form. The maximum tyrosine-phosphorylation occurred at 25 uM dimyristin, 30 seconds after treatment, the earliest time-point. TPA also induced phosphorylation on a 63,000 kd membrane-bound protein while 4alphaPDD, its analog inactive in tumor promotion, was also inactive in pp63 phosphorylation, suggesting both phorbol ester and fecal diglyceride tumor promoters utilized this intermediary.

Three other colon carcinoma cell lines, HT29, SW620 and LS174T, exhibited constitutive tyrosine phosphorylation of pp63. An adenoma in primary culture was induced to tyrosine phosphorylate pp63 by dimyristin. In contrast, normal colonocytes from two subjects exhibited no constitutive tyrosine phosphorylation of pp63, and this phosphorylation could not be induced by dimyristin.

Several control experiments were performed (Marian et al, 1989). Since pp63 was constitutively phosphorylated on tyrosine in HI-1 cells, it might play a role in carcinoma cell growth such as responding to autocrine mitogens or to PDGF in fetal calf serum. To test this hypothesis, HI-1 cells were incubated for one cell cycle in the presence of a phosphatase inhibitor, sodium orthovanadate. This led to a two-fold increase in pp63 tyrosine phosphorylation indicating that cells continually phosphorylate and dephosphorylate pp63 during cell growth, even in the absence of diglycerides. To further demonstrate that the phosphorylation was on tyrosine, phosphotyrosine or its analog, phenylphosphate, was added to the immunoblotting reaction. Both greatly inhibited binding of the phosphotyrosine monoclonal to pp63 by competition with the phosphotyrosine in pp63.

7. CONCLUSION

Diglycerides are endogenous mitogens selective for tumor cells, stimulating proliferation of premalignant colonocytes and of one class of carcinoma cells, but not affecting normal colonocytes. Since diglycerides are found in abundance in the feces of individuals on unrestricted western diets, both lines of evidence suggest that fecal diglycerides have the properties of endogenous promoting agents. Diglycerides at in vivo concentrations induce tyrosine phosphorylation of a membrane-bound pp63 protein within 30 seconds of application. TPA, but not its inactive analogs, also induce this phosphorylation, suggesting both phorbol ester and fecal diglyceride promoting agents use this mechanism for signal transduction. pp63 is constitutively phosphorylated in every carcinoma cell line and adenoma examined, suggesting that fecal diglycerides use a signal pathway already in use by the cell, possibly to respond to other mitogens.

REFERENCES

Baker SJ, Fearon ER, Nigro JM, Hamilton SR, Presinger AC, Jessup JM, vanTuinen P, Ledbetter DH, Barker DF, Nakamura Y, White R, Vogelstein B. (1989) Chromosome 17 deletions and p53 gene mutations in colorectal carcinomas. Science 244:217-221.

Bodmer WF, Bailey CJ, Bodmer J, Bussey HJR, Ellis A, Gorman P, Lucibello FC, Murday VA, Rider SH, Scambler P, Sheer D, Solomon E, Spurr NK.(1987) Localization of the gene for familial adenomatous polyposis on chromosome 5. Nature 328:614-616.

Bos JL, Fearon ER, Hamilton SR, Verlaan-de Vries M, van Boom JH, van der Eb AJ, Vogelstein B. (1987) Prevalence of ras gene mutations in human colorectal cancers. Nature 327:293-297.

Dotto GP, Parada LF, Weinberg RA (1985) Specific growth response of ras-transformed embryo fibroblasts to tumour promoters. Nature 318:472-475.

Friedman E. (1981) Differential response of premalignant epithelial cell classes to phorbol ester tumor promoters and to deoxycholic acid. Cancer Res.41:4588-4599.

Friedman E, Gillin S, Lipkin M. (1984a) TPA stimulation of DNA synthesis in cultured preneoplastic familial polyposis colonic epithelial cells but not in normal colonic epithelial cells. Cancer Res. 44:4078-4086.

Friedman E, Urmacher C, Winawer S. (1984b) A model for human colon carcinoma evolution based on the differential responses of cultured preneoplastic, premalignant and malignant cells to TPA. Cancer Res. 44:1568-1578.

Friedman E, Lightdale C, Winawer S. (1988) Effects of psyllium fiber and short-chain organic acids derived from fiber breakdown on colonic epithelial cells derived from high-risk patients. Cancer Letts. 43:121-124.

Friedman E, Isaksson P, Rafter J, Marian B, Winawer S, Newmark H. (1989) Fecal diglycerides as selective endogenous mitogens for premalignant and malignant human colonic epithelial cells. Cancer Res. 49:544-548.

Forrester K, Almoguera C, Han K, Grizzle WE, Perucho M. (1987) Detection of high incidence K-ras oncogenes during human colon tumorigenesis. Nature 318:298-303.

Glenney JR, Zokas L, Kamps MP (1988) Monoclonal antibodies to phosphotyrosine J. Immunol. Methods 109:277-285.

Marian B, Winawer S, Friedman E. (1989) Tyrosine phosphorylation of a M_r 63,000 protein induced by an endogenous mitogen in human colon carcinoma cells, but not in normal colonocytes. Cancer Res. 49:4231- 4236.

Sefton B and Hunter T. (1984) Tyrosine protein kinases. In :P. Greengard and G.A. Robison (eds). Advances in Cyclic Nucleotide and Protein Phosphorylation Research 18:pp195-219, New York, Raven Press.

Schroy PC, Cohen A, Winawer S, Friedman E (1988) New chemotherapeutic drug sensitivity assay for colon carcinomas in monolayer culture. Cancer Res. 48:3236-3244.

Vogelstein B, Fearon ER, Kern SE, Hamilton SR, Presinger AC, Nakamura Y, White R. (1989) Allotype of colorectal carcinomas. Science 244:207-211.

Overview and Epilogue

HENRY T. LYNCH and JOJI UTSUNOMIYA

This international meeting has provided a unique opportunity for authorities representing diverse disciplines to come together in Kobe, Japan to discuss their data and ideas dealing with a common theme; namely, colorectal cancer genetics. Possibly for the first time, an opportunity became available for clinicians and basic scientists to discuss concomitantly familial adenomatous polyposis (FAP), hereditary nonpolyposis colorectal cancer (HNPCC), and other variants of familial and hereditary colorectal cancer to an almost unparalleled intensity. Indeed, so far as we can determine, these meetings represent the first attempt at a comprehensive coverage of the genetic aspects of virtually all forms of colorectal cancer.

The sessions were opened by a series of plenary reports dealing with differing facets of colorectal cancer genetics. This exchange enabled the channeling of the best posits of information about virtually all conceivable facets of colorectal cancer genetics so that it could be marshalled toward the goals of the conference; namely, maximum elucidation of etiology, carcinogenesis, and control.

While this overview is directed toward the scientific aspects of these sessions, it is important to realize that the pervasive collegial atmosphere created through the graciousness of the Japanese people will undoubtedly bear fruit through many anticipated collaborations. Indeed, this was unquestionably an important stimulus to the prolific and cogent information flow which took place throughout these meetings.

Plenary Sessions

Hereditary colorectal cancer was identified as a major public health concern. The plenary talks focused on differing facets of this problem. Joji Utsunomiya covered many of the underlying clinicogenetic concepts of hereditary colorectal cancer and emphasized FAP, its heterogeneity, particularly with respect to extracolonic polyps and cancer. He stressed the importance of effective tumor registries in the interest of improved cancer control. Registries developed by him in Japan have provided models for implementation of systematic logistical strategies which are now being replicated in many areas of the world.

Jerome DeCosse reviewed the recently held Leeds Castle polyposis meeting and discussed the increasing interest by this group in biomarker studies. Indeed, it was noted that eventually, biomarkers may play an exceedingly important role in case identification. The question which logically followed pertained to "How important will registries of FAP families be once biomarker data becomes widely available to the practicing physician community?" This group has also become concerned with the more difficult diagnostic problem of HNPCC, given the lack of any premonitory clinical signs and/or biomarkers of cancer susceptibility in this disease.

Henry Lynch discussed HNPCC and emphasized its history, dating back to Warthin's observations of Family G, initiated in 1895. HNPCC was characterized as a hereditary (autosomal dominant) cancer susceptibility syndrome by Lynch in 1966. The historical evolution of the genetic, clinical, and pathological features of the syndrome were discussed. Primary attention was given to the cardinal facets of the syndrome, particularly proximal colonic cancer excess, thereby mandating colonoscopy or double air-contrast barium enema for screening. No less than a subtotal colectomy for management of colorectal cancer, given the marked excess of synchronous and metachronous cancer in this disease was put into its appropriate perspective. Problems in HNPCC's heterogeneity, particularly with respect to its tumor spectrum and other facets of natural history, were addressed.

Paul Rozen reviewed strategies for surveillance of patients with a familial risk for colorectal cancer. He described the inordinately increased risk for colorectal cancer which he observed in families with two or more colon cancer affecteds. This colon cancer excess was highly significant when compared to the risk to sporadic patients. The value of family history, a problem often neglected in the usual clinical practice setting, was once again stressed.

Chemoprevention of colorectal cancer became a rather pervasive subject throughout these meetings. Indeed, an entire workshop was devoted to this subject. In his plenary talk, Philip Bralow defined chemoprevention as the use of chemical or pharmacologic agents capable of interrupting the carcinogenic process at various phases between initiation, promotion, and progression to neoplasia and malignancy. Primary chemoprevention was said to involve the addition of anti-carcinogens to our diet to prevent the initiation phase of cancer. However, it was pointed out that no such single agent is currently available. Secondary chemoprevention would employ agents to curtail the promotional or progression stages in the carcinogenic process. Secondary chemoprevention would benefit high risk individuals such as those from kindreds with FAP, HNPCC, or even in cases with sporadic polyps. The most likely candidate agents include supplemental calcium, prostaglandin inhibitors, and possibly Vitamins C, E, and wheat bran in high doses. Calcium may be ineffective when adenomas have already developed. Prostaglandin inhibitors, such as Sulindac and piroxicam, may be preferable in selected high risk individuals.

Jeremy Jass discussed juvenile polyposis and emphasized the need to consider this as a precancer disorder. The diagnosis rests on the demonstration of at least 5 juvenile polyps and/or juvenile polyps throughout the gastrointestinal tract and/or any juvenile polyps in concert with a positive family history.

C. Richard Boland discussed glycoconjugates, lectins, and mucin expression in familial colorectal cancer with particular emphasis on FAP and HNPCC. Interestingly, in the Lynch syndromes, he has identified a subset of patients at 50% risk for this disorder who have reduced binding by the lectin Dolichos biflorous agglutinin (DBA) in the colonic tissues, suggesting the possibility that addition of the terminal sugar (GalNAc) is deficient in the premalignant tissue. Previously, he had demonstrated that DBA preferentially binds to goblet cell mucin present in the mature epithelial cells at the top of the colonic crypt, but not at the bottom of the crypt, where cell proliferation takes place. Finally, he has recently developed a new lectin, amaranthin, that appears to recognize glycoconjugates synthesized by the proliferative cell pool. This lectin binds to normal colonic epithelial cells at the base of the crypt of Lieberkuhn and in adenomas and cancers.

Levy Kopelovich discussed the role of cultured skin fibroblasts and the convenience of these for studies of susceptibility to colorectal cancer. He has found expression of the transformation-associated p53 antigen in FAP cells. In general, no immediate differences were detected in the coding segment of the human p53 gene between normal and FAP cells by either southern or northern blot analysis. Apparently, over-expression of the p53 antigen is due in part to an increased stability of the p53 antigen in FAP cells. The increased expression of p53 antigen prior to any alternations in expression of the c-*ras* family of oncogenes indicates that it is an early event associated with cancer initiation. The localization of the p53 gene to human chromosome 17p is of interest because of the findings of chromosome 17p allele loss in colorectal cancer. Clearly, this observation is cogent, given the keen interest in the p53 gene and chromosome 17 throughout these meetings.

Bert Vogelstein depicted colonic tumorigenesis to result from accumulative changes in both oncogenes and tumor suppressor genes wherein mutations of at least 4-6 genes appear to be required. Most of these mutations are thought to involve tumor suppressor genes. Two chromosomal regions (17p and 18q) are lost in more than 75% of colorectal carcinomas, and at least six additional loci are lost in more than a fourth of the carcinomas. Chromosome 5 markers are lost in over a third of sporadic adenomas, but surprisingly, they are deleted infrequently in the adenomas of FAP. The predominant oncogene has been *ras*. DNA is consistently hypomethylated in colorectal tumors of all stages, with the suggestion that hypomethylation represents a very early event in colorectal neoplasia. This hypomethylation could promote aberrant segregation of chromosomes, leading to the loss of wild-type tumor suppressor genes. Hypomethylation appears to be early, *ras* gene mutations in chromosome 5q allelic losses generally precede 18q allelic losses which, in turn, precede 17p allelic deletions. He reasoned that the total accumulation of changes, not their order with respect to one another, is crucial. Accumulation of genetic alterations in individual tumors appears to be directly correlated with their biologic behavior and provides the basis for prognostic tests. Those carcinomas with greater than the median number of allelic deletions are much more likely to metastasize to distant organs than those tumors with less than the median number, irrespective of the size or histopathological stage of the tumor. The accumulation of genetic alterations is clearly shown during the evolution of adenomas. A combination of mapping and sequencing studies in colorectal carcinomas has shown that the p53 gene is probably located on chromosome 17p. This gene may play a role in the development of most common adult cancers, including those of the colon. Current studies are aimed at defining the chromosome 18q locus that is lost in colorectal carcinomas. This region appears to be of particular interest in light of the previous linkage (Kidd blood group) of HNPCC to markers on chromosome 18q.

Ray White described a large kindred with a history of early onset colon cancer which occurred in the absence of typical diffuse polyposis, although several members had a small number of colonic polyps. Colon cancer was not accompanied by diffuse polyposis and it showed early onset. It is of interest that he has linked this kindred to the FAP locus. Since this presentation at Kobe, Leppert working with Ray White observed linkage to the FAP locus in a family with a strikingly similar phenotype. This family, in addition, has flat adenomas and has been under investigation by Henry Lynch, Thomas Smyrk, Stephen Lanspa, Patrice Watson, and Jane Lynch. The family is not a Lynch syndrome kindred. Of further interest is the fact that to date, the Salt Lake City group (Ray White and Mark Leppert) has not identified linkage of the Lynch syndrome to chromosomes 5, 17, or 18, although this search for linkage remains intensified. Thus, it appears that these new findings of linkage at the FAP locus in these two families is consonant with the hypothesis that heterogeneity may be extant in these colorectal cancer-prone disorders. It should also be noted that Gardner's syndrome has recently been mapped to the FAP locus on the long arm of chromosome 5. The findings in these two interesting families (Ray White's and Henry Lynch and colleagues) suggest that mutations within this FAP locus may be responsible for the inherited colon cancers in some families, even when the florid polyposis coli phenotype is lacking. Characterization of this FAP gene should therefore provide important insights into the mechanism of tumorigenesis in colon cancer in extra-FAP clinicogenetic settings.

Workshops

FAP

A workshop was devoted to the identification, surveillance, and management of polyposis syndromes. This had a strong international flavor wherein experience from FAP registries in Denmark (Steffen Bulow), The Netherlands (Garrit Griffioen), Japan (Yoshio Mishima), Poland (Piotr Krokowicz), and Australia (Finlay Macrae) was represented. In accord with some of the earlier comments from the plenary papers, the Danish investigators addressed concerns that recent identification of a specific FAP gene would change the logistics of screening programs. Thus, in families with informative gene markers, decisions for performing proctosigmoidoscopy would be restricted to FAP genotype-positive (based on marker identification) first degree relatives of an FAP affected. By enabling a high degree of sensitivity and specificity to FAP's genotype identification in any individual's risk status, those patients who were not genotypically affected would be spared entry into the costly and time consuming surveillance program. Physicians could then concentrate their surveillance and management efforts on those patients who were FAP genotype positive and who thereby harbor an enormous cancer risk.

Data from the Danish registry provided proof that screening would lead to early detection of FAP patients, thereby leading to a decrease in the incidence of colorectal cancer in at-risk patients. Experience from Japan showed the importance of extracolonic malignant tumors in FAP. These included thyroid, gastric, periampullary, and small bowel cancer, in addition to desmoid tumors. Clearly, control of colonic cancer in FAP, through surgical prophylaxis, would lead to added years of risk for extracolonic malignant tumors, including desmoids. It is therefore mandatory that closer attention be given to the potential for extracolonic tumors in patients at risk for FAP.

The role of a hospital-based registry for management of FAP was discussed. In the absence of active surveillance of at risk family members, lethal delays in diagnosis were likely to be encountered. Failure of early detection can be ameliorated through a dedicated registry system. This must entail the notification of clinicians and patients about the requirements, timing, and type of surveillance procedures for their at risk patients. To this end, the Victorian ESSO Familial Polyposis Register was established by the Anti-Cancer Counsel of Victoria in April 1988.

A pedigree analysis model for estimating the polyp and colorectal cancer risk of family members at high risk for FAP was discussed by Joan Slack. She stressed the need for screening by sigmoidoscopy beginning at about 10 years of age. The cumulative risk of developing polyps with advancing age, as calculated in 34 relatives at 50% risk, who were negative at the first screen, and who were subsequently found to be affected, was assessed. By age 15, 50% had developed polyps, while 75% manifested polyps by age 22. If sigmoidoscopy was negative at age 22, the chance of developing FAP was only 15% and the chance of having an affected child was reduced to only 7.5%. Finally, for those at risk of inheriting FAP, the probabilities of being affected in the presence of a negative sigmoidoscopy and negative gene markers, could be combined, and by age 22, if the probability was 1:2, the risk was found to be less than 1%. Indeed, this was less than the lifetime population risk of developing sporadic colorectal cancer.

The recently described phenotypic marker for FAP; namely, congenital hypertrophy of the retinal pigment epithelium (CHRPE) was discussed. This phenotypic sign was shown to have important clinical utility. It is important to note that CHRPE is not restricted to so-called Gardner's syndrome, in that it has been identified in patients with FAP in the absence of Gardner's extracolonic phenotypic stigmata.

HNPCC

Stephen Lanspa presented the Creighton resource's experience dealing with prevalence of adenomas in HNPCC. He noted that initially, a statistically significant excess of adenomas was found. However, of extreme interest was the observation that when a single family with flat adenomas was excluded from the analysis, the frequency of adenomatous polyps in the Lynch syndrome kindreds was found to be the same as that observed in the general population. Attention must now be focused on flat adenomas since their occurrence in families may reflect a new heterogeneous subset of colorectal cancer. Note the previous comments on this matter.

Stig Kullander discussed findings based on a prospective interview study of all newly diagnosed cases of endometrial carcinoma in Malmo, Sweden during a two year period (51 cases) with a comparison of male consorts as controls. From these data, he observed an excess of colorectal cancer among the endometrial cancer cases and identified three Lynch syndrome II families. Mitsuro Chiba and colleagues from Japan presented a striking Lynch syndrome II kindred which included three siblings with urologic (transitional cell) cancer. The pedigree demonstrated early onset of cancer, including carcinoma of the right colon and endometrium, which fulfilled the criteria of Lynch syndrome II. Hans Vasen and colleagues from The Netherlands stressed the importance of screening in HNPCC and its value for early detection of colorectal carcinomas and adenomas among asymptomatic members of these kindreds. The need for initiation of screening at age 20 and the necessity of continuing this throughout the life of the individual was emphasized. The Finnish group (Jukka-Pekka Mecklin) have enunciated this same logic.

The MD Anderson Cancer Center experience with hereditary colorectal cancer, emphasizing HNPCC was discussed by Patrick Lynch. A prospective, multicenter, international early detection program was proposed which will adopt the following operational definition for HNPCC: three or more relatives with colon cancer, with at least one such member being a first degree relative to the other two. At least two such members should have, in addition, at least one of the following clinical features - colon cancer onset before age 45, right-sided colonic involvement, multiple primary colon cancer, or the presence of endometrial, breast, other GI or GU malignancy before age 45.

Medical/legal concerns in the management of patients from Lynch syndrome kindreds was discussed with particular attention to tumors observed following incomplete medical evaluation. The disaster of 'a missed lesion' in each of these settings, and the importance of preventive implications, including the potential for litigation when such preventive measures have been ignored were described by Giuseppe Cristofaro. These issues will undoubtedly become more troublesome in direct proportion to advances in knowledge about cancer genetics in general and with carcinoma of the colorectum in particular.

Jane Lynch described the role of the nurse and/or other paramedicals in the workup of patients at risk for all forms of hereditary colorectal cancer, inclusive of the Lynch syndromes. Attention was given to responsibilities of this "team player" in the areas of research, with the need for coordination of field visits to families, data organization, and their entry into computer programs, patient and physician education, and cancer control pursuits. The registered nurse has an ideal background as a family contact person for compiling and coordinating family history. In short, the nurse is seen as a liaison between patient, physician, and researcher.

Robert Fitzgibbons Jr has recommended that patients presenting with colorectal cancer in the Lynch syndromes undergo a subtotal colectomy. This recommendation is based on the known increased occurrence of synchronous and metachronous colorectal cancers in this disease. Specifically, metachronous colon cancer was found to be 40% by 10 years. He noted that the overwhelming majority of patients with colorectal cancer in the Lynch syndromes are not receiving subtotal colectomy and, indeed, present to us frequently with metastatic cancer secondary to metachronous colorectal cancer. Thus, he suggested that a real challenge to the profession is to improve the surgical treatment of patients with Lynch syndrome by better education of surgeons, indicating the possibility of the existence of the disease and the need for this surgical recommendation.

Chemoprevention

Participants in the workshop pertaining to chemoprevention appeared to share the following considerations: Assumption 1 - based on epidemiologic clues, colon cancer risk in humans is related to the presence of harmful environmental/dietary agents (e.g., dietary fat, prostaglandins) or to the absence of protective agents (e.g., dietary calcium, fiber, antioxidants); Assumption 2 - laboratory markers exist that correlate with colon cancer risk; Assumption 3 - manipulation of dietary agents decreases colon cancer risk, as measured by these laboratory markers; and Assumption 4 - given the validity of testing carcinogen/anticarcinogen interactions in animal models, the evaluation of high risk groups for colorectal cancer would have a greater yield than would clinical trials of chemopreventive agents in average risk populations.

The validity of currently held epidemiologic suppositions as to the role of the mentioned dietary agents was not seriously challenged. These concerns were pioneered with respect to oral calcium supplementation by Martin Lipkin. Most attention was directed toward those ongoing clinical trials concerned with the testing of various oral agents, in high risk groups, with intermediate markers serving as endpoints for statistical evaluation.

Several problem areas emerged with respect to the intermediate markers themselves. In three calcium intervention series presented by David Earnest, Paul Rozen, and Bernard Levin, it was found that calcium was only effective in reducing tritiated thymidine labeling in patients with the highest baseline values. While this may indicate a real treatment effect in a subset of patients characterized by the increased labeling index, the possibility of statistical artifact must be entertained. Problems of intermediate marker assay reproducibility under various conditions must be considered, particularly since a study by Hartley Stern and colleagues failed to show a significant calcium effect. Notably, their study had less variation in baseline labeling, which may account for some of the discrepancy with the other studies.

None of the chemoprevention studies evaluated clinical endpoints (adenomas, carcinomas). The need for such prospective studies was repeatedly emphasized. Arguments focused on the unknown relationship between in vitro marker modulation and clinical disease, as well as the lack of consistent findings in the mentioned studies. Essentially, all investigators anticipate participation in prospective trials designed to assess the effect of various interventions, alone or in combination, on disease processes. These could be done with or without monitoring of intermediate markers, though most favor their inclusion.

So far, we have concentrated primarily on calcium as the chemopreventive agent and proliferative markers in the colon as endpoints. However, other interventions and markers were discussed. Bran cereal was found by David Earnest to decrease tritiated thymidine labeling in patients with elevated baseline activity in a fashion very similar to that noted for dietary calcium. Piroxicam was also found to reduce the proliferation index, though to a lesser extent, and PgE2 was decreased as well.

Ornithine decarboxylase (ODC), the rate limiting enzyme in the polyamine pathway, was considered to be a significant regulator of cell proliferation. Indomethecin was found by Tomio Narisawa to decrease ODC in the mucosa of patients with previously resected colon cancer. Hideho Takada found that in rats given AOM, co-treatment with Eicosapentanoic acid (EPA) resulted in lower tumor burden, ODC activity, and PgE2 levels than was seen in rats on a relatively higher linoleic acid diet only.

Clearly, more work needs to be done in both animal and human models, using a range of potentially protective agents. These should perhaps be offered in combination, ideally under circumstances where individual agents protect by differing mechanisms.

Molecular Genetics

The discussants at the workshop dealing with molecular genetics considered the role of suppressor gene loss to be as important as oncogene activation in carcinogenesis. The model most generally discussed pertained to multiple steps in the evolution of normal colonic mucosa to carcinoma. Colon carcinogenesis may be initiated by gene inactivation at the FAP locus on chromosome 5q in the normal colonic cell, with formation of the early phases of an adenoma. Other molecular changes may occur, including hypomethylation of DNA and *ras* gene mutation. Chromosome 17 and 18 loss may then be responsible for the adenoma proceeding to an even more advanced stage of progression to carcinoma. Finally, additional chromosome losses may be necessary for metastasis to take place. It is clear from this model of colon carcinogenesis that many hits may accumulate in the cell prior to malignant transformation. These DNA changes may then activate cellular oncogenes, leading them to increased cell growth with progression to those characteristic abnormalities that typify malignancy.

The thesis of a stepwise accumulation of mutations involving suppressor genes, as well as oncogenes, in colon carcinogenesis was proposed for both hereditary (FAP) and so-called sporadic forms of colorectal cancer. In the case of HNPCC, attention was focused on the possibility that loss of a locus at chromosome 18 may be playing an important etiologic role in carcinogenesis.

Bert Vogelstein espoused an hypothesis that those cancers which involve a greater number of DNA changes are the ones most likely to be aggressive, metastasize, and ultimately lead to the patient's demise. This hypothesis harbors important implications to medical oncologists. Specifically, a different therapy may be indicated for those patients who show a greater number of gene alterations in their colorectal tumors. For example, small benign adenomas may have only a single, recognizable gene change, with accumulation of several such mutations as they increase in size.

To date, only one of the suspected suppressor genes believed to be important in colorectal carcinogenesis has been identified; namely, the p53 gene localized on the deleted segment of chromosome 17. This gene may encode a protein that suppresses tumor formation because it can act as a suppressor of neoplastic transformation [see Finlay et al; Cell 57:1083-93, 1989]. The loss or inactivation of the p53 gene, in addition to its putative role in colorectal cancer, may also be involved in other common cancers, including carcinoma of the lung and breast.

Bruce Boman reported a new colorectal cancer cell line (DiFi) from a patient with the Gardner syndrome. The molecular analysis of these cells revealed several molecular alterations, including allelic loss on chromosomes 17p and 18, amplification of the EGF receptor gene, and expression of transforming growth factor-alpha, c-*myc*, and p53 transcripts. This cell line should be useful to study how these molecular alterations give colorectal cancer cells a selective growth advantage. Dr. Boman also reported that the retinoblastoma gene is overexpressed in colorectal cancers relative to normal mucosa. Southern blot analysis of DNA from colorectal carcinomas showed an increase in gene copy number in 40% of tumors. These results are consistent with karyotype studies showing that nonrandom gains of chromosome 13 occur in approximately 50% of colorectal cancers. Southern blot analysis also shows that none of the colorectal cancers examined had allelic loss at the Rb locus. These results suggest that the Rb gene is not lost or transcriptionally inactivated in colorectal cancers.

In conclusion, several intriguing biomolecular/genetic theories of carcinogenesis were advanced by the participants. It is clear that while steady progress is being made in tracking events at the biomolecular level of carcinogenesis, we are nevertheless still at the early portion of the learning curve. The prospects for the future are exciting and it is in this discipline that many of us have hope that the research will lead to improvement in cancer control and possibly even cure.

Pathology

Stanley Hamilton discussed the importance of experimental models of carcinogenesis, with attention to the identification of potential chemopreventive agents. Extrapolation was made from these animal models to intervention in humans. The occurrence of hepatic activation of systemic carcinogens was found to be an important consideration in the appropriate use of these models. Modulating factors which affect only hepatic metabolism appeared to be irrelevant to human colorectal neoplasia. Fecal carcinogens were found to have the advantage of direct exposure of the luminal portion of the colonic mucosa, which may be more pertinent to the pathogenesis of human colorectal neoplasia.

Stanley Hamilton also presented data on 12 cases of Turcot's syndrome, along with an analysis, of 58 additional cases from the literature. It was concluded that medulloblastoma or glial cell tumor may occur as a pleiotropic extra-intestinal manifestation of Turcot's syndrome in a patient affected by or destined to develop adenomatous polyposis.

Hidenobu Watanabe described the pathology of upper gastrointestinal lesions in FAP. He suggested that a higher incidence of gastroenteric lesions occur in FAP than had been previously appreciated. This observation mandates that further attention be given to the stomach and small intestine, in addition to the colon and rectum, in FAP affecteds.

Takeo Iwama described 19 of cases of Peutz-Jegher's syndrome and summarized some 420 cases of this disorder reported in the Japanese literature. Four cases of cancer were found in their 19 cases, which included a patient with jejunal polyps wherein one of the resected polyps from this patient showed marked cellular atypism and mucus-producing components. Peritoneal dissemination of the tumor was identified three years later and was responsible for the patient's death. A second patient had a mucin-producing carcinoma of the jejunum; a third underwent hysterectomy for uterine endometrial carcinoma; and a fourth had a mucus-producing cervical adenocarcinoma and a tumor in the head of the pancreas. Of the 420 literature reports, there were 70 examples of gastrointestinal cancer with a mean age of 34.4. It is clear that the Peutz-Jegher's syndrome is <u>not</u> a benign disorder, but rather, should be included as a significant hereditary precancerous disease which is inherited as an autosomal dominant.

Tetsuichiro Muto described the clinical/pathological features of flat adenoma of the large bowel. Histologically, all of the tumors were tubular adenomas, with different grades of atypia. It was noted that adenomatous tubules tend to spread laterally instead of growing towards the lumen, to develop polypoid adenoma, and the adenomatous component of "flat adenoma," which was less than twice as thick as surrounding normal mucosa. It was concluded that a flat adenoma with severe atypia should be considered a new type of precursor of colonic carcinoma and its biologic behavior should be carefully investigated for further understanding of colonic carcinogenesis. Data on the familial aspects of flat adenoma are now under investigation by Muto and colleagues.

Thomas Smyrk described the histologic features of HNPCC in 65 tumors from 52 patients who were members of 10 HNPCC kindreds. Colonic tumors among 40% of HNPCC cases were graded as poorly differentiated, based on the absence of gland lumens, compared to 14% of tumors from sporadic cases. Other features more commonly seen in the hereditary group included an expanding growth pattern (63% vs. 39%), marked lymphocytic response (37% vs. 20%), and marked Crohn's reaction (44% vs. 25%). There was no difference in tumor stage between the two groups. The finding of expanded growth pattern, lymphocytic response, and Crohn's reaction, all of which were more common in the HNPCC tumors, were thought to confer improved prognosis.

Pantaleo Bufo reported pathology findings of crypt atrophy of colorectal mucosa in Lynch syndrome I and II patients. The study is preliminary but he recommends that patients who show crypt atrophy in HNPCC be followed prospectively to investigate whether or not they are more likely to develop carcinomas of the colorectum. Silvano Senatore investigated cellular immune response in Lynch syndrome II. This study was based on gastrointestinal biopsies from 18 members of the original Lynch syndrome II kindred reported by Giuseppe Cristofaro and colleagues from Italy. Activation of both B and T cell functions which appeared to be an M-dependent process was described.

Young Kim discussed carbohydrate-associated antigens as potentially useful tools in yielding further knowledge on colon carcinogenesis and colon cancer cell biology. He noted that changes in carbohydrates of colonic mucin glycoproteins, which have been observed in premalignant and malignant colonic mucosa, can be divided into three categories: 1) inappropriate expression which may occur as a result of reactivation of fetal genes; 2) deletion of normally expressed antigens which arise as a result of incomplete carbohydrate side chain; and 3) neosynthesis which occurs as a result of either extension or modification of an existing carbohydrate structure. He concluded that while the precise biochemical and molecular basis of these alterations in colonic mucin are not well understood, nevertheless, they provide potentially useful tools for the study of colon carcinogenesis as well as for developing strategies for the diagnosis and management of colorectal cancer.

Mitsuro Chiba discussed the possibility that mental retardation may be another complication of FAP and emphasized the need for large-scale study. Cases were appropriately described.

Common Polyps

The importance of adenomas and their significance in all forms of hereditary colorectal cancer was discussed by Randall Burt. A reasonable assumption was that host factors, in concert with environmental perturbation, may be of major importance in polyp formation in so-called sporadic occurrences of this disease. Based on research, particularly in population studies, he suggested that common familial clustering of polyps and cancer might occur on the basis of: 1) polygenic inheritance; 2) Mendelian inheritance with decreased gene penetrance; or 3) environmental factors common to family members. Furthermore, he suggested that acquired mutations in the FAP locus might be found at 'random' in adenomatous polyps, especially large polyps, and in colorectal cancers. Several additional acquired genetic mutations also are consistently observed in such neoplastic tissues. These include mutations on chromosome 17p and 18q as well as mutations of the K-*ras* oncogene. These loci of acquired mutations are also candidate loci for the investigation of the purported gene or genes which give rise to inherited susceptibility to common adenomatous polyps. This entire subject merits priority attention, particularly at the biomolecular level, given the public health impact of colonic polyps.

D. Timothy Bishop discussed research involving pedigree analysis and a statistical technique based on likelihood theory in order to examine the evidence for inherited susceptibility to adenomas. Pedigree analysis incorporates information on both frequency of adenomas within the pedigrees and the pattern of affection (i.e., the genetic relationships of affected individuals) to distinguish between genetic models. The likelihood analysis suggested that the parsimonious genetic model is a dominantly inherited susceptibility with a gene frequency of 0.19. The interesting aspect of the model is that the maximum likelihood solution indicates that all adenomas are attributable to this allele; no phenocopies are expected. He is now examining more complex models which assume both polygenic and major genetic inheritance; in this case, he anticipates that some of the familial resemblance will be attributable to polygenic factors but initial suggestions are that this is a small contribution.

Gloria M. Petersen provided preliminary studies on genetic linkage of juvenile polyposis and found that it is not linked to the gene for FAP. Carli M.J. Topps, in a study of linkage and FAP in The Netherlands, suggested that C11p11 and Pi227 are located on the same side relative to FAP, with C11p11 somewhat telomeric to Pi227 and closer to FAP. Based on the known linkage data and the available information on the physical map, he proposes the following provisional orientation for the loci on chromosome 5q:
5cen--M4--Pi227-C11p11--FAP--YN5.48--5qter.

General Commentary

Alcohol and Colon Cancer

Takeshi Hirayama discussed his 17-year followup of some 265,118 Japanese adults over age 40 years who showed a close association between cancer of the sigmoid colon (n=91) and alcohol consumption. The relative risk (RR) for drinkers vs. nondrinkers was 4.38 (90% CI, 1.75-10.97) in men and 1.92 (1.13-3.26) in women. The combined effect of alcohol and smoking was evident for cancers of the upper digestive tract, as has been previously reported, but interestingly, this synergism was absent for the lower digestive tract.

Diagnostic Concerns

Each of the workshops covered specialized areas of colorectal cancer genetics; e.g., pathology, biomolecular genetics, surveillance/management, registries, and chemoprevention. The coverage of each topic was broadly based but certain themes did emerge. Foremost was the high potential yield of useful information which is likely to be derived through the study of patients at high genetic risk for colorectal cancer, with appropriate comparison made with patients showing well-verified evidence of sporadic colorectal cancer. It was deemed mandatory that there be a high degree of confidence in the accuracy of the cancer genetic diagnoses of the specific patients undergoing investigation. However, it was readily appreciated that cancer genetic classification was likely to become blurred in many of these patients, due to genetic heterogeneity and the clinical overlap of phenotype. These concerns clearly enunciated the need for priority attention to biomolecular strategies for identification of the deleterious genotype(s).

A prime example of cancer genetic classification pitfalls was given by Yusuke Nakamura's published findings involving linkage analysis on six pedigrees, three having the FAP phenotype in the absence of Gardner's stigmata and three having so-called Gardner's syndrome. He discovered linkage for all of these kindreds to the FAP locus on chromosome 5q. There was no evidence of genetic heterogeneity between the two phenotypes. Although the possibility that two different, defective genes located close together on chromosome 5 could not be eliminated, the simplest interpretation was that separate mutations within the same gene were generating the differences between the phenotypes. Clearly, Nakamura's observations might have been anticipated given the evidence of Bulow from Denmark and Utsunomiya from Japan on a large number of patients with FAP who underwent orthopantomography. Specifically, a significant number of these patients showed evidence of osteomas as well as other extracolonic manifestations which had heretofore been considered as cardinal aspects of Gardner's syndrome, yet they had not been classified as having Gardner's. Further evidence for the "lumpers" as opposed to the "splitters" comes from the more recently described phenotype of congenital hypertrophy of the retinal pigment epithelium (CHRPE), initially thought to be restricted to Gardner's syndrome, but which has now been observed in patients with FAP who lack the extracolonic phenotypic manifestations of Gardner's syndrome.

An even more vexing cancer genetic diagnostic dilemma pertains to the status of patients with one or more adenomatous polyps of the colorectum. Are some of these patients with isolated adenomatous polyps of the colorectum representative of the extreme end of the FAP phenotype? Do some fit the HNPCC classification and if so, is the presence of an adenomatous colonic polyp, particularly in a patient less than 40 years of age, who is a member of a pedigree showing convincing evidence of HNPCC, genotypically affected? In other words, is the presence of an adenomatous polyp in that specific setting sufficient to conclude that the patient is eventually destined to manifest colorectal cancer because he/she harbors the deleterious genotype? Thus, in that particular setting, the adenomatous polyp might serve as a marker for the hereditary trait. A consensus on this point did not seem to emerge. Again, the discussants harkened back to the importance of biomarker investigations in an attempt to lend confidence to the diagnostic reliability and validity of assumptions about the genetic significance of isolated adenomatous polyps.

In the case of HNPCC, mounting evidence for cancer of diverse anatomic sites, inclusive of the stomach, small bowel, pancreas, and urologic system (particularly transitional cell carcinoma of the ureter and adenocarcinoma of the kidney), were found independently by several investigators from differing parts of the world. Do these observations indicate pleiotropy of the HNPCC genotype? Does this represent heterogeneity of HNPCC? Do we require reclassification of certain kindreds which fulfill the cardinal findings of HNPCC; namely, a predominance of early onset cancer of the colorectum with an excess of proximal involvement, an increased frequency of synchronous and metachronous colonic cancer (Lynch syndrome I), and in kindreds with these same features but showing an excess of carcinoma of the endometrium and ovary (Lynch syndrome II), all in the absence of diffuse polyposis? When showing an integral genetic association of cancer of some of these diverse sites, should we consider these kindreds to be showing an entirely distinctive cancer genetic syndrome? These considerations are extremely important since they may mandate additional surveillance/management strategies for some of these cancers sites. They are also reminiscent of problems in FAP, a disease which had been thought (at least historically) to have concerned <u>only</u> the colorectum but which has now been abundantly shown to harbor cancer of extracolonic sites, particularly gastric (as in Japan), small bowel, periampullary carcinoma, papillary carcinoma of the thyroid, adrenocortical carcinoma, brain tumors, and possibly cancer of other anatomic sites, which are believed to be pleiotropic manifestations of the FAP genotype.

An important problem pertained to the role of environmental interaction on the FAP genotype and its cancer phenotype, which may have been contributory to cancer of these extracolonic sites. This was seen in most high relief when considering the excess occurrence of gastric carcinoma in the Japanese general population, and the fact that a greater predilection to this anatomic site was found in patients with FAP from Japan when compared to its frequency in patients with FAP from other areas of the world.

Future Projections

Walter Bodmer discussed the high mutation rate for FAP. He suggested that most families will be new mutants and that local drift may give rise to clusters of families in a given area with the same mutation. The high mutation rate also suggests that the gene for FAP may be a large one. He noted that the 5q allele loss to date has been limited to colorectal cancer. This contrasts to many of the other chromosome changes which occur in differing types of tumors.

Chromosome 5 allele loss in colorectal carcinomas focuses on the 5q21 region, with a maximum frequency of over 60%, implying that APC is the gene which explains chromosome 5 allele loss. In contrast to sporadic adenomas, it was generally agreed that allele loss in polyps from FAP patients is low. Bodmer did not believe that there was evidence for any additional genetic event for polyp formation in FAP, a phenomenon which fits with the threshold model for a stochastic event in polyp development which he had originally hypothesized. On the preventive side, he speculated that the loss or inactivation of the APC may switch on a growth factor mechanism and lead to polyp formation, then agents which block the activity of such a growth factor may result in control of this disease process. A question of concern, however, is whether or not this would lead to to the total eradication of cancer risk since, in our opinion, the entire colonic mucosa in FAP may have a propensity to malignant transformation.
Bodmer suggested that the majority, "if not all," of the 17p allele losses are due to mutations at the p53 gene, as had been shown by Bert Vogelstein. In his own laboratory, he found that about 50% of colorectal carcinomas on immunoperoxidase staining show reactivity which is presumed to represent a mutant form of p53. However, none of 10 adenomas from both FAP and sporadic patients showed staining, suggesting that even the first step in alteration of p53 is indeed a relatively late event. He suggested however that the p53 mutation has a dominant effect which is most probably enacted through blocking the normal p53 activity which is followed secondarily by additional selection against the presence of the remaining alleles.

Particular interest was expressed regarding the gene described by Vogelstein on chromosome 18 which explained 18q allele loss. This may represent a cell adhesion molecule, a phenomenon which fits data suggesting an important role for extracellular matrix receptors in the control of differentiation.

The findings at the molecular genetic level led Bodmer to suggest that they may strongly influence the pathology of the future and that pathologists will necessarily have to match what they observe histologically to the genetic diagnosis rather than vice versa. It appeared that this premonition was shared by many of the attendees.

Interest was given to the finding of chromosome 22 allele loss as being seemingly observed only in Japan, and thereby representing an example of geographic variation in the pattern of genetic change in colorectal cancer. Such geographic variation was postulated as representing an effect of the microenvironment; namely, diet. Conceivably, this could differentially pose selective advantage to certain mutants.

Bodmer considered the HNPCC syndromes to be a heterogeneous collection, and that herein, the heterogeneity will ultimately be sorted out by genetic linkage studies in addition to careful clinical descriptions. However, he noted that the clinical picture may exaggerate the genetic heterogeneity. This is certainly a logical supposition. Such genetic linkage studies are ongoing in the Creighton resource in collaboration with Ray White and Mark Leppert. Explanations for phenotypic variation in the Lynch syndromes may be explained by genetic background in concert with environmental effects, including diet, sex, occupational exposures, and potentially myriad unknown carcinogenic exposures, as well as chance variations. In addition, differing mutations of the same gene could have different effects which, collectively, could lead to clinical heterogeneity associated with mutations at a single gene locus.

Bodmer commented about studies on colon cancer prevention, including increased fiber, decreased fat, and increased calcium, prostaglandin synthetase inhibitors, unsaturated fatty acid components, vitamins D, C, and A, and retinoids as well as inhibitors of ornithine decarboxylase. He believes that until the molecular genetics and biology provide convincing clues as to the directions to go, it may be difficult to argue for a systematic prevention trial. Furthermore, there is the question as to whether high risk situations, and in particular, polyposis, provide an appropriate model for testing potential preventive approaches for the majority of sporadic colorectal carcinomas. We believe they may do so, even at the level of preventing primary development of polyps, but the situation will undoubtedly become clearer once the polyposis gene itself has been identified." We share this conviction and once again urge that priority consideration be given to molecular genetic studies among high risk colorectal cancer populations. This concern should be addressed immediately and put in perspective so that expensive preventive dietary trials will not be unduly promoted at the expense of biomolecular genetic research.

HNPCC International Study Group

The final portion of the program included an informal discussion of the newly formed HNPCC International Task Force. The objective of this group is to pool data on the natural history aspects of HNPCC and to define its diagnostic features in a uniform manner. This would then enable meaningful strategies for collecting and pooling DNA for linkage studies and for developing targeted screening programs for high risk patients. It is clear that the pervasive nature of HNPCC, including its complex heterogeneity, as evidenced in part by its variable tumor spectrum in certain kindreds, warrants investigation of as large a number of well-defined kindreds as possible through research by colleagues throughout the world who might be willing to contribute to these pursuits. Considerable enthusiasm for participation in this new movement was evidenced by the attendees.

1991 Meeting in Torino, Italy

Finally, an announcement for the next meeting; namely, the 5th International Workshop on Colorectal Cancer, which will take place in Torino, Italy in September 1991, was made. Henry Lynch will be Chairman, P. Meera Khan will be Cochairman, and Giuseppe Cristofaro will be Secretary General.

Author Index

FSC
www.fsc.org
MIX
Papier aus verantwortungsvollen Quellen
Paper from responsible sources
FSC® C105338

If you have any concerns about our products,
you can contact us on
ProductSafety@springernature.com

In case Publisher is established outside the EU,
the EU authorized representative is:
Springer Nature Customer Service Center GmbH
Europaplatz 3, 69115 Heidelberg, Germany

Printed by Libri Plureos GmbH
in Hamburg, Germany